Health Psychology

Third Edition

Sara Miller McCune founded SAGE Publishing in 1965 to support the dissemination of usable knowledge and educate a global community. SAGE publishes more than 1000 journals and over 800 new books each year, spanning a wide range of subject areas. Our growing selection of library products includes archives, data, case studies and video. SAGE remains majority owned by our founder and after her lifetime will become owned by a charitable trust that secures the company's continued independence.

Los Angeles | London | New Delhi | Singapore | Washington DC | Melbourne

Health Psychology

Understanding the Mind–Body Connection

Third Edition

Catherine A. Sanderson
Amherst College

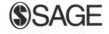

Los Angeles | London | New Delhi
Singapore | Washington DC | Melbourne

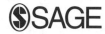

FOR INFORMATION:

SAGE Publications, Inc.
2455 Teller Road
Thousand Oaks, California 91320
E-mail: order@sagepub.com

SAGE Publications Ltd.
1 Oliver's Yard
55 City Road
London EC1Y 1SP
United Kingdom

SAGE Publications India Pvt. Ltd.
B 1/I 1 Mohan Cooperative Industrial Area
Mathura Road, New Delhi 110 044
India

SAGE Publications Asia-Pacific Pte. Ltd.
3 Church Street
#10-04 Samsung Hub
Singapore 049483

Acquisitions Editor: Lara Parra
Content Development Editor: Emma Newsom
Editorial Assistant: Zachary Valladon
Production Editor: Tracy Buyan
Copy Editor: Rachel Keith
Typesetter: C&M Digitals (P) Ltd.
Proofreader: Rae-Ann Goodwin
Indexer: Beth Nauman-Montana
Cover Designer: Michael Dubowe
Marketing Manager: Katherine Hepburn

Printed in the United States of America

Library of Congress Cataloging-in-Publication Data

Names: Sanderson, Catherine Ashley, 1968- author.

Title: Health psychology : understanding the mind-body connection / Catherine A. Sanderson, Amherst College, Massachusetts.

Description: Third edition. | Thousand Oaks, California : SAGE, [2019] | Includes bibliographical references and indexes.

Identifiers: LCCN 2017049103 | ISBN 9781506373713 (hardcover : alk. paper)

Subjects: LCSH: Clinical health psychology. | Health—Psychological aspects. | Medicine and psychology.

Classification: LCC R726.7 .S26 2019 | DDC 616.001/9—dc23
LC record available at https://lccn.loc.gov/2017049103

This book is printed on acid-free paper.

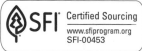

Certified Sourcing
www.sfiprogram.org
SFI-00453
SFI label applies to text stock

18 19 20 21 22 10 9 8 7 6 5 4 3 2 1

BRIEF CONTENTS

CONTENTS

LIST OF FEATURES

Focus on Diversity

Test Yourself

When I agreed to write the first edition of this textbook in 2001, I was in my fourth year as an assistant professor, had a two-and-a-half-year-old son, and was in my eighth month of pregnancy with my second son. As I now complete the third edition of this book, I am struck by the changes that have occurred in the field of health psychology during this time, such as growing awareness of how genes impact virtually all aspects of health-related behavior, how chronic pain and pain medication contribute to the opioid epidemic, and how behavioral choices—from texting and driving to intentional self-harm—cause many injuries and fatalities each year. I am also vividly aware of how changes in my own life influence my perspective on health-related issues. My two sons are now teenagers, and thus I write about alcohol-related injuries and car accidents with considerable understanding of the prevalence of such behaviors in teenage boys. My daughter just turned 13, and thus I'm mindful of the pressures related to body image and disordered eating facing many teenage girls. Since writing the first edition of this book, I've also experienced the death of my mother, from cancer, and my mother-in-law, from a stroke, and thus I now view the leading causes of mortality and the challenges families face in confronting terminal illness and bereavement from a very personal perspective. On a national level, as I'm finishing this third edition, Congress is debating various revisions to the Affordable Care Act, which could have a lasting impact on Americans' access to health care. I therefore approach the material described in this book from both a professional and personal perspective.

THE GOALS OF THIS TEXT

I have several goals for this third edition. First, I want students to understand the methods that researchers use to test particular questions within this field and the importance of critically thinking about how a specific research method could influence the conclusions we draw. In turn, the second chapter includes a comprehensive review of research methods used in this field to help students understand the strengths and weaknesses of different approaches to conducting research (e.g., sometimes people overreport their exercise behavior and underreport their smoking, which is a concern with using self-report surveys). In addition, each chapter will include a Research in Action box that describes the methods and findings of a recent study in health psychology to help students understand how research questions are tested using the scientific methods. The research reviewed in each box was specifically chosen to be of interest to students, such as how an alcohol tax reduces rates of STDs, why later school start times reduce car crashes, and why women forget the pain of childbirth. Each chapter will also include two data figures that illustrate specific research findings to help students understand how scientific findings are presented.

Second, the third edition of this book includes a larger, and more inclusive, focus on the role of diversity in influencing health-related behavior. Each chapter will include a specific box that describes how ethnicity/race and/or culture influence that particular topic in some way. Once again, the material presented in these boxes will be chosen specifically to be engaging to students, such as differences between cultures in their preference for the thinness norm in women, the impact of patients' race on doctors' nonverbal communication, and the role of acculturation in predicting rates of smoking in Latinos. In addition, each chapter will describe how race/ethnicity, gender, culture, and/or sexual orientation are associated with that particular health-related topic.

The third edition of this book also adds a new feature called Focus on Neuroscience, in which cutting-edge information on the role of genes, hormones, and the brain on health will be described in a clear and accessible way. This distinct feature is not present in any of the current health psychology books, although a growing amount of research points to the substantial impact of biological factors—including genes, hormone levels, and patterns of brain activity—on health as well as responsiveness to health-related messages and interventions. These boxes will include a number of highly engaging topics, including how mindfulness meditation changes the brain, why the presence of moms improves teenagers' driving (by activating a particular part of the brain), and how genetic screening can save people's lives.

Finally, because ultimately this book is designed to be read by students, I have included a number of features to help students understand how the theories and findings described apply directly to their own lives. These features include the Test Yourself measure (so that students can examine their own scores on the same measures used by researchers) and an Information YOU Can Use feature at the end of each chapter (that provides a specific and relatively easy way for students to use the information presented in their own lives). This book also includes updated real-world examples and photos, such as the prevalence of drug overdose deaths in celebrities such as Prince, Brittney Maynard's decision to end her life following diagnosis with cancer (and the right-to-die movement), the lasting consequences of concussions among NFL players, and the serious impact of PTSD among survivors of mass school shootings. My hope is that students will enjoy reading this textbook, in part because they will see its relevance for helping them live long and healthy lives. The third edition of this book will also maintain traditional features to help students master the material in each chapter. These include key terms in bold, an outline with two levels of heading at the start of each chapter, and, at the end of the chapter, a bulleted chapter summary.

⑤SAGE edge™

Give your students the SAGE edge!

SAGE edge offers a robust online environment featuring an impressive array of free tools and resources for review, study, and further exploration, keeping both instructors and students on the cutting edge of teaching and learning. Learn more at **edge.sagepub.com/sandersonhealthpsych3e**.

ACKNOWLEDGMENTS

Writing a book is a long and sometimes lonely process, and this book is substantially better thanks to the assistance of many people. I am particularly grateful to the numerous reviewers commissioned by SAGE, who shared with me their thoughts on the challenges they face in teaching health psychology and made numerous (large and small) suggestions for improving this book. Their wise suggestions were extremely helpful in guiding my revisions, and I am particularly grateful that they took time out of their own teaching and research activities to provide such thoughtful feedback. These reviewers include the following:

- Jane Austin, William Paterson University
- Karen Linville Baker, University of Memphis—Lambuth
- Michael Berg, Wheaton College
- Walter Chung, The Chicago School of Professional Psychology
- Marie-Joelle Estrada, University of Rochester

- Erin M. Fekete, University of Indianapolis
- Kristel Gallagher, Thiel College
- Olya Glantsman, DePaul University
- Erica Hart, American University
- Kristin Hoffner, Arizona State University
- Joel Hughes, Kent State University
- Dulcinea Kaufman, Great Bay Community College
- Lorna London, Midwestern University
- Shannon Lupien, Daemen College
- Angie MacKewn, University of Tennessee at Martin
- Deborah Majerovitz, York College, City University of New York
- Saadia McLeod, California State Polytechnic University, Pomona
- Erin L. Merz, California State University, Dominguez Hills
- Tamara J. Musumeci-Szabo, Rider University
- Dorie Richards, University of La Verne
- Sarah Savoy, Stephen F. Austin State University
- Sangeeta Singg, Angelo State University
- Cinnamon Stetler, Furman University

I also need to acknowledge the considerable assistance from numerous people at SAGE, who worked diligently to bring this book to fruition. First, my editor, Lara Parra, deserves substantial credit for convincing me that SAGE was the right publisher for this third edition and then providing prompt advice and guidance at virtually every stage of this process. I feel fortunate to have worked under the direction of such a supportive, thoughtful, and patient editor. I also appreciate the considerable efforts of Zachary Valladon, who helped me stay on track for assorted deadlines, assisted with gathering and summarizing reviews, and provided consistent editorial support throughout. Thanks also go to Emma Newsom, who provided helpful guidance on preparing the final manuscript, and Rachel Keith, who worked diligently to copyedit the manuscript and ensure stylistic consistency throughout. Finally, I want to acknowledge Danny Meldung's assistance with locating photographs to really bring the material alive as well as Michael Dubowe's design and creation of the fabulous new cover.

I also want to thank several student research assistants who contributed to this book in various ways. Nicholas Marsh, JP Miller, Chris Roll, and Olivia Vayer all provided valuable assistance in gathering articles, providing updated statistics, and compiling references. Their work over two summers helped me stay (mostly) on deadline, and is much appreciated.

Finally, I want to thank the professors who have chosen to use this text for their own classes and, especially, the students who have made the wise decision to take a health psychology class. One of the most rewarding aspects of teaching health psychology is the opportunity to give students information they will really use: perhaps they will turn off their phone before driving, learn effective strategies for managing stress, and/or decide to adopt healthier eating and exercise habits. My hope in teaching health psychology—and now in writing a health psychology textbook—is that students will not only learn the essential theories and research in this field but will also learn practical skills and strategies they can put to use in their own lives.

Best wishes for the semester,

Catherine A. Sanderson
Amherst College

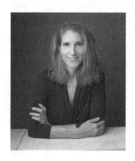

Catherine A. Sanderson is the Manwell Family Professor of Life Sciences (Psychology) at Amherst College. She received a bachelor's degree in psychology, with a specialization in Health and Development, from Stanford University, and received both master's and doctoral degrees in psychology from Princeton University. Professor Sanderson's research examines how personality and social variables influence health-related behaviors such as safer sex and disordered eating, the development of persuasive messages and interventions to prevent unhealthy behavior, and the predictors of relationship satisfaction. This research has received grant funding from the National Science Foundation and the National Institute of Health. Professor Sanderson has published over 25 journal articles and book chapters in addition to four college textbooks, middle and high school health textbooks, and a popular press book on parenting. In 2012, she was named one of the country's top 300 professors by the *Princeton Review*. Professor Sanderson speaks regularly for public and corporate audiences on topics such as the science of happiness, the power of emotional intelligence, the mind–body connection, and the psychology of good and evil. You can watch the talks (for free!) on her website: SandersonSpeaking.com.

1

INTRODUCTION

Learning Objectives

1.1 Describe how psychological factors influence health, pain, disease, and health care utilization

1.2 Summarize the history of the field of health psychology

1.3 Explain factors leading to the development of health psychology

1.4 Describe the influence of health psychology on other fields

1.5 Compare different training pathways and careers in health psychology

What You'll Learn

1.1 How getting daily hugs helps prevent colds

1.2 Why having support shortens pain during childbirth

1.3 Why happy teenagers become healthy adults

1.4 How doctors' rudeness hurts medical care

1.5 Why slamming doors may be good for health (at least in Japan)

Preview

Have you ever snacked on junk food when feeling stressed about a romantic relationship, checked your phone for a text while driving, or tried to distract yourself while receiving a shot at the doctor's office? These are all examples of how psychological factors influence physical well-being, for better or for worse. In this first chapter, you'll learn about the field of health psychology, how it has changed over time, and its link to other disciplines. You'll also learn about training pathways and career options in this exciting field.

UNDERSTANDING HEALTH PSYCHOLOGY

LO 1.1

Describe how psychological factors influence health, pain, disease, and health care utilization

The field of **health psychology** examines how biological, social, and psychological factors influence health and illness. This field developed in part due to a growing recognition of the substantial role psychological factors play in influencing health. As described in Table 1.1, every 10 years the surgeon general of the United States sets specific goals for improving health (Friedrich, 2000). Health professionals then work toward achieving these goals and researchers measure progress. As you can see, many of these goals involve people's behavioral choices, such as whether they engage in physical activity, use tobacco, or drive safely.

The field of health psychology uses theory and research in psychological science to promote health, prevent illness, and improve health care systems. Specifically, and as described in this first section, health psychology examines how psychological factors influence

Table 1.1   Examples of Healthy People 2020 Goals

Physical Activity

- Increase the proportion of adults who engage in aerobic physical activity of at least moderate intensity for at least 150 minutes/week.
- Increase the proportion of the nation's public and private schools that require daily physical education for all students.

Overweight and Obesity

- Reduce the proportion of adults who are obese.
- Reduce the proportion of children and adolescents who are considered obese.

Tobacco Use

- Reduce the initiation of tobacco use among children, adolescents, and young adults.
- Increase smoking cessation attempts by adult smokers.

Substance Abuse

- Decrease the proportion of adults reporting any use of illicit drugs during the past 30 days.
- Reduce the proportion of adolescents engaging in binge drinking during the past month.

Responsible Sexual Behavior

- Increase the proportion of sexually active persons aged 15 to 19 years who use condoms and hormonal or intrauterine contraception to both effectively prevent pregnancy and provide barrier protection against disease.
- Increase the proportion of adolescents aged 17 years and younger who have never had sexual intercourse.

Injury and Violence

- Reduce motor vehicle crash–related deaths.
- Reduce homicides.

Immunization

- Increase the proportion of children aged 19 to 35 months who receive the recommended doses of DTaP, polio, MMR, Hib, hepatitis B, varicella, and PCV vaccines.

- Increase the proportion of children and adults who are vaccinated annually against seasonal influenza.

Access to Health Care

- Increase the proportion of persons with health insurance.

- Increase the proportion of pregnant women who receive early and adequate prenatal care.

health-related behaviors and physiological reactions, the management of pain and disease, and health care utilization (Matarazzo, 1980).

Impact on Behavior and Physiology

Psychological factors have a substantial impact on health behaviors and on health outcomes. As shown in Figure 1.1, these psychological factors include environmental stressors, personality factors, and social influences, which in turn influence illness and disease through their impact on physiological responses in the body as well as health-related behaviors (Adler & Matthews, 1994).

Figure 1.1 The Impact of Psychological Factors on Health

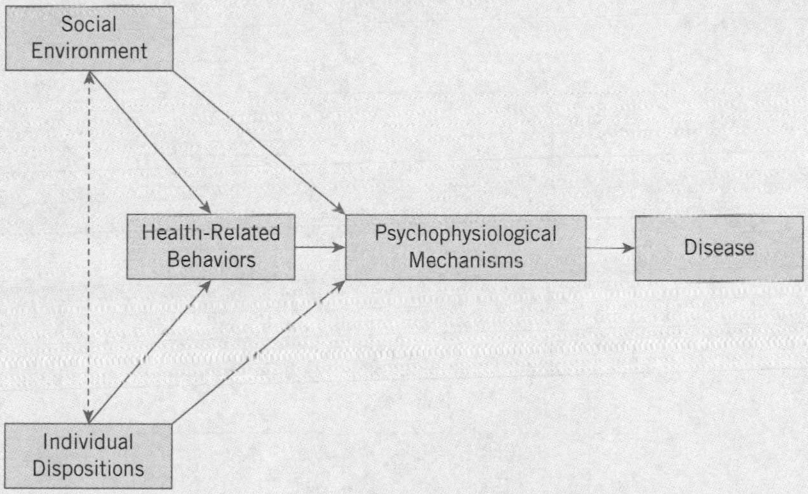

Psychological factors, including stress, personality, and social influences, impact people's physiological responses as well as their health behaviors, which in turn impact incidence of illness and disease. However, the relationship between psychological factors and physical health is bidirectional: physiological responses, health behaviors, and disease can also influence psychological factors.

Source: Taken from p. 231 of Adler, N., & Matthews, K. (1994). Health psychology: Why do some people get sick and some stay well? *Annual Review of Psychology, 45,* 229–259.

First, people who experience higher levels of stress are at greater risk of experiencing both minor and major illnesses, in part because stress weakens the immune system (Cohen & Herbert, 1996). For example, after exposure to a cold virus, people who experience higher levels of stress are more likely to develop a cold than those who are experiencing less stress (Cohen, Tyrrell, & Smith, 1991). Long-term stress can therefore lead to more severe health-related problems. In line with this view, people who reported feeling high work stress—meaning feeling overwhelmed by job demands; or low work stress—meaning feeling bored and unchallenged—were more likely to develop diabetes, even when researchers took into account other risk factors, such as age, family history, and BMI (Toker, Shirom, Melamed, & Armon, 2012). However, people who are able to see stress as a challenge—and have resources to manage stress—experience fewer health problems than those who find such experiences overwhelming.

People who are under stress also tend to engage in behaviors that weaken the body's ability to fight off infections. Just think about the typical behaviors of a college student during exam period. Many students stop exercising, eat more junk food, drink more caffeine, and get less sleep. In other words, the stress of exams leads people to engage in unhealthy behavior, which in turn decreases the body's resistance to illness. For example, and as shown in Figure 1.2, people who get less sleep are more likely to develop a cold (Prather, Janicki-Deverts, Hall, & Cohen, 2015).

Personality traits, such as optimism, hostility, and conscientiousness, are also associated with people's physiological responses to various situations as well as their health-related behaviors (Winett, 1995). For example, people who are high in hostility exhibit higher blood pressure and heart rate when they are in virtually any type of "competitive situation" (which could include even a game of Ping-Pong with a friend) (Miller, Smith, Turner, Guijarro, & Hallet, 1996). Over time, experiencing constant high levels of physiological arousal leads

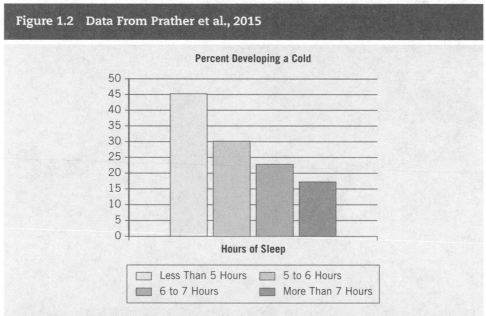

Figure 1.2   Data From Prather et al., 2015

Percent Developing a Cold

Hours of Sleep

Less Than 5 Hours   5 to 6 Hours
6 to 7 Hours   More Than 7 Hours

Researchers measured people's sleep habits, and then exposed them—through nasal drops—to a cold virus. People who slept on average less than six hours a night were more than four times as likely to develop a cold as those who got more than seven hours of sleep a night, even when researchers took into account factors that could predict susceptibility to a cold, such as stress, education, and income.

Source: Data from Prather, Janicki-Deverts, Hall, & Cohen (2015).

to cardiovascular damage, which may explain why people who are hostile are more likely to experience heart disease. On the other hand, people who are high in positive emotions, such as happiness, joy, enthusiasm, and optimism, experience better health, including lower rates of getting the common cold, experiencing a stroke, and having an accident, than those with lower levels of such emotions (Boehm & Kubzansky, 2012; Lyubomirsky, King, & Diener, 2005; Scheier & Carver, 1987). You can test your own level of optimism using **Table 1.2: Test Yourself.** Personality variables also influence the types of health-related behaviors people engage in on a regular basis. People who are high in hostility, for example, may ignore doctor recommendations for treatment and thereby fail to recover—or at least recover more slowly—from illnesses, whereas those who are conscientious tend to engage in health-promoting behaviors, such as eating a healthy diet, engaging in regular physical activity, and avoiding substance use.

Similarly, social factors are associated with individuals' physiological reactions and health-related behaviors. Individuals with high levels of social support have lower blood pressure and a more active immune system compared to those with less support (Cohen & Herbert, 1996; Uchino, Cacioppo, & Kiecolt-Glaser, 1996). In turn, people who have more social support may be better able to fight off minor illnesses and avoid major ones. In line with this view, researchers in one study first asked people how many hugs they received each day over a two-week period, and then—with the people's permission—exposed them to a cold virus (S. Cohen, Janicki-Deverts, Turner, & Doyle, 2015). As predicted, people who reported receiving more frequent hugs were less likely to show signs of infection and illness. Why? Researchers believe that a hug by a trusted person may be a strategy for conveying support, which in turn helps reduce feelings of stress. People who have high levels of social support may also engage in more health-promoting behavior (e.g., eating nutritiously, exercising regularly), in part because their loved ones encourage such activities. Moreover, because people learn about health behaviors from watching others' behavior, the attitudes and behaviors of family members and friends also influence health-related behavior. Children who have a parent, sibling, or friend who smokes, for example, are much more likely to start smoking themselves later on.

What You'll Learn
1.1

Table 1.2   Test Yourself: Are You an Optimist?

The following statements express how you may generally feel. Respond to these statements using a scale of 1 (strongly disagree) to 5 (strongly agree).

1. In uncertain times, I usually expect the best.

2. If something can go wrong for me, it will.

3. I'm always optimistic about my future.

4. I hardly ever expect things to go my way.

5. Overall, I expect more good things to happen to me than bad.

6. I rarely count on good things happening to me.

First, reverse your answers on items 2, 4, and 6 (meaning you give yourself a 5 if you put a 1, 4 if you put a 2, 3 if you put a 3, 2 if you put a 4, and 1 if you put a 5). Then sum up your answers using the new score for items 2, 4, and 6 and the original score for items 1, 3, and 5. Higher numbers indicate greater optimism.

Source: Scheier, Carver, & Bridges (1994).

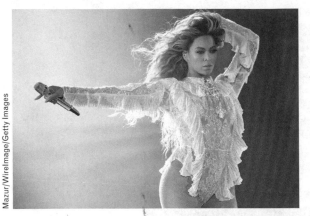

Mazur/WireImage/Getty Images

Even people we don't know, such as movie stars or professional athletes, can serve as models that influence our health-related behavior. After the announcement that singer Beyoncé would receive $50 million to promote Pepsi products, public health researchers expressed concern that her endorsement would increase soda consumption, a leading contributor to today's obesity epidemic.

What You'll Learn
1.2

Impact on Pain and Disease

Psychological factors, including environmental stress, personality, and social support, influence the development and treatment of pain (Winett, 1995). Have you ever developed a severe headache or felt nauseous before taking an important exam? This is a simple example of how stress can create physical pain. Pain is also influenced by other psychological factors, such as the rewards received for experiencing pain (e.g., a child who complains about a stomachache gets to miss school), people's thoughts about the results of the pain (e.g., a tattoo or body piercing may feel less painful than immunizations), and modeling (e.g., cultural norms about expressing pain vary substantially).

Psychological factors can also help reduce the experienced of pain. For example, considerable research points to the benefits of having support during labor in reducing pain and medical complications. For example, women who receive support during labor experience fewer complications, are less likely to undergo a cesarean section, require fewer drugs, and have a shorter labor (Kennell, Klaus, McGrath, Robertson, & Hinckley, 1991; Sosa, Kennell, Klaus, Robertson, & Urrutia, 1980). On the other hand, women who are more afraid of childbirth experience a longer labor, regardless of whether or not they choose epidural pain relief (Adams, Eberhard-Gran, & Eskild, 2012).

Psychological factors contribute to the development of many types of chronic and life-threatening diseases, such as coronary heart disease, cancer, and AIDS. Many of these diseases are influenced at least in part by behavioral choices that people make, such as whether to smoke, exercise, maintain a healthy weight, engage in unsafe sex, or drink alcohol. Other psychological factors, including personality and coping style, also impact whether people develop particular chronic and life-threatening illnesses as well as the progression of such diseases. For example, people who are depressed have an increased risk of developing diabetes and experiencing a heart attack or stroke, and among those with diabetes or coronary heart disease, higher levels of depression are associated with an increased risk of mortality (Herbert & Cohen, 1993; Pan, Sun, Okereke, Rexrode, & Hu, 2011).

Finally, the link between psychological factors and both pain and illness is clearly bidirectional. A person who is constantly in physical pain, for example, may feel depressed and anxious, avoid many social settings, and even withdraw from close family members and friends. People who experience chronic diseases, such as diabetes, cancer, and coronary heart disease, may experience similar negative emotions. Finally, and not surprisingly, many people who are diagnosed with a terminal illness experience depression and anxiety, and survivors often experience lower levels of psychological and physical well-being.

Impact on Health Care Utilization

Health psychology also examines how psychological factors influence whether people take steps to identify and treat illnesses early, whether they adhere to medical recommendations, and how they respond to health-promotion messages (Winett, 1995). Behavior that involves detecting illness at an early stage as a way of reducing the illness's potential effects is called **secondary prevention** and can include checking cholesterol, having a mammogram, and following an insulin-taking regimen in the case of diabetes. Secondary prevention is very important because in many cases people have more treatment options and a better likelihood of curing their problem if it is caught early. For example, detecting a small cancerous lump in the breast during a routine mammogram may allow a woman the option of having this lump removed in a simple operation before cancer spreads to other parts of her body, whereas a woman who is found to have a lump in her breast only after the cancer has spread has unknowingly delayed treatment, has decreased her treatment options, and will undergo much more difficult treatment, such as invasive surgery (possible removal of both breasts), chemotherapy, and/or radiation. However, psychological factors such as fear and anxiety influence whether someone engages in prevention and health-promotion behavior. For some people, getting tested for HIV is simply too frightening to contemplate.

In addition, psychological factors influence the effectiveness of various treatments to manage pain as well as chronic and terminal disease. Treatments that can help minimize or slow the damage caused by a disease are known as tertiary prevention actions and can include taking medicine, engaging in regular physical therapy, and following a recommended diet (Winett, 1995). Patients with chronic conditions, such as cancer, AIDS, and heart disease, need to regularly manage their illnesses, cope with pain, and comply with medical regimens. However, some studies suggest that as many as 93% of patients fail to adhere to recommended treatments (Taylor, 1990). Why do some people follow doctor recommendations and others ignore these messages? Psychological factors, including people's thoughts about their symptoms and illnesses as well as interactions with health care providers and the medical system in general, influence how people react to treatment plans, and thus whether they recover from illness. Psychosocial factors even influence how quickly people are diagnosed with cancer, how they manage this diagnosis, and even how long they live following the diagnosis (Antoni & Lutgendorf, 2007). For example, and as you'll learn more about in *Chapter 11: Leading Causes of Mortality*, early-stage breast cancer patients who write about their feelings regarding their diagnosis later report fewer physical symptoms and have fewer medical appointments than those who write simply about the facts of their illness (Stanton et al., 2002). This research suggests that writing about positive feelings may lead to better health outcomes even in patients who have been diagnosed with cancer, revealing a powerful mind–body connection.

THE HISTORY OF HEALTH PSYCHOLOGY

Health psychology is a relatively new field. In 1973, a task force was created by the American Psychological Association (APA) to study the potential for psychology's role in health research. Although the final report of this task force in 1976 found little evidence that psychologists were examining health-related issues, the task force noted that the potential for psychological factors to influence health was clear (American Psychological Association, 1976). In turn, this report led to the creation in 1978 of a Health Psychology division with the goal of providing "a scientific, educational, and professional organization for psychologists interested in (or working in) areas at one or another of the interfaces of medicine and psychology" (Matarazzo, 1984, p. 31). The development of this division was followed in 1982 by the creation of the journal *Health Psychology*, in which many research articles on issues in health psychology are published. This section examines various factors that led to the development of the exciting new field of health psychology.

LO 1.2

Summarize the history of the field of health psychology

Early Views on the Mind–Body Connection

Although health psychology is a relatively new discipline, the idea that the mind influences the body is a very old one—in fact, historically, most cultures have recognized some type of a connection between how we think, feel, and behave and our health (Ehrenwald, 1976). Many early cultures viewed illness and disease as caused by evil spirits—and there is some evidence

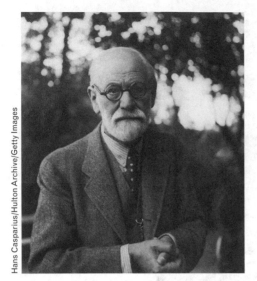

Freud's theory about the role of unconscious conflict in leading to physical symptoms, including paralysis, sudden loss of hearing and sight, and muscle tremors, is clearly based in the theory that physical problems may represent manifestations of unconscious symptoms as opposed to a true medical disorder.

that early medical procedures, at least in some cases, involved such methods as drilling holes in people's skulls to "let out the evil spirits." As early as 400 B.C., Hippocrates described health as the interaction between mind and body, stating, "Health depends on a state of equilibrium among the various internal factors which govern the operation of the body and the mind; the equilibrium in turn is reached only when man lives in harmony with his environment" (Dubus, 1959, p. 114). In line with this view, Hippocrates's humoral theory described disease as caused by an imbalance in the different fluids he believed were circulating in the body: phlegm, blood, black bile, and yellow bile. Despite the faulty theory of the four humors, the emphasis on the interrelation between mind and body is clear.

However, during the 17th century this holistic view of health changed, and, for the first time, health was seen as purely caused by bodily processes. What led to this change? First, René Descartes's development of the doctrine of mind–body dualism, namely, the view that the mind and body are two separate entities with little interaction, led to the view that the body was basically a machine. Disease was seen as resulting from the physical breakdown of the machine, and it was believed that the physician's job was to fix the machine. Second, advances in other scientific fields such as physics led to the view that science could be used to determine precise physical principles. For example, Isaac Newton's demonstration of an apple falling to the earth because of gravitational pull led other theorists to believe that all physical phenomena could be observed with such ease and explained by concrete laws. Third, various scientific advances, including Giovanni Battista Morgagni's work in autopsy, Rudolf Virchow's work in pathology, and Louis Pasteur's work in bacteriology, led to a focus on how microorganisms cause disease. All of these factors facilitated the focus on a biomedical model.

The Failure of the Biomedical Model

The biomedical model, which was formed in the 19th and 20th centuries, proposes that health problems are rooted in physical causes, such as viruses, bacteria, injuries, and biochemical imbalances (Engel, 1977; Schwartz, 1982; Wade & Halligan, 2004). This model therefore explains illness in terms of the pathology, biochemistry, and physiology of a disease—diabetes is caused by an imbalance in blood sugar, polio is caused by exposure to a virus, and cancer is caused by genetic mutations. In turn, the biomedical model proposes that medical treatment is needed to cure or manage the physical complaint and thereby return a person to good health. The biomedical model therefore focuses on physical treatments for disease, such as a vaccine to prevent measles, medication to manage high blood pressure, and chemotherapy to delay the spread of cancer.

Although the biomedical model has led to a number of benefits for our society, including advancements in immunology, public health policy, pathology, and surgery, increasingly evidence is showing that biological factors alone cannot account for health. First, and as described previously, psychological and behavioral factors are associated with the development of many of the leading causes of death, such as cancer and heart disease. People who are high in neuroticism are at increased risk of developing an ulcer, chronic fatigue syndrome, and coronary heart disease (Charles, Gatz, Kato, & Pedersen, 2008; Suls & Bunde, 2005). Similarly, people who are experiencing high levels of stress—at home and/or work—are at greater risk of experience a heart attack (Rosengren et al., 2004). The biomedical model also fails to take into account how psychological factors, such as personality, cognitive beliefs, social support, and the relationship between the patient and the health care practitioner, can influence development of and recovery from illness and disease. Why do placebos, drugs, or treatments that influence health outcomes, purely because of people's expectations of them, lead to improvement of symptoms in a sizable proportion of patients? Why do surgery patients who get more visitors leave the hospital sooner? These are just some of the questions that the biomedical model really cannot answer.

The Creation of the Biopsychosocial Model

Given the considerable evidence that the biomedical model alone can't explain physical health, researchers have turned to a biopsychosocial model in which the mind and body are seen as inherently connected (Ray, 2004; Suls & Rothman, 2004). The biopsychosocial model was developed in the late 1970s and posits that health is affected by both biology and social factors (Engel, 1977, 1980). In this perspective, the physical body is seen as only one aspect of a person; other aspects, such as personality, family, and society, also influence the person and his or her health. In contrast, the biomedical model, which was formed in the 19th and 20th centuries, describes health as a function only of physical attributes and sees physical health as completely separate from psychological health.

The biopsychosocial model, which was developed by psychiatrist George Engel, views health and illness as the consequences of the complex interplay between biological factors (e.g., genetics, physiology), psychological factors (e.g., personality, cognition), and social factors (e.g., culture, community, family, media) (Engel, 1977, 1980; Schwartz, 1982). As described by Engel,

> To provide a basis for understanding the determinants of disease and arriving at rational treatments and patterns of health care, a medical model must also take into account the patient, the social context in which he lives and the complementary system devised by society to deal with the disruptive effects of illness, that is, the physician role and the health care system. This requires a biopsychosocial model. (p. 132)

The biopsychosocial model is holistic in that it considers the mind and body as inherently connected. In addition, it acknowledges that biological factors can and do influence health and illness, but that social, cultural, and psychological factors also exert an effect. The biopsychosocial model therefore contributes to the biomedical model by helping to explain the impact of psychological factors on the development and progression of chronic conditions as well as how people cope with pain, illness, and disease. **Research in Action** describes how people with high-quality social relationships live longer, which is a vivid example of the biopsychosocial model's ability to explain health outcomes.

Let's take, as an example, a patient, Melanie, who arrives at her doctor's office complaining of recurring heart pain. A physician utilizing the biomedical model would focus almost entirely on physical causes of such pain and would rely primarily on diagnostic tests, such as heart monitor results, temperature, pulse, and so forth, to determine the cause of this symptom. Although the physician might ask Melanie a few questions (when did you last eat? how long have you felt this pain?), the physician would base the diagnosis on the (more objective) test results. Once a physical diagnosis was established, the physician would prescribe a treatment regimen for the patient. In contrast, a physician using the biopsychosocial model might start by gathering personal data, such as symptoms, activities, recent behaviors, and social/family relationships. The physician might, for example, ask Melanie whether she was experiencing any particular stressors at home or work or whether she had experienced significant life changes in the past few months (e.g., loss of a job, death of a loved one). Although the physician would also use standard diagnostic tests, more emphasis would be placed on eliciting psychological factors that could contribute to the symptoms. During this information-gathering

RESEARCH IN ACTION

How Good Friendships May Extend Your Life

Researchers in this study examined how people's social relationships predict physical well-being and longevity (Yang, Boen, Gerken, Li, Schorpp, & Harris, 2016). Using data from four national surveys of Americans from adolescence through old age, they examined three distinct aspects of people's social relationships: the size of their social networks, their level of social support, and the degree of social strain they were experiencing (meaning demands, criticism, and disappointments in their relationships). In addition, they measured four physical factors that predict overall health and longevity: body mass index (BMI), waist size, blood pressure, and level of C-reactive protein (a measure of inflammation). Their findings revealed consistent links between people's social relationships and indicators of physical health. However, different aspects of social relationships predicted health for people across the lifespan. Specifically, for both adolescence and older adults, having more social relationships was associated with better health outcomes. In fact, for people in these two age groups, lacking social relationships was as detrimental for health as being physically inactive or having diabetes. For people in middle age, the quality of people's social relationships, meaning their levels of social support and social strain, was a better predictor of health than the presence of a large social network. For people in mid-adulthood, who may already have multiple relationships to manage as a spouse and parent, additional relationships may provide more opportunities for strain and thus not be beneficial in reducing stress and thereby improving health. These findings are particularly important since the markers of physical well-being studied are predictors of long-term health problems, including heart disease, stroke, and cancer. In sum, developing strong social relationships is a very important way of having good health.

phase, the physician would also provide information about what was happening and for what reasons to minimize the stress Melanie experienced with the various medical procedures. Once a diagnosis was made, the physician would discuss the treatment options with Melanie, and she would have a voice in selecting her own treatment plan. The physician would not only work with Melanie to develop a treatment plan but would also pay attention to aspects of Melanie's daily life that could influence her adherence to the plan.

THE DEVELOPMENT OF HEALTH PSYCHOLOGY

LO 1.3

Explain factors leading to the development of health psychology

The creation of the biopsychosocial model was an essential step in creating the field of health psychology. A number of other factors also contributed to its development, including a change in the meaning of health, an increase in the prevalence of chronic conditions, the rising cost of health care, and advances in scientific and medical technology.

A Change in the Meaning of Health

Over the last 100 years, the meaning of health has changed in several ways. We used to think of health as simply the absence of illness or disease, but we now see health and wellness in a much broader way. The World Health Organization now defines health as "a state of complete physical, mental and social well-being, and not merely the absence of disease and illness" (World Health Organization, 1964). So, people who are physiologically healthy but who are very depressed might be viewed as unhealthy under the new definition. Similarly, most college students seem healthy—generally they exercise with some regularity and exhibit few obvious signs of disease or serious illness. But can they be viewed as healthy if you look at their eating habits or, even worse, their drinking habits? By the new standard, many college students suddenly seem as if they are in worse health. Along the same lines, consider someone who has no obvious signs of illness or disease but who has a mother and two aunts who died of breast cancer. Is she healthy? In sum, researchers now see health as a continuum, ranging from a healthy level of wellness on one end and illness and even death on the other, and they have found that this continuum is viewed in different ways by different people (Antonovsky, 1987).

This change in perspective is also reflected in a relatively new focus within psychology on studying the predictors of happiness and well-being as opposed to the predictors of depression and poor health (Seligman & Csikszentmihalyi, 2000). The newly developed field of positive psychology, which examines how psychological factors influence positive human functioning and flourishing, focuses on helping people achieve physical and psychological well-being. Considerable research demonstrates that people who are high on positive personal traits, such as optimism and positive affect, engage in more health-promoting behaviors and are less likely to develop chronic and life-threatening diseases. For example, people who are high on optimism are more likely to engage in regular exercise, less likely to smoke, and less likely to experience a stroke (Kim, Park, & Peterson, 2011; Steptoe, Wright, Kunz-Ebrecht, & Iliffe, 2006). Similarly, people with coronary heart disease who experience more positive emotions—such as *proud*, *enthusiastic*, and *inspired*—report engaging in more health-promoting behaviors, including exercising, avoiding smoking, and greater adherence to medication, which, in turn, should reduce the risk of experiencing subsequent cardiac events (Sin, Moskowitz, & Whooley, 2015).

**What You'll Learn
1.3**

Researchers in one study examined whether teenagers with good emotional health and well-being developed into healthier adults later on (Hoyt, Chase-Lansdale, McDade, & Adam, 2012). First, more than 10,000 teenagers answered questions about their overall emotional health, including happiness, enjoyment of life, self-esteem, and hopefulness for the future. They then examined rates of health-related behavior in these same teenagers—now young adults—seven years later. Their findings revealed that teenagers who generally felt happy and positive were less likely to engage in unhealthy behaviors, such as smoking, binge drinking, using drugs, and eating unhealthy foods, later on. This link between experiencing positive emotions during the teenage years and engaging in healthier behaviors in young adulthood remained even when researchers took into account other variables that could explain better health, including socioeconomic status, gender, ethnicity, and depression. These findings suggest that helping teenagers feel positive may have lasting benefits for health.

An Increase in Chronic Conditions

Until the early 1900s, most people in the United States died from acute infectious diseases, such as tuberculosis, smallpox, measles, pneumonia, and typhoid fever (see Table 1.3). These diseases were caused by viruses or bacteria and were typically the result of eating or drinking contaminated water or food, interacting with infected people, or living in unhealthy conditions. Moreover, although people sought treatment for these disorders, doctors often had little knowledge or resources to treat or even manage these illnesses.

Today, in contrast, relatively few people (at least in the United States) die from the major infectious diseases that previously caused such high rates of death. What led to the decrease in the incidence of such diseases? First, changes in technology and lifestyle, such as the development of sewage treatment plants, water purification efforts, and better overall nutrition, led to better overall hygiene. Second, because of the development of vaccines and antibiotics, very few people contract (and even fewer die from) diseases such as smallpox, tuberculosis, and polio (see Figure 1.3). Most children are vaccinated against many of the major infectious

Table 1.3	The 10 Leading Causes of Death in 1900 Versus 2015	
Major Causes of Death		
In 1900	**In 2015**	
1. Cardiovascular diseases (strokes, heart disease)	1. Heart disease	
2. Influenza and pneumonia	2. Cancer	
3. Tuberculosis	3. Chronic lower respiratory disease	
4. Gastritis	4. Unintentional injuries	
5. Accidents	5. Stroke	
6. Cancer	6. Alzheimer's disease	
7. Diphtheria	7. Diabetes	
8. Typhoid fever	8. Flu and pneumonia	
9. Measles	9. Kidney disease (nephritis)	
10. Chronic liver disease and cirrhosis	10. Suicide	

Note: In 1900, many people died from infectious diseases; today, many of the leading causes of death are chronic conditions that are at least partially caused by lifestyle choices.

diseases, and other diseases can be effectively treated with antibiotics. **Focus on Development** describes the important role parents play in promoting health in their children, and in other children, by following recommended immunization schedules.

This shift in the pattern of illnesses from acute or infectious diseases to chronic conditions has focused attention on the role of psychological factors in predicting health. Specifically, the major health problems in the United States today are chronic conditions, such as cancer, cardiovascular disease, obesity, diabetes, and pulmonary diseases, which are caused at least in part by behavioral, psychosocial, and cultural factors. As shown in Table 1.3, heart disease is currently the most common cause of death in the United States. However, the likelihood of developing heart disease is influenced by many behavioral choices—smoking, high-fat diet, physical inactivity, obesity, and alcohol use (all behavioral choices) as well as psychological variables (e.g., stress) and environmental factors (e.g., social support). Similarly, the major cause of lung cancer—which is the leading cause of cancer deaths for men and women—is cigarette smoking. Smoking contributes not only to heart disease and cancer but also to strokes (the third leading cause of death), chronic lower respiratory disorder (the fourth leading cause of death), pneumonia (the eighth leading cause of death), and diabetes (the seventh leading cause of death). In sum, people's own behavior contributes to many of the leading causes of death today. Specifically, the five leading causes of death among people younger than 80 cause 63% of deaths each year in the United States; these causes are heart disease, cancer, stroke, chronic

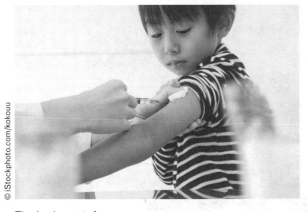

The development of penicillin, which treats previously untreated bacterial illnesses such as pneumonia and cholera, had a substantial impact on life expectancy.

FOCUS ON DEVELOPMENT

How Immunizations Save Lives

One of the most significant factors leading to the increase in life expectancy over the last century is the development of vaccinations, which help the immune system fight infections and thereby prevent diseases. Vaccines are now able to prevent many diseases that used to be common in the United States and around the world, including polio, measles, rubella (German measles), and pertussis (whooping cough). Although getting vaccinations is one of the best ways people can stay healthy, 27% of American preschool-age children do not have full immunization against currently controllable diseases (National Center for Health Statistics, 2017). Unfortunately, when children don't get vaccinated, they can develop very serious, and even life-threatening, illnesses. For example, after the development of the varicella vaccine, which prevents chicken pox, in 1995, deaths from varicella dropped 88% in a six-year period (Marin, Zhang, & Seward, 2011). Children who aren't vaccinated are at risk not only of developing a potentially life-threatening disease but also of infecting others. In 2010, 10 babies in California died from whooping cough. Although these babies were younger than three months, which means they were too young to have been vaccinated against this disease, they clearly had come in contact with someone who wasn't vaccinated. Thus, parents have a responsibility to make sure their children have all recommended vaccinations to protect not only their children but also those with whom their children come in contact.

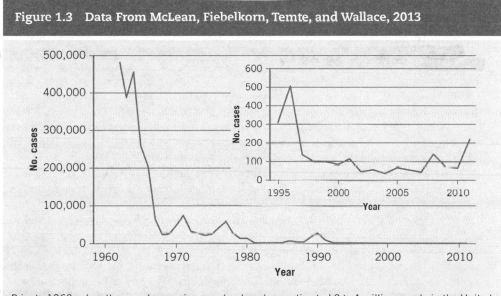

Figure 1.3 Data From McLean, Fiebelkorn, Temte, and Wallace, 2013

Prior to 1963, when the measles vaccine was developed, an estimated 3 to 4 million people in the United States were infected each year, and 450 to 500 of these people died. In 2016, only 70 people in the United States were diagnosed with measles, and not a single person died.

Source: McLean, Fiebelkorn, Temte, & Wallace (2013).

lower respiratory diseases, and unintentional injuries (García, Bastian, Rossen, et al., 2016). But roughly one-third of these deaths could be prevented through changes in people's behavior, such as not smoking, maintaining a healthy weight, and safer driving.

Given the role of individuals' behavior in contributing to health problems, principles of psychology can be used to try to change people's behavior to prevent health problems from ever developing, such as to increase health-promoting behavior (e.g., wearing seat belts, engaging in regular exercise, using sunscreen) and decrease health-damaging behavior (e.g., smoking, using drugs, eating a diet high in fat). This type of preventive behavior is known as primary prevention, meaning behavior designed to prevent or diminish the severity of illnesses and diseases. Researchers in one study examined the influence of smoking and obesity on life expectancy (van Baal, Hoogenveen, de Wit, & Boshuizen, 2006). Men who smoke die on average 7.7 years sooner, and women who smoke die 6.3 years sooner. Similarly, obese men die 4.7 years earlier and obese women die 4.4 years earlier. This research provides powerful evidence that the behavioral choices we make have a major impact on how long we live.

Yet influencing people's behavior is complex, as you will see throughout this book; many people engage (or fail to engage in) behaviors that they know impact their health, such as smoking, getting too little sleep, not exercising, and failing to have that recommended colonoscopy. As physician John Knowles (1977) noted, "over 99 percent of us are born healthy and made sick as a result of personal misbehavior and environmental conditions. The solution to the problems of ill health in modern American society involves individual responsibility, in the first instance, and social responsibility through public legislation and private volunteer efforts, in the second instance" (p. 58).

The Rising Cost of Health Care

Health care costs have risen sharply in the last 50 years. The U.S. population currently spends nearly $3.8 trillion a year on health care, which represents 17.8% of the gross domestic product (Centers for Disease Control and Prevention, 2017h). In contrast, health care costs represented only 5.1% of the gross domestic product in 1960.

One reason for the rise in health care costs is the dramatic increase in life expectancy that has occurred over the last century. In the early 1900s, people lived to an average age of 47.3 years; today the mean life expectancy is nearly 79 years (Kochanek, Murphy, Xu, & Tejada-Vera, 2016). This increase in life expectancy is partially a result of a substantial drop in the rate of infant mortality. Specifically, in 1960, 47 infant deaths occurred for every 1,000 live births, whereas fewer than 6 infant deaths occur for every 1,000 live births today. Moreover, infants who are born two or three months premature now have a very good chance of surviving, whereas even 10 years ago their odds were significantly worse.

This increase in life expectancy contributes to the high cost of health care; people are living longer, so they develop more chronic, long-term diseases that require ongoing care, possibly for years. AIDS, Alzheimer's disease, coronary heart disease, and cancer are all examples of very common diseases that people may live with for many years—sometimes requiring extended and expensive treatment (e.g., bypass surgery, drug regimens, chemotherapy, and radiation). More than half of all spending on health care costs in the United States is on 20 conditions; the most expensive of these is diabetes (Dieleman et al., 2016). Other costly health conditions include heart disease, back and neck pain, injuries from falls, and hypertension.

Another factor contributing to the rising cost of health care is increasing technological advancements, such as new surgical techniques and medical procedures, which require specialized equipment and are very expensive. Doctors are now able to perform truly remarkable procedures to save and improve lives, including transplanting organs, performing surgery on fetuses prior to birth, and tailoring cancer treatments to patients' particular genetic profiles. These advances in medical technology also mean that in some cases people are now able to live with serious conditions that in the past would have killed them. Although such treatments are partially responsible for the increase in life expectancy, they have also greatly increased the cost of health care.

Concern about the high cost of health care has led to increasing acceptance of psychologists and their research by physicians and other health care professionals for several reasons. First, principles in health psychology can be used to prevent health problems from developing, which is much more cost-effective than diagnosing and treating illness and disease (Fries, 1998; Winett, 1995). For example, preventing premature birth by ensuring that pregnant women have prenatal care reduces medical costs considerably (Brown, 1985)—babies who weigh as little as 1 pound at birth can be saved, but it costs about $350,000 per baby for four months of care in the neonatal intensive care unit, and these babies often have ongoing struggles and disabilities. In contrast, it would cost about $600 per pregnant woman to provide prenatal care to 583 women, which substantially reduces the likelihood of premature birth (Butter, 1993). Although this type of prevention program would reduce the demand for medical services and thereby reduce health care costs, the vast majority of funds devoted to researching health issues each year are devoted to treating illness, not preventing it (DeLeon, 2002). Principles in health psychology can also be used to persuade people to seek medical care in order to detect health problems at an early stage, when there are more treatment options available and these options are less expensive. For example, people who learn they are HIV positive are able to start antiretroviral therapy (ART), which slows the growth of the virus in the body.

Although many chronic conditions cannot be cured, people can often live with them for many years. Health psychologists can therefore contribute to the design of treatment programs that help people manage these illnesses, such as ones that encourage patients with heart disease to adopt healthier eating habits and to stop smoking. Moreover, in many cases psychological treatments may help people cope with pain and recover from medical problems at a lower cost. For example, women who have a "doula" (a trained supportive companion to assist with labor and delivery) have shorter labors, use less epidural anesthesia, and are less likely to have a cesarean section than women without such support (Kennell, Klaus, McGrath, Robertson, & Hinkley, 1991). They are also less likely to have babies that require neonatal hospitalization, which is a tremendous cost savings. Similarly, surgical patients who receive high levels of social support show less anxiety, receive lower doses of narcotics, and are released from the hospital faster than those with lower levels of support (Krohne & Slangen, 2005). All of these psychologically based strategies for improving health can lead to decreases in health problems and/or minimize the pain and disability caused by such problems, and thereby reduce health care costs.

Advances in Technology

Another factor that has contributed greatly to the development of health psychology, and our understanding about the link between psychological factors and physical health, is scientific advances. For example, the field of genetics has grown substantially over the last few decades, enabling researchers to examine how particular genes are associated with health and behavior. We now know that genes influence health-related behaviors, such as obesity, substance abuse, and even risk of experiencing an injury. In part through its influence on health-related behaviors, genetics also plays a role in the development of many chronic diseases, including diabetes, cancer, coronary heart disease, and Alzheimer's disease.

Advances in technology have also enabled researchers to examine the link between brain activity and particular health-related behaviors. Neuroscience research now illustrates that activation

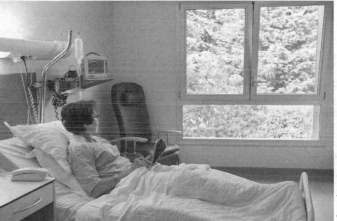

© Eric Audras/Getty Images

Even subtle shifts in the environment, such as having a room overlooking nature, can speed up recovery from surgery, and thereby reduce medical costs.

in specific parts of the brain may provide insight into various health behaviors, such as how people with anorexia respond to food, why certain people really crave alcohol, and why people prefer high-calorie foods (Foerde, Steinglass, Shohamy, & Walsh, 2015; Frye et al., 2016; Tang, Fellows, & Dagher, 2014). This type of technology can also provide valuable information about the effectiveness of fear-based appeals for helping smokers quit and mindfulness meditation for reducing pain (Falk, O'Donnell, Tompson, et al., 2015; Zeidan et al., 2011). The contributions of neuroscience to health psychology are highlighted in special Focus on Neuroscience boxes in each chapter of this book. For example, **Focus on Neuroscience** describes how obese people continue to respond to food cues, even when they are not hungry.

THE BROAD INFLUENCE OF HEALTH PSYCHOLOGY

LO 1.4

Describe the influence of health psychology on other fields

The growing awareness of the link between psychological states and physical health has influenced not only the field of psychology but also other disciplines. In this section you'll learn about the link between health psychology and the fields of medicine, sociology, and anthropology.

Medicine

Although this section has focused on the development of the distinct field of health psychology, several branches of medicine have also described the role of psychological factors in influencing physical health. **Psychosomatic medicine**, which developed in the 1930s, studies how emotional, social, and psychological factors influence the development and progression of illness (Lipowski, 1986). For example, researchers might study how psychological factors such as anxiety, depression, and stress may lead to physical problems such as ulcers, migraine headaches, arthritis, and asthma.

FOCUS ON NEUROSCIENCE

Why Some People Respond to Food Cues, Even When Not Hungry

Researchers in one study examined how people's brains respond to pictures of food, and whether such responses vary depending on both level of hunger and level of obesity (Puzziferri et al., 2016). Half of the women in the study were lean (they had a BMI under 25), whereas the others were obese (they had a BMI over 35). All women, who had fasted for nine hours before the study to make sure they were hungry, looked at photos of food while they were in an MRI machine, which measures brain activity. Next, all participants ate the same meal in the lab, so that they were no longer hungry, and then once again viewed photos of food while in an MRI machine. Their findings revealed that both hunger and obesity influenced patterns of brain activation in response to food cues. First, all women showed the same type of brain activity when they were hungry, indicating that hunger activates particular parts of the brain that process rewarding experiences. After eating a full meal, lean women's brains showed a substantial decrease—15%—in brain activity in response to photos of food, indicating that these women aren't particularly responding to cues of food once they are no longer hungry. In contrast, women who were obese showed only a very slight decline—4%—in brain activity in response to photos of food, indicating that even after they've eaten and thus are no longer hungry, their brain is still responding to food cues. These findings, which suggest that obese people continue to respond to food cues even when no longer full, demonstrate why it is so difficult for obese people to lose weight.

Similarly, behavioral medicine is an interdisciplinary field that developed in the 1970s and that focuses on the integration of behavioral and biomedical sciences. Specifically, behavioral medicine focuses on developing and applying behavioral techniques to the treatment, management, and rehabilitation of patients (Gentry, 1984). Such techniques are used widely to help people overcome various types of health-damaging behaviors. Correspondingly, the discipline of behavioral health, a subdiscipline of behavioral medicine, emphasizes enhancing health and preventing disease in currently healthy people (Matarazzo, 1980). Researchers in this field focus on general strategies of health promotion.

Although the medical community has often resisted collaborating with psychologists (or other non–medically trained personnel), this resistance has faded substantially given the growing evidence that psychological factors improve patient outcomes and reduce costs. As of July 1, 2001, the Accreditation Council for Graduate Medical Education required that residency programs teach skills in such collaboration, and residency programs must now demonstrate that residents have these skills prior to graduation. Moreover, as of 2015, the American Association of Medical Colleges added a section to the Medical College Admission Test (MCAT) that tests people's understanding of human behavior and psychology. These changes in medical school admissions and training reflect a growing awareness that doctors' behavior has a substantial impact on patients' health outcomes. For example, and as described in **Focus on Diversity**, doctors interact with patients differently as a function of their race/ethnicity, which could in turn influence patients' decision making regarding end-of-life care.

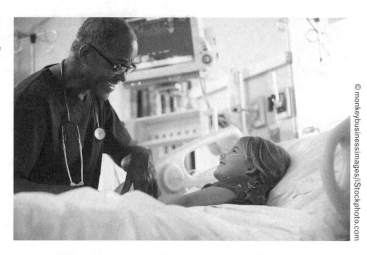

© monkeybusinessimages/iStockphoto.com

Theories and principles in health psychology are now used regularly in medical settings, largely because of a greater understanding and acceptance of how psychological factors influence physical health.

FOCUS ON DIVERSITY

The Impact of Patients' Race on Doctors' Nonverbal Communication

Doctors may behave differently when interacting with patients from different ethnic and racial backgrounds, which in turn could influence patients' health outcomes. Researchers in one study asked physicians—who were mostly White men—to participate in realistic simulations about how they would convey information to patients and their family members regarding end-of-life care (Elliott, Alexander, Mescher, Mohan, & Barnato, 2016). Physicians were given specific information about the patient's medical condition, such as poor vital signs for someone with late-state cancer, and were told to convey this information to the patient and their family and to determine what type of lifesaving measures, if any, they wanted. Researchers then watched videotapes of these doctor–patient interactions and measured both verbal and nonverbal communication (e.g., body position, eye contact, proximity, and touch). Although physicians gave similar verbal messages to both Black and White patients, their nonverbal cues differed substantially as a function of the patient's race. Specifically, when talking with a White person about next steps for care, the physicians were more likely to stand right beside the patient's bedside and touch them than when talking with a Black person. These unconscious nonverbal behaviors, in turn, could have a substantial impact on Black patients' trust and confidence in their physicians as well as on the medical decisions they make.

Doctors' interactions with other medical professionals also impact the quality of medical decision making in hospitals. Researchers in one study examined whether rudeness between medical professionals impacts the care people receive in a hospital (Riskin et al., 2015). Teams of doctors working in neonatal intensive care units (NICUs) participated in an exercise in which they had to decide how to care for a premature infant suffering from a relatively common, but severe, medical complication. They were told that an expert on "team reflexivity" would be observing them through a live video and would make suggestions. Half of the teams received suggestions from a "neutral" expert, whereas the others received suggestions from a "rude" expert, who started the observation by noting that he was not very impressed by the quality of medical care offered at this hospital. Three independent judges—who were not told about the initial statements made by the expert—then viewed the videotaped discussions to evaluate the teams' performance. As predicted, teams who were exposed to the rude expert scored lower on diagnostic performance, meaning their ability to appropriately identify key aspects of the infant's condition, as well as on procedural performance, meaning the technical skills used to provide care to the infant. These findings suggest that even relatively low levels of rudeness in a medical setting may lead to an overall lower quality of care, which clearly could have substantial implications for health outcomes.

Sociology

Medical sociology examines how social relationships influence illness, cultural and societal reactions to illness, and the organization of health care services (Adler & Stone, 1979). For example, researchers in this field might examine the effects of social stress on health and illness, how attitudes and behaviors influence health and illness, and the negative consequences of labeling someone a "patient."

Sociologists also examine how social and cultural factors—such as race, socioeconomic status, religion, and sexual orientation—influence health and health care utilization. For example, research consistently finds that people with lower levels of education experience overall worse health outcomes, in part because they are more likely to engage in detrimental health behaviors, such as smoking (Conti & Heckman, 2010). Lower levels of education are also associated with an increased risk of experiencing chronic pain, meaning pain that interferes with the ability to function in daily life; in fact, people who didn't finish high school are 370% more likely to experience severe chronic pain than those with graduate degrees (Grol-Prokopczyk, 2017). Similarly, both race and income are associated with a greater risk of developing chronic and life-threatening health conditions. A recent large-scale study of over 12,000 children living in Houston, Texas, found that asthma was more prevalent in Black children than in White children, and was also more prevalent in children living in poor neighborhoods—meaning those with a median income of less than $34,000—than in middle-class or affluent ones (Kranjac et al., 2017).

Furthermore, social and cultural factors influence health care utilization. For example, data from a large national survey revealed that Latinos and Blacks are more likely than Whites to feel their doctors didn't see them as equals and aren't concerned for their well-being, which in turn could influence comfort in seeking health care (Sewell, 2015). Similarly, certain religious groups believe illnesses are caused by mental and spiritual processes, and thus rely entirely on prayer and other nonmedical interventions to treat disease.

Anthropology

The field of **medical anthropology** examines the differences in how health and illness are viewed by people in different cultures. Cultures, in fact, vary tremendously in how they define health, how they view disease, and, in turn, how they treat illness. People in different cultures vary in how they describe health and even in the behaviors that they view as healthy. People vary considerably, for example, in how they interpret and express physical symptoms, as well as in their willingness to rely on medical professionals as opposed to a "lay referral system" of family and friends for advice regarding medical issues (Bates, Edwards, & Anderson, 1993; Burnam, Timbers, & Hough, 1984; Landrine & Klonoff, 1994; Sanders et al., 1992).

Interestingly, the predictors of health may also differ across cultures. Researchers in one study examined the link between expressing anger, such as "slamming doors" and "saying nasty things," and physiological responses in people from the United States and Japan (Kitayama et al., 2015). Greater anger expression was associated with increased physiological responses, including cardiovascular functioning and inflammation, for people from the United States, indicating that expressing anger was linked to increased health risks. But for people from Japan, expressing anger was associated with lower levels of physiological response, indicating that expressing anger was actually good for health. Researchers believe that for Americans, anger is a manifestation of frustration in response to daily life stress, which negatively impacts health. But for Japanese people, the ability to express anger reflects power and dominance over others, and such feelings of entitlement are beneficial to health. In sum, the predictors of health may well differ substantially for people from different cultures.

Culture may also play an important role in how people respond to health-promoting messages and interventions. For example, interventions that emphasize increasing connection to and support from family and friends are particularly effective at decreasing substance use among Blacks living in low-income communities (Cheney, Booth, Borders, & Curran, 2016). Although many approaches to treating addiction focus on the use of formal drug treatment programs, many people of color living in high-poverty communities are best able to recover from addiction by connecting to and obtaining support from social networks and resources within their own community.

What You'll Learn
1.5

WORKING IN HEALTH PSYCHOLOGY

Given the growing evidence of the impact of psychological factors on physical well-being, many opportunities are available to work in the field of health psychology. In this section, you'll learn about various training pathways and career options.

LO 1.5

Compare different training pathways and careers in health psychology

Training Pathways

What should you do if you are interested in a career in health psychology? First, you should enroll in a range of courses in psychology. The field of health psychology draws on a number of parts of the field of psychology; hence, students who are interested in this field should try to get a broad background. Taking courses in anatomy and physiology may also be beneficial, as would courses in statistics and research methods (which are required for some graduate programs). Second, many students find that getting hands-on experience in health psychology is a great way to learn more about the field, as well as a good résumé builder! You might be able to assist one of your professors with his or her research in health psychology, find a summer internship in a hospital, or volunteer with a social service agency.

After receiving an undergraduate degree in psychology, training in health psychology can involve a number of different programs, depending on your career goals. The majority of health psychologists obtain a PhD (a doctorate degree) in some discipline within psychology. Graduate school consists of coursework as well as training in research, which culminates in the completion of a dissertation (an original research project). Graduate programs in health psychology typically provide training in biology (e.g., anatomy, physiology, psychopharmacology, epidemiology, neuropsychology), the broad domains of psychology (e.g., social, developmental, personality, cognitive, neuroscience), and social factors (e.g., family, ethnicity, culture, race). They also include training in statistics and research methods. Many health psychologists also choose to do postdoctoral training or an internship, often in a hospital, clinic, or university setting, for a year or two after graduate school to gain additional experience and skills.

Depending on your specific interests, you could pursue training in a specific area within health psychology. For example, the field of *clinical* health psychology focuses on using knowledge gained in the discipline of psychology to promote and maintain physical health, including preventing and treating injury and disease, identifying causes of health problems, and improving health policy and the health care system (Belar, 1997). *Occupational* health psychology focuses on using theory and research in psychology to protect and promote worker safety, health, and well-being (Quick, 1999). People with this type of focus explore how work-related factors influence stress, injury, and violence as well as strategies for encouraging workers to participate in wellness programs, effectively balance home and work life, and maintain overall health and well-being (see Table 1.4).

Career Options

Health psychologists work in a variety of settings, including medical schools, government agencies, universities, and private practice (Enright, Resnick, DeLeon, Sciara, & Tanney, 1990; Frank, Gluck, & Buckelew, 1990; Robiner, Dixon, Miner, & Hong, 2014). Some health psychologists conduct research in academic settings and may also teach courses to undergraduate and/or graduate students. They might also do research and teach in medical, dental, and nursing schools. Other health psychologists work directly with patients to prevent and/or improve psychological and physical well-being, such as by providing diagnostic and

Table 1.4   Occupational Health Psychology in Action
Occupational health psychology is an emerging area of health psychology that focuses specifically on healthy workplaces, namely, ones in which people produce high-quality work and achieve great personal satisfaction (Quick, 1999). This field blends issues in public health, clinical psychology, organizational behavior, and industrial/organizational psychology. For example, research results of occupational health psychologists suggest that people who are able to have some control and flexibility in their jobs experience better health and satisfaction, that workers benefit from having effective ways of reducing stress (e.g., exercise, social support), and that workers can be more effective when they are not concerned about family issues. These psychologists could work directly with a business and in this capacity advise employers on ways to improve employee health (e.g., smoking cessation interventions, exercise facilities, stress management), as described in the following two examples.
U.S. Air Force
In 1993, Joyce Adkins of the U.S. Air Force Biomedical Sciences Corps started an organizational health center at the McClellan Air Force Base in Sacramento, California (Quick, 1999). The goals of this center included improving working conditions; monitoring psychological disorders and risk factors; providing information, training, and education; and providing psychological health services to all employees. Within the first year of the project, several substantial changes were noted. First, the total cost of worker's compensation

payments (given to employees who were injured) decreased 3.9%, leading to a savings of $289,099. Second, medical visits and health care utilization for job-related injury and illness decreased by 12%, leading to a cost savings of $150,918. Finally, there was a decrease in death rates, suggesting that perhaps 10 deaths caused by behavioral-related events were avoided. In turn, this decrease in premature mortality was associated with a tremendous savings in terms of productive years gained (e.g., recruiting, hiring, training new employees).

Johnson & Johnson

In 1978, Johnson & Johnson developed a comprehensive health-promotion program titled Live for Life (Quick, 1999). This program included health assessments, materials promoting health behavior change, and the development of a physical fitness program. In turn, the addition of this program led to increases in workers' psychological and physical well-being (Bly, Jones, & Richardson, 1986). First, employees showed improvements in their attitudes toward many aspects of their jobs, including commitment, supervision, working conditions, job competence, pay and benefits, and job security. These increases should lead to lower turnover and thereby reduce the considerable costs associated with hiring and training new employees. The company also experienced lower health care costs, partly because of lower rates of hospital admissions and fewer hospitalized days. Specifically, inpatient health care costs for workers in this program were only $42 to $43 per employee as compared to $76 for those without this program.

Source: Quick (1999).

counseling services, preparing patients for surgery and other medical procedures, and designing programs to help patients adhere to medical recommendations and cope with chronic pain. These positions often involve working in a hospital, medical school, HMO, pain and rehabilitation clinic, or independent practice. Still other health psychologists work on forming health policies and finding funding research on health-related issues, often in a government agency such as the National Institutes of Health or the Centers for Disease Control and Prevention.

Other people who are interested in the broad topic of health psychology choose a career in a health-related field, such as medicine or nursing, physical or occupational therapy, nutrition, or social work. These different careers involve different training paths, as described in Table 1.5. The specific career you choose should be determined by your major interests and goals for your work life. Do you prefer working directly with people and personally helping people make changes in their behavior or manage their pain? If so, you may want to pursue a degree in counseling or clinical psychology, social work, or nursing and work in an applied setting.

Do you especially enjoy working on research projects and forming and testing different hypotheses to find the answer to a particular question? If so, you may want to pursue a degree in psychology or public health and work in a research setting. Are you primarily interested in people's physical and physiological responses and in exploring how their bodies work? In this case, you should consider pursuing a degree in medicine, physical therapy, or occupational therapy.

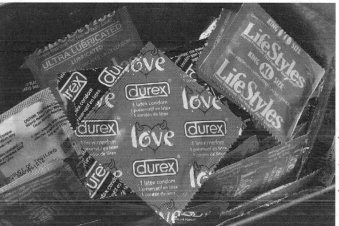

© jdwfoto/iStockphoto.com

Health psychologists work in many different settings and on many different health-related issues. For example, research in health psychology has examined whether providing free condoms in schools increases rates of sexual activity and reduces rates of teenage pregnancy.

Table 1.5   Careers in Health-Related Fields

When you think of people working as health professionals, what types of jobs come to mind? Probably doctors, nurses, and perhaps dentists. But there are many types of careers in health-related fields, and virtually all of them involve and use principles and research of health psychology in some way. Most of these careers require an undergraduate degree in the field and often some type of additional training or education for a year or two after college.

Job Title	Job Functions	Work Setting
Physical Therapist	Help people with diseases of or injuries to muscles, joints, nerves, or bones; evaluate a patient's capabilities, including muscle strength, coordination, endurance, and range of motion, and design a treatment to address the person's limitations; may also work to increase people's mobility and decrease their pain; provide training in using adaptive devices, such as crutches, canes or walkers, or prostheses (artificial limbs).	Hospitals, nursing homes, rehabilitation clinics
Occupational Therapist	Work with patients who have physical, mental, or emotional disabilities and try to help them learn the skills they need to function in a productive way; evaluate a patient's capabilities and then design a treatment program.	School, work, or community setting
Dietitians and nutritionists	Help people create and manage healthy diets; work with patients and their families on making and adhering to dietary changes.	Hospitals, clinics, or nursing homes
Social worker	Help individuals and their families cope with psychological and social issues; serve as therapists; connect people with various community services.	Hospitals, community agencies, clinics, nursing homes
Public health researcher	Work directly with people in a given community to improve their health; develop and implement interventions to prevent health problems or evaluate programs that are currently in use.	Academic settings, government agencies, hospitals, social service agencies, clinics

Source: Created by Catherine A. Sanderson.

Table 1.6   Information YOU Can Use

- Stress has a negative impact on psychological and physical well-being, but coping with stress in positive ways—such as relying on social support and maintaining a positive attitude—can improve health outcomes.

- Many health problems are caused at least in part by behaviors we choose to engage in, so make sure to choose health-promoting behaviors—wear a seat belt, engage in healthy eating and exercise, avoid smoking and excessive alcohol use—whenever possible.

- Writing about traumatic events can help people express their feelings and, in turn, reduce physical symptoms and improve health outcomes. So, keeping a journal may in fact help you be healthy!

- Psychological factors—such as level of social support and neuroticism—influence the experience of pain, the likelihood of becoming ill, and the speed of recovery from surgery, so try to surround yourself with loved ones and maintain a positive outlook.

- Treating health problems at an early stage is far easier than treating them later on, so make sure to engage in recommended screenings for illness, such as checking cholesterol and performing regular breast and testicular self-exams.

Understanding Health Psychology

- Psychological factors, including environmental stressors, personality, and social influences, have a substantial impact on health behaviors and on health outcomes. People who experience higher levels of stress are at greater risk of experiencing both minor and major illnesses, in part because stress weakens the immune system, and tend to engage in behaviors that weaken the body's ability to fight off infections. Personality traits as well as social factors (social support, modeling) are also associated with people's physiological responses to various situations as well as their health-related behaviors.

- Psychological factors influence the development and treatment of pain as well as chronic and life-threatening illnesses. Pain is influenced by psychological factors, and psychological factors can help reduce the experience of pain. Psychological factors impact whether people develop particular chronic and life-threatening illnesses and the progression of such diseases.

- Health psychology examines how psychological factors influence whether people take steps to identify and treat illnesses early, whether they adhere to medical recommendations, and how they respond to health promotion messages. Behavior that involves detecting illness at an early stage as a way of reducing the illness's potential effects is called secondary prevention. Treatments that can help minimize or slow the damage caused by a disease are known as tertiary prevention actions. Psychological factors influence how people react to treatment plans and whether they recover from illness.

The History of Health Psychology

- Many early cultures viewed illness and disease as caused by evil spirits and described health as the interaction between mind and body. However, during the 17th century, this view of health changed, and health was seen as purely caused by bodily processes. This change was caused by Descartes's development of the doctrine of mind–body dualism as well as advances in other scientific fields.

- The biomedical model proposes that health problems are rooted in physical causes, such as viruses, bacteria, injuries, and biochemical imbalances, and explains illness in terms of the pathology, biochemistry, and physiology of a disease. This model therefore proposes that medical treatment is needed to cure or manage physical complaints. Although the biomedical model has made some contributions, evidence shows that biological factors alone cannot account for health.

- The biopsychosocial model views health and illness as the consequences of a complex interplay between biological factors (e.g., genetics, physiology), psychological factors (e.g., personality, cognition), and social factors (e.g., culture, community, family, media). The biopsychosocial model acknowledges that biological factors can and do influence health and illness, but that social, cultural, and psychological factors also exert an effect. The biopsychosocial model contributes to the biomedical model by helping to explain the impact of psychological factors on the development and progression of chronic conditions as well as on how people cope with pain, illness, and disease.

The Development of Health Psychology

- We used to think of health as simply the absence of illness or disease, but researchers now see health as a continuum, ranging from a healthy level of wellness on one end and illness and even death on the other. This change in perspective is also reflected in a relatively new focus within psychology on positive psychology, which examines how psychological factors influence positive human functioning and flourishing.

- Changes in technology and lifestyle as well as the development of vaccines and antibiotics have led to dramatic decreases in deaths from infectious diseases caused by viruses or bacteria. Most health problems are now caused by chronic conditions, which are influenced by people's own behavior. Principles of psychology can be used to try to change people's behavior to prevent health problems, which is known as primary prevention.

- Health care costs have risen sharply due to increases in life expectancy and subsequent increases in chronic diseases as well as various technological advancements. Principles in health psychology can help prevent health problems from developing, persuade people to seek medical care in order to detect health problems at an early stage, and develop treatment programs that help people manage these illnesses; these are all cheaper approaches than treating chronic diseases.

- Scientific advances have also contributed to the development of health psychology. We now know that genes influence health-related behaviors and play a role in the development of many chronic diseases. Advances in technology have also enabled researchers to examine the link between brain activity and particular health-related behaviors.

The Broad Influence of Health Psychology

- Several branches of medicine include the role of psychological factors in influencing physical health. Psychosomatic medicine studies how emotional, social, and psychological factors influence the development and progression of illness. Behavioral medicine integrates behavioral and biomedical sciences and focuses on developing and applying behavioral techniques to the treatment, management, and rehabilitation of patients. The discipline of behavioral health, a subdiscipline of behavioral medicine, emphasizes enhancing health and preventing disease in currently healthy people.

- Medical sociology examines how social relationships influence illness, cultural and societal reactions to illness, and the organization of health care services. Sociologists also examine how social and cultural factors—such as race, socioeconomic status, religion, and sexual orientation—influence health and health care utilization.

- The field of medical anthropology examines the differences in how health and illness are viewed by people in different cultures. Cultures, in fact, vary tremendously in how they define health, how they view

disease, and, in turn, how they treat illness. People in different cultures vary in how they describe health and even in the behaviors they view as healthy. Culture may also play an important role in how people respond to health-promoting messages and interventions.

Working in Health Psychology

- Students interested in a career in health psychology should enroll in a range of courses in psychology as well as courses in anatomy, physiology, statistics, and research methods. Hands-on experience in health psychology is a great way of learning more about the field. Following an undergraduate degree in psychology, training in health psychology can involve a number of different programs, such as a PhD (a doctorate degree) in some discipline within psychology or specific training in an area within health psychology.

- Some health psychologists conduct research in academic settings and may also teach courses to undergraduate and/or graduate students. Other health psychologists work directly with patients to prevent and/or improve psychological and physical well-being. These positions often involve working in a hospital, medical school, HMO, pain and rehabilitation clinic, or independent practice. Other health psychologists work on forming health policies and conducting research on health-related issues, often in a government agency such as the National Institutes of Health or the Centers for Disease Control and Prevention. People who are interested in the broad topic of health psychology can also choose a career in a health-related field, such as medicine or nursing, physical or occupational therapy, nutrition, or social work.

RESEARCH METHODS

Learning Objectives

2.1 Describe the scientific method

2.2 Compare different types of descriptive research methods

2.3 Summarize the features of experiments and quasi-experiments

2.4 Describe different types of epidemiological research methods

2.5 Compare internal and external validity

2.6 Summarize ethical issues in conducting research in health psychology

What You'll Learn

2.1 Why living near a park helps reduce the risk of developing diabetes

2.2 Whether people who are married live longer

2.3 Why exercising with a friend is a good idea

2.4 Why people who *believe* they are engaging in physical activity lose weight

2.5 Why divorce is sometimes bad for children's health

Preview

Students sometimes approach learning about research methods with concern, believing this material will be boring, or difficult to master, or hard to apply to their own lives. But the information covered in this chapter is an essential part of understanding the rest of this book, because it provides tools for understanding and evaluating

(Continued)

(Continued)

the findings in health psychology described throughout this book. And the examples chosen throughout this chapter all have real-world implications, such as whether Google searches can predict suicide risk, whether women's dissatisfaction with their weight changes with age, and whether college students who join fraternities or sororities drink more alcohol. First, you'll learn the steps involved in conducting research in general. The chapter then describes three different types of research methods used in the field of health psychology, including descriptive, experimental, and epidemiological. The chapter ends with a description of the ethical issues involved in conducting research in this field.

UNDERSTANDING THE SCIENTIFIC METHOD

Health psychology is an empirical science, and hence research in this field is based in the **scientific method** (see Figure 2.1). The general goals of research using the scientific method are to describe a phenomenon, make predictions about it, and explain why it happens. All research in health psychology as well as in other scientific fields starts with a question. Sometimes researchers form these questions based on what they observe in the world. For example, you might notice that you always seem to get a cold right after exam period. Sometimes researchers form questions based on intuition or a "gut feeling." You might have a feeling that people who are happier tend to get sick less often than those who are depressed. These are both examples of a **hypothesis**, which is a testable prediction about the conditions under which an event will occur.

In other cases, researchers generate hypotheses to test a specific **theory**, an organized set of principles used to explain observed phenomena. Although hypotheses are specific predictions about the association between two events (such as exam period and illness, for example), they do not explain how or why these two events are connected. Theories provide potential explanations for particular phenomena and therefore generate specific ideas for future research. For example, you could have a theory that students don't take care of themselves well during exam period (e.g., they don't sleep enough, don't eat balanced meals) and that these poor health behaviors in turn lead to illness. And if you had this theory, you'd be right (as you'll learn in *Chapter 4: Understanding Stress*).

Once you have formed the particular question that you will attempt to answer through experimentation, you need to form an *operational definition* of how you will study this problem. For example, you need to decide how you will classify illness (is it sneezing and coughing? is it a diagnosed medical health problem?) and how you will classify exam period (is it only the time during final exams? or the time before any test?). Researchers can define their variables in very different ways, which in turn can influence the findings, so it's important to standardize definitions.

Next, you *collect data*. Data could be collected in a number of different ways, including by observation, surveys, or experiments. For example, you could ask people about various symptoms they are experiencing at the beginning of the semester and then ask them the same questions again during exam week. Alternatively, you could track the number of students who visit the health center during the beginning of the semester and then at the end of the semester. If you are really adventurous, you could go to local stores and count how many people standing in line are buying cold medicine or go through students' trash cans and count used tissues!

Figure 2.1 Steps in the Research Process

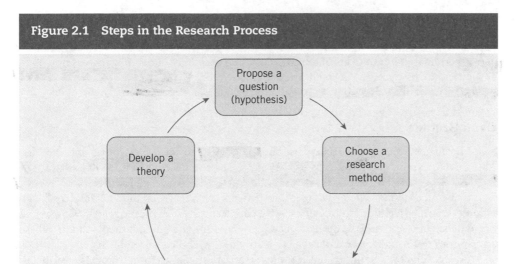

Although the specific research method used may vary, all research studies use these steps to answer questions.

Source: Created by Catherine A. Sanderson.

After the data is collected, the next step is to *analyze the data.* This step is often one of the most exciting parts of conducting research because you get to find out the answers to your questions and write up those responses. (Although issues of data analysis are not covered in this textbook, you can learn more about different approaches to analyzing research findings by taking a statistics class.) This is my favorite part of conducting research because I get to see whether my hypothesis is right.

The next step in the research process is developing or revising a *theory* based on the findings of the research. If your data supports what you predicted in your hypothesis, you may decide to develop a theory to explain what you found. In other cases your findings may provide additional support for a theory, which gives you confidence that the theory is indeed accurate. However, all researchers sometimes get findings that are unexpected. When this happens, the findings may lead to a revision of the hypothesis or theory, which then of course must be tested again in another research study.

DESCRIPTIVE RESEARCH METHODS

Descriptive research, in which behavior and/or thoughts are systematically observed and recorded, is commonly used in health psychology. In this approach, researchers describe their observations but do not manipulate or interfere with behavior. This section reviews the various types of descriptive research methods used to test questions in health psychology, and then how these methods show correlations between variables but not causation.

In this section, you'll learn about several different types of descriptive research methods and then the strengths and limitations of such approaches. These methods include qualitative research, archival research, surveys, developmental studies, behavioral genetics research, and meta-analyses.

LO 2.2

Compare different types of descriptive research methods

Qualitative Research

Qualitative research, which focuses on understanding and interpreting behavior in a natural setting, originated in the fields of anthropology and sociology but is now increasingly used in the field of psychology. As you'll learn in this section, qualitative research methods can provide important insights about the predictors of health-related behavior.

Case Studies

Some health psychology researchers use the case study to form hypotheses and theories. This research technique relies on studying one or more individuals in great depth to determine the causes of the person's behavior and to predict behavior in others who are similar. Sigmund Freud's famous descriptions of his patients, such as Dora and "Little Hans," who suffered from psychological difficulties, are examples of case studies (Freud, 1963). Freud wrote detailed descriptions of his patients' experiences and dreams and then examined these descriptions to form theories about the causes of their psychological problems.

One of the most famous examples of the use of case studies to form hypotheses related to health occurred in the early 1980s, when the first documented cases of a strange new syndrome were reported in the *Morbidity and Mortality Weekly Report* (*MMWR*) of June 5, 1981 (Foege, 1983). Five young men in Los Angeles were treated for *Pneumocystis carinii* pneumonia, a rare type of pneumonia that typically affects those with suppressed immune systems. These previously healthy men had developed severe symptoms, including nausea, weight loss, night sweats, and general tiredness. Interestingly, all of these men were gay. At just about the same time, doctors in New York City diagnosed a rare skin cancer, Kaposi's sarcoma, in 20 gay men. Given these unusual cases affecting a particular population, a task force was created by the Centers for Disease Control and Prevention to interview all patients with these symptoms to determine what factors might have led to these illnesses. By the fall of 1981, epidemiologists had determined that patients with these diseases reported having many sexual partners. Researchers then hypothesized that some type of disease was spreading in the gay population, possibly through sexual contact. Although the first cases of this strange type of pneumonia were found in gay men, doctors soon began seeing similar symptoms in other populations. Doctors in New York noticed similar symptoms in heterosexual men and women who used intravenous drugs. State health departments in New York and New Jersey also reported finding symptoms in prisoners. Nearly one year later, in the summer of 1982, three patients with hemophilia, a blood disorder that requires frequent blood transfusions, had developed similar symptoms. This finding finally led public health officials to recognize that this disorder could be transmitted via blood as well as through sexual contact.

Case studies are typically used to examine relatively rare events or unique populations. For example, in-depth studies of professional athletes who experienced concussions while playing their sport and later committed suicide provided evidence that head trauma may have lasting effects on psychological well-being (Omalu et al., 2006; Omalu, Hamilton, Kamboh, DeKosky, & Bailes, 2010).

Although case studies can be very valuable in generating hypotheses and theories, their usefulness is limited because it is always possible that the person (or persons) who was studied

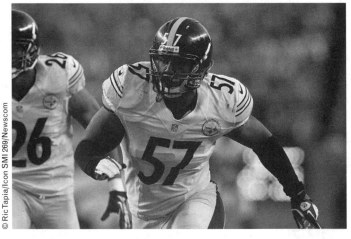

Former National Football League (NFL) linebacker Adrian Robinson was 25 years old when he committed suicide in May 2015. Following his death, it was found that he had the degenerative brain disease chronic traumatic encephalopathy (CTE), which occurs following repeated concussions.

is atypical in some way and hence the information cannot be *generalized*, or assumed to apply, to a larger population. Moreover, case studies can be very vivid in sensory detail and hence overwhelm more objective data recorded with other methods. For example, you might have a friend who became quite depressed following his parents' divorce and therefore believe strongly that divorce causes depression even if large scientific surveys show no such association.

Observational Approach

Another type of qualitative research method is naturalistic (or participant) observation, in which researchers observe and record people's behavior in everyday situations and interactions, and then systematically measure that behavior in some way. For example, if you were interested in examining the association between obesity and activity level in children, you might observe children at a playground and, after operationally defining the variables, count the amount of physical exertion obese versus nonobese children engaged in (e.g., running, climbing, throwing). If you found that obese children were less active than nonobese children, based upon further analysis, you might conclude that there is a link between activity and obesity.

One problem with the observational approach is that the presence of the observer is likely to influence people's behavior. Specifically, people are likely to behave differently when they know they are being watched. You might, for example, load your cafeteria tray with healthier foods if you knew that a health psychologist would be rating the nutritional content of your food as part of her study on eating behavior in college students. Also, observers' own biases can influence how they perceive the behavior they observe. To help limit the problems of observer bias, researchers often have at least two people complete the behavior ratings independently, and then they measure how often the raters' data agrees.

Archival Research

Another type of descriptive approach is archival research, in which researchers use already-recorded behavior, such as rates of illness or disease. To examine the link between positive emotion and health, researchers analyzed the smiles of 230 Major League Baseball players from the 1952 register of all players (Abel & Kruger, 2010). Photos of some of these men showed no smile at all, others showed a slight smile, and still others showed a big smile. The researchers examined how old each player was when he died (as well as other variables that could impact life expectancy, such as year of birth, BMI, career length, marital status, and college attendance). Players with no smiles lived an average 72.9 years; those with partial smiles lived an average of 75 years; and those with big, authentic grins lived an average of 79.9 years. These findings illustrate the link between positive affect (as measured by facial expression) and longevity.

Researchers in one study examined the rate of chronic illnesses in 250,000 older adults living in the Miami-Dade County area as a function of whether they lived close to nature (Brown et al., 2016). Nature was measured by observing—using NASA satellite imagery—green space, such as trees and parks. As predicted, people who lived in neighborhoods with more green space were less likely to develop chronic illnesses, including diabetes (14% lower risk), hypertension (13% lower risk), and lipid disorders (10% lower risk). As you'll learn more about in **Chapter 5: Managing Stress**, spending time in nature reduces feelings of stress, which in turn leads to better health.

What You'll Learn 2.1

Many research studies in health psychology now collect data from various sources of social media, such as Facebook, Twitter, and Google searches. For example, an examination of people's Facebook likes can accurately predict a number of health-related behaviors, including use of alcohol, cigarettes, and drugs (Kosinski, Stillwell, & Graepel, 2013). Similarly, counties in which people tweet more positive statements, such as "opportunities, overcome, and weekend," show lower rates of heart disease than those with more negative tweets

(Eichstaedt et al., 2015). In fact, positivity of Twitter posts is a better predictor of disease likelihood in a county than more traditional measures, such as education, obesity, and smoking. In some cases, this method of data collection can provide important information for improving public health. Researchers in one recent study compared nationwide responses to questions on suicidal thoughts and behaviors to Google searches for suicide-related search terms in all 50 states (Ma-Kellams, Or, Baek, & Kawachi, 2015). The Google search data was a better estimate of suicide deaths than other survey methods, suggesting that this type of data may be helpful in developing suicide-prevention programs.

Surveys

Surveys rely on asking people questions about their thoughts, feelings, desires, and actions and recording their answers. These questions may be asked directly by the experimenter in a face-to-face or a phone interview, or participants may complete written surveys. For example, the Rosenberg Self-Esteem Scale is one commonly used measure that assesses whether people generally have positive feelings about themselves (Rosenberg, 1965; see **Table 2.1: Test Yourself** for an example). Researchers may give people this scale as well as a measure of health behaviors to determine whether people with high self-esteem engage in more healthy behaviors than those with low self-esteem.

Researchers in one recent survey study asked nearly 2,000 heterosexual married couples to rate their own happiness and their health, including level of physical impairment, level of physical activity, and chronic illnesses, over a six-year period (Chopik & O'Brien, 2016). People in this study ranged in age from 50 to 94. Their findings revealed that people with happy spouses were much more likely to report better health themselves. In fact, having a happy spouse led to better health even after researchers took into account people's own level of happiness (which was also linked to health).

Table 2.1   Test Yourself: How Do You Feel About Yourself?

Indicate whether you strongly agree, agree, disagree, or strongly disagree with each of these statements.

1. I feel that I'm a person of worth, at least on an equal plane with others.

2. On the whole, I am satisfied with myself.

3. I wish I could have more respect for myself.

4. I certainly feel useless at times.

5. At times I think I am no good at all.

6. I feel that I have a number of good qualities.

7. All in all, I am inclined to feel that I am a failure.

8. I am able to do things as well as most other people.

9. I feel that I do not have much to be proud of.

10. I take a positive attitude toward myself.

Source: Rosenberg (1965).

Note: For statements 1, 2, 6, 8, and 10, give yourself 4 points for strongly agree, 3 points for agree, 2 points for disagree, and 1 point for strongly disagree. For statements 3, 4, 5, 7, and 9, give yourself 1 point for strongly agree, 2 points for agree, 3 points for disagree, and 4 points for strongly disagree.

Using surveys enables researchers to collect data from many people at the same time, and hence is a very inexpensive way to gather data. Researchers could, for example, recruit many college students to complete a written survey on their exercise habits and illness rates to gather data on the link between physical fitness and health. Surveys also allow researchers to ask questions about a range of topics, including actions, feelings, attitudes, and thoughts, that could not be assessed simply by observing people's behavior. Finally, because surveys are often completed anonymously, researchers do not have to be concerned about the effects of observer bias, which can be a problem with some types of studies using naturalistic observation.

Although surveys are useful, they have a number of potential problems. First, survey methods introduce the possibility of bias through the use of *leading questions*. Leading questions are those that provide some evidence of the "right answer" based on how the question is phrased. For example, experimenters should ask "Do you examine your breasts for cancer?" as opposed to "How often do you examine your breasts?" which implies that everyone engages in this behavior. Similarly, let's say that you want to examine the frequency of drinking and driving in college students. If you ask students, "How often have you ever driven after having an alcoholic drink?" you will get more accurate estimates than if you asked students, "How often have you gotten behind the wheel of your car when you have had too much to drink, thereby putting your own and others' lives in danger?" This is an extreme example, but it is not far from what actually happens in some surveys that contain leading questions.

Similarly, when researchers provide different *response options*, they must be careful to phrase them in such a way as to avoid getting biased results. The provided responses give people an idea of what the "normal" or "typical" behavior is, and people often don't want to appear very different from others. (And they *really* don't want to appear worse than others.) Respondents are therefore likely to choose one of the midlevel choices as opposed to one of the more extreme (high or low) choices no matter what their actual behavior is. So, if you ask people if they smoke less than 1 cigarette a day, 1 to 2 cigarettes a day, 3 to 5 cigarettes a day, or more than 5 cigarettes a day, they will give lower estimates about their cigarette smoking than if you ask if they smoke fewer than 10, 10 to 20, 20 to 30, or more than 30 cigarettes a day. In this first example, regardless of their actual smoking behavior, people will tend to report smoking between 1 and 5 cigarettes a day (the two midlevel choices in this set of answers), whereas in the second example, people are likely to report smoking 10 to 30 cigarettes a day, again, because these responses are the midlevel options and many respondents wish to report their behavior in a way that seems to fall within the norm.

Although we assume that people can accurately report on their own beliefs, attitudes, and behaviors, people are less accurate than we might think. Thus, survey methods are also limited by the possibility of *inaccurate reporting*. In some cases, people might believe they are telling the truth, but they simply may not be able to accurately recall the necessary information. For example, people may actually not remember when they last visited the dentist, when they first noticed a given symptom, or how long pain lasted. One study found that asking people to report on their sexual behavior over the last two weeks led to more reliable estimates than asking people to report over the last three months, presumably because it is easier to recall more recent behavior as well as behavior that occurred over a shorter period of time (Bogart et al., 2007).

In other cases, people may be motivated to give inaccurate information, such as when they are asked about highly personal or sensitive attitudes or behavior. In **Chapter 13: Managing Health Care**, you'll learn that people often provide inaccurate information to their health care provider about how well they follow a prescribed medical regimen. For example, rates of adherence to medication are different when adherence is measured through self-report versus electronic monitoring of how often a pill bottle is opened (Levine et al., 2006).

Developmental Studies

**What You'll Learn
2.2**

Developmental studies examine whether and how people change over time. The two distinct types of research methods used to answer developmental questions are longitudinal and cross-sectional studies, which each have particular strengths and weaknesses.

In longitudinal studies, a single group of people is followed over time. These studies are expensive to conduct because they require following many people over a considerable period of time. They can, however, provide valuable information about how specific variables influence health over time within the same person. Researchers in one longitudinal study gathered data starting in 1960 from a sample of over 1,300 adults to examine the impact of marital separation or divorce on early mortality (Sbarra & Nietert, 2009). They then collected data from the same people over the next twenty-five years. As predicted, participants who were separated or divorced at the start of the study experienced significantly higher rates of early mortality. Whereas 65% of those who had stayed married, were widowed, or had never married were alive 25 years later, only 50% of those who had divorced or separated were still living. Moreover, this association between separation/divorce and life expectancy remained even when researchers took into account other factors, including initial health status and various demographic variables (age, sex, race) that could be associated with life expectancy.

In cross-sectional studies, researchers compare people of different ages at the same point in time. You could, for example, compare the rate of cancer in 20-year-olds, 40-year-olds, and 60-year-olds to assess whether older people have higher rates of cancer than younger people in a cross-sectional study. Researchers in one study explored the association between age and body weight dissatisfaction in young (22–34), middle-aged (35–49), and older (50–65) women (Siegel, 2010). All women completed questionnaires measuring the discrepancy between their current and ideal body, ratings of different parts of their body, and the extent to which weight affected their self-concept. The results revealed no significant differences by age, indicating that body weight dissatisfaction among women is (unfortunately) consistent across the lifespan.

Although developmental studies can provide important information about how people's health-related behavior changes over time, each of these approaches also has strengths and limitations. Cross-sectional studies provide quick information about age differences and typically include relatively large samples. However, the findings from cross-sectional studies are sometimes the result of changes in society over time and not revealing of changes that reflect aging. *Cohort effects*, meaning differences that result from the specific histories of people in different age groups, can cause differences in one set of people that won't necessarily apply to other people growing up in different periods. For example, one study comparing well-being in younger people and older people found that well-being was lower in older adults than in younger ones, suggesting that well-being declines with age (Sutin et al., 2013). However, when researchers also examined longitudinal data testing this same question, they found that older people—who had experienced major societal stresses during their younger years, including the Great Depression and major world wars—had started out with lower levels of well-being than younger adults were experiencing at the same age. After taking into account these initial differences in well-being, the findings now revealed that well-being increases with age for all cohorts.

Longitudinal studies also have distinct strengths and limitations. Such studies provide more in-depth information about how people change over time, since they study the same people, and thus can give researchers more confidence in their findings. However, longitudinal studies, by design, are very expensive and time-consuming and thus don't provide quick answers to research questions. Moreover, although researchers attempt to study the same people over time, all longitudinal studies have some attrition, meaning some people drop out of the study (e.g., they move away, stop responding, lose interest, or even die). This means that researchers are drawing conclusions from a more restricted, self-selected sample, and such findings may or may not generalize, or apply more broadly, to other people.

Behavioral Genetics

Given tremendous advances in the field of genetics over the last decade, researchers are now able to assess the impact of particular genes on people's behavior and health outcomes. Specifically, the field of behavioral genetics examines the relative impact of genetic factors versus environmental factors on health and behavior. Researchers using this technique may study differences between identical and fraternal twins. Identical and fraternal twins who grow up together in the same family should experience a relatively similar environment. However, since identical twins share all of their genes whereas fraternal twins share only half of their genes, identical twins should show more similarities than fraternal twins if particular traits or behaviors are rooted in genes. For example, researchers used data from 600 twins (some identical, some fraternal) to examine how different people respond to potentially stressful work environments (Judge, Ilies, & Zhang, 2012). Their findings revealed that people's genes had a stronger impact on work stress, job satisfaction, and health problems than did the environment in which they were raised. In fact, genes were four times as important as environment in terms of predicting health problems.

Similarly, researchers may also compare adopted children's health and behavior to that of their biological parents—who are responsible for their genes—versus that of their adoptive parents—who are responsible for their environment. As shown in Figure 2.2, findings consistently show a stronger link between obesity and biological relatives than adoptive ones, suggesting that genetics has a stronger role in predicting weight than environment does (as you'll learn more about in *Chapter 8: Obesity and Disordered Eating*). When interpreting the results of these, and other, studies examining associations between children's biological families and adoptive ones, keep in mind that adoption is not a random process, and thus other factors may also influence such findings. For example, people who adopt children often differ from those who have biological children; given the process involved in becoming an adoptive parent, people who adopt tend to be older, wealthier, and more educated, which in turn influences their children's environment. Similarly, children who are placed for adoption

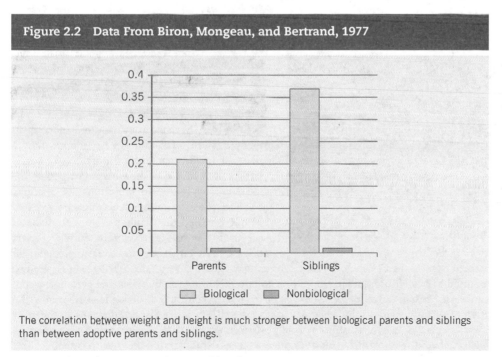

Figure 2.2   Data From Biron, Mongeau, and Bertrand, 1977

The correlation between weight and height is much stronger between biological parents and siblings than between adoptive parents and siblings.

Source: Data from Biron, Mongeau, & Bertrand (1977).

may differ from those who are not. Because biological parents typically choose adoption for their babies when they lack the resources to care for and raise a child, these babies are at greater risk of experiencing distinct types of prenatal conditions, including higher levels of stress as well as exposure to alcohol and tobacco.

An interesting, and relatively new, field of study within health psychology is that of epigenetics, which examines how heritable changes in gene function are influenced by environmental factors (Provencal & Binder, 2015). Specifically, environmental factors, such as stress, diet, and exposure to chemicals, can cause changes in gene expression. For example, even among people with the same genetic predisposition to obesity (such as occurs with identical twins), environmental factors may influence whether the gene triggering obesity is turned on or off (Dalgaard et al., 2016). This finding helps explain why even in the case of identical twins, one twin may be obese while the other is not. Epigenetic factors help predict the development of diabetes (Multhaup et al., 2015), chronic pain (Manners, Ertel, Tian, & Ajit, 2016), and cancer (Hassler et al., 2016).

Moreover, epigenetic changes can be passed on through generations. In one particularly remarkable study, researchers examined women who were pregnant and near the World Trade Centers on the day of the 9/11 terrorist attacks (Yehuda, Engel, Brand, Seckl, Marcus, & Berkowitz, 2005). First, they tested these women's levels of cortisol, a stress hormone, shortly after the attack, and then they examined rates of posttraumatic stress disorder (PTSD) in these women about a year later. In line with prior research, women who developed PTSD during the year after the attack had lower levels of initial cortisol than those who did not develop this disorder. More importantly, children who were born to women who developed PTSD also had lower levels of cortisol. Cortisol levels were particularly low for children whose mothers had been in the third trimester of pregnancy at the time of the 9/11 attack. These findings provide substantial evidence that environmental stressors cause genetic changes, which in turn are passed on to subsequent generations.

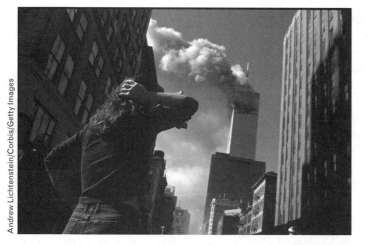

Children born to women who were pregnant at the time of the 9/11 terrorist attacks and later developed PTSD are at increased likelihood of developing PTSD themselves due to epigenetic changes.

Andrew Lichtenstein/Corbis/Getty Images

Meta-Analysis

A meta-analysis is a type of statistical procedure in which researchers combine data from multiple studies examining the same topic to determine overall trends. This approach allows the strengths and weaknesses of particular studies to even out, which helps researchers draw clearer overall conclusions. Because they combine data from many studies, meta-analyses have large sample sizes and include data from a more diverse population. They may also allow researchers to examine data from particular subgroups; for example, a meta-analysis including data from over 850,000 people revealed that while people with diabetes are at greater risk of developing coronary heart disease, this effect is substantially stronger in women than in men (Peters, Huxley, & Woodward, 2014). Meta-analyses have been used to examine a number of issues in health psychology, including the link between peer norms and adolescent sexual behavior (Van de Bongardt, Reitz, Sandfort, & Deković, 2015); how the amount of time spent sitting each day affects the risk of heart disease, diabetes, and cancer (Biswas et al., 2015); burnout in medical professionals; and patient care (Salyers et al., 2017). As described in **Focus on Diversity,** a meta-analysis demonstrated that health care providers prescribe pain medication differently as a function of patients' ethnicity.

FOCUS ON DIVERSITY

The Impact of Ethnicity on Pain Medication Prescribed

Considerable research in psychology suggests that health care providers respond in different ways to patients as a function of their ethnicity, and in particular that doctors prescribe lower amount of pain medication to patients of color than to Whites. To examine this issue, researchers conducted a meta-analysis, which included 34 studies examining how ethnicity is associated with the prescription of pain-relieving drugs (Meghani, Byun, & Gallagher, 2012). These findings revealed that Hispanics/Latinos were 22% less likely than Whites to receive treatment with opioids for similar painful conditions and that Blacks were 29% less likely to receive treatment with opioids. Although there were no differences as a function of race in pain medication received for managing surgical pain, when the cause of the pain was less verifiable, such as back pain, migraine, or abdominal pain, Blacks were 22% less likely than Whites to receive pain medication. These findings indicate that compared to Whites, Hispanics and especially Blacks are less likely to receive adequate pain relief.

Distinguishing Correlation and Causation

Descriptive research methods have many advantages and thus are commonly used to collect information about the link between people's attitudes and behaviors. These methods therefore all indicate correlations, or relationships, between variables. The direction and strength of the relationship between two variables is measured using a correlation coefficient, meaning a number ranging from -1.00 to +1.00. As shown in Figure 2.3, as the number of friends

Table 2.2 Types of Descriptive Research Methods

Type of Descriptive Research Method	Description	Example
Qualitative Research (case study, observational)	Examines behavior in a natural setting	Measures whether children who are obese are less physically active on the playground
Archival	Uses already-recorded behavior	Measures whether rates of obesity changed after implementation of a tax on soft drinks in a particular city
Survey	Asks people questions about thoughts, feeling, and/or behavior	Measures whether people who are high in self esteem engage in healthier eating habits
Developmental (cross-sectional, longitudinal)	Examines whether and how people change over time	Measures whether children who are overweight are more likely to be overweight as adults
Behavioral Genetics	Examines the relative impact of genetic versus environmental factors	Compares adopted children's weight to that of their biological versus adoptive parents
Meta-analysis	Combines data from multiple studies	Examines whether people who participate in a weight-loss intervention are able to maintain weight loss over time

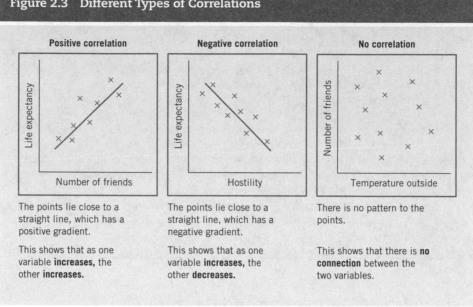

Figure 2.3   Different Types of Correlations

Positive correlation	Negative correlation	No correlation
The points lie close to a straight line, which has a positive gradient.	The points lie close to a straight line, which has a negative gradient.	There is no pattern to the points.
This shows that as one variable **increases,** the other **increases.**	This shows that as one variable **increases,** the other **decreases.**	This shows that there is **no connection** between the two variables.

Source: Created by Catherine A. Sanderson.

increases, life expectancy increases, which illustrates a positive correlation. On the other hand, as hostility increases, the number of friends decreases, which illustrates a negative correlation.

Although correlations can tell us about the strength of the association between two variables, they cannot prove that one variable causes the other. For example, if you find that people with more friends live longer than those with few friends, you still cannot determine which of these two variables causes the other. There may be many possible explanations, and one possibility is that having friends helps buffer people from stressful events and thereby leads to fewer illnesses and hence a longer life. However, it is also possible that people who are generally healthy have more opportunities to participate in social events, which then leads them to have more friends. Similarly, if you find that people who are more hostile have fewer friends (an example of a negative correlation), you can't tell whether people who are mean to others have trouble making friends or whether people who don't have many friends grow to be hostile over time.

Descriptive research methods also do not eliminate the possibility of a *third variable* that explains the observed association. For example, in men, hair loss and the death of one's spouse are positively correlated: men who are bald are more likely to experience the death of their spouse. However, it would be inaccurate to say that balding *causes* one's spouse to die because both balding and becoming a widow are actually the result of getting older (the "third variable" in this example). Thus, while observational methods are very useful in describing the association between two variables, they do not allow researchers to determine which variable causes the other.

One study widely reported in the press revealed that adolescents who frequently had dinner with their families reported lower levels of smoking, drinking, drug use, and depressive thoughts (Eisenberg, Olson, Neumark-Sztainer, Story, & Bearinger, 2004). These adolescents also had better grades. Many media outlets urged parents to have dinner with their kids as a way of preventing drug use and increasing grades. But let's think about whether this study demonstrates that having dinner as a family really has such a strong impact. Can you think of other explanations for this finding?

First, remember that this study shows that two things are *related* to each other, but it doesn't demonstrate that one thing—such as eating dinner together—*causes* another—such as less smoking and higher grades. One possibility is that parents who eat dinner with their children differ in some other way from those who don't eat dinner with their children, and that this other factor leads to this relationship. For example, maybe parents who are wealthier, or more religious, or more conscientious, spend more time with their children, and these other factors (wealth, religiosity, conscientiousness) lead to better grades and less smoking.

Another possibility is that simply spending time with children is associated with better outcomes, regardless of whether that time is during dinner specifically. In turn, research might show that parents who spend more time with their children each day, or each week, have children who have better grades and healthier behavior. In this case, it would be the amount of time that would influence these behaviors, not whether that time was during dinner.

Still another possibility is that children who engage in unhealthy behavior and show poor academic performance are less interested in or less willing to eat dinner with their families. Perhaps children who are "acting out" in some way refuse to eat dinner with their parents, even if their parents are home during the dinner hour. This example illustrates the principal of reverse causality, in which two factors are related in precisely the opposite direction than is hypothesized.

Although descriptive studies are all limited in their ability to determine causation, this approach is the best, and potentially only, way to examine some questions. For example, it is ethically impossible to force some people to smoke and others not to smoke to determine whether smoking causes cancer. However, when multiple studies using various types of descriptive methods all point to the same conclusion, we can be more confident that causal relationships likely do exist.

EXPERIMENTAL RESEARCH METHODS

LO 2.3

Summarize the features of experiments and quasi-experiments

Given the limitations of descriptive research methods in determining the causal direction of associations between variables, many researchers use experimental methods to prove how two variables are associated. This section describes the features of experimental design, the related technique of quasi-experimental design, and strategies for improving the validity of experiments.

Features of Experimental Design

In conducting an **experiment**, researchers randomly assign people to receive one or more **independent variables**, namely, the factors being studied to see if and how they will influence attitudes and/or behavior. A particular type of education (e.g., fear-based messages versus neutral messages) or treatment (e.g., group therapy for cancer survivors versus individual therapy) could serve as the independent variable. Then experimenters measure the effect of the independent variable on one or more **dependent variables**, the measured outcome of the experiment. The dependent variable could be an attitude or a behavior, such as frequency of condom use or blood pressure.

Another key feature of experiment design is the use of **random assignment** to conditions. Random assignment means that every participant has an equal chance of being subjected to either of the conditions; the participants do not choose which condition they want, nor does the experimenter use any type of nonrandom selection process to assign people to conditions. For example, to test whether exercising with a partner increases the amount of

What You'll Learn 2.3

exercise people do, researchers randomly assigned half of the people at a gym to go find a new "gym buddy" to exercise with for the next eight weeks, whereas the others continued with their normal gym exercise routine (Rackow, Scholz, & Hornung, 2015). Can you predict what they found? (Here's a hint: go find an exercise partner.)

Random assignment improves the likelihood that there is not a third variable causing some association between the independent and dependent variables, therefore explaining your seemingly significant findings. Imagine, for example, that instead of using a truly random method to assign people to conditions, researchers simply put the first 10 people to show up for a study into the treatment condition and the next 10 people into the control condition. Although this method would create groups of equal size, it is distinctly possible that people who show up earlier for a study differ in some way from those who show up later. Perhaps they are more conscientious, or are more interested in the study. In turn, it would be impossible to determine whether any significant differences between the conditions resulted from differences caused by the conditions or preexisting differences between people.

Let's take a real-world example of the importance of experimental methods in drawing conclusions. As we will discuss in *Chapter 8: Obesity and Disordered Eating*, losing weight is a challenge for many people, and thus many people try different dieting plans. Imagine you wanted to test whether Jenny Craig or Weight Watchers is a more effective approach to losing weight. Ideally, you could gather a representative sample of a population, obtain their informed consent, weigh them all, and then enroll half of them in the Jenny Craig diet plan and the other half in the Weight Watchers diet plan. If you then weighed these people again one month later, you could see whether those in one group had lost more weight than those in the other. Because experiments contain multiple conditions or groups (e.g., those who got a video or attended a workshop and those who did not), they can show causality, namely, that the independent variable (having the videotape or attending the workshop) leads to the dependent variable (the loss of weight or decrease in alcohol consumption) and not the other way around. This is therefore an advantage experiments have over the other research methods, which show correlation but not causation.

FOCUS ON NEUROSCIENCE

The Power of Mindfulness Meditation

Growing evidence points to the benefits of meditation for reducing stress and thereby improving psychological and physical well-being. To examine the impact of mindfulness meditation on brain activity, researchers randomly assigned 35 highly stressed adults (they were all unemployed) to one of two intensive three-day programs (Creswell et al., 2016). One group of participants completed a mindfulness meditation program in which they learned strategies for increasing body awareness, meditation, and mindfulness. Participants in the other group completed a relaxation program, which included walking and stretching exercises. All participants underwent brain scans both before and after the three-day program and provided blood samples before the intervention and again four months later so that researchers could assess the longer-term impacts of such training. Their findings revealed that mindfulness meditation training, compared to relaxation training, reduced levels of inflammation. Moreover, brain scans revealed that mindfulness meditation training increased connections between parts of the brain responsible for attention and executive control (the dorsolateral prefrontal cortex). Participants who received the relaxation training did not show such changes in the brain. These findings provide important evidence that mindfulness meditation changes the brain in ways that help people manage stress, which in turn leads to better health.

Figure 2.4   Key Elements of Experimental Design

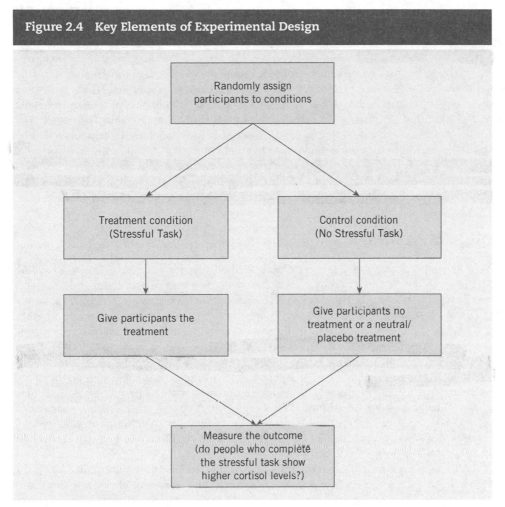

Source: Created by Catherine A. Sanderson.

Why is random assignment so important? Think about what would happen if you ran your experiment on the effects of these different diet plans, but instead of using random assignment, you let people choose whether they'd like to receive the Jenny Craig plan or the Weight Watchers plan. If you then find that those who received one of these plans lost more weight than those who didn't get a tape, can you be certain that receiving that plan caused the weight loss? No, because it is likely that people who *chose* to enroll in a given plan differ from those who chose the other plan. Perhaps those who chose the Weight Watchers plan, which requires people to count and keep track of the "point allotments" for what they eat all day, are more motivated to lose weight in general. Perhaps those who chose the Jenny Craig plan, which requires participants to eat (and pay for) particular meals, are wealthier, and thus have an easier time maintaining this plan over time. Perhaps those who chose the Weight Watchers plan were all heavier to start with than those who chose the Jenny Craig plan, which means any differences in weight loss could be a function of the diet plan or people's initial weight. Although we can't tell whether any of these factors influenced your findings, they are all possible. We therefore can't tell whether the independent variable (diet plan) influenced the dependent variable (weight loss). This is why random assignment is so important—to minimize the likelihood of a third variable influencing the results.

Despite their strengths, experiments also have some weaknesses. First, *artificial settings can influence behavior*. Because experiments typically take place in laboratory settings, the participants' attitudes and behavior can sometimes be influenced by such settings instead of by the independent variable. For example, people who are asked to do an unusual procedure in the study setting may act how they think they should act as opposed to how they normally would in a real-life situation. In **Chapter 7: Substance Use and Abuse**, you'll read about some studies in which participants are given alcohol to examine the impact of drinking on some type of intention or behavior. In this study design, it is certainly possible that people who are drinking in a laboratory setting—and know that their drinking is being watched by researchers—will not act the same in that environment as they would in the real world. To try to overcome this potential weakness, experimenters try to design experimental procedures that are high on *experimental/psychological realism*, namely, those that people are involved in and take seriously, which in turn leads them to behave naturally and spontaneously.

Quasi-Experiments

Although experiments are the only research method that allows researchers to determine whether one variable *causes* another, there are some cases in which practical and/or ethical concerns make it impossible to conduct true experiments. For example, you can't randomly assign some people to get divorced or to acquire cancer in order to determine whether these types of major stressors lead to illness and mortality. In these cases, researchers conduct quasi-experiments. These are research studies in which there are distinct groups of people in different conditions, but unlike in true experiments, the people are not randomly assigned to the groups. A study that compares rate of illness in people who are divorced versus married, for example, includes an independent variable (marital status) that may impact a dependent variable (illness), but people are of course not randomly assigned to the divorced and married groups. As described in **Focus on Development**, longitudinal research demonstrates that babies who are breastfed are less likely to become overweight or obese children.

Although quasi-experimental methods can provide useful information about the effects of an independent variable on a dependent variable, they suffer from some of the same limitations

FOCUS ON DEVELOPMENT

The Link Between Breastfeeding and Childhood Obesity

To examine the link between breastfeeding and childhood obesity, researchers collected data from over 40,000 parents of infants ages six to seven months on their primary method of feeding: exclusive breastfeeding, partial breastfeeding, or exclusive formula feeding (Yamakawa, Yorifuji, Inoue, Kato, & Doi, 2013). These families were then contacted again when their children were seven to eight years old and asked about their child's current weight. As predicted, children who had been exclusively breastfed at six to seven months were 15% less likely to be overweight and 45% less likely to be obese seven years later than babies who had been exclusively formula fed. These findings about the benefits of breastfeeding in terms of childhood weight took into account other variables that are linked with weight, such as how much time children spent watching TV and playing video games, their mother's level of education, and whether their mother worked outside the home. Given the link between obesity and various health-related problems, breastfeeding may therefore be a valuable strategy for reducing negative health outcomes.

as naturalistic, observational, and survey methods. First, these types of approaches do not randomly assign participants to different conditions or treatments, and hence they do not answer questions about correlation versus causation. If researchers using a quasi-experiment find that students in fraternities engage in more alcohol abuse than those not in fraternities, can they be sure that fraternity life leads to more drinking, or can they conclude that those who like to drink alcohol prefer to join fraternities?

Quasi-experimental approaches also do not eliminate the possibility of a *third variable* causing the observed association. For example, if breastfed babies are less likely to be obese than nonbreastfed babies, it is possible that a third

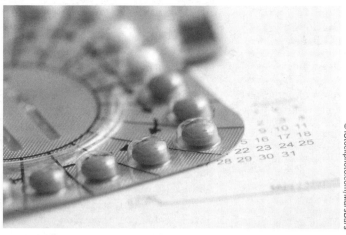

variable leads to both breastfeeding and a lower rate of obesity. Perhaps mothers who are obese are less likely to breastfeed and are also more likely to pass their genetic predisposition to obesity on to their children. Thus, it is possible that the link between breastfeeding and obesity is actually the result of another variable. Researchers typically try to control for potential third variables by matching participants in control and subject groups on other related variables. For example, researchers might match each woman who chose to breastfeed with a woman who had a similar BMI or income in the control group, and then compare infant IQs between these two groups. Although creating matched groups helps minimize the problem of third-variable effects, researchers obviously can match on only some, not all, variables. Quasi-experimental methods can therefore suggest associations between two or more variables, but researchers must conduct experiments to determine the precise association between the variables.

The challenges of drawing conclusions based on quasi-experimental research were clearly demonstrated over the last decade as researchers formed very different opinions about the costs and benefits of hormone replacement therapy for women experiencing menopause. In the mid-1990s, most doctors believed that taking hormones during menopause helped reduce heart disease and osteoporosis. This belief was based largely on the results of the Nurses' Health Study, a longitudinal study showing that women who took estrogen were much less likely to develop coronary heart disease (Grodstein et al., 1996; Stampfer et al., 1991). However, in 2002, the Women's Health Initiative study was published, showing that although hormone replacement therapy helped prevent osteoporosis, it was actually associated with an increased risk of heart disease, stroke, and breast cancer (Writing Group for the Women's Health Initiative Investigators, 2002).

How can these studies draw such dramatically different conclusions? One of the main problems is that these studies used different methods, which in turn led to dramatically different findings. Specifically, the Nurses' Health Study was an observational study in which women's behavior was simply measured over time. However, the women in this study may have engaged in particular behaviors other than taking hormones, which in turn led to their reduced risk of coronary heart disease. For example, perhaps the women engaged in more exercise, were more educated, or were wealthier; all of these factors could have led to a reduced risk of cardiovascular disease. On the other hand, the Women's Health Initiative study was a true experiment, in which some women received hormones and others received a placebo. Thus, the finding that women who took hormones actually experienced more health problems is particularly important, since random assignment was used to make sure that women in these two groups didn't differ in any particular way. This real-world example points to the value of conducting true experiments whenever possible.

The drawbacks of relying on quasi-experimental research are clearly shown in the quite different findings that have emerged about the effects of hormone replacement therapy over the last 20 years. Initial research based on quasi-experimental studies pointed to largely beneficial effects, whereas research using a true experimental design pointed to largely harmful effects.

EPIDEMIOLOGICAL RESEARCH METHODS

LO 2.4

Describe
different types of
epidemiological
research methods

Although the field of health psychology is rooted in research methods based in psychology, research in the field of **epidemiology**, a branch of medicine that studies and analyzes the patterns, causes, and effects of health and disease, also makes important contributions to knowledge in health psychology. Epidemiologists measure **morbidity**, meaning the number of cases of a specific disease, illness, or health condition, as well as **mortality**, meaning the number of deaths resulting from a specific cause. Epidemiologists also employ two measures: **incidence**, defined as the frequency of new cases of a disease, and **prevalence**, defined as the proportion of a population that has a particular disease. These rates are measured by dividing the number of people in a given population (e.g., those at risk) by those who have the disease (to calculate the prevalence) or those who have developed the disease in a set period of time (to find the incidence). Some diseases, such as asthma, may be very prevalent (e.g., many people in a population have asthma) but have a relatively low incidence (e.g., because new cases do not occur very frequently). On the other hand, other diseases, such as the flu, may have relatively low prevalence (e.g., not many people in a given community have the flu) but have a high incidence, at least at some point during the year (e.g., flu cases are frequently diagnosed in the winter, but people do recover). After assessing the incidence and prevalence of a given disease, epidemiologists then try to examine different behaviors and lifestyles that might lead to the development of a particular disorder or disease. For example, epidemiology studies first noted the relationship between smoking and lung cancer as well as the relationship between Type A behavior and coronary heart disease. This section will describe the three research methods used by epidemiologists: observational methods, natural experiments, and randomized controlled trials (RCTs).

Observational Methods

Observational methods in epidemiology are similar to the descriptive methods used in psychology; this approach reveals correlations between variables but does not determine whether one variable causes the other. The sociologist Émile Durkheim (1951) conducted naturalistic research by examining the records of people who had committed suicide between 1841 and 1872. He found that suicide was more frequent in people who were single than in those who were married and was more common during the week than on weekends. Through this investigation, he hypothesized that alienation from others was a predictor of suicide.

Two important types of observational methods used by epidemiologists are prospective and retrospective studies. In a **prospective study**, researchers compare people with a given characteristic to those without it to see whether these groups differ in their development of a disease. These studies, therefore, are prospective because they follow people over time. For example, one prospective study examined daily stress in 400 women who were trying to become pregnant to determine the effect of stress on likelihood of conception (Akhter, Marcus, Kerber, Kong, & Taylor, 2016). As predicted, women who reported feeling more stressed during ovulation were 40% less likely to conceive during that month than during other months and 45% less likely to conceive than women who weren't experiencing such stress.

In a **retrospective study**, researchers examine differences in a group after a disease has occurred and attempt to look back over time to examine what previous factors might have led to the development of the disease. For example, some studies compare those who have cancer to those without cancer in terms of the experience of major life events (e.g., death of a loved one, marital discord; Sklar & Anisman, 1981). This research indicates that those with cancer have experienced more significant life events, suggesting that life stressors can lead to the development of cancer.

However, research relying on retrospective reports is difficult to interpret, because it may reveal that stress and cancer are correlated but not whether stress in fact *causes* cancer. Specifically, it is possible that people with cancer report experiencing more major life events prior to the development of cancer because they are searching for an explanation for their cancer and/or are in a more negative state of mine, which leads to the recollection of more negative life events. Studies that use a prospective design, meaning they examine reports of stress at one time and then follow participants over time to see who develops cancer, provide a stronger test for whether the experience of stress can lead to cancer.

Natural Experiments

Epidemiologists often use natural experiments, in which the researchers compare people in two (or more) conditions but have not been able to randomly assign people to those conditions (Lilienfeld & Lilienfeld, 1980). In *Chapter 4: Understanding Stress*, you'll read about a study comparing psychological distress following the 9/11 terrorist attacks in those who lived in New York City and Washington, DC, which were targets of the attacks, versus those in other parts of the country (Schlenger et al., 2002). Similarly, and as described in **Research in Action**, researchers examined the impact of an alcohol tax by comparing changes in rates of sexually transmitted diseases (STDs) in one state to those in states that didn't make such a change.

Natural experiments are commonly used to test questions in health psychology since many of the issues of interest in this field cannot be tested practically and ethically using true experimental methods. For example, it is impossible to randomly assign people to get divorced to see how divorce impacts life expectancy, to assign women to attend single-sex versus coeducational schools to assess the impact of school type on rates of disordered eating, or to assign people to live in a fraternity house to measure the effect of housing on alcohol abuse. (These are all research studies you'll learn about in subsequent chapters.)

Randomized Controlled Trials (RCTs)

Epidemiologists who are examining the effectiveness of different drugs or therapies on medical problems often use **randomized controlled trials (RCTs)**, which are considered the gold

RESEARCH IN ACTION

How an Alcohol Tax Can Reduce STDs

To examine the impact of increasing state alcohol taxes, researchers in one study compared rates of sexually transmitted diseases (STDs) both before and after such a tax increase (Staras, Livingston, & Wagenaar, 2016). Specifically, the researchers assumed that raising taxes on alcohol would decrease alcohol consumption, which would in turn reduce the frequency of risky sexual behavior. To test this question, researchers compared rates of STDs in the state of Maryland before and after the increase in state alcohol tax went into effect in 2011. They also compared rates of STDs in other states. The findings from this study revealed that gonorrhea rates decreased by 24% following the tax increase, leading to an estimated 2,400 fewer statewide cases of gonorrhea during the first 18 months after the tax increase went into effect. Moreover, no such decrease was found in other states that didn't make such a change, suggesting that this increase in the cost of alcohol reduced rates of intoxication, which in turn reduced the frequency of unprotected sex.

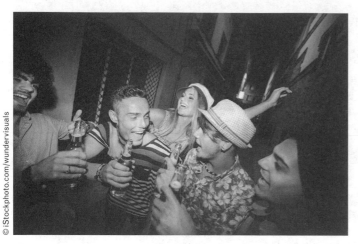
©iStockphoto.com/wundervisuals

Researchers could compare rates of alcohol abuse between men living in fraternities to those using other college housing options.

standard in clinical research. These methods are very similar to experiments in many ways in that they use random assignment to conditions and are often blind or even **double-blind** studies, meaning the participants or the participants and the experimenter are unaware of which conditions the participants are being subjected to and perhaps are unaware even of the hypothesis of the study (see Table 2.3). This type of research can provide valuable information about the effectiveness—or in some cases, lack thereof—of a particular drug or treatment. However, because these studies often involve patients who have actively sought help for a given disorder (such as cancer or depression), the practical and ethical issues involved in conducting this type of study can be complex.

Well-designed clinical trials must have clear *patient selection* criteria. In other words, researchers must set specific guidelines determining which participants are eligible for participation in the study. For example, if you are conducting a study on the effectiveness of a given therapy or drug on relieving back pain, you must make sure that all patients included in the study actually have back pain as defined for your study, not neck pain or joint pain.

Another issue to consider in conducting a clinical research study is whether participants have *comorbidity* and/or *concomitant treatment*. Clinical studies often involve people with comorbidity, namely, those who are suffering from more than one disease, which tends to add variability and make it harder to conduct a controlled experiment. For example, some people could have cardiovascular disease caused by diabetes, whereas others may have only cardiovascular disease. Similarly, people may be receiving ongoing treatment for diseases other than the target of the treatment they are currently participating in the study to assess. Any change in health could therefore be due to the other treatment they are receiving. Once again, random assignment helps to ensure that any findings will be caused by the effects of the intended treatment and not other factors. Some clinical studies may even exclude participants with comorbidity and/or concomitant treatment to avoid the potential impact of the factors.

Finally, researchers who are conducting clinical research must be sure they have *patient cooperation*. Specifically, researchers must involve patients who will precisely follow treatment recommendations. For example, if people are instructed to take a particular pill every morning, they must follow the instructions, because every deviation affects the accuracy of the study results. This matter of cooperation is a particularly important issue because patients often do not voluntarily disclose a lack of cooperation on their part, and so study design must

Table 2.3 Comparing Methods in Psychology Versus Epidemiology

Goal of Study	Psychology	Epidemiology
Correlation	Qualitative, Survey, Archival, Developmental, Behavioral Genetics, Meta-analysis	Observational Methods
Correlation	Quasi-experiment	Natural Experiment
Causation	Experiment	Randomized Controlled Trial (RCT)

encourage full cooperation as well as provide a way for participants to honestly report their conformance or nonconformance. (The issue of adherence is addressed in detail in *Chapter 13: Managing Health Care*.)

EVALUATING RESEARCH METHODS

Thus far, you've learned about different types of research methods used to examine questions in health psychology. However, all research studies—regardless of the method used—should be evaluated in terms of their internal and external validity. This section describes these two types of validity and explains why they are important.

LO 2.5

Compare internal and external validity

Internal Validity

One way of evaluating the quality of a research study is to examine whether it is high in **internal validity**, which means the degree to which researchers have reasonable confidence that the effects on the dependent variable were caused by the independent variable. For example, let's say we are conducting an experiment about the effects of a given drug on mood. We randomly assign some consenting participants to get the drug and others to not get the drug. If the results show that those who received the drug have a better mood (as we've defined it) than those who do not receive the drug, we must be sure that this effect is caused by the independent variable (i.e., the drug). Maybe those who didn't receive the drug were disappointed that they didn't get the drug and therefore felt worse. Maybe the experimenter assumed that those who received the drug would be in a better mood and therefore was nicer to those people, affecting their responses. Perhaps those people who received the drug felt better because they were treated well by the experimenter, not because of the effects of the drug. Maybe people who received the drug talked about how great it was to receive the drug, which made those who didn't get the drug feel bad. In other words, there could be a variety of alternative explanations for the findings, which therefore weakens the internal validity of the experiment. However, if all of these effects have been eliminated or minimized in the study design, it is highly likely that the drug actually caused the improvement in mood, and therefore, the design has high internal validity.

To increase internal validity, researchers must be sure that participants' expectations do not influence the dependent variable. Here are some of the strategies researchers can use to improve the internal validity of a study.

Use a Placebo

Experiments often use a **placebo**, meaning a neutral treatment added to a research study as a way of controlling for the effects caused by a person's expectations. Placebos are inactive substances that should cause no psychological effects inherently; any effect that they do have, then, may be assumed to be caused by the participant's mental processes. In fact, because people who believe they are receiving a drug that will reduce their symptoms often show improvements—even if they are given only an inert sugar pill—drug companies must demonstrate that the actual drug they are marketing is more effective than a placebo pill at relieving a particular symptom. Another way to minimize the effects caused by participants' expectations about a particular treatment is to keep the participants *blind*, namely, to avoid telling them which condition they are being subjected to (e.g., whether they will experience the "real" condition or the "placebo," or control, condition).

Although people commonly think of placebos as a type of inert drug (as in the preceding example), placebos can also be different types of conditions or procedures that some participants are exposed to in order to provide a comparison for participants in the test condition. For example, researchers in one study were interested in examining the effect of people's expectations on health (Crum & Langer, 2007). Eighty-four women who worked for hotels cleaning rooms were randomly assigned to one of two conditions. Women in the informed condition were told that their daily housekeeping work met the Centers for Disease Control and Prevention's recommendations for engaging in regular exercise. They were also given specific information about the number of calories burned performing various tasks (e.g., vacuuming, changing linens, cleaning bathrooms). Finally, they were told that the type of exercise they were already doing as part of their jobs met and even exceeded the recommendations. Women in the control (placebo) condition were given general information about the recommendations for engaging in regular exercise but were not told that their housekeeping work met these recommendations. Researchers also gathered physiological data from all women, including height, weight, blood pressure, and body fat. Four weeks later, all women completed self-report measures of health as well as these physiological measures again. Findings indicated that women who were informed about the health benefits of their jobs lost an average of 2 pounds (reducing both their body fat and BMI levels) and lowered their blood pressure by on average 10 points, whereas those in the control group showed no such changes. These findings indicate that people's mind-set, meaning how they think about their health-related behavior, influences physiological changes in the body, providing powerful evidence that how we think about something can have a real impact on our physical health.

Avoid Experimenter Expectancy Effects

Researchers must also protect experiments from experimenter expectancy effects to increase internal validity. *Experimenter expectancy effects* are produced when an experimenter's expectations about the results of the experiment influence his or her behavior toward the participants and thereby ultimately affect the results. For example, if you know which patients in a research trial are getting a real drug and which others are getting a placebo, you may treat participants in these two conditions differently in subtle ways that influence participants' behavior and responses. You might frame questions in particular ways, based on your expectations, which then may elicit your predicted response from participants. For example, you might ask some people, "How much of a lessening of pain have you experienced?" (a leading question) and others, "Did you experience any lessening of pain?" This may happen even if you are consciously attempting to treat all participants the same.

To examine the potential problems caused by experimental expectancy effects, researchers examined the safety reports of different drugs based on whether the research was funded by the manufacturer of the drug, who presumably would have a vested interest in the outcome of the research (Nieto et al., 2007). Studies funded by pharmaceutical companies were less likely to find adverse effects of the drug and more likely to make a favorable interpretation of any clinical effects than those receiving no funding from such companies. This study illustrates the importance of avoiding experimenter expectancy effects to ensure internal validity.

To protect against the biases of experimenter expectancy effects, some experiments are conducted double-blind, meaning neither the participants nor the experimenter knows which participants are in which condition. This approach decreases the possibility of experimenter expectancy effects influencing the data.

External Validity

External validity refers to the degree to which researchers have reasonable confidence that the same results may be obtained using the same experiment for other people and in other situations—in other words, that the experiment is repeatable. For example, magazines and television shows often feature truly amazing stories of celebrities quickly losing pregnancy weight and provide helpful tips for us noncelebrities on how to accomplish this goal. But the techniques provided by very wealthy celebrities—who likely are paying private chefs and personal trainers to assist with their efforts, as well as full-time nannies—may not be particularly useful for regular people. The results of these approaches probably would not be replicated widely and therefore would be considered to have low external validity.

This problem of low external validity is relatively common. For example, many studies on HIV prevention are conducted on college campuses. However, college students tend to be younger and more educated than the general population, so, if we learn that a given intervention is effective for college students, can we assume that this intervention would work in other populations? Similarly, can we assume that individuals on a college campus who care to attend an HIV prevention intervention are similar to those who do not come voluntarily? The findings from a self-selected sample may not generalize to other people in experiments with low external validity.

There are, fortunately, several ways of increasing external validity, as described below.

Just two months after giving birth, Gisele Bündchen posed for a swimsuit campaign. But the strategies she used to accomplish this weight loss would likely not be practical for many noncelebrities to use.

Use a Representative (Not Convenience) Sample

First, *use a representative sample*, meaning a sample that reflects the characteristics of the target population at large, including gender, race/ethnicity, age, and so on. If you are interested in examining the frequency of drinking alcohol on college campuses, it would be a mistake simply to survey students who live in a fraternity or sorority house, because research shows that these students drink more alcohol than those who live in residence halls or off-campus housing (Wechsler, Dowdall, Davenport, & Castillo, 1995). Instead, you would want to recruit a sample that truly reflects all the students on campus. In contrast, other studies use a *convenience sample*, meaning a sample that is selected because the members are readily accessible to the researcher (such as college sophomores who are taking a psychology course!). Using a convenience sample is not necessarily bad, but other researchers should be made aware of what sample is being used so they can better interpret the results. Results from a study that used only college students as participants, for example, are likely to be most accurate in predicting behavior in other college students, not the general population.

Researchers must also consider that those who take the time to participate in a study might differ from those who choose not to participate, and therefore participant responses may not generalize, or be applicable, to the general population (Bradburn & Sudman, 1988). For example, a study of sexual behavior was conducted by researchers at the University of Chicago (Michael, Gagnon, Laumann, & Kolata, 1994). It included a number of questions on personal topics, such as frequency of masturbation, marital affairs, and homosexual behavior. People who were relatively comfortable discussing such sensitive issues and revealing personal information to strangers were likely the ones to decide to participate in the study, knowing its topic at the screening phase; people who lacked this comfort might simply have refused to participate. Individuals who are comfortable discussing such topics may also be more likely to engage in such behaviors, and thus this type of survey approach may lead to an overestimation of the frequency of these behaviors in the general population if the composition of the participant group is not considered during interpretation of the results.

Similarly, those with particularly strong feelings about the topic of a study may be most likely to respond. Let's say you are asked to evaluate the quality of your Health Psychology course. If you really like your professor, you are probably highly motivated to complete the survey to let others know how great this class is. Similarly, if you really hate this course, you are likely to want to warn others away from this class and hence complete the survey. However, if you have mixed feelings about the class (you like some parts, you don't like other parts, but you don't generally feel strongly), you may not be very motivated to complete a survey at all.

Make Participation Convenient

Researchers can also increase external validity by *making participation in the study as convenient as possible*. If you recruit people to participate in a smoking cessation intervention that requires them to spend every Saturday for a month traveling to a faraway place, you are probably involving and influencing only those who are very motivated to quit, and thus the results may not generalize, or be applicable, to the average smoker (who likely lacks such extreme motivation). On the other hand, if you find that attending one two-hour workshop helps people stop smoking, this intervention may be very generalizable to other smokers. Many people would be willing to attend this type of program, and therefore the researchers should feel more confident that their approach could work with other people.

Replicate the Study

A third way of increasing external validity is to *conduct the same study in different populations or locations*. As you'll learn further in **Chapter 7: Substance Use and Abuse**, many studies testing the effectiveness of interventions to reduce alcohol abuse are conducted on college campuses; however, college students tend to be younger and more educated than the general population. If we learn that a given intervention is effective for college students, we cannot assume that this approach would work in other populations. However, if a program to reduce texting and driving was effective for newly licensed teenagers as well as older adults and for people driving in different locations, then researchers can be confident that the intervention would be effective for most people in the general population.

What You'll Learn 2.5

Researchers in one study examined whether children with divorced parents would experience worse health outcomes depending on how common divorce was where they lived (Smith-Greenaway & Clark, 2017). To test this question, they compared health outcomes in children living in regions of sub-Saharan Africa, where divorce is quite rare, to that of those living in regions in which divorce is a more common experience. In line with the researchers' predictions, children living in areas in which divorce is uncommon experience worse health outcomes, including coughs, fevers, and even mortality. These findings illustrate the importance of testing the same research questions in different populations or locations to determine if the findings from one study generalize more broadly.

Replicating studies across cultures is particularly important, since the findings observed in one culture may or may not extend to those in others. For example, and as you learned in **Chapter 1: Introduction**, expressing anger is associated with positive health outcomes for people in Japan but negative health outcomes for Americans (Kitayama et al., 2015). Similarly, expressive writing, meaning writing about one's deepest thoughts and feelings related to a traumatic experience, is consistently associated with greater psychological and physical well-being among people in the United States, but recent research suggests that this type of focus on emotions is not beneficial for Asian Americans (Lu et al., 2017). As you'll read more about in **Chapter 3: Theories of Health Behavior**, people show greater responsiveness to health-related messages that are portrayed in a culturally sensitive or tailored way, meaning messages that are designed to fit the unique values and needs of a person's cultural group. Such studies have led to increased rates of safer sex behavior as well as fewer rates of asthma-related illnesses (Borrelli, McQuaid, Novak, Hammond, & Becker, 2010; Kalichman, Kelly, Hunter, Murphy, & Tyler, 1993).

Create High Mundane Realism

Finally, researchers must *design studies with high mundane realism*, that is, studies that resemble places and events that exist in the real world, in order to be able to apply the findings from an experiment to the real world. For example, some research has examined how susceptible college students are to getting a cold during exam period (Jemmott & Magliore, 1988). Obviously, the exam period occurs several times during the academic year; therefore, findings from this type of research approach are likely to provide valuable information about how the regular college exam period impacts health. However, imagine an experiment in which students were asked questions and were given an electric shock each time they gave a wrong answer. Although getting shocked would probably be extremely stressful (as well as ethically questionable) to participants, the design setup has low mundane realism and hence might not give researchers accurate information about how stress can influence health in real-life situations. Figure 2.5 presents data from a study on the impact of bowl and spoon size on the amount of ice cream consumed, a method that clearly is high in mundane realism.

Conclusions

How do you decide which research technique to use to answer a particular question? There is no single best method, and all methods have strengths and weaknesses. Because experiments are the only technique that randomly assigns people to conditions, this approach is the best method for determining which variable definitively causes another. However, because experiments are necessarily somewhat artificial, this approach does not give us as much information about what actually happens in real-life situations. On the other hand, while naturalistic

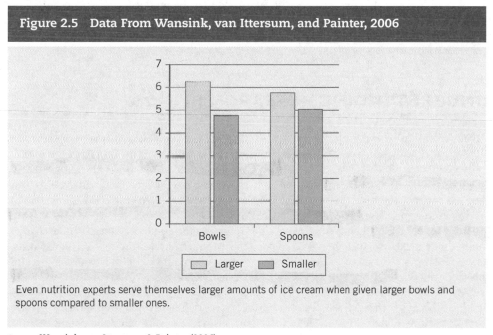

Figure 2.5   Data From Wansink, van Ittersum, and Painter, 2006

Even nutrition experts serve themselves larger amounts of ice cream when given larger bowls and spoons compared to smaller ones.

Source: Wansink, van Ittersum, & Painter (2006).

Table 2.4 Comparing Internal and External Validity

	Internal Validity	External Validity
Definition	The degree to which researchers have confidence that the effects on the dependent variable were caused by the independent variable	The degree to which researchers have confidence that the same results would be obtained for other people and in other situations
Strategies for Increasing	Use a placebo	Use a representative (not a convenience) sample
	Avoid experimental expectancy effects	Make participation convenient
		Replicate the study (in different populations and locations)
		Create high mundane realism

observation methods give us very accurate information about what happens in the real world, they tell us more about how two (or more) different variables are connected than they do about one variable causing the other. In sum, different methods are best for providing certain types of information and for answering particular questions. For example, you might use naturalistic observation or quasi-experimental methods to examine how experiencing the loss of a loved one influences depression, because obviously you could not answer this question using a true experimental design. On the other hand, if you are interested in examining the effectiveness of a particular type of smoking cessation program, conducting a true experiment is probably the best approach. Finally, we can be more confident about scientific findings if researchers using different types of research methods all produce the same results. For example, and as described in Table 2.4, if researchers using a variety of different approaches all examine the link between smoking and health and reach the same conclusion, we can be quite confident in those results.

UNDERSTANDING RESEARCH ETHICS

LO 2.6

Summarize ethical issues in conducting research in health psychology

Paying attention to the ethical issues involved in conducting research is now mandatory, in part because of some previous studies that were ethically questionable. For example, a study conducted in Tuskegee, Alabama, from 1934 to 1974 examined the effects of syphilis on 412 African American men. The researchers were aware that the men had syphilis, but they did not tell the men they were infected, nor did the researchers provide penicillin to cure them, because the researchers were interested in measuring the long-term effects of syphilis left untreated. The men were asked to return to the clinic periodically (in exchange for free hot meals) so that the researchers could conduct physical exams and blood tests. The researchers even asked local doctors not to provide treatment to these men. What did this study show? That, left untreated, syphilis causes blindness, insanity, and even death (Faden, Beauchamp, & King, 1986). Yet, the Tuskegee experiment is considered totally unethical because, through deception, the men were left untreated and suffered greatly from the effects of the disease. This experiment has had a lasting effect on perceptions of the health care system in general by many Black Americans. As you'll read more about in

Chapter 13: Managing Health Care and *Chapter 14: Conclusions and Future Directions*, people of color have a greater distrust of medical professionals than do Whites, in part due to prior unethical treatment. We now know that a number of other studies were conducted on various people, including prison inmates, pregnant women, and low-income children, who were unwittingly participants in experiments and suffered significant long-term health consequences.

Human Research Ethics

To avoid ethically questionable studies, there are now procedures researchers must follow when conducting scientific research (see Table 2.5). First, studies must undergo an extensive *institutional review* before they are implemented. This review by a panel of experts is required by virtually all organizations in the United States, including schools, hospitals, community organizations, and so forth. These boards review whether the potential benefits of the research are justifiable in light of possible risks or harms, and they may force experimenters to make changes in the design or procedure of the research to minimize negative effects. You might wonder about the effects of (falsely) telling your roommate he had cancer or that he had failed out of school, but a research review panel would never allow a study using this type of deception because of the high potential risk of harming your unsuspecting roommate.

Research studies require participants to give *informed consent*. This consent is an individual's deliberate, voluntary decision to participate in research based on the researcher's description of what such participation will involve. It is not necessary to describe every single

---

Table 2.5   APA Guidelines for Conducting Research With Humans

Informed Consent

- Using language that is reasonably understandable to participants, psychologists inform participants of the nature of the research; the researchers inform participants that they are free to participate or decline to participate or to withdraw from the research; the researchers explain the foreseeable consequences of declining or withdrawing; the researchers inform participants of significant factors that may be expected to influence their willingness to participate; and the researchers explain other aspects about which the prospective participants inquire.

- When psychologists conduct research with individuals such as students or subordinates, psychologists take special care to protect the prospective participants from adverse consequences of declining or withdrawing from participation.

- When research participation is a course requirement or opportunity for extra credit, the prospective participant is given the choice of equitable alternative activities.

Deception in Research

- Psychologists do not conduct a study involving deception unless they have determined that the use of deceptive techniques is justified by the study's prospective scientific, educational, or applied value and that equally effective alternative procedures that do not use deception are not feasible.

- Psychologists never deceive research participants about significant aspects that would affect their willingness to participate, such as physical risks, discomfort, or unpleasant emotional experiences.

Source: American Psychological Association (1992).

aspect of the research to potential participants, but they do need to hear enough to make an educated decision about whether they would like to be involved.

Third, patients' *confidentiality* must be protected from unauthorized disclosure; hence, surveys often use a code number instead of the person's name to preserve anonymity. Data also must be stored in a locked room with restricted access. Reports based on the data must contain only group-level information, not descriptions of results for individual people. You would say that "most students who received the alcohol prevention workshop drank less" instead of "most students who received the alcohol prevention workshop drank less, except for Brad Simpson who surprisingly doubled his beer intake over the following month."

Some research studies use *deception*, in which they give false information to participants in order to measure their responses to certain stimuli. For example, people may be told that they are receiving a drug when they are actually receiving a placebo. Why would researchers do this? As we discuss in **Chapter 9: Understanding and Managing Pain**, people who think they are getting a drug actually have more positive results along the trial's measurement scale than those who think they are not getting a drug. Using this type of deception allows researchers to compare the effects of actually getting a particular drug to the effects of people simply believing they are getting a drug (e.g., comparing the efficacy of the drug to the power of positive thinking). However, deception is used only in cases in which there is no other reasonable way of studying a particular research question and in which it is extremely unlikely that physical and/or emotional harm could result.

Following participation in a research study, participants are given a *debriefing*, a disclosure after research procedures are completed in which the researcher explains the purpose of the study, answers any questions, attempts to resolve any negative feelings, and emphasizes the contributions of the research to science. This is especially important in cases in which deception has been used.

Animal Research Ethics

Although the majority of psychological research uses humans as participants, a small minority of research studies (about 7% to 9%) are conducted on animals (Gallup & Suarez, 1985). Research is conducted with animals for both ethical and practical reasons (Miller, 1985). First, certain types of studies are impossible to conduct on humans, given ethical concerns. Researchers cannot, for example, randomly assign some pregnant women to drink alcohol to test the effects of this behavior on the fetus. Research with pregnant animals, however, provides convincing evidence that alcohol has negative effects on the fetus (Sutherland, McDonald, & Savage, 1997). Second, experimenters have much more control over animals' lives than over people's; using animals allows researchers to come to stronger conclusions about the nature of cause and effect since many extraneous factors can be controlled for. For example, in a trial examining whether people who are under greater stress experience more illness, it is impossible to examine all of the different variables that might lead to this association, such as poor health habits, genetic factors, and lack of social support. Research with animals, however, could control for all of these variables by using genetically similar rats (e.g., rats from the same litter) and providing all rats with the same exact living environment.

Although some animal rights activists believe that animals should never be used for research purposes, research with animals has given us important information helping to

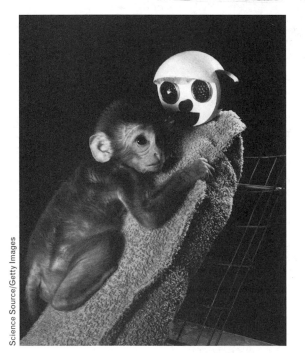

Research by Harry Harlow in the 1960s using rhesus monkeys led to significant change in hospital procedures to allow more sustained contact between mothers and their newborn infants.

Science Source/Getty Images

Table 2.6 Information YOU Can Use

- Your mind-set, meaning how you think about your behavior, has a substantial impact on your physical health, including your body fat, BMI, and blood pressure. This research provides powerful evidence for the mind–body connection.

- Even nutritionists eat less when using a smaller bowl and smaller spoon than larger ones. So, if you are trying to lose some weight, an easy strategy is to choose smaller dishes and utensils!

- Be wary of findings from studies funded by companies with a particular vested interest in the outcome. Data reported in such studies may well be influenced by experimenter expectancy effects, meaning we should be less confident in accepting their conclusions.

- Although research studies may find evidence of correlation, remember that correlation is not the same as causation. Make sure to think skeptically about scientific findings reported in the media and carefully evaluate whether evidence truly supports the often-made claims about the causal association between different variables.

- The best way to evaluate whether a particular treatment, drug, or procedure truly impacts health is by using a true experiment or clinical trial. So, when you are making decisions about your own health, such as which approach to use to stop smoking or what treatment to use when diagnosed with cancer, rely most heavily on results from experimental research (the "gold standard" of research design).

improve people's quality of life. Specifically, research with animals has provided insight into the link between stress and health, methods of treating drug addiction and eating disorders, and strategies for helping premature infants gain weight (Miller, 1985). Many people with incurable illnesses such as cancer and AIDS have benefited from drug treatments originally tested on animals.

Researchers who use animals in a study must adhere to a set of strict guidelines regarding the animals' ethical treatment. Researchers must be properly trained in providing care for the animals, must justify the scientific value of the research, and must attempt to minimize stress and harm to the animals whenever possible. Moreover, Miller (1985) points out that many, many animals who are *not* used in research often suffer much more than those who are used to advance scientific research. For example, at least 20 million dogs and cats are abandoned each year in the United States, and of these, approximately half are ultimately euthanized in pounds or shelters, while many others die in painful ways (e.g., are hit by cars, starve to death). Although some people remain strongly opposed to the use of any animals in psychological research, recent studies indicate that over 70% of both psychologists and psychology majors support the use of animals in research (Plous, 1996a, 1996b).

SUMMARY

Understanding the Scientific Method

- Health psychology is an empirical science, and hence research in this field is based on the scientific method, in which the goals are to describe a phenomenon, make predictions about it, and explain why it happens.

Research starts with a hypothesis, which is a testable prediction about the conditions under which an event will occur. Next, form an operational definition of how the variables will be measured, collect data, analyze data, and then form or revise a theory, meaning an organized set of principles used to explain observed phenomena.

Descriptive Research Methods

- Some health psychology researchers use qualitative research methods. These methods include the case study technique, which relies on studying one or more individuals in great depth to determine the causes of the person's behavior and to predict behavior in others who are similar, and naturalistic (or participant) observation, in which researchers observe and record people's behavior in everyday situations and interactions and then systematically measure that behavior in some way.

- Another type of descriptive approach is archival research, in which researchers use already-recorded behavior, such as rates of illness or disease.

- Surveys rely on asking people questions about their thoughts, feelings, desires, and actions. These questions may be asked in a face-to-face or phone interview or completed on paper or on a computer.

- Developmental studies examine whether and how people change over time. In longitudinal studies, a single group of people is followed over time, whereas in cross-sectional studies, researchers compare people of different ages at the same point in time.

- The field of behavioral genetics examines the relative impact of genetic factors versus environmental factors. Researchers using this technique may study differences between identical and fraternal twins and/or compare adopted children's health and behavior to that of their biological versus adoptive parents. The field of epigenetics examines how environmental factors can influence whether particular genes are expressed.

- A meta-analysis is a type of statistical procedure in which researchers combine data from multiple studies to determine overall trends. This approach allows the strengths and weaknesses of particular studies to even out.

- Descriptive research methods can describe the correlation between two variables but cannot prove that one variable causes the other. They also do not eliminate the possibility of a third variable that explains the observed association.

Experimental Research Methods

- In conducting an experiment, researchers randomly assign people to receive one or more independent variables, namely, the factor that is being studied, to see if and how it will influence attitudes and/or behavior. Then experimenters measure the effect of the independent variable on one or more dependent variables, the measured outcome of the experiment. Experiments use random assignment to conditions, meaning that every participant has an equal chance of being subjected to either of the conditions.

- In cases in which practical and/or ethical concerns make it impossible to conduct true experiments, researchers conduct quasi-experiments. These are research studies in which there are distinct groups of people in different conditions but the people are not randomly assigned to the groups. Quasi-experimental methods are unable to answer questions about correlation versus causation and do not eliminate the possibility of a third variable causing the observed association.

Epidemiological Research Methods

- Research in the field of epidemiology, a branch of medicine that studies and analyzes the patterns, causes, and effects of health and disease, measures morbidity, meaning the number of cases of a specific disease, illness, or health condition, as well as mortality, meaning the number of deaths resulting from a specific cause. Epidemiologists employ two measures: incidence, defined as the frequency of new cases of a disease, and prevalence, defined as the proportion of a population that has a particular disease.

- Observational methods in epidemiology reveal correlations between variables. These include prospective studies, in which researchers compare people with a given characteristic to those without it to see whether these groups differ in their development of a disease, and retrospective studies, in which researchers examine differences in a group after a disease has occurred and attempt to look back over time to examine what previous factors might have led to the development of the disease.

- Epidemiologists use natural experiments, in which the researchers compare people in two (or more) conditions but have not been able to randomly assign people to those conditions. Natural experiments are often used when research questions cannot be tested practically and ethically using true experimental methods.

- Epidemiologists who are examining the effectiveness of different drugs or therapies on medical problems often use randomized controlled trials (RCTs). These methods use random assignment to conditions and are often blind or even double-blind studies. Well-designed clinical trials must have clear patient selection criteria, consider whether participants have comorbidity and/or concomitant treatment, and have high patient cooperation.

Evaluating Research Methods

- High-quality research studies are high in internal validity, which means the degree to which researchers have reasonable confidence that the effects on the dependent variable were caused by the independent variable. Strategies for increasing internal validity include using a placebo (meaning a neutral treatment added to a research study) and avoiding experimenter expectancy effects (which are produced when an experimenter's expectations about the results of the experiment influence his or her behavior toward the participants and thereby ultimately affect the results).

- High-quality research studies are also high in external validity, which refers to the degree to which researchers have reasonable confidence that the same results may be obtained using the same experiment for other people and in other situations—in other words, that the experiment is repeatable. Strategies for increasing external validity include using a representative sample, making participation convenient, replicating the study in different locations and with different populations,

and designing studies with high mundane realism (meaning studies that resemble places and events that exist in the real world so that the findings from an experiment can be applied to the real world).

Understanding Research Ethics

- To avoid ethically questionable studies, researchers must follow specific procedures. First, studies must undergo an extensive institutional review by a panel of experts before they are implemented, obtain informed consent from participants, and protect participants' confidentiality. A study may use deception, in which false information is given to participants to measure their responses to certain stimuli, only if it is absolutely necessary to test the particular research question. If deception is used, participants must be given a debriefing in which the researcher explains the purpose of the study, answers any questions, attempts to resolve any negative feelings, and emphasizes the contributions of the research to science.

- A small number of research studies are conducted on animals for both ethical and practical reasons. Researchers who use animals in a study must adhere to a set of strict guidelines regarding the animals' ethical treatment. They must be properly trained in providing care for the animals, must justify the scientific value of the research, and must attempt to minimize stress and harm to the animals whenever possible.

3

THEORIES OF HEALTH BEHAVIOR

Learning Objectives

3.1 Describe the three continuum theories of health behavior

3.2 Compare the three distinct learning theories of health behavior

3.3 Explain the three stage models of health behavior change

3.4 Describe distinct strategies for creating health behavior change

3.5 Summarize the use of personalized health-promotion messages

What You'll Learn

3.1 How "friendship bracelets" may increase condom use

3.2 Why paying smokers to quit saves lives

3.3 Why CPR is less effective than you think

3.4 How reality television can prevent teen pregnancy

3.5 How personalized feedback reduces drinking during a 21st-birthday celebration

Preview

This chapter introduces the major theories used to examine health-related behavior, including models predicting when people will engage in particular types of behavior as well as what strategies can help people make changes in their behavior. Before reading this chapter, think about what factors influence whether or not you engage in a behavior related to health. Is it that you don't really think you are personally at risk of experiencing a negative consequence from your behavior (such as believing that because you are a good driver, you aren't going to get

(Continued)

in an accident even if sometimes you check your phone while driving)? Is it how confident you are that you could actually engage in the behavior? For example, maybe you know it's important to adopt healthier eating habits but don't have the willpower to stop eating junk food while studying. Is it that the negatives about doing the behavior seem more important than the positives (e.g., you know you should avoid binge drinking but worry about what your friends will say if you start drinking less)? Now read about the variables that each of these models includes and see how well they might predict your own behavior.

CONTINUUM THEORIES OF HEALTH BEHAVIOR

LO 3.1

Describe the three continuum theories of health behavior

Continuum theories identify some set of variables that are thought to influence people's behavior and then combine those variables to predict the likelihood that the person will engage in a given behavior (Weinstein, Rothman, & Sutton, 1998). As you will see, these theories share some common elements but also differ in terms of the specific components they use to predict behavior as well as how these components are combined.

Health Belief Model

The **health belief model** is one of the oldest and most widely used theories to explain people's health-related behavior. A group of social scientists originally developed this model in the 1950s to explain why people often fail to participate in programs to prevent or detect diseases (Rosenstock, 1960). For example, after the government provided free tuberculosis screening conveniently located in various neighborhoods, researchers were surprised that relatively few people took advantage of this opportunity for early detection and treatment. (Professors often feel a similar amazement when they sit waiting for students to stop by during office hours and have no visitors.) An examination of the factors that successfully led to more people using screening formed the basis of the health belief model (see Table 3.1).

Table 3.1	Sample Testing Components of the Health Belief Model
Susceptibility	The possibility of getting wrinkles or age spots worries me.
Severity	It would be terrible to look older than I really am because of too much sun exposure.
Benefits	Wearing sunscreen with an SPF of at least 15 regularly when I am in the sun would reduce my chances of getting skin cancer.
Barriers	How likely is it that the cost of sunscreen would keep me from using it?

Source: Taken from Jackson & Aiken (2000).

Components of the Health Belief Model

The health belief model posits that the likelihood that individuals will take preventive action is a function of four types of factors. First, individuals need to believe that they personally are *susceptible* to the condition. Perceived susceptibility can include beliefs about the general risks of engaging in a behavior (e.g., the likelihood of getting cancer if you smoke) as well as beliefs about how likely you personally would be to acquire an illness or disease. For example, you may be aware that driving after having a few drinks increases the chances of having a car accident, but if you've occasionally driven after drinking and never had an accident, you might not really worry that you personally will have an accident.

Next, individuals must believe that if they were to acquire a particular illness or disease, it would have *severe* consequences. For example, if you believe that having an STD would not be particularly bad ("Hey, I'll just go get some penicillin at the campus health center"), you will be less motivated to use condoms than if you believe that having an STD would be pretty unpleasant ("Hmm, it will hurt badly when I pee, it will be embarrassing to go to the campus health center for treatments, and I might infect someone I care about"). The evaluation of perceived severity can include the consequences we individually would face, such as pain, disability, and even death. For example, if you believe that having a baby as a teenager would hurt your chances of attending college, you will be highly motivated to either remain abstinent or use effective contraception if you really want to continue your education. The evaluation of severity can also include the consequences others in our social network would face if we were to experience an illness or disease. Parents who smoke, for example, may be motivated to try to stop this behavior to protect their children from the pain they would encounter in having to cope with the death of a parent.

Finally, people must believe that engaging in a particular behavior would have *benefits* in terms of reducing the threat of a particular illness and that the benefits of taking this preventive action outweigh the *barriers*. The benefits of stopping smoking are pretty clear (longer life expectancy, less expense, whiter teeth, etc.), but for some people, the barriers to quitting, such as the fear of being more tense or of gaining weight, could outweigh the benefits. Similarly, people who have cancer have to balance the benefits of various treatment options (e.g., chemotherapy, radiation, surgery) with the treatment option costs (e.g., losing hair, risk of death, severe illness).

Although the original version of the health belief model included only the four components of severity, susceptibility, benefits, and costs, a revised version of this model also includes cues to action (Janz & Becker, 1984). *Cues to action* refers to any type of reminder about a potential health problem that could motivate behavior change. These cues can be internal, such as experiencing a health symptom, or external, such as receiving a postcard reminder to get your teeth cleaned or watching a public service announcement on television about the dangers of smoking. These cues are just the final push that it sometimes takes to get people to act.

Researchers in one study were interested in testing the effectiveness of reminder cues on condom use (Dal Cin, MacDonald, Fong, Zanna, & Elton-Marshall, 2006). College students were randomly assigned to one of three interventions: a standard safe-sex intervention, a safe-sex intervention with a reminder cue, or a control intervention on drinking and driving. Both interventions consisted of a video (either stories of people living with HIV describing contracting the disease or, in the case of the control condition, a documentary about a young man killed by a drunk driver). Participants in the intervention with the reminder cue were given a "friendship bracelet" to wear at the conclusion of the intervention and were told to wear this bracelet until the end of the study period and to think about the stories of the people with HIV whenever they looked at it. All participants completed a follow-up questionnaire five to seven weeks later to assess the effects of these different interventions. As predicted, students in the reminder cue ("bracelet") condition were significantly more likely to report using condoms than those in the other two conditions. Specifically, participants in the reminder cue

**What You'll Learn
3.1**

intervention reported using condoms 58% of the time in the last month, compared to 34% of those in the standard safer-sex intervention and 40% of those in the control intervention. Similarly, 55% of those in the reminder cue intervention reported using a condom the last time they had sex, compared to only 27% of those in the standard safer-sex intervention and 36% of those in the control intervention. This research provides compelling evidence that reminding people to engage in a behavior can be a valuable strategy for changing behavior.

Evaluating the Health Belief Model

Overall, the health belief model is a good predictor of whether people engage in health-related behaviors as well as whether they participate in health-screening programs (Rosenstock, 1990). Specifically, the health belief model can predict behavior related to dental care, healthy eating, condom use, and adherence to medical recommendations (Abraham & Sheeran, 2015). One recent study examining parents' decisions about whether to vaccinate their daughters for human papillomavirus (HPV)—a leading cause of cervical cancer—found that parents who chose to vaccinate felt their daughters were more susceptible to acquiring HPV, saw more benefits and fewer barriers to the vaccine, and reported more cues to action, such as prompting by a health care provider (Krawczyk et al., 2015).

Although studies on the health belief model have generally found support for its ability to predict health-related behavior, researchers have raised some questions about its usefulness. First, this model does not include the component of self-efficacy, or a person's confidence that he or she can effectively engage in a behavior (Schwarzer, 1992). As you'll learn later in this section, self-efficacy is a consistently strong predictor of health-related behavior, and thus more recent theories include this component. Second, while perceived barriers and perceived susceptibility tend to be the best predictors of behavior, perceived severity is not a very strong predictor of behavior and may be a particularly poor predictor of health behavior in cases in which health problems are either hard to define in terms of severity (e.g., medical conditions with which people are unfamiliar) or are extremely severe for virtually everyone (e.g., cancer; Janz & Becker, 1984). Third, this model was originally developed to predict whether people would obtain immunizations, and it continues to be more useful in predicting one-time or limited behaviors than in predicting habitual behaviors (Kirscht, 1988). The health belief model may therefore be more useful in describing relatively simple behaviors, such as having a required immunization, than in describing complex behaviors, such as condom use (which requires negotiating that behavior with another person).

Social Cognitive Theory

According to **social cognitive theory**, people learn attitudes about particular behaviors by observing other people engaged in such behavior and by seeing the outcomes these people experience from such behavior (Bandura, 1977, 1986). For example, a young high school student could observe an older high school student drinking alcohol at a party and receiving positive attention from others for engaging in that behavior. However, whether that high school student in turn chooses to drink will depend, at least in part, on his or her confidence in being able to engage in such behavior.

Components of Social Cognitive Theory

Social cognitive theory emphasizes the power of observation in helping people form attitudes about particular behaviors (Bandura, 1986). *Direct modeling* occurs when people observe others in their social networks—such as parents, siblings, or peers—engaging in particular behaviors. In contrast, *symbolic modeling* occurs when people observe people portrayed in the media, including in magazines, in newspapers, and on television. These types of social modeling have a strong influence on various types of health-related behavior, including the types of health-promoting behaviors people engage in as well as how they respond to medicines and treatments (Faasse & Petrie, 2016). For example, and as described in *Chapter 13: Managing Health Care*, coverage of distinct health symptoms occurring in a given community or linked with taking a particular drug can lead people to believe they are experiencing similar effects (a phenomenon known as *mass psychogenic illness*).

However, whether these attitudes lead to behavior is a function of people's beliefs about their own ability to engage (or not engage) in a particular behavior as well as their beliefs about

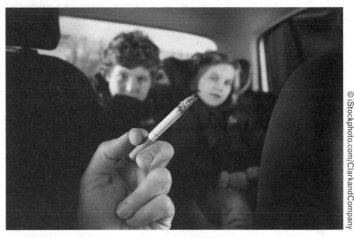

Children whose parents smoke are more likely to form positive attitudes and beliefs about this behavior than those whose parents don't smoke. Not surprisingly, these positive attitudes and beliefs about smoking increase the likelihood of that child eventually becoming a smoker.

the consequences of engaging (or not engaging) in a particular behavior. For example, when deciding whether to stop drinking alcohol, individuals might think about whether they realistically would be able to "just say no" and whether they think not drinking would have positive or negative consequences (on their health, social life, etc.). These two components of social cognitive theory are self-efficacy and outcome expectancies.

The term **self-efficacy** describes the extent to which a person believes he or she can engage in a particular behavior (see Table 3.2; Bandura, 1977, 1986). For example, people who strongly believe they will be able to follow through on their intentions to exercise four times a week will be more likely to successfully carry out this behavior than those who have doubts about their ability to follow through on such intentions. Self-efficacy is seen as a particularly powerful influence on health behavior because it is thought to influence people's behavior in two distinct ways (O'Leary, 1992). First, people who have a strong sense of self-efficacy for a given behavior are likely to exert considerable effort to perform the behavior. A person who has great confidence in her ability to stop smoking, for example, may try harder to resist offers of cigarettes from friends. She may also continue with her goal of quitting even if she experiences a brief lapse in judgment and smokes a cigarette on one occasion. In contrast, someone with low self-efficacy may show little resistance when confronted with tempting offers and may quickly return to regular smoking after smoking a single cigarette (Van Zundert, Ferguson, Shiffman, & Engels, 2010). Second, people with low self-efficacy have a greater physiological response to stressful situations (such as making difficult changes in their behavior), including higher heart rates and blood pressure, than those with high self-efficacy. This greater anxiety response may lead people with low self-efficacy to be less likely to even attempt to engage in behavior change than those with high self-efficacy. Finally, and perhaps most important, people with high self-efficacy show a higher correlation between knowledge and behavior: they are more likely to act on their knowledge (e.g., to eat healthy foods if they understand that healthy foods are good for them; Rimal, 2000).

Social cognitive theory also includes the component of **outcome expectancies**, an individual's beliefs about whether engaging in a particular behavior will have a desired outcome. For example, people who believe that eating healthy foods will make them feel good and be healthy are more likely to eat such foods than people who believe that nutritious foods taste bad and probably aren't going to help their health much anyway. Outcome expectancies can be learned through direct experience with a behavior, or by observing the consequence someone else experiences as a result of that behavior. You may learn, for example, that drinking alcohol leads to relaxation by watching the positive consequences your parents experience after drinking a glass of wine after a tough day at work. One study of overweight adults participating in a weight-loss program found that those who believed losing weight would

Table 3.2	Sample Items From the Condom Use Self-Efficacy Scale

- I feel confident in my ability to put a condom on myself or my partner.

- I feel confident in my ability to suggest using condoms with a new partner.

- I feel confident that I could remember to use a condom even after I have been drinking.

- I feel confident that I could stop to put a condom on myself or my partner even in the heat of passion.

- I feel confident in my ability to persuade a partner to accept using a condom when we have intercourse.

- I feel confident in my ability to use a condom correctly.

- I feel confident I could purchase condoms without feeling embarrassed.

- I feel confident that I could use a condom with a partner without "breaking the mood."

- I feel confident I could remember to carry a condom with me should I need one.

- I feel confident I could use a condom during intercourse without reducing any sexual sensations.

Note: This scale measures people's self-efficacy for using condoms.

Source: Brafford & Beck (1991).

lead to more positive consequences—in terms of self-esteem, health, and relationships—had successfully lost more weight 18 months later (Finch et al., 2005).

Evaluating Social Cognitive Theory

Social cognitive theory is a good predictor of many different types of behavior, such as quitting smoking, eating healthier foods, losing weight, and practicing safer sex (Bandura, 1998). This theory is also able to predict how people cope with pain and illness. For example, both self-efficacy and outcome expectancies are significant predictors of whether women use pain relief medication during childbirth. Researchers found that women who were more confident in their ability to withstand the pain of labor and delivery without medical relief, as well as those who had more positive expectances about childbirth, were less likely to use medication in general (Manning & Wright, 1983).

Given the success of social cognitive theory in predicting health-related behavior, many health-promotion interventions focus on increasing people's confidence in and expectancies for engaging in a particular behavior. For example, many HIV-prevention interventions use various techniques based on social cognitive theory to reduce unsafe sexual behavior, such as increasing confidence in negotiating safer sex as well as the expectations of such a discussion (Bandura, 1994). One school-based intervention in which students were taught strategies for avoiding infection with HIV and other STDs, including specific skills for refusing to have sex and insisting on condom use, led to lower rates of risky sexual behavior a year later (see Figure 3.1). Similarly, and as described in **Focus on Development**, children who learn cooking skills gain self-confidence for making nutritious food choices, which in turn leads to healthier eating patterns.

Theories of Reasoned Action and Planned Behavior

The **theory of reasoned action** is a general psychological theory that is useful in predicting the link between attitudes, intentions, and behavior across different domains, such as voting,

Figure 3.1 Data From Jemmott et al., 2010

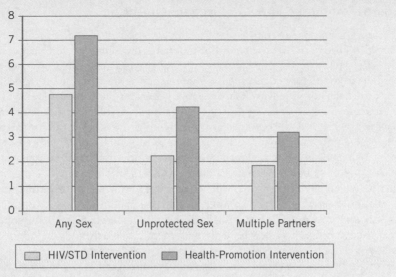

Compared to students who received a general health-promotion intervention, a smaller percentage of those who participated in an HIV/STD intervention had engaged in sexual intercourse, unprotected sex, or sexual activity with multiple partners in the last three months.

Source: Data from Jemmott et al. (2010).

FOCUS ON DEVELOPMENT

Why Kids Who Cook Eat More Vegetables

Several studies have examined how learning cooking skills improves children's self-efficacy for making healthy foods choices. For example, researchers in one study asked children how often they helped their parents with cooking at home and how confident they were in their ability to select healthy foods at home and at school (Chu et al., 2013). Children who reported helping to prepare and cook food at home more frequently showed greater preferences for eating fruits and vegetable as well as higher self-efficacy for selecting and eating healthy foods. Although this study examined the effects of cooking at home with parents, research on the effects of taking a cooking class with an instructor reveals similar findings. Specifically, children who participated in a ten-week cooking class at school showed higher levels of cooking self-efficacy as well as increased nutrition knowledge (Jarpe-Ratner, Folkens, Sharma, Daro, & Edens, 2016). Moreover, children who participated in this program reported increased vegetable consumption six months later. These findings suggest that teaching children how to cook—either at home or in school or community-based programs—may be a relatively easy way to increase their self-efficacy for healthy eating, which can have lasting health benefits.

donating money, and choosing a career (Fishbein & Ajzen, 1975). For example, if you want to know how likely someone is to start an exercise program, you must examine their attitudes toward exercise as well as their intentions to exercise. This theory emphasizes the role of individuals' beliefs about their social world and therefore includes components assessing individuals' beliefs about others' attitudes toward a given behavior (e.g., how do you think your friends will feel if you start an exercise program?).

Understanding the Theory of Reasoned Action

The theory of reasoned action posits that the key determinant of people's behavior is their *intention* to engage in that behavior. For example, your intention to brush your teeth every night is probably a very strong predictor of whether you actually do brush your teeth. In turn, according to the theory of reasoned action, intentions are determined by people's attitudes toward the behavior as well as their subjective norms for the behavior.

Attitudes are a person's positive or negative feelings about engaging in a particular behavior. You might have a positive attitude about eating breakfast every day but a negative attitude about avoiding your morning coffee. In turn, individuals' attitudes are a function of their beliefs about the consequences of engaging in a particular behavior as well as their evaluation of these outcomes. For example, a woman's attitudes about dieting will be formed by her beliefs about whether a diet will help her feel thinner and more attractive and her feelings about the benefits of having a thinner body (see Table 3.3).

Subjective norms refer to individuals' beliefs about whether other people would support them in engaging in a new behavior and whether they are motivated to follow the beliefs of these salient others (see Table 3.3). Who are these "other people," according to this theory? They might be family members, friends, and romantic partners. For example, an individual's intention to diet could be influenced by his beliefs about whether his family and friends would be supportive of his efforts to diet as well as by whether he is motivated to engage in behaviors these people encourage. In line with this theory, considerable evidence points to the influence of norms on health-related behavior. For example, a meta-analysis found that people who are told that others are making particular food choices (selecting low-calorie or high-calorie items) are much more likely to make similar choices themselves (Robinson, Thomas, Aveyard, & Higgs, 2014).

Understanding the Theory of Planned Behavior

A later version of this model, the **theory of planned behavior**, added one additional factor to the theory of reasoned action (Ajzen, 1985). This component of **perceived behavioral control** describes the extent to which a person believes that he or she can successfully enact a behavior. (The concept of perceived behavioral control is similar to that of self-efficacy.) Perceived behavioral control is a reflection of both past experience with the behavior as well as beliefs about one's ability to engage in a particular behavior in the future. For example, if you are trying to lose weight but have failed to resist eating Ben & Jerry's New York Super Fudge Chunk in the past and doubt whether your willpower is strong enough to resist eating it now, your perceived behavioral control will be low. According to the theory of planned behavior, attitudes, subjective norms, and perceived behavioral control all influence

Table 3.3 Sample Items Based in the Theory of Reasoned Action	
Attitude Items	**Social Norm Items**
If I eat fruits and vegetables regularly, I will improve my health.	My parents would like me to be healthier.
I would feel better about myself if I were healthier.	My friends think I should eat healthier food.

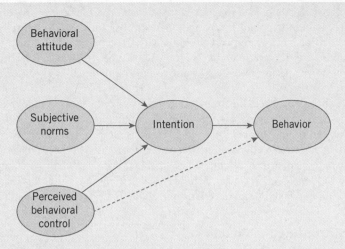

According to the theory of planned behavior, attitudes, subjective norms, and perceived behavioral control all influence behavior indirectly, through their impact on intentions. However, perceived behavioral control also exerts a direct impact on behavior.

Source: Ajzen (1991, p. 182).

intentions, which in turn predict behavior. Moreover, and as shown in Figure 3.2, perceived behavioral control is also described as having a direct impact on behavior.

Evaluating the Theories of Reasoned Action and Planned Behavior

The theories of reasoned action and planned behavior are successful in predicting a range of different types of health behaviors, including losing weight, engaging in physical activity, wearing seat belts, smoking cigarettes, using condoms, and undergoing health screenings (Albarracín, Johnson, Fishbein, & Muellerleile, 2001; Godin & Kok, 1996; Sieverding, Matterne, & Ciccarello, 2010). For example, a study of college students—over 70% of whom admitted to talking and texting while driving—revealed that attitudes, subjective norms, and perceived behavior control together predicted intentions to change this behavior (Bazargan-Hejazi et al., 2017). Moreover, intentions were a substantial predictor of willingness to both send and receive texts while driving. These studies all point to the value of these four components—attitudes, norms, perceived behavioral control, and intentions—in predicting health-related behavior.

Interventions developed based on components of these theories have led to improved health-related behaviors, including increased rates of condom use and healthy eating as well as decreased rates of smoking and tanning (Abar et al., 2010; Malek, Umberger, Makrides, & ShaoJia, 2017; Morisky, Stein, Chiao, Ksobiech, & Malow, 2006; Sheeran et al., 2016; Topa & Moriano, 2010). For example, people who receive training on how to identify warning signs of suicide and encourage people at risk to seek mental health treatment show more positive attitudes toward and greater self-efficacy for preventing suicides (Kuhlman, Walch, Bauer, & Glenn, 2017). They also reporter greater intentions to ask people about suicidal ideation, and, in turn, these increased intentions to intervene predict actual behavior, such as asking people about suicidal intentions and providing referrals to mental health care.

Finally, although these theories posit that individuals' intentions lead directly to behavior, people often intend to do a behavior but fail to actually follow through (Sheppard, Hartwick, & Warshaw, 1988). (You can probably think of many times in which your intentions to do a behavior did not successfully lead to enacting the behavior.) One strategy that helps increase the link between intentions and behavior is to form **implementation intentions**, meaning a specific plan of how, where, and when to perform a behavior (Gollwitzer, 1993). For example, if you intend to exercise regularly, you will be more likely to follow through on this intention if you form specific plans (e.g., I am going to join a gym and run on the treadmill 30 minutes right after work on Mondays, Wednesdays, and Fridays). For example, a study predicting whether people treated for substance abuse would seek further treatment found that those who formed specific plans, including the time and location for further treatment, were more likely to follow through on these intentions after undergoing detoxification than those without such plans (Kelly, Leung, Deane, & Lyons, 2016). Forming implementation intentions also helps people lose weight, reduce alcohol use, quit smoking, and increase exercise (Adriaanse, de Ridder, & de Wit, 2009; Armitage, 2004, 2009, 2015; Luszczynska, Sobczyk, & Abraham, 2007; Prestwich, Perugini, & Hurling, 2010; Tam, Bagozzi, & Spanjol, 2010).

Critiques of Continuum Models

Although the theories and models described in this section are widely used to predict health-related behaviors, they do have some limitations. First, these approaches all fail to include the person's current or past behavior, even though the best predictor of future behavior is often past behavior, and past behavior may influence behavior both directly and indirectly through its influence on intentions (Albarracin, Johnson, Fishbein, & Muellerleile, 2001; Manstead, Proffitt, & Smart, 1983). In line with this view, one recent study examining the predictors of various forms of distracted driving behavior (reading and sending text messages, making and answering cell phone calls, reading/viewing social media, and posting on social media while driving) found that past experience, in addition to the components of the theory of planned behavior, also had a significant impact on such behavior (Tian & Robinson, 2017).

These models also ignore other factors that may be quite strong predictors of behavior, including race, gender, and socioeconomic status (Rosenstock, 1990). Many of these models are largely based on studies with White people, and often only White men; therefore, they may not consider the different values that motivate behavior among members of other racial or ethnic groups (Cochran & Mays, 1993). For example, because the Black community places a stronger priority on interdependence and connection with extended family than does the White community, Black people may be more influenced in terms of their health-related behavior by the attitudes of their family. Similarly, people who have limited financial resources may be strongly motivated to engage in health-promoting behavior but simply lack the money to purchase healthy foods or receive preventative medical care.

Another concern about these theories is whether they simply show associations, or correlations, between various components versus predicting behavior over time. Specifically, studies that measure all of the components at a single time are unable to determine whether attitudes, norms, and perceived behavioral control predict behavior, or, alternatively, whether engaging in a behavior may change these other components. For example, engaging in unsafe sex leads to changes in attitudes and norms about such behavior over time (Huebner, Neilands, Rebchook, & Kegeles, 2011).

Finally, although each of the distinct theories described in this chapter includes specific components and models of how these components predict behavior, combining different components from several models may be the best way of predicting health-related behavior (Armitage & Arden, 2008; Reynolds, Buller, Yaroch, Maloy, & Cutter, 2006). In line with this view, susceptibility, subjective norms, and physicians' recommendation (a cue to action) are the best predictors of whether college women receive the HPV vaccination (Krawczyk et al., 2012). Similarly, a study predicting condom use found that planning, self-efficacy, and intentions were the best predictors of actual condom use one month later, again showing that constructs from different models of health-behavior may be particularly useful for predicting behavior (Teng & Mak, 2011). Different models may be most useful in describing particular types of behavior. For example, research generally shows that the health belief model is a better predictor of one-time or infrequent behavior, such as getting immunizations or having a mammogram, whereas other models are stronger predictors of more frequent behavior, such as quitting smoking and using condoms.

LEARNING THEORIES OF HEALTH BEHAVIOR

LO 3.2

Compare the three distinct learning theories of health behavior

Learning theories are based on the assumption that behavior is influenced by basic learning processes, such as association, reinforcement, and modeling (Bandura, 1977; Pavlov, 1927; Skinner, 1938; Thorndike, 1905). People learn health-related behaviors in the same way that they learn other behaviors. The three main types of learning approaches are classical conditioning, operant conditioning, and observational learning.

Classical Conditioning

Classical conditioning occurs when a previously neutral stimulus comes to evoke the same response as another stimulus with which it is paired. You may be familiar with a famous study on classical conditioning conducted by the Russian physiologist Ivan Pavlov (1927). At the start of the study, Pavlov noted that dogs normally salivate in response to the presentation of food but do not salivate in response to hearing a bell. For several days, he then rang a bell right before delivering food to hungry dogs. Over time, the dogs began to salivate merely at the sound of the bell before the food was presented. This research demonstrates the power of associative learning, in which dogs (and people!) understand that two events are linked (see Figure 3.3).

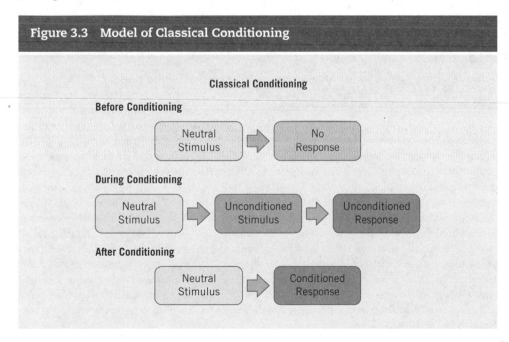

Figure 3.3 Model of Classical Conditioning

Classical Conditioning

Before Conditioning

Neutral Stimulus → No Response

During Conditioning

Neutral Stimulus → Unconditioned Stimulus → Unconditioned Response

After Conditioning

Neutral Stimulus → Conditioned Response

Classical conditioning can also influence people's health-related behavior. For example, imagine that you are reclining in a seat at your dentist's office hearing the sound of a dentist's drill coming from the next room. Even though the dentist is not anywhere near you (or your teeth), simply hearing the drill may produce feelings of arousal, anxiety, or pain because over time you have come to associate the noise of the drill with the pain in your mouth. Similarly, patients who have undergone chemotherapy, a treatment that often leaves people feeling nauseous and weak, sometimes develop anticipatory nausea even before they begin receiving a periodic dosage of the drugs. They may start to feel sick when they are sitting in the chair waiting for treatment or in the car as they are driving to the hospital. One study demonstrated that cancer patients who had previously received either chemotherapy or radiation reported experiencing nausea or vomiting in response to smells, sights, or tastes that reminded them of their treatment (Cameron et al., 2001). Thirty percent of the patients reported experiencing nausea in response to smells that reminded them of the treatment, and 17% reported experiencing nausea in response to sights that reminded them of the treatment.

Classical conditioning techniques can be used to create negative associations with unhealthy behaviors. For example, researchers in one study paired images of snack foods with images of adverse health consequences, such as a candy bar and a fat stomach (Hollands, Prestwich, & Marteau, 2011). Participants were then asked to select a snack food, as a reward for participating in the study, from choices of fruits or other less healthy snacks (e.g., cake, candy bar). In line with predictions, participants who saw the pairings of snack foods and images of adverse health consequences chose healthy foods more often than those who hadn't seen such pairings. Similarly, and as discussed in detail in *Chapter 7: Substance Use and Abuse*, aversion therapy is designed to eliminate substance abuse by pairing a given action, such as smoking or drinking alcohol, with a negative consequence, such as an electric shock or negative visual images (Kamarck & Lichtenstein, 1985). Over time, it is thought that this pairing should work to eliminate the undesired behavior.

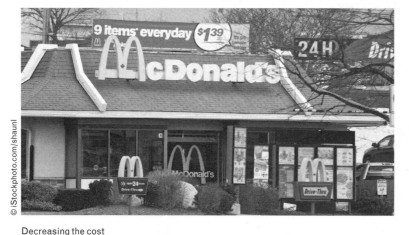

Decreasing the cost of healthy foods and increasing the cost of unhealthy foods may be an effective way to improve healthy eating. Unfortunately, in the real world, unhealthy foods are often much cheaper than healthy ones (think about the "value menus" at fast food restaurants with many unhealthy foods priced at just $1.00 compared to the price of many fresh fruits).

Operant Conditioning

Operant conditioning refers to the idea that behaviors can be increased or decreased as a function of the consequences of engaging in them (Skinner, 1938). On the one hand, desired behaviors can be positively reinforced through rewards, which should lead to their continuation. For example, if you are trying to stick to an exercise program, you might decide to give yourself a small reward each week that you run at least four days. On the other hand, the frequency of undesirable behaviors can be decreased through punishment. For example, people who are caught driving under the influence of alcohol typically receive severe punishments, including loss of their license, fines, and possibly even jail time. These negative consequences should motivate people to avoid drinking and driving.

Many health-promotion programs use rewards to increase healthy behaviors. For example, smokers who are offered gift cards to quit are more than twice as likely to successfully quit compared to those who are not offered this incentive (Kendzor et al., 2015). Similarly, obese children who are given rewards by their parents for engaging in physical activity later show increases in physical activity and, more importantly, decreases in weight (Epstein, Paluch, Kilanowski, & Raynor, 2004).

Researchers in one study compared the effectiveness of smoking cessation programs that created positive consequences for quitting to the effectiveness of those that created negative consequences for not quitting (Halpern et al., 2015). In the incentive condition (positive consequence for quitting), people received $200 for successfully quitting, whereas in the deposit condition (negative consequences for quitting), people received back their own $150 deposit if they successfully quit. People in the control group received information about local smoking cessation programs and a guide to help them quit. Six months after completing the program, 53% of those in the deposit condition had successfully quit, compared to only 17% of those in the incentive condition and 6% of those in the control condition. These findings suggest that creating negative consequences for not making behavior change (failing to quit smoking) may, at least in some cases, be more effective at creating behavior change than providing positive consequences.

Operant conditioning approaches are most effective when people receive rewards for making small steps toward behavior change. Changing behavior is often a long and difficult process; hence, if people receive rewards only after they have completely adopted the behavior, they will likely experience frustration. People should therefore receive rewards simply for taking steps toward adopting the behavior. For example, if you are trying to stop smoking, you might receive a reward for cutting down the number of cigarettes you smoke each day or for delaying smoking your first cigarette each morning. After you have mastered one of these steps toward smoking cessation, you will then receive rewards only for mastering the next step. For example, participants who set rewards for themselves for accomplishing their exercise goals (e.g., "will get my morning cup of coffee after I've finished my two-mile walk") are more likely to continue exercising over time than those without this incentive (Atkins, Kaplan, Timms, Reinsch, & Lofback, 1984).

Observational Learning

According to *social learning theory*, people do not need to directly experience the rewards or costs of engaging in a particular behavior to learn about its outcomes; learning can occur simply through *observational learning*, meaning watching someone else engage in a particular behavior and seeing or hearing about its consequences (Bandura, 1977, 1986). Children often form their beliefs about the consequences of various health-related behaviors by watching their parents and older siblings (Whitehead, Busch, Heller, & Costa, 1986). For example, the more younger siblings believed their older siblings drank, the more the younger siblings believed that positive outcomes would emerge from heavy drinking and the more the younger siblings themselves drank (D'Amico & Fromme, 1997).

People can even form such beliefs from observing the behavior of someone they do not personally know, such as a famous athlete, actor, or public figure. In turn, many health-promotion messages portray desirable role models promoting a particular behavior. Public service announcements on television, for example, often feature an actor urging people to avoid drug use, driving under the influence, or cigarettes. One study found that many people had heard a celebrity talk about the importance of cancer screening, and about a quarter of those who heard such an announcement reported they intended to get screened (Larson, Woloshin, Schwartz, & Welch, 2005). **Research in Action** describes how celebrities' public discussion of their own health issues can have a substantial impact on other people's health-related behaviors.

Observational learning from the media—including television shows, advertisements, and movies—can also influence health-related behavior. In some cases, such influence increases the prevalence of unhealthy behaviors. For example, teenagers who watch more sexual content in movies start having sex at an early age, have more sexual partners, and are less likely to engage in safe sex, even when taking into account participants' age, race, gender, and participation in religious activities (O'Hara, Gibbons, Gerrard, Li, & Sargent, 2012). Similarly, adolescents who are exposed to pro-alcohol images and messages through online social media websites (e.g., Facebook and Twitter) are more likely to engage in risky drinking (Moreno & Whitehill, 2014). Media portrayals of health-promoting behavior can also have beneficial effects, including increasing healthy eating and exercise behavior and decreasing rates of smoking and risky sexual behavior (Evans et al., 1981; Valente, Murphy, Huang, Gusek, Greene, & Beck, 2007; Vaughan, Rogers, Singhal, & Swalehe, 2000).

What You'll Learn
3.3

Although media portrayals can lead to improved health-related behaviors, they can also lead to inaccurate beliefs about medical procedures by presenting unrealistic examples. Researchers in one study examined the use of cardiopulmonary resuscitation (CPR) in medical dramas, such as *Grey's Anatomy* and *House*, and found 46 examples of their use over 91 episodes (Portanova, Irvine, Yi, & Enguidanos, 2015). In the real world, only 37% of people given CPR are brought back to life, whereas medical dramas portray CPR as lifesaving nearly twice as often (69.6%). Moreover, even in cases in which a person is brought back to life using CPR, only 13% of such patients ever recover enough to leave the hospital and thus survive long-term. But medical dramas show such a recovery in 50% of the cases. These overly optimistic portrayals may lead people to overestimate the likelihood of the success of CPR, as well as other medical procedures, which could impact people's ability to make realistic health care decisions for themselves and their loved ones.

Evaluating Learning Theories

Although learning theories are widely used to predict and influence behavior, these approaches have important limitations. First, although classical conditioning can be an effective way of influencing health-related behavior, it also has potential problems. As we examine in detail in *Chapter 7: Substance Use and Abuse*, one way to help alcoholics stop drinking is to give them a drug (e.g., Antabuse) that causes them to become violently ill when they drink alcohol. The theory behind this approach is that patients will grow to associate drinking alcohol with nausea and therefore stop drinking. However, patients typically understand that the Antabuse is causing the sickness; therefore, they may simply stop taking the drug instead of avoiding alcohol.

Second, operant conditioning can lead people to engage in a behavior simply to get the reward, but not because of any intrinsic changes in their intentions to engage in the behavior; once the reward is withdrawn, the behavior will stop. For example, children who receive small prizes (e.g., pencil, pen, yo-yo) for using a fluoride mouthwash daily are more likely to use the rinse, but once the prizes are eliminated, they no longer continue to use the rinse (Lund & Kegeles, 1984). In sum, learning theories may be effective at changing behavior but are less effective in maintaining behavior.

Finally, although media images clearly exert a strong influence on individuals' attitudes and behaviors, not all people are equally susceptible to such images. Children and teenagers who were high in self-control, meaning the ability to delay gratification, were less influenced by exposure to tobacco and alcohol use in movies and advertising than those who were lower in this trait (Wills et al., 2010). Specifically, although higher exposure led to more smoking and drinking as well as willingness to smoke and drink in the future, these results were seen only in those who were low in self-control. In sum, advertising had no influence on detrimental health behaviors among those with high levels of self-control.

STAGE MODELS OF HEALTH BEHAVIOR CHANGE

Although the models described thus far have all focused on describing the various components that predict whether people engage in a particular health-related behavior, some researchers believe these models are too simple because they focus only on the outcome behavior of interest (e.g., condom use, smoking cessation). Critics of these models believe that behavior change occurs gradually and in stages, and they have therefore proposed alternative models that focus on the process that leads to behavior change. In turn, these models specify a set of ordered categories, or stages, that people go through as they attempt to change their behavior.

LO 3.3

Explain the three stage models of health behavior change

Transtheoretical (Stages of Change) Model

According to the **transtheoretical (stages of change) model**, making changes in health-related behavior is a complex process, and individuals make such changes only gradually and not necessarily in a linear order (see Figure 3.4; Prochaska, DiClemente, & Norcross, 1992). People move from one stage to another in a spiral fashion, which can include movement to new stages as well as movement back to previous stages, until they have finally completed the process of behavior change. It is likely, for example, that a person who decides to stop smoking will experience several setbacks, or relapses, as he or she attempts to quit.

The first stage in this model is *precontemplation*. Individuals who are in this stage lack an awareness of the problem behavior and have no intentions or plans to change the behavior in the foreseeable future (e.g., "I have no intention to stop smoking"). Basically, they just aren't motivated to make any change in their own behavior, and they may underestimate the benefits of change and overestimate the costs to justify their inaction. People who smoke, for example, may believe that because they exercise regularly, they will not suffer the negative health effects of smoking, and that if they stop smoking, they will gain weight and hence suffer the (much worse) health consequences of obesity. They may also believe that although other people have suffered negative outcomes from the behavior, they have some unique personal invulnerability. I remember a friend in college telling me he actually believed he drove better while intoxicated. Individuals in this stage may also lack confidence in their ability to successfully engage in the new behavior.

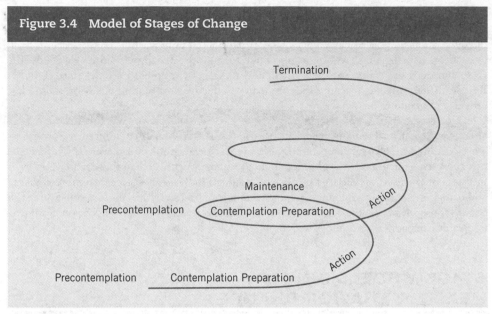

Figure 3.4   Model of Stages of Change

Termination

Maintenance

Precontemplation

Contemplation Preparation

Action

Precontemplation

Contemplation Preparation

Action

Source: Prochaska, DiClemente, & Norcross (1992).

Individuals who are beginning to consider making a change are in the *contemplation* stage (e.g., "I may start to think about how to quit smoking"). This stage is often characterized by a growing awareness of the costs of the negative behavior as well as of their personal susceptibility. People who are in this stage are out of the "ignorance is bliss" stage of precontemplation and are realizing that making a change would probably be a very good idea. People in the contemplation stage may start seeking information on the negative effects of their behavior and strategies for changing such behavior, although they may still lack confidence in their ability to make the change. This stage is often characterized by ambivalence as well as frustration.

Individuals who have made a commitment to change their behavior are in the stage of *preparation* (e.g., "I will stop smoking within the next 30 days"). They may start making small changes in an attempt to move toward the desired end point, such as decreasing the number of cigarettes they smoke each day or trying to delay the time they have their first cigarette each day. People in this stage are preparing to ultimately change their behavior but are starting by taking a series of small steps toward the desired behavior change. Although individuals in this stage are often highly motivated to change, they may vary in how confident they are of achieving success.

The stage of *action* is reached when they are actually engaging in a new behavior ("I have stopped smoking"). The behavior change is now public, and the criterion for successfully engaging in it is high. Although the risk of relapse is strong at this stage, people often receive a lot of support from their family and friends during this stage because they have made a public commitment to changing their behavior.

Finally, the *maintenance* stage is reached when people sustain the change over time, typically six months ("I will continue to not smoke"). The focus in this stage is on preventing relapse. People receive less social support during this stage because they have already engaged in action, but support is still an important predictor of maintaining the new behavior.

Early research using the transtheoretical model focused on its effectiveness in predicting smoking cessation (DiClemente et al., 1991; Prochaska et al., 1992). As this model predicts, people who are in different stages of change in terms of their smoking behavior differ in predicted ways on numerous variables, including self-efficacy for smoking cessation, perception of costs and benefits of smoking, and behavioral efforts toward quitting. People's stage of change at one point in time is also a pretty reliable predictor of whether (and when) they will quit. For example, only 6% of those in the precontemplation stage and 24% of those in the contemplation stage at one point in time reported having quit a month later, whereas 56% of those in the preparation stage had successfully quit by this point. The transtheoretical model can also predict the adoption of a variety of health-related behaviors, including fruit and vegetable consumption, condom use, exercise, sunscreen use, and screening for and treatment of cancer (Prochaska & Velicer, 1997; Prochaska et al., 1994).

What factors influence people to move from one stage to the next? Researchers believe that people go through specific processes of change as they progress through the various stages (Prochaska et al., 1992). At the earliest stages, people must become aware of the problem and learn effective ways of avoiding it. For some types of health behaviors, such as smoking, people typically already have exposure to information about their negative effects, but in other cases, such as getting a regular tetanus shot, people must be educated about the benefits of engaging in the behavior. External forces that facilitate change, such as smoking bans or higher taxes on alcohol or soft drinks, can also be effective in moving people through the stages. As people move along to the later stages of the models, they often examine the costs and benefits of changing their behavior. They might, for example, reflect on whether their desire to lose weight is really worth giving up late-night McDonald's trips. Perceived benefits of changing the behavior usually increase as people move from precontemplation to contemplation, and the costs of the new behavior usually decrease between the contemplation and action stages. So, behavior change messages should help people focus on the costs of continuing the old behavior (e.g., "I have stained teeth because of all my smoking") and the benefits of adopting the new behavior (e.g., "think about how much money I'll save by not smoking"). Finally, strategies that help people move from the action stage to the maintenance stage include substituting new behaviors for the old ones and providing rewards for continued behavior change. These methods might include treating oneself to dinner at a favorite restaurant after a week of not smoking or chewing gum instead of smoking. (Issues of preventing relapse following behavior change are discussed in detail in **Chapter 7: Substance Use and Abuse**.)

As with all theories of health behavior, the transtheoretical model has some limitations. First, although the processes of change by stage have been widely studied with respect to issues of smoking and substance abuse (DiClemente et al., 1991), some the cognitive processes involved in leading people to stop certain behaviors (e.g., smoking) may be different than those involved in leading them to start behaviors (e.g., exercise; Rosen, 2000). Specifically, while consciousness raising and social liberation are seen as most useful during the early stages of change toward ceasing a behavior, these processes are used frequently during later stages of change toward adopting a new behavior. Second, although this model describes how cognitive processes should lead people to move forward in the stages, most of the research testing this model has examined people only at one point in time. However, some research indicates that people who are weighing the costs and benefits of smoking at one time are *not* more likely to move to a higher stage one or two years later (Herzog, Abrams, Emmons, Linnan, & Shadel, 1999). These researchers believe that thinking about the costs and benefits of a behavior is not a good predictor of whether people will move further toward change. Third, some researchers have questioned whether these stages are in fact distinct categories, and whether they are

© iStockphoto.com/cigmusic

External cues that remind people about the costs of engaging in a given behavior, such as smoking bans and higher taxes on particular products, can help move people through the stages of change.

in correct order (Herzog, 2008; Herzog & Blagg, 2007). Relatedly, are the specific stages described in this model the right ones? As described next, other stage models describe health behavior change as occurring in a somewhat different way.

Precaution Adoption Process Model

The **precaution adoption process model** is similar in some ways to the transtheoretical model—it also proposes that when individuals consider engaging in new health-related behaviors, they go through a series of stages (Weinstein, 1988). As with the transtheoretical model, people do not necessarily move directly from one stage to another but rather can move backward or forward between stages. For example, you may decide on New Year's Eve that your resolution for the upcoming year is to stop drinking alcohol, but by February 1, you may have changed your intention to follow through with this behavior. The precaution adoption process model differs from the transtheoretical model, though, in the number of stages it proposes as well as the process by which it predicts how people progress through the stages (see Figure 3.5).

The precaution adoption process model includes seven stages (see Table 3.4). In *stage 1*, people are not even aware of the disease or problem. For example, many adolescent girls do not get enough calcium in their daily diet but often are unaware that this greatly increases their risk of osteoporosis in the future. In *stage 2*, people are generally aware of the health risk and believe that others might be at risk, but they do not believe that they personally are at risk. So, you might know that speeding increases the risk of having a car accident, but you may believe that because you are a safe driver, you will never experience an accident anyway. In sum, whereas the transtheoretical model groups all people who are not currently thinking about behavior change into one stage (precontemplation), this model separates these people into those who are unaware of a health issue (stage 1) and those who are aware of an issue but do not see themselves as personally vulnerable to it (stage 2) (Weinstein et al., 1998).

Next, people move along to *stage 3*, the decision-making stage, in which they have acquired a belief in their own personal risk but still have not decided to take action to protect themselves from that risk. You may know people who understand that lack of exercise puts them at greater risk of developing heart disease, for example, but they haven't decided whether they are going to exercise. From stage 3, people may move to *stage 5*, in which they decide to take action (e.g., finally do exercise), but they may also move to *stage 4*, in which they decide that action is unnecessary (e.g., they plan to continue being inactive, at least for the time being). Thus, the precaution adoption process model includes a specific stage for those who have thought about making a change but have decided against it, at least for the time being.

Figure 3.5   Precaution Adoption Process Model

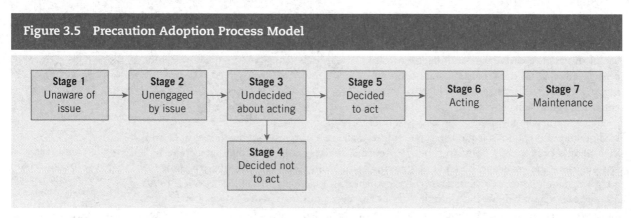

Source: Based on Weinstein (1988).

Table 3.4 Examples of the Seven Stages of the Precaution Adoption Process Model

Statement	Stage Classification
I have never seriously thought about trying to increase the amount that I currently exercise.	Stage 1
I have seriously thought about trying to increase the amount that I exercise but decided against it.	Stage 2
I have seriously thought about trying to increase the amount that I currently exercise, but I have not thought about it in the past 6 months.	Stage 3
I am seriously thinking about trying to increase the amount that I exercise sometime within the next 6 months.	Stage 4
I plan to increase the amount that I exercise within the next 6 months.	Stage 5
I am currently doing things to increase the amount that I exercise.	Stage 6

(Women who were already engaging in exercise for at least 45 minutes three times a week and who reported that they had been engaging in exercise for the last 6 months were classified as stage 7.)

Source: Blalock et al. (1996).

The final two stages of this model are very similar to those seen in the transtheoretical model. In *stage 6*, people have begun to change their behavior (similar to the stage of action). Finally, in *stage 7*, people maintain the behavior change over some period of time (similar to the stage of maintenance).

In line with the predictions of the precaution adoption process model, people at different stages of making health behavior changes report different beliefs about their own risks and intentions to adopt new behaviors. For example, although few smokers are at stage 1 (probably because virtually everyone is aware of the health hazards of smoking), many smokers are at stage 2, in which they see smoking as generally dangerous but still possess an optimistic view of their own risk, meaning they see themselves personally as less at risk than "typical smokers" of developing smoking-related consequences (McCoy et al., 1992). However, smokers who have joined a smoking cessation clinic are typically one or two stages further along: they recognize their own vulnerability to smoking-related health problems and have made a decision to try to quit. This model is also a useful predictor of engaging in contraceptive use, mammography, exercise, and home radon testing (Blalock et al., 1996; Clemow et al., 2000; Emmett & Ferguson, 1999; Weinstein & Sandman, 1992).

As with the other models we've discussed, the precaution adoption process model has some important implications for designing health behavior change interventions. First, individuals who are at different stages should be influenced by different types of information. When someone is deciding whether to take action (stage 3), for example, perceptions of vulnerability should predict whether he or she moves to stage 5 (decides to engage in behavior change) or stage 4 (chooses not to engage in behavior change). On the other hand, when someone has decided to engage in behavior change (stage 5), whether that person actually does so (moves to stage 6) should be influenced by obstacles and barriers to such change. Moreover, and as described in **Focus on Diversity**, people who receive culturally relevant messages designed to increase their perception of risk are more likely to change their behavior.

Health Action Process Approach

The **health action process approach** is the most recent stage model to predict health-related behavior (Schwarzer, 1992). According to this model, people making changes in their behavior undergo two distinct stages. First, they must form an intention to change their behavior in some, such as by starting to exercise or stopping drinking alcohol. In this *motivation stage*, people evaluate the risk of the behavior, the outcomes they expect to result from such a change, and their self-efficacy for making such a change.

Next, if a person does form an intention to make a change in their behavior, he or she then enters the *volition phase*, which involves making specific plans to carry out these intentions. This stage includes developing specific plans and strategies for enacting the desired behavior change. (Such planning is similar to developing implementation intentions, as described earlier in this chapter.) It also involves developing self-efficacy for being able to make this change, even when urges, emotions, and/or environmental factors may occur. Finally, this stage includes a focus on developing confidence that they can recover if they experience relapses during this process of behavior change.

Although this is the most recently developed model predicting health behavior, research already provides support for its applicability, including its ability to predict changes in eating and exercise, smoking, and condom use (Lippke & Plotnikoff, 2014; Parschau et al., 2014; Teng & Mak, 2011; Williams, Herzog, & Simmons, 2011). For example, researchers in one recent study examined whether the health action process approach could be used to predict avoiding future drunk driving among people currently appearing in court following a drunk-driving arrest (Wilson, Sheehan, Palk, & Watson, 2016). First, people who were higher in self-efficacy for avoiding drunk driving, held positive outcomes about avoiding this behavior, and saw the risks of drunk driving as severe report greater intentions to avoid such behavior (in line with the motivation stage). Furthermore, people who had greater confidence in their ability to plan to avoid drunk driving in the future were more likely to report successfully avoiding drunk driving at the six-month follow-up. These findings provide support for the effectiveness of the health action process approach in predicting health-related behavior.

CREATING HEALTH BEHAVIOR CHANGE

LO 3.4

Describe distinct strategies for creating health behavior change

One of the biggest challenges facing health professionals is how to effectively persuade people to change their health-related behavior. Early efforts designed to create behavior change simply provided the facts about a given behavior with the hope that giving people the information would motivate change. According to this view, people who understand that smoking causes cancer or that a lack of physical activity increases the risk of obesity, for example, will be motivated to change their behavior to avoid these negative consequences.

Unfortunately, and as you might imagine, in most cases information is not a sufficient motivator of behavior change. In fact, we all engage in behaviors (sometimes frequently) that we know are not great for our health (e.g., texting and driving, failing to use sunscreen, eating high-fat foods). Research studies provide additional support for the view that information alone is rarely a sufficient motivator of behavior. For example, attitudes that are based in how people *feel* about something are more predictive of behavior than attitudes that are based in what people *think* about something (Lawton, Conner, & McEachan, 2009). In sum, although providing people with information about healthy behaviors does, not surprisingly, increase their knowledge about such behavior, it is rarely sufficient to lead to behavior change. Health professionals have therefore turned to strategies in an attempt to help people change their health-related behavior.

Fear-Based Appeals

Fear-based appeals, meaning messages that use negative stimuli in some way, are designed to create the threat of impending danger or harm caused by engaging in particular types of behavior (e.g., drug use, smoking) or failing to engage in other types of behavior (e.g., not using a condom, not using sunscreen). Fear-based appeals sometimes use scary verbal statements and may show graphic, even disgusting, images. For example, one television ad promoting the use of seat belts showed a young man backing his car out of the driveway to go pick up ice cream for his pregnant wife, but he didn't put on his seat belt and was then hit by a speeding car. In some other countries, such as Australia and Canada, television ads may include even more graphic images, such as dead bodies and crash survivors learning how to walk again.

These messages are designed to increase people's feelings of vulnerability to various health problems and thereby motivate them to change their behavior (Freimuth, Hammond, Edgar, & Monahan, 1990; Higbee, 1969; Janis, 1967; Leventhal, 1970; Rogers, 1975). Moreover, as compared to positive messages, negative ones are thought to be more primary, easier to understand, more quickly processed, and more accurately remembered (Reeves, Lang, Thorson, & Rothschild, 1989). Moreover, and as described in **Focus on Neuroscience**, fear appeals activate particular parts of the brain that process emotion, memory, and decision making, which may explain why such messages can be particularly effective.

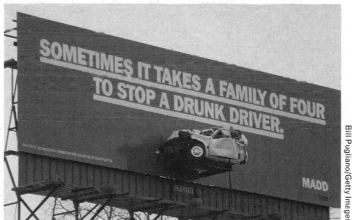

Bill Pugliano/Getty Images

Fear-based appeals are commonly used to motivate health-related behavior change. However, some research calls into question whether such approaches are really effective.

In one of the earliest studies on the effectiveness of fear appeals, people were randomly assigned to receive one of three smoking cessation messages (Leventhal & Watts, 1966). The low-fear message consisted of a color film describing the threat of lung cancer using charts and diagrams; the medium-fear message consisted of the same film plus an additional segment documenting how a small-town newspaper editor discovered he had lung cancer; and the high-fear message consisted of the same film and additional segment plus a 10-minute color sequence showing an operation in which a lung is removed. Not surprisingly, people who watched the high-fear film showed many signs of distress, including looking away, groaning, and even crying. This study revealed that low- versus high-fear ads have a different impact on behavior at different times. First, those in the low-fear condition were the most likely to immediately get an x-ray of their lungs at a nearby booth (53% in low fear versus 44% in medium fear, 6% in high fear), indicating that high-fear messages were the least effective in motivating short-term behavior. However, a follow-up questionnaire five months later revealed significant differences in the opposite direction: 57% of those in the low-fear and moderate-fear conditions reported cutting down on smoking compared to 79% of those in the high-fear condition. In sum, high-fear messages may be ineffective in the short term, as people react defensively to these upsetting and personally relevant messages, but may be quite effective over time.

Critiques of Fear-Based Appeals

However, more recent research suggests that fear-based appeals often create increases in anxiety but have little, if any, effect on actual behavior (Evans, 1988; Jarlais, Friedman, Casriel, & Kott, 1987; Rigby, Brown, Anagnostou, Ross, & Rosser, 1989; Sherr, 1990). For example, Project DARE (Drug Abuse Resistance Education), a commonly used fear-based drug prevention program for children, has little effect on preventing or reducing drug use, and it is often less effective than programs that focus simply on social skills (Ennett, Tobler, Ringwalt, & Flewelling, 1994). Ironically, people who receive high-fear messages often report that they are very influenced but in reality show lower levels of attitude and behavior change than those who receive positive approaches (Evans, Rozelle, Lasater, Dembroski, & Allen, 1970; Janis & Feshbach, 1953). In line with this view, one meta-analysis examining the effects of fear-inducing arguments about HIV revealed that such messages increased perceptions of the risk of HIV but led to decreased knowledge about HIV as well as decreased condom use (Earl & Albarracin, 2007).

One of the problems with fear appeals is that they create considerable anxiety, which can interfere with cognitive processing, including learning, attention, and comprehension (Janis, 1967). For example, smokers who received a strong fear message showed more tension and concern about lung cancer but less attitude change (Janis & Terwilliger, 1962), and high school students who received a strong fear message about decayed teeth and gum disease remembered fewer arguments from the message and showed less attitude change than those who received a milder argument (Janis & Feshbach, 1953). Research in neuroscience provides further evidence that fear-based appeals interfere with cognitive processing, demonstrating that people show lower levels of brain activity in response to threatening health-related messages (Kessels, Ruiter, & Jansma, 2010).

Another factor that helps explain why fear-based appeals may fail to elicit behavior change is that people protect themselves from the anxiety caused by such appeals by denying and/or minimizing the information presented in such appeals (Chaiken, 1987; Freeman, Hennessy, & Marzullo, 2001; Halpern, 1994; Kunda, 1990). For example, heavy coffee drinkers are more critical of a study supposedly showing a link between caffeine consumption and disease than those who don't drink coffee, presumably because coffee drinkers really don't want to believe they are engaging in a health-damaging behavior (Liberman & Chaiken, 1992; Sherman, Nelson, & Steele, 2000). Similarly, smokers may see anti-smoking messages as biased and unconvincing (Rhodes, Roskos-Ewoldsen, Edison, & Bradford, 2008). Another way to minimize the effects of a fear-based appeal is by seeing the problem as more common—a strategy of "well, if everyone else is doing it, it must not be that bad" (Croyle, Sun, & Louie, 1993). For example, as compared to students who are told their cholesterol is at a low level, students who receive information that their cholesterol is at a somewhat risky high level perceive high cholesterol as a less serious threat, view the test as less accurate, and see high cholesterol as more common.

This tendency to deny, or minimize, personally relevant health information occurs even in the case of very serious illnesses, such as cancer. For example, smokers who are told they have a gene that places them at greater risk of experiencing negative consequences from smoking are more likely to inaccurately recall the level of risk and to misinterpret the meaning of the result (Lipkus, McBride, Pollak, Lyna, & Bepler, 2004). In line with this view, people who had a parent with hypertension and who hence already saw themselves as vulnerable to this problem were much less likely to attend a blood pressure screening after receiving a message that emphasized the dire consequences of hypertension than after receiving a message that emphasized the benefits of acting to maintain well-being (Gintner, Rectanus, Achord, & Parker, 1987). On the other hand, those without a family history of hypertension were more likely to receive screening after they received threatening information.

Finally, and perhaps most important, people may even respond defensively to messages that try to change their behavior and thus increase their levels of unhealthy behavior (Rhodes et al., 2008). For example, college students who hear anti-drinking messages may want to drink more, and smokers who hear anti-smoking messages may show an increase in intentions to keep smoking. All of this evidence suggests that fear-based appeals can have some unintended—and even dangerous—side effects.

Improving Fear-Based Appeals

However, fear-based appeals can at times influence health-related behavior. When are such messages effective? Research demonstrates that the following strategies all increase the effectiveness of such messages in leading to behavior change.

CREATE MODERATE LEVELS OF FEAR. Messages need to create a moderate level of fear (Janis, 1967; Janis & Feshbach, 1953; Leventhal, 1970; Soames Job, 1988; Witte & Allen, 2000). At very low levels of fear, the danger is not seen as very important or very severe, and hence the average person will be relatively unmotivated to seek help. On the other hand, and as described previously, at high levels of fear, people try to deny or minimize the threat to cope with their anxiety. However, at moderate levels of fear, people will be motivated to protect themselves because the threat seems relatively likely and relatively severe, but they will not be paralyzed by anxiety and hence unable to act.

PROVIDE SPECIFIC STRATEGIES. Because fear appeals create considerable anxiety, people must be given a specific strategy for handling the anxiety to avoid the motivation to minimize or deny the threat (Leventhal, Singer, & Jones, 1965; Sturges & Rogers, 1996). Students who receive highly threatening messages but who are told that they can take some specific action to manage the threat show stronger intentions to change their behavior than those who receive messages that frighten them but don't give strategies for coping (Self & Rogers, 1990). So, fear-based drug prevention campaigns are probably not an effective approach to attitude and behavior change, but programs that give teenagers specific techniques for managing peer pressure to use drugs without alienating friends may be quite effective. For example, the Midwestern Prevention Project, a moderately successful drug prevention program for middle and junior high school students, provides students with information about drugs coupled with training in strategies for resisting social pressure, such as assertiveness training, modeling, and role play (MacKinnon et al., 1991). Participation in this program leads to more negative attitudes toward drugs and decreases in intentions to use drugs as well as decreased reported drug use.

FOCUS ON SHORT-TERM CONSEQUENCES. Fear appeals are often more effective when they focus on the short-term, as opposed to the long-term, consequences (Klohn & Rogers, 1991; Pechmann, 1997)—many people, especially teenagers, just aren't concerned about long-term consequences. Similarly, people might learn that tanning can cause skin cancer but still feel that they'd like to be tan because they look healthier and more attractive (Broadstock, Borland, & Gason, 1992; Leary & Jones, 1993). In fact, Jones and Leary (1994) found that college students were more persuaded to use sunscreen after reading an essay describing the short-term negative effects of tanning on appearance (e.g., increased wrinkles, scarring, aging) than after reading an essay describing the long-term negative effects (e.g., the health risks of tanning, the prevalence of different types of skin cancer). Similarly, although teenagers who watched a video describing how exposure to UV light increases skin cancer and those who watched a video describing how exposure to UV light harms appearance (by causing wrinkles and premature aging) showed equivalent levels of increased knowledge about the importance of sun-protective behavior, only those who watched the appearance-based video showed increases in actual sunscreen use (Tuong & Armstrong, 2014).

What You'll Learn 3.4

Researchers in one study examined whether the reality television programs *16 and Pregnant*, which show the less-than-glamorous reality faced by teenage parents, had positive effects on adolescent sexual behavior (Kearney & Levine, 2015). The researchers first collected data assessing the popularity of this program, including Nielsen ratings as well as measures of Google and Twitter searches. They then examined national rates of births to teenagers in the 18 months after the show first started airing. First, and as predicted, this show was very popular, as measured by both national ratings and Internet searches. Interestingly, searches for topics raised in the show, such as birth control and abortion, spiked precisely when these shows were on and in parts of the country in which they were most popular. These findings suggest that watching *16 and Pregnant* leads teenagers to seek out relevant information. Most important, the findings revealed that the national teenage birth rate decreased by an estimated 4.3% in the first 18 months after the show was first broadcast. The rate of abortions to teenagers also fell during this period, indicating that this show does not lead to increases in abortion but rather to decreases in sexual activity and/or increases in birth control use.

ENHANCE VULNERABILITY. Fear appeals may also work when they force people to actually imagine having a particular disease or problem and thereby lead to a heightened sense of vulnerability (Janis & Mann, 1965). One public service announcement designed to enhance people's perceived vulnerability to HIV featured an attractive Hispanic man saying the following: "Do I look like someone who has AIDS? Of course not. I am Alejandro Paredes. I finished school. I have a good job. I help support my family. My kind of guy doesn't get AIDS, right? Well, I have AIDS, and I don't mind telling you it's devastating. If I had a second chance, I'd be informed. Believe me" (Freimuth et al., 1990, p. 788). This appeal is clearly designed to increase people's vulnerability to HIV and to eliminate the use of various cognitive defenses against this information (e.g., only poor people get HIV, only people who look unhealthy have HIV). Similarly, college students who heard a personal account by someone who became infected with the hepatitis B virus showed stronger intentions to get vaccinated than those who were given statistical information about the prevalence of this disease (De Wit, Das, & Vet, 2008).

Messages that increase perceptions of personal vulnerability to a particular health problem may be especially effective. For example, college students who see photographs of themselves that illustrate the damage of sun exposure (e.g., wrinkles, age spots) show decreases in indoor tanning and increases in sun-protective behaviors, such as fewer hours tanning and more use of sunscreen (Gibbons, Gerrard, Lane, Mahler, & Kulick, 2005; Mahler, Kulik, Gerrard, & Gibbons, 2007). Compared to those who did not receive personalized photos, students who received photos also had lighter skin later on, indicating that these photos were effective in changing tanning behavior.

PROVIDE SELF-AFFIRMATION. As described previously, people have a tendency to react against messages that threaten their well-being and hence may tune out fear-based appeals. One strategy for reducing this tendency to engage in defensive processing is to provide some type of self-affirmation along with the threatening messages (Sherman & Cohen, 2002). This strategy can increase people's receptivity to messages that potentially threaten the self because buffering people's feelings of self-worth increases their ability to accept information that is seen as threatening in terms of maintaining a positive self-concept. For example, coffee drinkers who are given information about the risks of caffeine but also have the opportunity to self-affirm by writing about their most important value show more accessibility of the message, more positive beliefs about message quality, and more intentions to change their behavior (van Koningsbruggen, Das, & Roskos-Ewoldsen, 2009). Self-affirmation also leads to increases in fruit and vegetable consumption and condom use as well as lower levels of alcohol use and smoking (Epton & Harris, 2008; Harris & Napper, 2005; Harris, Mayle, Mabbott, & Napper, 2007; Sherman et al., 2000).

How exactly does self-affirmation lead to greater behavior change? Apparently, self-affirmation increases our receptivity to information that is hard to hear. In fact, research using fMRI reveals that people who engage in self-affirmation show greater activity in a part of the brain (the ventromedial prefrontal cortex) that processes self-relevant information (Falk, O'Donnell, Cascio, et al., 2015). Moreover, greater activity in this part of the brain while listening to potentially threatening messages (such as "According to the American Heart Association, people at your level of physical inactivity are at much higher risk for developing heart disease") predicts greater reductions in sedentary behavior in the following month.

Message Framing

Another factor that influences the persuasiveness of messages promoting health behavior change is how such messages are presented, or framed (Rothman & Salovey, 1997). Subtle shifts in wording—such as describing condoms as 90% effective versus as having a 10% failure rate—influence how people make health-related decisions. In line with this view, students rate a medical treatment with a 50% success rate as more effective and as one they are more likely to recommend to members of their immediate family than a treatment with a 50% failure rate (Levin, Schnittjer, & Thee, 1988), and students feel more optimistic about a person with a 90% chance of survival than a 10% chance of dying.

Health-promotion messages generally are framed in one of two ways. Gain-framed messages focus on the positive outcomes that can be attained—or the negative outcomes that can be avoided—by adopting a particular type of health-related behavior (see Table 3.5). Loss-framed messages, on the other hand, focus on the negative outcomes that may occur from failing to adopt a particular type of health-related behavior. Interestingly, these different types of message framing are more effective at promoting different types of health-promoting behaviors.

Gain-framed messages tend to be more effective than loss-framed messages in helping people to engage in behavior that prevents a health problem from developing (Rothman & Salovey, 1997). In turn, gain-framed messages are indeed more effective than loss-framed ones at increasing people's intentions to use condoms and protect themselves from the sun

Table 3.5 Comparison of Sample Gain- Versus Loss-Framed Persuasive Statements	
Gain-Framed	**Loss-Framed**
We will show that detecting breast cancer early can save your life.	We will show that failing to detect breast cancer early can cost you your life.
Although all women are at risk for breast cancer, there is something you can do to increase your chances of surviving it.	Although all women are at risk for breast cancer, there is something you can do that increases your risk of dying from it.
For this reason, when you get a mammogram, you are taking advantage of the best method for detecting breast cancer early.	For this reason, when you avoid getting a mammogram, you are failing to take advantage of the best method for detecting breast cancer early.
If a cancer has not spread, it is less likely to be fatal.	If a cancer has spread, it is more likely to be fatal.
Another advantage of finding a tumor early is that you are more likely to increase your treatment options and may need less radical procedures.	Another disadvantage of failing to find a tumor early is that you may have fewer treatment options and may need more radical procedures.
The bottom line is, when you get regular mammograms, you are doing your best to detect breast cancer in its early stages.	The bottom line is, when you fail to get regular mammograms, you are not doing your best to detect breast cancer in its early stages.

Note: These statements provide examples of gain- versus loss-framed persuasive statements.

Source: Banks et al. (1995).

(Detweiler, Bedell, Salovey, Pronin, & Rothman, 1999; Kiene, Barta, Zelenski, & Cothran, 2005). For example, 85% of students who were told that a particular brand of condoms had a 90% success rate intended to use this type of condom, whereas only 63% of those who learned that this brand had a 10% failure rate intended to use that type (Linville, Fischer, & Fischhoff, 1993). Another study found that 71% who received the gain-framed messages about skin cancer requested free sunscreen with a sun protection factor (SPF) level of 15 as compared to only 46% of those who got the loss-framed messages about skin cancer (Rothman, Salovey, Antone, et al., 1993).

Loss-framed messages, on the other hand, tend to be more effective for helping people seek medical care regarding a potential health problem. Loss-framed messages therefore can push people to have mammograms, HIV testing, or skin cancer detection exams (Gallagher, Updegraff, Rothman, & Sims, 2011; Kalichman & Coley, 1995; Rothman et al., 1993; Schneider et al., 2001). For example, 66.2% of women who received a loss-framed message about mammograms had obtained a mammogram 1 year later as compared to 51.5% of those who had received a gain-framed message (Banks et al., 1995). In sum, loss-framed messages are more effective than gain-framed messages at encouraging people to engage in behaviors to detect a symptom of illness.

The way health practitioners describe different treatment options also influences patients' preferences (Levin et al., 1988; Marteau, 1989; McNeil, Pauker, Sox, & Tversky, 1982). The risks of a particular surgical procedure, for example, can also be described in terms of the likelihood of living (a gain frame) or the likelihood of dying (a loss frame). For example, physicians, patients, and medical students in one study were given information that described the consequences of having surgery versus radiation to treat lung cancer using either gain-framed or loss-framed wording (McNeil, Pauker, Sox, & Tversky, 1982). The gain-framed message read, "*Of 100 people having surgery, 90 will live during treatment, 68 will be alive at 1 year, and 34 will be alive at 5 years. Of 100 people having radiation therapy, all will live during treatment, 77 will be alive at 1 year, and 22 will be alive at 5 years.*" The loss-framed message read, "*Of 100 people having surgery, 10 will die during treatment, 32 will have died by 1 year, and 66 will have died by 5 years. Of 100 people having radiation therapy, none will die during treatment, 23 will die by 1 year, and 78 will die by 5 years.*" As predicted, more people chose surgery when information was presented in terms of likelihood of living (a gain frame) than when information was presented in terms of likelihood of dying (a loss frame).

Messages that emphasize the benefits of using sunscreen to prevent skin cancer tend to be more effective at encouraging people to adopt sun-protective behaviors than those that emphasize the costs of not using sunscreen.

PERSONALIZED HEALTH-PROMOTION MESSAGES

Although traditional health education messages have used a "one-size-fits-all" approach by giving the same information to everyone, both theory and research suggest that different people respond in different ways to different types of information (Kreuter & Holt, 2001; Kreuter & Skinner, 2000; Kreuter, Strecher, & Glassman, 1999; Skinner, Campbell, Rimer, Curry, & Prochaska, 1999; Skinner, Strecher, & Hospers, 1994). According to the

LO 3.5

Summarize the use of personalized health-promotion messages

interactionist perspective, people are much more responsive to personally relevant information. Specifically, people are more likely to read, remember, comprehend, and discuss personally relevant messages, and they perceive these messages as more interesting, likable, and in line with their attitudes (Brug, Steenhuis, van Assena, & de Vries, 1996; Campbell et al., 1994; Kalichman, Carey, & Johnson, 1996; Kreuter, Bull, Clark, & Oswald, 1999; Peterson & Marin, 1988). They also have more positive thoughts about the material, make more personal connections to the material, develop stronger intentions to change their behavior, and, most important, are more likely to be successful in their behavior change efforts. In turn, different people should find different types of health-promotion information most convincing and, most important, show greater behavior change in response to personally relevant messages.

Given these findings, researchers in the field of health psychology are increasingly creating different types of messages for different people. In some cases, these messages are *targeted* to a specific group of people and/or specific characteristics of a group of people. For example, teenagers might be most convinced by information about the negative effects of smoking on appearance (e.g., smelly clothes, yellow teeth, bad breath), whereas women who smoke may be most convinced by information about preventing weight gain. In sum, health-promotion messages should be most effective when they provide people with personally relevant information. In other cases, researchers have created messages that are *tailored* to an individual's particular needs and goals. A message that is created to address a specific woman's concerns about mammography (e.g., fear of pain, anxiety about learning she has cancer) is a tailored message. This section examines the benefits of receiving both types of personally relevant materials on a number of health-related topics, including adopting healthier behaviors, managing pain and illness, and screening for health conditions.

Adopting Healthier Behaviors

Personalized messages—including letters, interventions, and treatments—are consistently more effective than generic ones at helping people adopt healthier behaviors. This section describes the benefits of personalized messages for helping people engage in a variety of health-promoting behaviors, including quitting smoking, reducing alcohol use, improving eating and exercise behavior, and increasing condom use.

Quitting Smoking

Considerable research on smoking cessation programs suggests that these programs are more effective when they provide personally relevant information than when they provide generic information (Prochaska, DiClemente, Velicer, & Rossi, 1993; Solomon, Secker-Walker, Skelly, & Flynn, 1996). For example, smokers who were given a generic letter about the general benefits of and barriers to quitting were less likely to quit than those who received a personally tailored letter that addressed the specific benefits and barriers they had personalized described experiencing (Strecher et al., 1994). Specifically, four months later, only 7.4% of those who had received a generic letter had stopped smoking compared to 20.8% of those who had received the personally tailored letter.

Similarly, people with different motivations for smoking also respond differently to particular types of smoking cessation interventions. For example, to examine the effectiveness of different types of smoking cessation interventions for different people, smokers were randomly assigned to one of two interventions, which each met six times over a two-week period (Zelman, Brandon, Jorenby, & Baker, 1992). The rapid-smoking intervention required subjects to inhale from cigarettes every 6 seconds for a 60-minute period, during which time they consumed an average of 4.7 cigarettes; they were to refrain from smoking outside the sessions. Those in the nicotine gum intervention were given prescriptions for gum, and they were encouraged to use the gum whenever they wanted to. Although there were no long-term overall differences in the effectiveness of these two conditions, different people responded to these interventions in different ways. Specifically, and as predicted, the nicotine gum intervention was most effective when used with people who were high on physical dependence, whereas the rapid-smoking intervention was most effective when used with people who were low on physical dependence. This study provides further evidence that treatments must be matched to people's preferences and individual needs to maximize their effectiveness.

Reducing Alcohol Use

People who receive personalized information regarding their drinking behavior show greater behavior change than those who receive more general information (Neighbors et al., 2010; Neighbors, Lewis, Bergstrom, & Larimer, 2006). Heavy-drinking college students who received personalized feedback about how much they drank reported drinking about five drinks less per week at a six-month follow-up than those who hadn't receive such information (Walters, Vader, Harris, Field, & Jouriles, 2009). They also reported lower scores on an alcohol problem survey and lower levels of blood alcohol concentration when they did drink.

Researchers in one study examined the effectiveness of providing personalized feedback about students' drinking intentions regarding their 21st birthday celebration (a time in which many students are encouraged to drink dangerous amounts of alcohol; Neighbors, Lee, Lewis, Fossos, & Walter, 2009). College students who reported intending to drink at least two drinks on their 21st birthday were randomly assigned to either receive Web-based personalized feedback about their drinking two days before their birthday or simply complete a survey about their own drinking. This feedback included information about the blood alcohol concentration (BAC) that would result from drinking as much alcohol as they intended to drink, as well as the effects of such a BAC on the body, and specific strategies to help them engage in moderate alcohol consumption. When students were contacted one week later, those who had received the personalized feedback reported consuming less alcohol than those who had only completed the survey. Most important, the personalized feedback was particularly impactful for students who had initially reported intentions to consume the most alcohol and were thus most at risk of experiencing alcohol-related problems.

What You'll Learn
3.5

People in treatment for alcohol addiction may also benefit more from receiving particular types of treatment. For example, people who experience strong physiological cravings for alcohol benefit more from receiving medication that reduces the cravings, whereas those who are high in verbal skills really benefit from relapse prevention training (e.g., training in self-monitoring, stress management, modeling, role plays; Jaffe et al., 1996). Similarly, patients who score high on measures of psychopathology and sociopathy benefit much more from training in coping skills related to alcohol use than group-based, interactional therapy, presumably because they lack the social skills to benefit from the group experience (Kadden, Cooney, Getter, & Litt, 1989). These findings suggest that alcohol treatment programs need to carefully consider the factors that drive individuals' drinking in order to maximize their effectiveness.

Improving Eating and Eating-Disordered Behavior

Tailored messages can also influence eating and exercise behavior. For example, compared to patients who received general information on dietary and nutrition guidelines, participants who received an individually tailored letter (e.g., based on their beliefs about the benefits of changing their diet and their susceptibility to diet-related diseases) were more likely to remember receiving the letter, were more likely to have read all of the message, and reported eating less total fat four months later (Campbell et al., 1994). Tailored messages also lead to increases in fruit and vegetable consumption and recreational physical activity (Campbell et al., 2004). This type of personally relevant message may be more effective at least in part because people who get tailored messages promoting nutrition pay more attention to these than general messages (Ruiter, Kessels, Jansma, & Brug, 2006). Similarly, adults who received print-based individualized feedback promoting physical activity showed more minutes of moderate-intensity exercise one year later than those who received individualized feedback on the phone or those in a control condition (Marcus et al., 2007).

However, personality variables can also influence how people respond to particular messages promoting healthy eating and exercise behavior. For example, obese people who feel that their weight is outside their control (e.g., influenced by luck, genetics) actually respond more negatively to tailored than generic information: they counterargue the messages that provide personally relevant strategies for taking control of their eating and exercise behavior (Holt, Clark, Kreuter, & Scharff, 2000). In contrast, obese people who believe they are in control of their weight respond more favorably to messages that provide personally relevant strategies for weight loss than to generic information. Similarly, college students at varying levels of risk for developing an eating disorder benefit from distinct types of health-promotion messages (Mutterperl & Sanderson, 2002). For women at low risk of developing an eating disorder, receiving information about the signs, symptoms, and dangers of eating disorders reduces the desire for thinness, presumably because such information helps women understand the real risks posed by such behaviors (Sanderson & Holloway, 2003). For women who are already showing signs and symptoms of eating disorders, on the other hand, such information leads to an even stronger focus on achieving a very thin ideal; these messages may unintentional reinforce women's views about the importance of thinness and provide strategies for achieving this ideal. These findings provide some important information about how best to target eating disorders on college campuses—and strongly suggest that different women will benefit from receiving different types of health-promotion messages.

Finally, interventions for treating eating disorders are more effective when they take into account individuals' stage of change. Specifically, women who were at the stage of precontemplation preferred a treatment group that provided only general listening support, whereas those who were in the stage of preparation preferred a group that worked on setting specific goals for decreasing the frequency of bingeing and purging; those who were in the stage of maintenance preferred a group that focused on how to prevent relapse (Levy, 1997). Once again, people particularly benefit from receiving health-promotion information that matches their specific needs: "one size" clearly does not "fit all."

Increasing Condom Use

Gender, not surprisingly, influences people's response to different types of condom-promotion messages. As you might imagine, women and men often have different concerns about using condoms; hence, condom-promotion ads may be more effective when they present different types of information to men and women (Amaro, 1995; Marin & Marin, 1992; Mays & Cochran, 1988). For example, condom-promotion ads for women might be most effective if they portray condom use in romantic, committed relationships, in part because women are often concerned that buying and carrying condoms makes them appear promiscuous or "loose" (Struckman-Johnson, Gilliand, Struckman-Johnson, & North, 1990). In contrast, condom-promotion ads for men, who are generally more concerned about condom use reducing their own sexual pleasure, might be more effective if they use sexually arousing content and emphasize that condoms can lengthen sex and thereby enhance both partners' experiences.

Personality variables, such as a person's desire for intimacy and closeness in a relationship, also influence people's responsiveness to different types of messages that promote safer sex behavior. For example, college students who were strongly focused on intimacy in their dating relationships and received training in how to effectively communicate with their partner about condom use showed more positive attitudes toward condom use, as well as greater self-efficacy for and intentions to use condoms (Sanderson & Cantor, 1995). In contrast, college students without such a focus on intimacy were more responsive to interventions that stressed technical skills, such as how to put on a condom and how to eroticize condoms. Most important, students who received a "matching" condom use intervention also reported engaging in lower levels of risky sexual behavior as long as one year later.

Managing Pain and Illness

Another contribution of research on the importance of personalized health care messages is in the area of helping people manage pain—a topic that is very important to most people at one time or another. For example, people vary considerably on the amount of information they want to receive about medical procedures (Carpenter, Gatchel, & Hasegawa, 1994; Litt, Nye, & Shafer, 1995; Ludwick-Rosenthal & Neufeld, 1993; Miller & Mangan, 1983). Specifically, some people prefer to receive detailed information about the proposed management procedure and to learn as much as possible about what to expect, whereas others strongly prefer to not think about the procedure and to adopt an "ignorance is bliss" approach. Neither of these styles seems to be "better"; what appears to be important is that people get the type of information they want. Specifically, people who desire high levels of control and information about their upcoming surgical procedure show lower levels of arousal, stress, and anxiety when they receive such information than when they receive

Table 3.6 Test Yourself: How Much Information Would You Want?

Please rate your agreement (yes or no) with each of these statements.

1. I usually don't ask the doctor or nurse many questions about what he or she is doing during a medical exam.

2. Instead of waiting for them to tell me, I usually ask the doctor or nurse immediately after an exam about my health.

3. I'd rather have doctors and nurses make the decisions about what's best than for them to give me a whole lot of choices.

4. I usually ask the doctor or nurse lots of questions about the procedures during a medical exam.

5. It is better to trust the doctor or nurse in charge of a medical procedure than to question what he or she is doing.

6. I'd rather be given many choices about what's best for my health than to have the doctor make the decisions for me.

7. I usually wait for the doctor or nurse to tell me the results of a medical exam rather than asking for the results immediately.

Give yourself a point for each time you answered "no" to an odd-numbered item and each time you answered "yes" to an even-numbered item, and then sum up those points to get your total score. This questionnaire measures people's desire to ask questions and desire to get information regarding medical decisions; higher scores indicate a desire for more information.

Source: Krantz, Baum, & Wideman (1980).

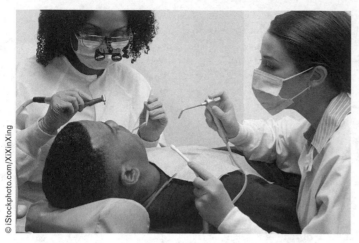
People who receive the amount and type of information they prefer show lower levels of anxiety, arousal, and pain.

little information, whereas those who prefer to know as little as possible show the reverse pattern. For example, people who want high levels of control experience less pain when they first see a video of a woman seeking dental treatment and receive training in coping and relaxing as compared to when they see a neutral film (on local areas of interest) and engage in a neutral conversation (Law, Logan, & Baron, 1994). You can measure your own preferences regarding how much information you want to hear using **Table 3.6: Test Yourself.**

People benefit not only from receiving different amounts of information prior to medical procedures but also from receiving different types of information. For example, people who were highly fearful of dental procedures benefited most in terms of distress (e.g., tension, nervousness, edginess) from distraction (Litt, Kalinowski, & Shafer, 1999). In contrast, those who were fearful only in response to specific cues (e.g., the sound of the drill, the sight of the dentist) benefited most from receiving desensitization training. Similarly, researchers in one study randomly assigned patients about to undergo oral surgery to one of three different stress management interventions (Martelli, Auerbach, Alexander, & Mercuri, 1987). Some of the patients received a problem-focused intervention, which provided information about the specific steps involved in the surgery as well as training on how to think about the surgery in a new way, whereas others received an emotion-focused intervention, which included training in relaxation, distraction, and other strategies to calm arousal. Can you predict the findings? For patients who wanted lots of information, the problem-focused intervention led to the lowest levels of pain and anxiety. In contrast, for those who wanted little information, the emotion-focused intervention was the most effective. In sum, an intervention's effectiveness in reducing stress, arousal, and pain is enhanced when it is in line with people's distinct preferences.

Finally, people vary in their responsiveness to different strategies for managing the stress of having a chronic disease. For example, newly diagnosed cancer patients who believe they have control over their health outcomes benefit more from receiving a decision aid to help them make choices regarding cancer treatment than those who feel they have less control over their health (Vodermaier et al., 2011). Those who believe they have high control over their health find using this tool to make a decision helpful in terms of reducing uncertainty, whereas those without such feelings of control don't find having more information about treatment options particularly helpful. Similarly, men with prostate cancer who are low in self-esteem particularly benefit from participating in a psychoeducational group, perhaps because men who are the least confident in themselves benefit the most from learning about side effects and how to cope from others (Helgeson, Lepore, & Eton, 2006). These findings point to the importance of tailoring interventions designed to help people who are struggling with a chronic disease.

Screening for Health Conditions

People who receive personally tailored message are more likely to engage in screening behaviors (Kreuter & Strecher, 1996; Rakowski et al., 1998; Skinner et al., 1999; Williams-Piehota,

Figure 3.6   Data From Lustria et al., 2016

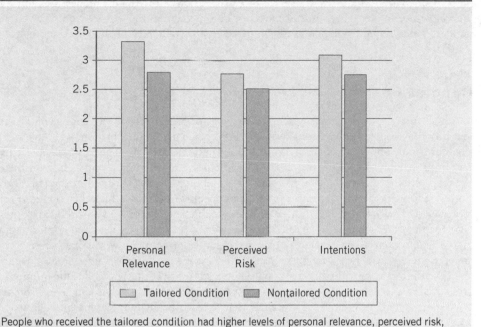

Tailored Condition   Nontailored Condition

People who received the tailored condition had higher levels of personal relevance, perceived risk, and intentions to get tested than those who received the non-tailored condition.

Source: Data from Lustria, Cortese, Gerend, Schmitt, Kung, & McLaughlin (2016).

Pizarro, Schneider, Mowad, & Salovey, 2005). For example, letters from physicians encouraging mammography that were tailored to a woman's particular risk factors (e.g., age, family history) were more effective in increasing screening than standardized letters (Skinner et al., 1994). Tailored messages are particularly effective at increasing screening in both Black and low-income women, who are at particular risk of not getting screened. Tailored messages are also more effective than standard messages at increasing skin cancer exams (Manne et al., 2010). In fact, people who receive the tailored intervention promoting skin cancer exams are nearly twice as likely to have a skin exam than those who receive a generic message. Similarly, and as shown in Figure 3.6, sexually active college students who receive personally tailored information about their STD risk, meaning information based specifically on their gender and relationship status, show increased perceptions of personal relevance and risk of acquiring an STD (Lustria et al., 2016). They are also more likely to actually order an at-home STD test kit.

Other messages to promote screening specifically target a given population through the use of particular narrators, language, or music, which is a more cost-effective approach than personally tailoring messages (Kreuter & Skinner, 2000). For example, a message designed to promote mammograms could focus on the rationale for such screening for young women, who may be less likely to see themselves as at risk for developing breast cancer. In one study, Black women were randomly assigned to watch one of three videotapes on HIV risk reduction (Kalichman et al., 1993). One tape simply presented information about the importance of risk reduction delivered by a White broadcaster, another gave the same information presented by a Black woman, and a third gave the same information presented by a Black woman and included culturally relevant themes, including cultural pride, community concern, and family responsibility. Two weeks later, women who had seen either of the videos featuring Black women were more likely to have discussed AIDS with friends, request condoms at the follow-up, and have been tested for AIDS. Fifty percent of the women who received the standard video requested condoms as compared to 88% and 91% of those in the other two conditions.

Conclusions

Although many research studies on different types of health-related behavior demonstrate that different people benefit from receiving different types of information, we don't know whether people know what type of information is best for them. This question obviously has great practical importance—if people know what type of information would be best for them, health-promotion programs could simply offer a choice of messages and media (e.g., brochures, videos, intervention groups) and then ask people to choose which they prefer. If this view were correct, it would be easy to give people the "matching," and most effective, message. On the other hand, in some cases people may not really know what type of information they would find most beneficial. A smoker, for example, may not know whether her cigarette use is triggered more by psychological factors (e.g., stress reduction) or physiological factors (e.g., nicotine cravings). In turn, if people don't know what they need, health-promotion programs have to develop a quick way to sort people into different groups, such as through a brief questionnaire or interview. Future research is clearly needed to examine whether people do in fact know what they need, or, alternatively, to develop appropriate strategies for sorting people into their "matching" group.

Table 3.7 Information YOU Can Use
• Your own outlook influences your health behavior, so to make changes in your health-related behavior, focus on improving your own self-efficacy for making changes, your own attitudes toward the behavior, and your outcome expectancies.
• Social factors, including images in the media and the norms in our environment, exert a strong influence on our health-related behavior. Try to avoid exposing yourself (or your children) to images of detrimental health-related behavior and seek out friends who support health-promoting behaviors.
• Although common sense might suggest that people would be less likely to engage in a particular health-diminishing behavior if they were scared about the consequences of this behavior, fear appeals can backfire. Thus, fear-based appeals to promote behavior change need to be designed very carefully in order to be effective.
• How you present, or frame, health-related information can have a remarkable influence on how people think about a given behavior. Framing can influence people's willingness to engage in different health-related behaviors and even people's choices regarding medical treatments.
• One size clearly does not fit all in terms of persuading people to engage in health-related behavior. People are more responsive in terms of attitude and behavior change to messages that are personally relevant. Thus, whenever possible, design messages to be highly relevant for the characteristics, such as the age or gender, of the intended audience. Messages need to consider the background and personality of the recipients to maximize their effectiveness.

Continuum Theories of Health Behavior

- The health belief model posits that the likelihood that individuals will engage in a behavior depends on four factors: susceptibility, severity, benefits, and barriers. In addition, this model describes the role of cues to action, which refers to any type of reminder about a potential health problem.

- Social cognitive theory emphasizes the power of observation in helping people form attitudes about particular behaviors. However, whether these attitudes lead to behavior change is a function of people's self-efficacy and outcome expectancies for that behavior.

- The theory of reasoned action posits that the key determinant of people's behavior is their intention to engage in that behavior. In turn, intentions are determined by people's attitudes as well as their subjective norms. A later version of this model, the theory of planned behavior, adds the component of perceived behavioral control. However, the link between intentions and behavior is stronger for implementation intentions.

- These theories have been critiqued for failing to include the person's current or past behavior as well as other factors that may be quite strong predictors of behavior. It is also not clear whether they show associations, or correlations, between various components, versus predicting behavior over time. Combining different components from several models may be the best way to predict health-related behavior.

Learning Theories of Health Behavior

- Classical conditioning occurs when a previously neutral stimulus comes to evoke the same response as another stimulus with which it is paired. This is a type of associative learning. Classical conditioning techniques can be used to create negative associations with unhealthy behaviors and thereby decrease such behaviors.

- Operant conditioning refers to the idea that behaviors can be increased or decreased as a function of the consequences of engaging in them. Desired behaviors can be positively reinforced through rewards, which should lead to their continuation, and undesired behaviors can be punished, which should lead them to stop. Operant conditioning approaches are most effective when people receive rewards for making small steps toward behavior change.

- According to social learning theory, people do not need to directly experience the rewards or costs of engaging in a particular behavior to learn about its outcomes; learning can occur simply through observational learning, meaning watching someone else engage in a particular behavior and seeing or hearing about its consequences. People can form such beliefs from observing the behavior of someone they do not personally know, and from the media.

Stage Models of Health Behavior Change

- According to the transtheoretical (stages of change) model, changes in health-related behavior occur in a gradual and spiral fashion. These stages are precontemplation, contemplation, preparation, action, and maintenance. Researchers believe that people go through specific processes of change as they progress through the various stages, such as becoming aware of the problem and reflecting on the costs and benefits of behavior change. External cues may also move people along the stages.

- The precaution adoption process model proposes that when individuals consider engaging in new health-related behaviors, they go through a series of seven stages. This model includes stage 1 (people are not even aware of the disease or problem), stage 2 (people are generally aware of the health risk and believe that others might be at risk, but they do not believe they personally are at risk), stage 3 (they believe they are personally at risk but have not decided to take action), stage 4 (they decide that action is not necessary), stage 5 (they decide to take action), stage 6 (they have begun to change their behavior), and stage 7 (they maintain the behavior change over some period of time). People at different stages of making health behavior changes report different beliefs about their own risks and intentions to adopt new behaviors.

- According to the health action process approach, people making changes in their behavior undergo two distinct stages. First, in the motivation stage, they must form an intention to change their behavior in some way. Next, they enter the volition phase, which involves making specific plans to carry out these intentions.

Creating Health Behavior Change

- Fear-based appeals are designed to create the threat of impending danger or harm caused by engaging in particular types of behavior or failing to engage in other types of behavior. These messages increase people's feelings of vulnerability, which should motivate behavior change, and are thought to be easier to understand, more quickly processed, and more accurately remembered. However, fear-based appeals often have little effect on actual behavior. These messages create considerable anxiety, which can interfere with cognitive processing, lead people to deny and/or minimize the information presented, and respond defensively. Fear-based appeals are most effective when they create moderate levels of fear, provide specific strategies, focus on short-term consequences, enhance vulnerability, and provide self-affirmation.

- Another factor that influences the persuasiveness of messages promoting health behavior change is how such messages are presented, or framed. Gain-framed messages focus on the positive outcomes that can be attained—or the negative outcomes that can be avoided—by adopting a particular type of health-related behavior. Loss-framed messages focus on the negative outcomes that may occur from failing to adopt a particular type of health-related behavior. Gain-framed messages tend to be more effective than loss-framed messages in helping people to engage in behavior that prevents a health problem from developing. Loss-framed messages tend to be more effective for helping people seek medical care regarding a potential health problem.

Personalized Health-Promotion Messages

- Both theory and research suggest that different people respond in different ways to different types of information. Specifically, people are much more responsive to personally relevant information. In some cases, these messages are *targeted* to a specific group of people and/or specific characteristics of a group of people. In other cases, researchers have created messages that are *tailored* to an individual's particular needs and goals.

- Personalized messages are consistently more effective than generic ones at helping people adopt healthier behaviors. Personalized messages are more effective at helping people quit smoking, reducing their alcohol use, improving their eating and exercise behavior, and increasing their condom use.

- Personalized health care messages help people manage pain. Some people prefer to receive detailed information about medical procedures and what to expect, whereas others strongly prefer to not think about the procedure and receive little information. People benefit not only from receiving different amounts of information prior to medical procedures but also from receiving different types of information. Finally, people vary in their responsiveness to different strategies for managing the stress of having a chronic disease.

- People who receive personally tailored message are more likely to engage in screening behaviors. Other messages to promote screening specifically target a given population through the use of particular narrators, language, or music, which is a more cost-effective approach than personally tailoring messages.

4

UNDERSTANDING STRESS

Learning Objectives

4.1 Describe different sources of stress

4.2 Compare methods of measuring stress

4.3 Summarize models of the stress response

4.4 Explain the physical consequences of stress on different body systems

4.5 Describe effects of stress on well-being, memory and cognition, and behavior

What You'll Learn

4.1 Why parenting causes more stress for moms than for dads

4.2 Why spending time on Facebook could increase stress

4.3 Why hiding your sexual orientation may be bad for your health

4.4 Why fighting with your spouse can lead to heart problems

4.5 Why not getting enough sleep can literally make you sick

Preview

Everyone has experienced stress (you may be feeling it as you read this chapter), and we know what people mean when they say they are "stressed." But what exactly is stress? In the field of health psychology, **stressor** describes any type of physically or psychologically challenging event or situation, and **stress** describes the process by which we perceive and respond to stressors. This chapter examines the link between stress and health, including factors that cause stress, the physiological impact of stress on the body, explanations for the link between stress and health, and the behavioral and psychological consequences of stress.

SOURCES OF STRESS

Stress is, unfortunately, a reality of life. We experience stress whenever we feel unable to manage the challenges in our daily lives. In everyday language, "stress" has become a catch-all phrase that describes the demands we face in our professional and personal lives, such as an upcoming exam, an important work deadline, a fight with a friend, or concern about paying the credit card bill. As you'll learn in this section, all of these—and more—experiences can lead to stress.

Relationships

Although most of us think about personal relationships as providing support (and this topic is addressed in the next chapter), they are also a major source of stress. In fact, one third of the stressful events college students experience are caused by relationships (Ptacek, Smith, & Zanas, 1992). Moreover, interpersonal conflicts account for as much as 80% of the stress experienced by married couples (Bolger, Delongis, Kessler, & Schilling, 1989). These conflicts can focus on how to spend money, the balancing of work and family time, and the fair distribution of childcare and household tasks. Even online social interactions can lead to stress: people who spend a lot of time on Facebook may feel stress due to feeling their own lives aren't as good as those of their friends (Steers, Wickham, & Acitelli, 2014).

More serious family issues, such as an illness or divorce, can also lead to stress, in part because these problems can lead to emotional and financial pressures. For example, caring for a loved one who has a chronic illness can cause financial burdens, such as the cost of in-home nursing care, and emotional problems, such as depression, anxiety, and sadness (Kiecolt-Glaser, Glaser, Shuttleworth, Dyer, Ogrocki, & Speicher, 1987). (In *Chapter 10: Understanding and Managing Chronic Illness*, we examine the particular stresses that are caused by having a chronic illness, and in *Chapter 12: Terminal Illness and Bereavement*, we examine the stress associated with experiencing the loss of a loved one.)

Although one might expect that only negative events would cause stress, positive events can also cause stress, in part because these events cause change that most people find unsettling. For example, when students start college, they may experience this change as an exciting and positive event, yet it is often accompanied by stress—stress over which classes to take, concerns about managing a heavy workload, uncertainty about living arrangements, fear of being away from home, and so on. Similarly, a couple with a new baby is likely to experience financial pressure, sleep deprivation, and challenges in balancing time, which are all stressful.

Interestingly, although parents in general experience stress from raising children, mothers experience higher levels of stress than do fathers. To explain this finding, researchers in one study examined gender differences in the experience of parenting, and in particular how mothers and fathers spent time with their children (Musick, Meier, & Flood, 2016). This research revealed that most of the time fathers spent with their children involved so-called leisure activities, such as relaxing, eating, and watching television. Mothers, on the other hand, spent most of their parenting time taking care of their children and managing their activities. As you can imagine, these differences in types of typical activities completed with children help explain why parenting is more stressful for mothers than for fathers.

Work

Work pressures, including long hours, constant deadlines, and substantial responsibility, can create considerable stress (Spector, 2002). The stressful period that hits most college students at the end of the semester when they must take exams and complete term papers is a good example of this type of stress. Other aspects of jobs that can create stress include relationships with colleagues or supervisors, lack of resources (e.g., defective equipment, few supplies), and the physical environment (e.g., noise, heat). In fact, chronic underemployment, meaning having a job that is below one's level of skills or education or that provides fewer hours than preferred, also causes stress (Butterworth et al., 2011).

People who have jobs that involve a responsibility for saving people's lives, such as doctors, firefighters, and air traffic controllers, often experience particularly high levels of stress because making a mistake can have dire consequences (Shouksmith & Taylor, 1997). In turn, and as we'll discuss in more detail in *Chapter 13: Managing Health Care,* doctors and nurses who spend more time providing direct patient care experience higher levels of stress (Rutledge et al., 2009).

People who have little control over their jobs, such as when, where, and how they complete their work, also experience considerable stress (Spector, 2002). For example, restaurant servers often experience high levels of stress because they must satisfy both customers and their employers, but they have very little control over their work environment (e.g., they do not prepare the food, set prices, or determine how fast food is ready; Theorell et al., 1990). Physicians whose work schedule (including number of hours worked as well as when those hours are worked) is not what they prefer experience more burnout (Barnett, Gareis, & Brennan, 1999). In line with these findings, many models predicting health-related behavior include the role of perceived control over one's environment, as described in *Chapter 3: Theories of Health Behavior.*

Environmental Factors

People may experience stress from environmental pressures, such as noise, crowding, and pollution. People who work in noisy conditions experience increased stress, as do those who live in busy cities (Evans, Bullinger, & Hygge, 1998; Levine, 1990). But shorter-term environmental factors can also create stress. For example, a recent survey found that more than half of all Americans reported that the current political climate was a very or somewhat significant source of stress (American Psychological Association, 2017). The outcome of the 2016 United States presidential election was an especially significant source of stress for people of color; 69% of Blacks, 57% of Asians, and 56% of Latinos reported that the election was a very or somewhat significant source of stress.

Although many Americans report that money, jobs, and the economy cause stress, people with lower incomes experience more stress than those with higher income (American Psychological Association, 2017). Moreover, people living in poverty often experience other stressors, such as crime, overcrowded housing, pollution, and noise (Johnson et al., 1995; Myers, Kagawa-Singer, Kumanyika, Lex, & Markides, 1995). In one study, researchers examined the level of stress in new parents who were living in poverty (Dunkel Schetter et al., 2013). As you might expect, the vast majority of these parents were experiencing very high levels of stress as they tried to manage taking care of a young baby (and sometimes other children as well) on very little money.

Cataclysmic Events

Major cataclysmic events, such as natural disasters, clearly cause considerable stress. These events cause substantial physical damage and often lead to both injuries and deaths. Not surprisingly, major natural disasters cause lasting symptoms of stress. For example, the 2005 Hurricane Katrina off the coast of New Orleans was a costly natural disaster in the

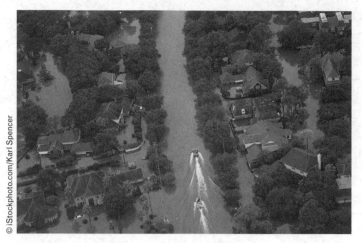

© iStockphoto.com/Karl Spencer

In August 2017, Hurricane Harvey hit Texas, damaging nearly 50,000 homes and businesses. This type of cataclysmic event can lead to lasting stress.

United States, killing over 1,000 people, forcing 500,000 people to leave their homes, and causing more than $100 billion in damage. Six months after the storm, 31.2% of people living in areas affected by the storm reported having some type of anxiety or mood disorder (Galea et al., 2007).

Other cataclysmic events that cause stress include terrorist attacks and mass shootings. In fact, about one third of Americans report that these fears about violence have increased their overall level of stress over the last decade (American Psychology Association, 2017). Experiencing violent cataclysmic events can have lasting consequences, as you'll read more about later in this chapter. For example, an estimated 15.4% of Virginia Tech students continued to experience high levels of posttraumatic stress three to four months following a school shooting in which 49 faculty members and students were shot (and 32 killed) (Hughes et al., 2011). These symptoms were particularly likely for students who had someone close to them who was injured or killed, and for those who were unable to reach particular friends immediately following the shooting and were anxious about their safety. Cataclysmic events occur suddenly, often without any warning, which can be particularly stressful.

Even watching media coverage of terrorist attacks can lead to stress. Researchers in one study measured level of stress in a national sample two to four weeks after the 2013 Boston Marathon bombings (Holman, Garfin, & Silver, 2014). People who watched high levels of media coverage of the bombings—defined as six or more hours a day—were nine times more likely to report experiencing high stress than those who watched fewer than one hour a day. These findings illustrate that cataclysmic events may lead to stress even among those who are not directly affected.

Internal Pressures

Pressures within ourselves, such as when we are torn between two different goals, is another factor that can cause stress (Lewin, 1935). For example, you may want to take a trip with your friends over spring break, but you may also want to earn money by working. This type of conflict is called an *approach-approach conflict*, because you are torn between wanting to do two desirable things that are incompatible. In other cases, people experience *approach-avoidance* or *avoidance-avoidance conflicts*. These types of conflicts might include wanting to eat tempting foods (approach) but also wanting to lose weight (avoid), and choosing between chemotherapy (avoid) and radiation (avoid) to treat cancer.

Conclusions

This section has described different sources of stress as distinct from one another. But in reality, many of these stresses are interrelated. Having greater pressure at work can make it more difficult to manage and maintain close relationships. Similarly, experiencing cataclysmic events, such as a major natural disaster, can lead to environmental stressors, such as overcrowding, pollution, and poverty. Learning skills for managing stress is therefore particularly important for people experiencing multiple different types of stressors (which you'll learn more about in *Chapter 5: Managing Stress*).

MEASURING STRESS

LO 4.2

Compare methods
of measuring stress

Although people commonly use the term *stress* in their daily lives (e.g., "I'm feeling very stressed about my upcoming exams"), it is difficult to measure precisely how much stress a person is experiencing. This section describes the different approaches researchers have used to assess stress, including several different types of self-report inventories as well as various physiological measures.

Self-Report Inventories

Many research approaches to examining stress simply ask people to report how frequently they experience various challenging events. Researchers can then evaluate whether people who face more stressors experience worse health.

Major Life Events

Early research on stress focused on identifying life events, or stressors, that require people to adapt to change, tolerate some discomfort, or deal with some threat. Researchers who use this approach simply ask people to list the number of major life events they have experienced in a given period of time.

One of the most commonly used self-report approaches for measuring stress is the Social Readjustment Rating Scale, or SRRS, which assesses the number and types of major events that have happened in a person's life in the past year (Holmes & Rahe, 1967). It includes both negative events—getting divorced, being fired from one's job, experiencing the death of a loved one—and positive events—getting married, having a baby, receiving a promotion. You can evaluate your own level of stress using **Table 4.1: Test Yourself.**

The SRRS scale was developed based on data from more than 5,000 patients revealing that significant life events seemed to precede illness (Rabkin & Struening, 1976; Rahe, Mahan, & Arthur, 1970). For example, in one of the earliest tests of this model, 2,664 male naval personnel completed a life-change questionnaire six to eight months prior to embarking on a navy cruise (Rahe et al., 1970). Researchers then measured number of reported illnesses throughout their time at sea. These findings indicated that men who reported more life events experienced more reported illnesses while at sea, suggesting that the experience of these types of stressors could lead to health problems. In line with this view, those who experience more life events (both prospectively and retrospectively) are more likely to experience heart attacks, diabetes, accidents, injuries, and tuberculosis (Rabkin & Struening, 1976; Rahe & Arthur, 1978; Rahe, Biersner, Ryman, & Arthur, 1972).

Some research even points to a link between experiencing more life stressors and the development of cancer (Jacobs & Charles, 1980). For example, one meta-analysis of 46 studies revealed that women who have experienced more stressful life events are somewhat more likely to develop breast cancer (McKenna, Zevon, Corn, & Rounds, 1999). The specific life events that are associated with the greatest increase in risk are divorce/separation, death of a husband, and death of a close friend or relative (Lillberg et al., 2003).

However, the SRRS has been criticized for several reasons (Schroeder & Costa, 1984). First, it does not take into account the subjective experience of an event for the person. Getting divorced, for example, may be very upsetting for someone whose religion forbids divorce, whereas someone who is leaving an abusive marriage may see divorce as a welcome relief. Similarly, a pregnancy could be a very positive and exciting event for a stable married couple hoping to start a family but could be extremely negative and upsetting for a high school student. In line with this view, measures of stress that assess people's appraisal or

Table 4.1 Test Yourself: Social Readjustment Rating Scale

Life Event	Mean Value
1. Death of spouse	100
2. Divorce	73
3. Marital separation	65
4. Jail term	63
5. Death of a close family member	63
6. Personal injury or illness	53
7. Marriage	50
8. Fired at work	47
9. Marital reconciliation	45
10. Retirement	45
11. Major change in the health of family member	44
12. Pregnancy	40
13. Sex difficulties	39
14. Gain of a new family member	39
15. Business readjustment	39
16. Change in financial state	38
17. Death of a close friend	37
18. Changing to a different line of work	36
19. Change in the number of arguments with spouse	35
20. Mortgage over $10,000	31
21. Foreclosure on a mortgage or loan	30
22. Change in responsibilities at work	29
23. Son or daughter leaving home	29
24. Trouble with in-laws	29
25. Outstanding personal achievement	28
26. Spouse beginning or stopping work	26
27. Begin or end school	26
28. Change in living conditions	25

Life Event	Mean Value
29. Revision of personal habits	24
30. Trouble with boss	23
31. Change in work hours or conditions	20
32. Change in residence	20
33. Change in schools	20
34. Change in recreation	19
35. Change in church activities	19
36. Change in social activities	18
37. Mortgage or loan for less than $10,000	17
38. Change in sleeping habits	16
39. Change in number of family get-togethers	15
40. Change in eating habits	15
41. Vacation	13
42. Christmas	12
43. Minor violation of the law	11

This scale measures the number of major life events that a person has experienced over the last few months and assigns each life event a point value that expresses the severity of the event. People who experience more stressful life events tend to have poorer health. The scale was developed in the 1960s and hence may be less appropriate for assessing stress today. Certain items, such as "mortgage over $10,000," may be quite dated.

Source: Adapted from Holmes & Rahe (1967).

perception of a particular life event are more strongly correlated with mental and physical health than measures of assessing simply whether a particular life event took place (Hayman, Lucas, & Porcerelli, 2014; Vasunilashorn, Lynch, Glei, Weinstein, & Goldman, 2015).

Moreover, some of the events included in this scale are objectively positive (e.g., marriage, outstanding personal achievement, vacation), whereas others are objectively negative (e.g., death of a spouse, foreclosure of a mortgage, jail term), and still others are ambiguous (e.g., change in job responsibilities, spouse beginning or stopping work, revision of personal habits). But experiencing positive personal events, while they may cause some stress, is typically less problematic than experiencing objectively negative events (Sarason, Johnson, & Siegel, 1978). Because this scale assumes that change in general is stressful, regardless of whether it is positive or negative, someone who gets fired gets the same score as someone who gets promoted!

Finally, some researchers have criticized this scale for focusing on stressful events that are likely to affect those in the middle or upper classes and for ignoring those that may affect people who are poor or members of minority groups (Jackson & Inglehart, 1995). Poverty and racism, for example, may be very stressful, but are not included in this scale (you'll learn more about this later in this chapter).

Daily Hassles and Uplifts

Although the SRRS is a widely used approach to measuring stress, some researchers have argued that many stressors come not from major life events but instead from *daily hassles* (Lazarus, Kanner, & Folkman, 1980). These more typical types of stressful daily life events could include losing one's keys, having difficulty paying bills, or having too many things to do. One study found that simply checking email frequently increases stress (Kushlev & Dunn, 2015)!

Researchers have also explored whether small uplifting events predict positive outcomes (Kanner, Coyne, Schaefer, & Lazarus, 1981). According to this perspective, experiencing even small events that bring you pleasure, such as spending time with friends, having a good night's sleep, and reading a good book, may have beneficial effects on physical health and psychological well-being (Lazarus et al., 1980).

Both hassles and uplifts are associated with health, although in distinct ways. Hassles are a strong predictor of both psychological and physical well-being; in fact, hassles are more highly correlated with psychological and physical symptoms than are major life events (Kanner et al., 1981; Zarski, 1984). As shown in Figure 4.1, men who experience fewer hassles in their daily lives live longer (Aldwin, Jeong, Igarashi, Choun, & Spiro, 2014). Although the frequency of uplifts is not a particularly good predictor of physical health, people who experience more uplifts have more positive moods (Kanner et al., 1981).

Although some research suggests that measures of daily hassles (and possibly uplifts) are a better predictor of health than measures of major life events, these self-report measures have some of the same limitations as the SRRS. One problem is that someone who

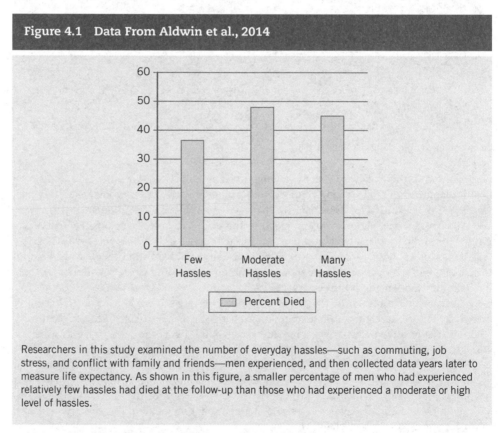

Figure 4.1 Data From Aldwin et al., 2014

Researchers in this study examined the number of everyday hassles—such as commuting, job stress, and conflict with family and friends—men experienced, and then collected data years later to measure life expectancy. As shown in this figure, a smaller percentage of men who had experienced relatively few hassles had died at the follow-up than those who had experienced a moderate or high level of hassles.

Source: Data from Aldwin, Jeong, Igarashi, Choun, & Spiro (2014).

experiences a major life event is also likely to experience many daily hassles. For example, someone who gets divorced may struggle with daily financial pressures, conflicts with the ex-spouse, and increased household responsibilities.

Another problem with these measures is that some scales assessing hassles and uplifts include items that refer to health-related behavior (e.g., drinking, smoking, feeling healthy). Thus, if studies find a correlation between frequency of hassles or uplifts and health, it may be due to the link between a given behavior (such as smoking) and health as opposed to the link between stress and health.

Finally, because simply asking people whether they have experienced a given life event or daily hassle does not take into account that different people evaluate such experiences in different ways, other researchers have developed a measure that assesses individuals' perceived stress (Cohen, Kamark, & Mermelstein, 1983). The Perceived Stress Scale (PSS) does not ask people whether they have experienced a particular event but simply asks how frequently they have felt stressed or upset in the last month. For example, items on this scale include, "In the last month, how often have you found that you could not cope with all the things you had to do?" and "In the last month, how often have you felt nervous and 'stressed'?" The PSS predicts psychological and physical symptoms (Hewitt, Flett, & Mosher, 1992) as well as changes in the immune and endocrine systems (Harrell, Kelly, & Stutts, 1996; Maes et al., 1997).

Physiological Measures

Given the various limitations of self-report measures of stress, some researchers have instead relied on measures of physiological measures to assess stress (Baum, Grunberg, & Singer, 1982; Speisman, Lazarus, Mordkoff, & Davison, 1964; Uchino, Cacioppo, Malarkey, & Glaser, 1995). Because a central aspect of stress is the stimulation of the sympathetic nervous system, stress can be measured through various measures of *physiological arousal*, including heart rate, blood pressure, respiration, and changes in the skin's resistance to electrical current (galvanic skin response, or GSR).

Biochemical measures can also be used to assess the presence of particular hormones, such as norepinephrine, epinephrine, and cortisol (Baum et al., 1982). These hormones can be detected in blood or urine tests and are reliable indicators of an individual's experience of stress. Increases in corticosteroids and catecholamines (two types of chemicals, or neurotransmitters, in the body) are found in many different types of stressful situations, including in astronauts during splashdown (Kimzey, 1975), people who are doing challenging mental arithmetic (Uchino et al., 1995), and snake phobics who see a snake (Bandura, Taylor, Williams, Mefford, & Barchas, 1985).

In one recent study, researchers examined how spending time on Facebook could lead to increases in cortisol (Morin-Major et al., 2016). Researchers asked adolescents, ages 12 to 17, about how frequently they used Facebook, how many friends they had on this site, and whether they supported these friends (by "liking" their posts). The researchers also collected saliva samples from these participants four times a day for three days to measure the presence of cortisol. As predicted, more Facebook friends—anything above 300—was associated with higher levels of cortisol, indicating a link between more friends and more stress.

Physiological measures have some limitations. First, some people find the use of physiological measures in and of themselves very stressful. If a person is nervous about having blood taken or being hooked up to a machine that is measuring sweat or heart rate, he or she will show higher levels of stress simply because of the use of these techniques. Second, physiological measures can be influenced by factors other than stress, including gender, weight, and physical activity level. Researchers therefore need to be aware of these complicating

What You'll Learn
4.2

factors and must interpret the results accordingly. Finally, because physiological measures of stress rely on either equipment or laboratory testing, the use of these measures is very expensive and time-consuming. They also require trained technicians to perform the tests and interpret the results.

MODELS OF THE STRESS RESPONSE

LO 4.3

Summarize models of the stress response

Our understanding of how exactly stress influences health has evolved considerably over time, as you'll learn in this section. First, this section describes two long-standing theories about how stress leads to physiological reactions, which in turn can impact physical well-being. Then, it summarizes some limitations and revisions to these initial models describing the stress–health relationship.

Cannon's Fight-or-Flight Response

Imagine that you are walking in a forest with some friends on a sunny afternoon. As you are talking to them, not really paying attention to where you are walking, you suddenly notice movement just in front of your right foot. You quickly glance down and see a large striped snake, coiled and seemingly ready to strike. What is your immediate physiological reaction? Like most people who are afraid of snakes, your heart will start to pound, your muscles will become tense, and you will start to sweat. In fact, you may have experienced mild forms of these reactions while reading this description of the snake.

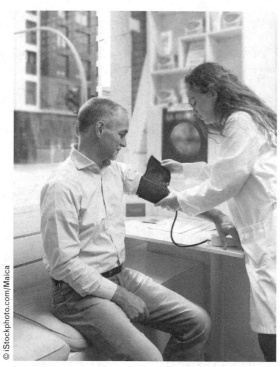

© iStockphoto.com/Maica

Although physiological measures of stress, such as blood pressure, avoid the inherent problems associated with self-report measures of stress, interpreting the results of such tests has its own challenges.

This type of physiological reaction in response to threat, called the **fight-or-flight response**, was first described by Walter Cannon, a physiologist at Harvard Medical School in the early 1900s. According to Cannon (1932), people are normally in a state of internal physiological equilibrium or balance called *homeostasis* (Chrousos & Gold, 1992). When a person (or animal) is threatened, the immediate response is to either fight off the stressor or escape from it. To prepare for either alternative, energy is shifted from the nonessential body systems to those systems necessary to respond to the challenge. So, when someone first notices a threat (such as the snake), the person's sympathetic nervous and endocrine systems are stimulated, which causes a dramatic rise in two types of hormones: *epinephrine* (or *adrenaline*) and *norepinephrine* (*noradrenaline*). The increase in these hormone levels in the bloodstream leads to a number of other physiological responses that prepare someone to either fight off a threat (unlikely, in the case of the snake) or run from it (very likely, in the case of the snake), including increases in heart rate, blood pressure, and breathing, widening of the pupils, and movement of blood toward the muscles. Similarly, the cardiovascular system is activated so that blood is directed to the brain and muscles. Processes that do not help fight off a threat, such as digestion and reproduction, are stopped or slowed down. This increase in some types of physiological responses and decrease in others allows the body to focus its resources where they are most needed to respond to the challenge.

General Adaptation Syndrome

Hans Selye (1956), an endocrinologist, extended Cannon's work by describing the stages the body goes through when reacting to a stressor. He conducted a series of tests in which laboratory rats were exposed to different types of stressors, such as heat, starvation, and electric shock. Interestingly, he found that regardless of what type of stress the rats were exposed to, they developed similar physiological reactions, including enlarged adrenal glands, shrunken lymph nodes, and bleeding stomach ulcers. This observation led to the development of his **General Adaptation Syndrome** (GAS), a model to describe how stress can lead to negative health consequences over time (see Figure 4.2).

First, there is the **alarm stage**, in which the body mobilizes to fight off a threat. When a threat is perceived, the hypothalamus (a structure in the brain) activates both the sympathetic nervous system and the endocrine system. The sympathetic nervous system signals the adrenal glands (endocrine glands on the top of each kidney) to release *catecholamines*, such as epinephrine and norepinephrine. As epinephrine and norepinephrine circulate in the bloodstream, they lead to a number of physiological changes, including increases in heart rate, blood pressure, and breathing rate. These changes all help to prepare the body to react to a threat: oxygen is brought to the muscles (to let you run or fight), pupils dilate (allowing more light to enter so you can see more clearly), and palms sweat (for better gripping). This stage is similar to Cannon's fight-or-flight response. At the same time, the pituitary gland releases adrenocorticotropic hormone (ACTH), which causes the adrenal glands to produce glucocorticoids, such as cortisol. Cortisol increases the production of energy from glucose and inhibits the swelling around injuries and

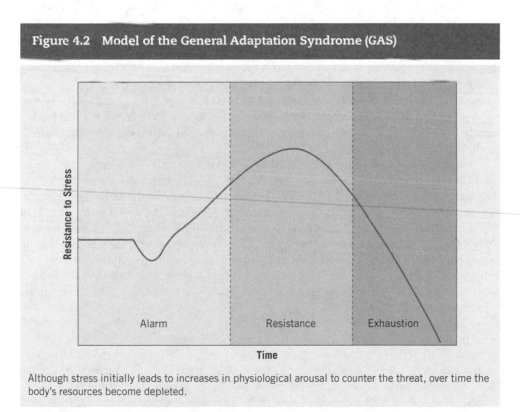

Figure 4.2   Model of the General Adaptation Syndrome (GAS)

Although stress initially leads to increases in physiological arousal to counter the threat, over time the body's resources become depleted.

Source: Based on data from Selye, H. (1950). Stress and the General Adaptation Syndrome. *British Medical Journal, 1*(4667), 1383–1392.

infections. Thus, the body has more energy to respond to threats and is protected from injuries. In this stage, the body is mobilizing all of its resources to do whatever is necessary to fight off (or escape from) the threat, and longer-term functions, such as growth, digestion, reproduction, and operation of the immune system, are inhibited. (You may now be wondering why the immune system, which protects the body from illness and disease, would be inhibited during times of danger. But remember, illness and disease may kill you, but they do so slowly—the alarm stage serves to protect you from immediate threats that could kill you quickly.)

Next, there is the **resistance stage**. After the body mobilizes to fight off the initial threat, it will continue trying to respond. This stage still requires energy, so heart rate, blood pressure, and breathing are still rapid in order to help deliver oxygen and energy quickly throughout the body. Nonessential functions, such as digestion, growth, and reproduction, may operate but at a slower pace than normal, and no new energy is stored during this time. After all, why waste energy where it is not needed? (This is one reason why menstruation may stop in women who are under severe stress.) Although there is less of a drain on energy during this stage than during the alarm stage, the body continues to work very hard to resist the stressor on a long-term basis. If the threat is brief, the body will have enough resources to respond to the threat. However, if the threat lasts for some time and the body stays in a state of physiological arousal for a long time, problems can begin to emerge. Essentially, the body neglects many normal physical and psychological functions during times of stress; over time, this neglect takes its toll on the body's resources.

Finally, when the threat continues for a long time, occurs repeatedly, or is very severe, the **exhaustion stage** may set in. For example, you may feel okay initially under conditions of high stress, but over time it can be damaging to your body since all of its resources are consumed. Continuing or particularly strong stress therefore creates a situation of imbalance that results in considerable wear and tear on the body. In the exhaustion stage, the body's resources are depleted and thus it becomes very susceptible to physiological damage and disease. Moreover, if epinephrine and cortisol stay at high levels over time, they can damage heart and blood vessels and suppress the immune system. These changes leave the body very susceptible to illness, such as heart disease, high blood pressure, arthritis, and colds and flu (McEwen, 1998). As described in **Research in Action**, world leaders may have shorter lives, precisely because of the impact of the stress of such a job on their health.

Stressors can also build up over time and lead to more significant outcomes. Particularly difficult life events may thus lead to chronic stress over time, with consequences for psychological as well as physical well-being. For example, people who assisted with recovery efforts at the World Trade Center following the 9/11 terrorist attacks reported more difficulty coping with other life stressors later on (Zvolensky et al., 2015). Even as long as six years following the devastating Hurricane Katrina, hospitals in New Orleans saw increases in heart attacks compared to before the storm (Peters et al., 2014). These findings suggest that chronic stress, as well as unhealthy behaviors used to manage that stress, such as smoking and substance abuse, may linger for years after a major natural disaster.

According to Selye, the GAS is *nonspecific*, which means that all stressors produce the same physiological response. In other words, people will go through this three-stage process in response to any type of stressful event, including taking final exams, losing a loved one, or living in a crowded situation. In fact, although he believed positive stresses (e.g., getting married) would be less harmful than negative ones (e.g., getting divorced), both types of events are seen as causing some stress, potentially leading to the same negative physiological responses.

Updates to the Fight-or-Flight and GAS Models

Cannon's fight-or-flight model and Selye's GAS have received considerable attention in the field of health psychology and clearly demonstrate the impact of stress on physical health. However, more recent research findings have challenged some of the tenets of these models and led to important revisions. For example, Cannon's model does not describe situations in which we become immobile in the face of stress and thus has now been revised from a two-option (fight-or-flight) response to a three-option response: fight-flight-freeze (Friedman, 2015).

Types of Stressors

First, and contrary to these original models proposing nonspecificity, we now know that different types of stressors are associated with different types of physiological reactions (Pacak et al., 1998). Researchers in one study exposed rats to different types of stressors, including cold, immobilization, and hemorrhage, and then measured various physiological reactions, such as level of epinephrine and norepinephrine. This research revealed that different hormones are released depending on the specific type and intensity of emotion experienced in response to a stressor (Mason, 1975). These differences may relate to the type of threat a given stressor presents, meaning that different stressors require different responses (e.g., fighting off a physical attack requires a difference reaction than staying warm). Similarly, research with humans finds that interpersonal stressors, such as relationships with family members and friends, are more strongly linked with depression than are noninterpersonal stressors, such as academic and work pressures, financial problems, and health (Sheets & Craighead, 2014).

Duration of Stressors

More recent research has also updated Seyle's model by showing that the duration of the stressor influences the physiological response (Segerstrom, 2007; Segerstrom & Miller, 2004). Some stresses are acute or time-limited, meaning they are stressful for only a brief period. These types of stresses, such as passing a driving test, going on a blind date, or being interviewed for a job, are examples of acute stress. The body is immensely resilient and thus is typically able to handle such stresses with little or no impact on physical well-being. In the face of such stresses, the body is able to meet the challenges of the demands of a given situation (McEwen, 1998, 2000; McEwen & Stellar, 1993). This physiological response could include a number of systems in the body, such as increases in blood pressure, the release of hormones, and the mobilization of energy mobilization, and is shut off as soon as the stress is over.

However, in other cases the stresses are chronic, meaning they continue over a long period of time. These stresses could include financial pressures, work pressure, and interpersonal conflict. In the case of long-term, cumulative stress, the body experiences wear and tear on multiple systems, including cardiovascular, neuroendocrine, and immune. This physiological response to long-term stress is known as **allostatic load** (Oken, Chamine, & Wakeland, 2015; Seeman, Singer, Rowe, Horwitz, & McEwen, 1997). For example, people who are experiencing stress at work coupled with providing caregiving to an elderly or disabled relative—two distinct types of ongoing stressors—show high levels of allostatic load (Dich, Lange, Head, & Rod, 2015). This type of ongoing stress suppresses immune function and increases cardiovascular hyperreactivity, which in turn increases susceptibility to disease (Kelly & Ismail, 2015; Segerstrom & Miller, 2004; Steptoe et al., 2014).

The Role of Individual Differences

Research suggests that people may vary in how they respond to stress; in other words, even in response to the exact same stressor, people differ in how their body responds (Stoney, Davis, & Matthews, 1987; Stoney, Matthews, McDonald, & Johnson, 1988). According to the **stress reactivity hypothesis**, people who recover more quickly from stress are less at risk for developing a stress-related illness than those who take longer to recover (Lovallo, 2015; Wright, O'Brien, Hazi, & Kent, 2014).

Moreover, because the vast majority of research on the stress response has studied men (or male rats!), it is not clear whether women show a similar response to stressful situations (Taylor et al., 2000). First, men tend to have higher blood pressure than women in general and also have a greater change in blood pressure during stressful situations. For example, in one study, researchers asked men and women to perform three different types of challenging tasks, including computing a series of math problems, giving a speech, and evaluating their own speech (Matthews, Gump, & Owens, 2001). Men showed higher blood pressure increases in each case. This greater physiological responsiveness to stress may partially explain why the rate of coronary heart disease is so much greater for men than women. Specifically, if men are constantly reacting to stress more than women, their hearts are likely to undergo much more wear and tear.

Men and women may also use different strategies to cope with stress. In fact, some research with humans suggests that women prefer to affiliate with others during times of stress, suggesting a **tend-and-befriend** response to stress, whereas men prefer less social interaction (Taylor et al., 2000). For example, when women expect that they will be given painful electric shocks, they prefer to wait with other women, whereas men often prefer to wait alone. However, more recent research suggests that men may also affiliate with others during times of stress (Berger, Heinrichs, Von Dawans, Way, & Chen, 2016).

The Role of Appraisal

Because Selye's theory was developed using animals, it does not address the psychological or cognitive responses that humans may have to stressful situations (Scherer, 1986). However, according to the **transactional**, or **relational**, **model**, the meaning a particular event has for a person is a more important predictor of the experience of stress than the actual event (Lazarus & Folkman, 1984). People can interpret or appraise stressors in different ways; a woman who is married and desperately trying to have a baby may react to conception differently than a woman who is single and still trying to finish college. Because people's cognitive interpretations of stressful events influence their reactions, people vary in how stressful they find different experiences. For example, one day when I was a college student, I was driving in a car with my boyfriend when we got a flat tire. Because I had no idea how to change a tire, I immediately appraised the situation as a real emergency and panicked ("How much will it cost us to get the car towed? How late will we be for class?"). My boyfriend, however, calmly got the spare tire out of the trunk and within 10 minutes had replaced the bad tire. For me, a flat tire equaled an emergency. For him, a flat tire equaled a minor inconvenience.

Lazarus and Folkman (1984) suggest that the cognitive appraisal of a stressful event includes two distinct parts (see Table 4.2). According to their transactional, or relational, model, whether people experience stress is influenced both by their initial reaction to the particular challenge and the resources they have to cope with this challenge. First, people engage in **primary appraisal** in which they assess the situation. In this stage, people are interpreting the situation and what it will mean for them (e.g., "Am I in danger?"). For example, a person who is fired from his or her job may see it as a stressful event (e.g., "My family will starve") or as a positive opportunity (e.g., "Now I can explore new career options").

People then engage in **secondary appraisal** in which they assess the resources available for coping with the situation. In this stage, people examine their ability to cope with the event based on their resources (e.g., "What can I do about this?"). For example, an individual who has a working spouse may appraise the loss of a job less negatively because he or she has more financial resources to rely on than someone who is the sole wage earner in a family. In line with this view, women with chronic ongoing life stressors who experience a stressful event show high levels of cortisol (a marker of stress), whereas women with supportive environments who experience a stressful event show no such increases (Marin, Martin, Blackwell, Stelter, & Miller, 2007). Similarly, and as you'll learn more about in *Chapter 5: Managing Stress*, people who approach stressors with a positive mind-set about stress tend to see such events as challenging, whereas those with a negative mind-set about stress see such events as threatening. The impact of a particular event may therefore have very different consequences depending on how individuals appraise it as well as the resources available for them to cope with it.

Table 4.2 Examples of the Transactional Model

Type of Stress	Primary Appraisal	Secondary Appraisal—Positive	Secondary Appraisal—Negative
Getting a C in a course	This grade makes it harder for me to get into medical school.	I can do better in other classes and bring up my GPA; I could pursue a different health-related career.	I will never get into medical school or have a good-paying job.
Breaking up with a dating partner	I am really sad this relationship ended.	Now I have a better sense of what I'm looking for in a dating partner; I am going to try harder to work through conflicts well in my next relationship.	No one will ever want to date me again; I probably won't even ever get married.
Having a car accident	Getting my car repaired is going to be really expensive.	I am really glad no one was hurt; maybe my parents could loan me the money.	I am a terrible driver; this will likely happen again.

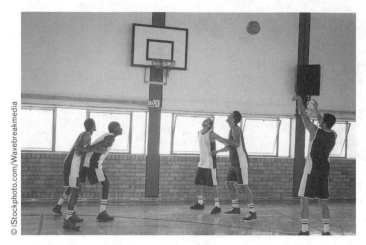

© iStockphoto.com/Wavebreakmedia

Athletes often want to feel somewhat excited as they compete, because this feeling of "getting up for a game" can enhance their performance.

One factor that influences how people appraise different events is their culture. For example, men who come from a "culture of honor" show higher rates of physiological arousal, as measured by increases in testosterone and cortisol, following an insult than do men from other cultures (Cohen, Nisbett, Bowdle, & Schwarz, 1996). These findings suggest that men from such a culture appraise insults as more threatening, and thus find them more stressful, than do other men. Similarly, immigrant Chinese American families who have a relative with schizophrenia, a serious and disruptive mental disorder, appraise this experience as more stressful, due both to the greater stigma attached to mental disorders within their culture and to the lack of a support system within the United States (Kung, 2016).

The Benefits of Stress

Finally, although this section has focused on the negative physiological consequences of stress, some researchers have examined the benefits that can come from experiencing stress. Selye (1974) used the term *eustress* to describe beneficial stresses. Moderate levels of stress can actually cause people to experience small amounts of arousal, providing extra energy, and can help them perform at their best. In contrast, very low and very high levels of arousal can be detrimental to performance, either because they do not motivate us sufficiently (in the case of low levels) or because they create too much anxiety (in the case of high levels). In line with this view about the potential benefits of at least some stress, some research suggests that individuals who experience some adverse life events may in fact have greater physical and psychological well-being than those who experience many or very few stressors (Seery, Holman, & Silver, 2010). Researchers hypothesize that overcoming some difficult events may make people more resilient later on, and thus they are better able to handle future stressors.

PHYSICAL CONSEQUENCES

LO 4.4

Explain the physical consequences of stress on different body systems

In a nutshell, stress is damaging to your health. People who are under stress have a greater risk of experiencing a number of illnesses and diseases, including ulcers, diabetes, colds and flu, arthritis, appendicitis, gastrointestinal disorders, herpes, asthma, sports injuries, headaches, migraines, eczema, hives, back pain, gastrointestinal disorders, hernias, cancer, and cardiovascular disease (Glaser & Kiecolt-Glaser, 1994). Experiencing stress is even associated with accelerated human aging (Zahran et al., 2015).

How exactly does stress lead to so many health problems? The physiological stress reaction characterized by Cannon's fight-or-flight response and Selye's General Adaptation Syndrome is designed to help humans (and animals) respond to extreme, life-threatening stressors, such as occurs when you are chased by a large barking dog or when you are in combat during war. These physiological reactions may also be adaptive during other "high-pressure" situations, such as during a job interview or on a first date. However, people often show a physiological stress reaction to situations that are not actually life-threatening in any way. Neuroscientist Robert Sapolsky believes that humans experience more stress (and more illness) because we generate all sorts of stressful things in our heads. Sapolsky (1998) writes, "Stress-related disease emerges, predominantly, out of the fact that we so often activate a physiological system that have evolved for responding to acute physical emergencies, but we turn it on for months on end, worrying about mortgages, relationships, and promotions." (p. 7). In turn, this ongoing activation of the stress response even to non-life-threatening events may lead to physiological reactions, which may help explain the high rate of stress-related illnesses, including headaches, ulcers, and coronary heart disease. This may be why, as Sapolsky cleverly writes, "zebras don't get ulcers" but humans often do. The following section examines the direct impact of stress on several systems within the body, as well as the interaction of these systems (as described by the field of **psychoneuroimmunology**).

Nervous System

The **nervous system**, which includes the **central nervous system** as well as the **peripheral nervous system**, controls the body's overall reaction to stress in several ways (see Figure 4.3). The central nervous system consists of the brain and spinal cord, where information processing occurs (e.g., "That's a bear—it could hurt me!").

Figure 4.3 Model of the Nervous System

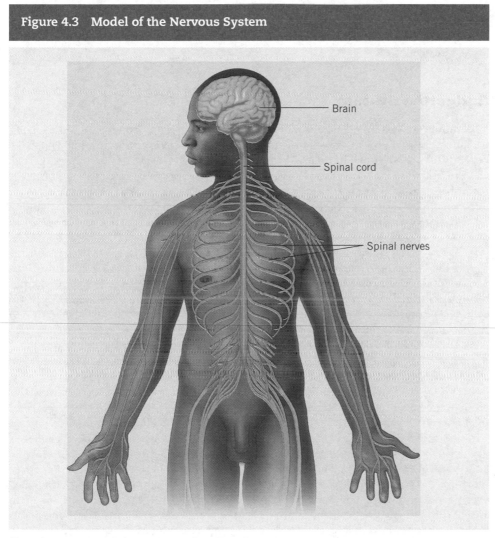

Brain

Spinal cord

Spinal nerves

Illustration: © SAGE Publishing. All Rights Reserved. Created by Body Scientific International.

The peripheral nervous system consists of the neural pathways that bring information to and from the brain. Specialized cells called **neurons** transmit this information, although the **neurotransmitters**, or chemical messengers, released by a particular neuron influence whether the information is transmitted (some neurotransmitters inhibit transmission and others facilitate it).

The peripheral nervous system includes the *somatic nervous system* and the *autonomic nervous system*. Both of these systems carry messages throughout the body, but they differ in the types of messages they transmit. The somatic nervous system transmits messages regarding sensation, such as touch, pressure, temperature, and pain, and messages regarding the voluntary movement of the body. In contrast, the autonomic nervous system, which consists of the *sympathetic* and *parasympathetic divisions*, carries information that is directly related to survival (for organs that are not under voluntary control). The sympathetic division mobilizes the body to react in the face of a threat, much like the response that occurs in Cannon's fight-or-flight response. This response includes increases in respiration, heart rate, and pulse; decreases in digestion and reproduction; dilation of pupils (for far vision); and movement of blood to the muscles to prepare for action. The parasympathetic division demobilizes the body to conserve energy, which includes increasing digestion; decreasing heart rate, respiration, and pulse; and constricting pupils. These physiological reactions occur because the autonomic nervous system triggers the endocrine system to react in the face of stress, as described in the next section.

Endocrine System

The **endocrine system** regulates a number of different physiological processes in the body, including physical growth, sexual arousal, metabolism, and stress response. The endocrine system works by releasing hormones from endocrine glands, such as the pituitary, thyroid, and pancreas, into the bloodstream (see Figure 4.4). These hormones then travel though the bloodstream to influence a particular body tissue or organ. For example, when the hormone estrogen is released from a young woman's ovaries, it causes the uterus to grow in preparation for carrying an embryo, the breasts to enlarge in preparation for nursing, and the brain to increase in interest in sexual activity.

During times of stress, the sympathetic nervous system activates two core systems within the endocrine system: the **sympathetic adrenomedullary (SAM) system**, which is responsible for the immediate fight-or-flight response to stress, and the **hypothalamic-pituitary-adrenal (HPA) axis**, which puts into motion a slower neuroendocrine response to stress (Chrousos & Gold, 1992; Cohen, Janicki-Deverts, & Miller, 2007). When the SAM system is activated, the hypothalamus triggers the adrenal glands to release epinephrine (adrenaline) and norepinephrine (noradrenaline). These hormones act very quickly and lead to a number of physiological effects, including increases in heart rate, blood flow, and sweat. The slower HPA system is also activated during times of stress. The HPA system starts by secreting corticotropin-releasing hormone (CRH), which in turn triggers the anterior pituitary gland to release adrenocorticotropic hormone (ACTH). Finally, the presence of ACTH leads the adrenal gland to release glucocorticoids, including cortisol (an important stress hormone that circulates back to the brain). As stress hormones circulate, rising levels of cortisol become a signal to the brain to shut off the fight-or-flight response, allowing the body to recover from stress. This is an important feedback system that protects the organism from the physiological harm of chronic sympathetic activation. If stress is maintained over time, the resulting high levels of cortisol can lead to damage in the hippocampus, an area of the brain involved in memory (you'll learn more about this in the final section of this chapter). During times of stress, the endocrine system also inhibits the secretion of growth hormones as well as hormones associated with reproduction (Chrousos, 1998). This is one

Figure 4.4   Model of the Endocrine System

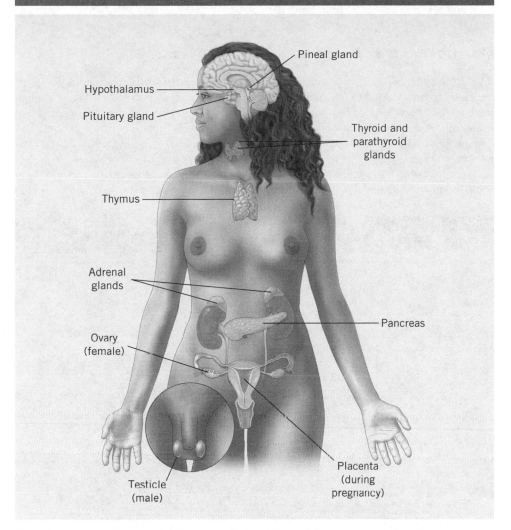

Hypothalamus

Pituitary gland

Pineal gland

Thyroid and parathyroid glands

Thymus

Adrenal glands

Ovary (female)

Pancreas

Testicle (male)

Placenta (during pregnancy)

Illustration: © SAGE Publishing. All Rights Reserved. Created by Body Scientific International.

reason why women may experience the loss of their menstrual cycle (amenorrhea) during times of high stress.

Several studies have demonstrated the powerful effects of stress on the endocrine system (Frankenhaeuser, 1975, 1978; Ursin, Baade, & Levine, 1978). One early study by Ursin and colleagues (1978), for example, examined how young military recruits reacted physiologically to the stressful situation of their first parachute-training jump. In this first stage of training, recruits climbed to the top of a 40-foot tower and then slid down a wire to the ground, which feels similar to free fall. Most people find this experience stressful, and, not surprisingly, levels of epinephrine, norepinephrine, and cortisol were significantly higher on the day of the jump than the day before. Although the type of stress experienced in this situation was obviously quite unique (and extreme), similar increases in stress-related hormones occur following other, more typical stressful situations, including taking exams, giving a speech, and having a repetitive and low-control job (Frankenhaeuser, 1975, 1978; Sumter, Bokhorst, Miers, Van Pelt, & Westenberg, 2010). For example, lesbian, gay, and bisexual people who are open about

What You'll Learn
4.3

their sexual orientation have lower levels of the stress hormone cortisol than people who are still in the closet; living with such a big secret is a chronic stressor that exerts tremendous wear and tear on the body (Juster, Smith, Ouellet, Sindi & Lupien, 2013).

Cardiovascular System

The primary function of the **cardiovascular system** is for the heart to generate the force necessary to pump blood to transport oxygen to and remove carbon dioxide from each cell in the body (see Figure 4.5). The blood travels initially through the larger blood vessels (such as the *aorta*), which in turn branch into smaller and smaller vessels, and eventually into capillaries. Two major measures to evaluate cardiovascular activity are *heart rate*, the number of beats per minute, and *blood pressure*, the force of blood against the artery walls.

Unfortunately, prolonged periods of high blood pressure can lead to a buildup of fatty acids and glucose on blood vessel walls, which forces the heart to work even harder to pump

Figure 4.5　Model of the Cardiovascular System

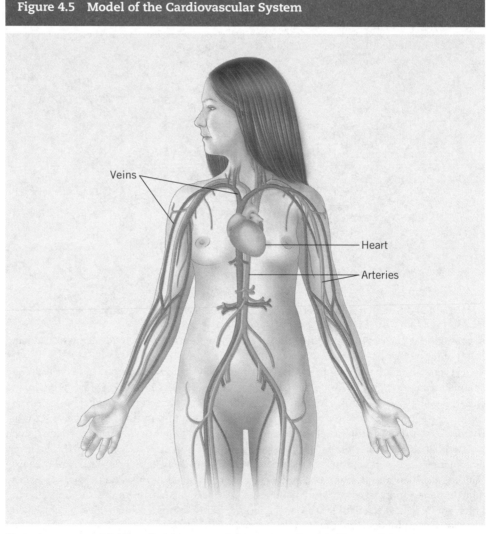

Veins

Heart

Arteries

Illustration: © SAGE Publishing. All Rights Reserved. Created by Body Scientific International.

blood through narrowing arteries. Over time, this wear and tear caused by long-term, or chronic, stress can lead to considerable damage to the heart and arteries.

The impact of stress on the cardiovascular system is well established; people under stress show heightened cardiovascular reactivity, including high blood pressure and increased heart rate (Kamarck, Muldoon, Shiffman, Sutton-Tyrrell, Gwaltney, & Janicki, 2004). For example, people who take a stressful math test in a psychology laboratory show faster heart rates and higher blood pressure after this stressor than before, and show a similar elevation in blood pressure when they are in stressful situations in daily life (Matthews, Owens, Allen, & Stoney, 1992; Uchino, Cacioppo, Malarkey, & Glaser, 1995). More routine types of stressors, such as interpersonal conflict, also impact the cardiovascular system; couples with low marital satisfaction show higher heart rates during conflicts than those with greater satisfaction (Kiecolt-Glaser et al., 1988; Manne & Zautra, 1989). In fact, married people who show outbursts of anger when talking about a marital conflict are at greater risk of developing chest pain, high blood pressure, and other cardiovascular problems over time (Haase, Holley, Bloch, Verstaen, & Levenson, 2016).

In turn, greater cardiovascular activity can contribute to both minor and major health problems. For example, stress can cause the dilation of arteries surrounding the brain and tension in muscles in the head, neck, and shoulders, both of which may lead to headaches (Turner & Chapman, 1982). In turn, only 7% of those who experience low stress report experiencing frequent headache pain, as compared to 17% of those with moderate stress and 25% of those with high stress (Sternbach, 1986). Moreover, higher levels of adrenaline—which result from stress—cause blood to clot more rapidly, which can lead to heart attacks (Strike et al., 2006). In fact, one large-scale study in over 52 countries revealed that individuals with high rates of stress—at home and/or work—were at greater risk of experience a heart attack (Rosengren et al., 2004). Sadly, and as described in **Focus on Diversity**, the ongoing stress of racial discrimination can increase the risk of experiencing cardiovascular problems.

Lacking control over a particular situation also contributes to the development of serious, and even fatal, cardiovascular problems. In line with this view, people who report feeling low levels of ability to exercise control over their work lives—including scheduling their work activities and changing work activities—have higher levels of atherosclerosis, a risk factor associated with cardiovascular disease, and are more likely to experience a heart attack than those who feel they have higher levels of control (Bosma et al., 1997; Kamarck, Muldoon, Shiffman, & Sutton-Tyrrell, 2007). Moreover, employees with high job strain, meaning they experience high demands at work and low control, are over twice as likely to die from cardiovascular-related causes than those without such strain (Kivimaki et al., 2002). Lacking control over one's personal life is also associated with negative cardiovascular outcomes. For example, people who provide in-home care to a spouse with Alzheimer's disease, a very stressful situation for virtually all caregivers, are at increased risk of developing coronary heart disease (von Känel et al., 2008).

What You'll Learn
4.4

Immune System

The **immune system**, which is the body's major line of defense against infections and diseases, provides three levels of protection: external barriers, nonspecific responses, and specific responses (Simpson, Hurtley, & Marx, 2000). Initially, the skin serves as an external barrier to protect the body from bacteria and viruses. However, if any type of foreign material, such as a bacteria or virus, invades this barrier, the immune system begins an immediate nonspecific response (any foreign material that activates this immune response is called an *antigen*). It works to eliminate foreign, "nonself" materials, such as bacteria, viruses, and parasites, that contact or enter the body. If you get a splinter in your hand, the immune system will trigger

FOCUS ON DIVERSITY

How Racial Discrimination Hurts Health

Racial discrimination is a type of chronic stressor that can have a significant impact on health. Specifically, feeling constantly mistreated based on one's ethnicity or race is a chronic stressor that may lead to higher blood pressure as well as damage to the cardiovascular system (Clark, Anderson, Clark, & Williams, 1999; Krieger & Sidney, 1996; Merritt, Bennett, Williams, Edwards, & Sollers, 2006; Smart Richman, Pek, Pascoe, & Bauer, 2010; Tomfohr, Pung, & Dimsdale, 2016). In line with this view, cardiovascular reactivity, including greater blood pressure, higher heart rate, and increased plaque in the arteries (an early sign of coronary heart disease), is more likely for people who have experienced past acts of discrimination, and this association is stronger for Blacks than Whites (Smart Richman, Bennett, Pek, Siegler, & Williams, 2007; Troxel, Matthews, Bromberger, & Sutton-Tyrrell, 2003). Experiencing discrimination also speeds up the biological aging process, which helps explain the persistent gap in life expectancy as a function of race (Lee, Kim, & Neblett, 2017). Although the majority of this research has focused on the influence of ongoing stress on health in Blacks, Latinos who believe they are discriminated against due to their ethnicity show higher rates of anxiety and depression as well as blood pressure, which may lead to greater risk of cardiovascular disease (Moody, Waldstein, Tobin, Cassells, Schwartz, & Brondolo, 2016; Salomon & Jagusztyn, 2008; Sirin et al., 2015). These findings illustrate the substantial health consequences of experiencing ongoing discrimination and may at least partially explain why Black people tend to have higher rates of hypertension and coronary heart disease than do White people. Sadly, data from over a million people living across the United States finds that Blacks who live in overtly racist communities are more likely to die from heart disease and other related illnesses, even when researchers take into account age, education, income, and living environment (Leitner, Hehman, Ayduk, & Mendoza-Denton, 2016). On a more positive note, Latina/o college students who live in ethnically based theme houses show lower levels of immune system activation, suggesting that such environments reduce the negative physiological responses associated with discrimination.

a response to fight against this invader (in this case, wood). The blood vessels will dilate to increase blood flow to the site of the injury, which leads to warmth, redness, and swelling and allows tissue repair to begin. A group of cells called *lymphocytes* finds and then destroys *antigen*s in the bloodstream.

As shown in Figure 4.6, the body's third line of defense against foreign matter is the specific immune system, which consists of specialized types of white blood cells called lymphocytes, including B cells and T cells. These cells differ from nonspecific lymphocytes in that they find and attack only very specific antigens. The B cells, which originate in the bone marrow, control the *humoral immune response system*, in which proteins called antibodies, which bind to foreign toxins and inactivate or destroy them, are produced. The T cells, which originate in the thymus, control the *cell-mediated immune response system*, in which they bind to foreign cells to kill them. Other immune system cells include the *natural killer (NK) cells*, which detect and then destroy damaged cells, such as precancerous cells before they develop into tumors, and *macrophages*, which engulf and digest foreign cells, such as bacteria.

Although you may think of the immune system as fairly abstract, it impacts your life in a variety of ways. For example, vaccinations for diseases such as polio and chicken pox were created based on knowledge of how the immune system works. When you get a vaccination, you are actually introducing a weakened form of a virus or bacterium into

Figure 4.6   Model of the Immune System

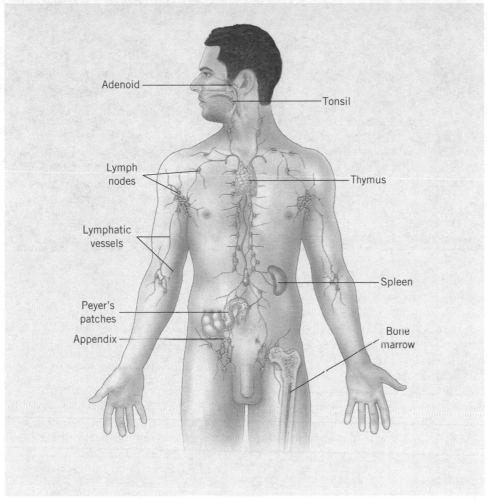

Adenoid

Tonsil

Lymph nodes

Thymus

Lymphatic vessels

Spleen

Peyer's patches

Appendix

Bone marrow

your body. The body then reacts to this threat by producing antibodies to fight it. When and if you are exposed to the actual disease, your body already has the antibodies ready to respond and thereby protect you from illness—it is like having a head start on fighting an illness.

Considerable research with both animals and humans demonstrates that stress has a number of negative effects on the immune system (Segerstrom & Miller, 2004). Individuals who experience a variety of different types of stressors, including divorce, loneliness, unemployment, bereavement, marital conflict, and exams, have fewer B, T, and NK cells (Cohen & Herbert, 1996; Kiecolt-Glaser, McGuire, Robles, & Glaser, 2002). For example, people who experience *stereotype threat*, in which they feel pressure to perform well due to negative expectations about their group membership, show increases in cortisol (Levy, Heissel, Richeson, & Adam, 2016; Townsend, Major, Gangi, & Mendes, 2011). As described in **Focus on Development**, children who experience high levels of family stress show weakened immune systems and hence are at greater risk of becoming sick.

FOCUS ON DEVELOPMENT

Why Family Stress Makes Kids Sick

High levels of family stress can weaken children's immune systems and therefore increase their risk of getting sick. For example, researchers in one study asked parents of five-year-old children questions about current stressors that were impacting the family, such as divorce, unemployment, or the death of a relative (Carlsson, Frostell, Ludvigsson, & Faresjö, 2014). The researchers then compared immune system functioning in children from families with high versus normal levels of stress. As predicted, children in families experiencing high levels of stress showed higher rates of cortisol, indicating greater physiological stress in the body. Given the considerable research showing that high cortisol levels indicate a weakened immune system, these children are unfortunately at increased likelihood of becoming sick. Experiencing this type of stress during childhood can have lasting effects on physical health, in part because early childhood stress increases the risk of obesity and depression (Wickrama, Kwon, Oshri, & Lee, 2014; Wickrama, Lee, O'Neal, & Kwon, 2015).

Although studies with humans often have difficulty showing that stress—as opposed to some third variable such as personality—causes such physiological reactions, experimental research with animals reveals such findings. For example, rats who are exposed to stressors, including noise, overcrowding, and inescapable shock, show less immune cell activity as well as a faster rate of tumor growth compared to rats not under such stress (Ben-Eliyahu, Yirmiya, Liebeskind, Taylor, & Gale, 1991; Moynihan & Ader, 1996).

Because chronic stress diverts resources away from the immune system and toward more urgent physiological needs, people who experience stress over long periods of time have a greater risk of developing an infectious disease, which the body would typically be able to fight off. In a series of studies, Sheldon Cohen has recruited healthy volunteers who are willing to be exposed to a cold virus (the virus is inserted using nasal drops) (Cohen, Doyle, Skoner, Rabin, & Gwaltney, 1997; Cohen, Tyrrell, & Smith, 1991; Cohen et al., 2012). Participants are quarantined (in separate living accommodations) for a few days, complete a series of measures (of such things as psychological stress, social support, personality, and health status), and are then exposed to the cold virus. Researchers then examine participants daily for signs and symptoms of a cold, such as sneezing, sore threat, sinus pain, and coughing, in order to determine how psychosocial factors may influence who develops a cold and who is able to fight off this virus and remain healthy. As predicted, people who experience more stress in their daily lives have a greater rate of infection with the cold, even after controlling for other factors (e.g., age, gender, personality variables).

Although this research is conducted in a laboratory setting, studies in more real-world settings reveal similar findings. For example, one study comparing the health of caregivers of Alzheimer's patients, who are undergoing a chronic stress, to a matched control group (people of a similar age but without such responsibility) found that caregivers had a weaker immune response and were more likely to develop infectious diseases (Kiecolt-Glaser, Dura, Speicher, Trask, & Glaser, 1991). Similarly, people who are unemployed show higher levels of inflammation, indicating an increased risk of infection or disease, even when researchers take into account other health-related factors, such as smoking, BMI, and alcohol consumption (Hughes, McMunn, Bartley, & Kumari, 2015). Older job seekers, who likely experience greater stress from unemployment than younger ones, are particularly likely to show such effects. This research provides strong evidence for the impact of psychological factors on physical well-being.

Psychoneuroimmunology

So far, you've learned about the impact of stress on the nervous, endocrine, cardiovascular, and immune systems as separate and distinct effects; in reality, these different body systems all interact to influence health. You may have noticed, for example, that when the endocrine system is activated, it in turn leads to cardiovascular changes, such as increases in heart rate and blood pressure (see Table 4.3). Activating the endocrine system also leads to the release of glucocorticoids, which hinder the formation of some white blood cells, including NK cells, and kill other white blood cells (Cohen & Herbert, 1996; Jemmott & Locke, 1984; Kiecolt-Glaser & Glaser, 1986).

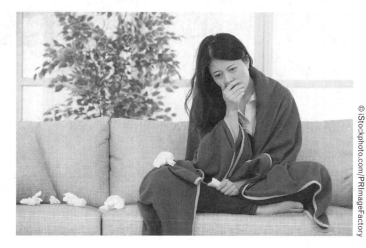

People who experience high levels of stress are at greater risk of developing all types of major and minor illnesses—including the common cold.

The field of psychoneuroimmunology examines the complex connection between psychosocial factors, such as stress, and the nervous, cardiovascular, endocrine, and immune systems (Adler, 2001). Moreover, and as shown in Figure 4.7, appraising particular life events as stressful leads to arousal as well as harmful health-related behaviors, which both in turn create physiological responses that increase the risk of illness and disease (Cohen, Gianaros, & Manuck, 2016). Thus, the association between stress and health is clearly complex and multifaceted.

Although we now fully accept the idea that the mind and body interact in complex ways to influence health, this finding was originally discovered by accident. In 1974, psychologist Robert Ader was working on a series of studies designed to show that rats could learn to avoid a sugar-flavored drinking water by using classical conditioning techniques (see **Chapter 3: Theories of Health Behavior** for a quick refresher). First, he gave rats a sugar-flavored water to drink, which, not surprisingly, the rats enjoyed. Then he injected the rats with an immune-suppressing drug that caused them to feel nauseous. The rats quickly learned that the drink would make them ill; hence, they developed an aversion to the taste that was associated through conditioning with the injection. However, several weeks later Ader found that many of the rats involved in this study on taste aversion became sick and ultimately died. Testing revealed that the immune system in these rats was impaired, apparently due to the drug they had received. But, amazingly, the immune system was also impaired in rats that had received the immune-suppressing drug on only one occasion and on all future trials had received only the sugar water (which obviously should have had no effect on their immune system). Apparently, the

Table 4.3 Physical Effects of Stress on Health

Body System	Effect on Health During Stress
Nervous System	Increase in respiration, heart rate, pulse; movement of blood to muscles
Endocrine System	Increases in heart rate, blood flow, sweat; increases in cortisol
Cardiovascular System	Increases in blood pressure and heart rate
Immune System	Decreases in cells that fight off infection
Psychoneuroimmunology	All of the above effects occur, as body systems are all activated and interact with one another

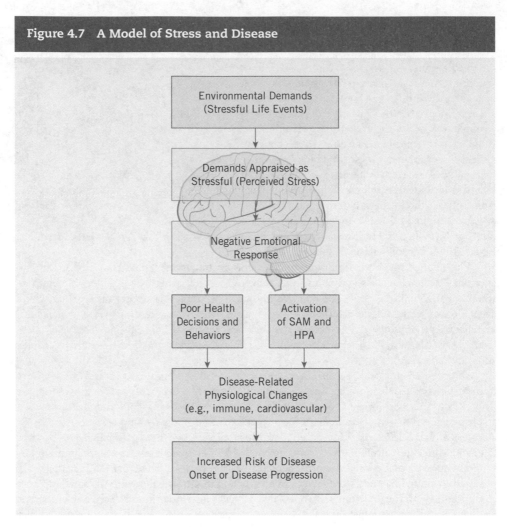

Figure 4.7　A Model of Stress and Disease

Environmental Demands
(Stressful Life Events)

↓

Demands Appraised as
Stressful (Perceived Stress)

↓

Negative Emotional
Response

↓

Poor Health
Decisions and
Behaviors

Activation
of SAM and
HPA

↓

Disease-Related
Physiological Changes
(e.g., immune, cardiovascular)

↓

Increased Risk of Disease
Onset or Disease Progression

Source: Cohen, Gianaros, & Manuck (2016).

animals' immune systems associated the taste of the sugar water with the experience of immune suppression, and hence they developed a conditioned response to this taste in later trials that led to a suppression of their immune response. Ader then conducted a series of studies with Nicholas Cohen, an immunologist, to replicate his surprising findings (Ader & Cohen, 1975, 1985). These studies again demonstrated that immune responses can be conditioned. These studies, which demonstrate that psychological, neural, and immunological processes interact in complex ways, led to the development of the field of psychoneuroimmunology.

LO 4.5

Describe effects of stress on well-being, memory and cognition, and behavior

ADDITIONAL EFFECTS OF STRESS

Although stress has a direct impact on all body systems, stress also impacts health in other ways. In this section, you'll learn how stress impacts psychological well-being and the development of **posttraumatic stress disorder (PTSD)**, an anxiety disorder that may occur after experiencing severely traumatic events, such as serving in a war, being the victim of a crime, or living through a natural disaster or terrorist attack. You'll also learn how stress impacts memory and cognition. Finally, this section will describe how behavioral choices may help explain the stress–health link.

Psychological Well-Being

In addition to impacting physical health, stress can impact psychological well-being. Specifically, stress can lead to a variety of negative emotions, such as fear, anxiety, and sadness (Rubonis & Bickman, 1991). Routine stresses, such as constant pressure at work, can eventually lead to frustration and apathy (Maslach, 1982). This state of emotional exhaustion, or burnout, is particularly common in people who work in helping professions, such as doctors, nurses, police officers, and social workers.

Ongoing, or chronic, stress, is particularly likely to lead to negative psychological consequences. For example, lesbian, gay, and bisexual teenagers often experience considerable stress regarding the decision to "come out" (Baams, Grossman, & Russell, 2015). Not surprisingly, feeling victimized based on their sexual orientation is associated with higher levels of depression as well as suicidal ideation. Similarly, people of color who have experienced specific acts of racial discrimination, such as being shouted at, physically acted upon, or made to feel unsafe due to their ethnicity, show higher rates of mental health problems than those who do not report such experiences (Wallace, Nazroo, & Bécares, 2016). The term *acculturative stress* describes the particular stress experienced by many immigrants who must adjust to a new culture, which can include learning a new language, facing discrimination, and feeling socially isolated. Not surprisingly, acculturative stress is associated with lower levels of psychological and physical well-being (Fang, Ross, Pathak, Godwin, & Tseng, 2014).

Moreover, considerable evidence suggests that depression is directly linked with poorer overall health, including lower levels of immune function (Kiecolt-Glaser & Glaser, 2002). Individuals who are depressed show compromised immune function, which can lead to prolonged infection and delayed wound healing. Depression also increases the risk of developing serious health problems, including heart disease and stroke (Gilsanz et al., 2015; Péquignot et al., 2016). In fact, one recent study found that depression increases the risk of a heart attack as much as high cholesterol and obesity (Ladwig et al., 2017).

Posttraumatic Stress Disorder (PTSD)

Posttraumatic stress disorder (PTSD) is a particular type of anxiety disorder caused by exposure to some type of extreme stressor, such as war, a natural disaster, or physical assault (American Psychiatric Association, 2013). Although many people who experience such a stressor develop disruptive symptoms, including intrusive thoughts about the event and difficulty sleeping, these symptoms typically fade with time. However, some people develop PTSD, in which these symptoms continue for months and cause significant distress and difficulty functioning in daily life. Symptoms of PTSD include reliving the event through memories, flashbacks, and nightmares; avoiding any reminders of the event; and having severe anxiety. For example, war veterans often experience severe behavioral symptoms, including sleeplessness, nightmares, and startle reactions (Sutker, Davis, Uddo, & Ditta, 1995). In cases of extreme stress, these reactions can last for many years. For example, survivors of Nazi concentration camps sometimes report continuing anxiety and fear as long as 50 years after their internment (Valent, 2000).

PTSD is more likely among those who are more affected by a particular event, such as those who live in close proximity or lose friends or loved ones (Ironson et al., 1997). One

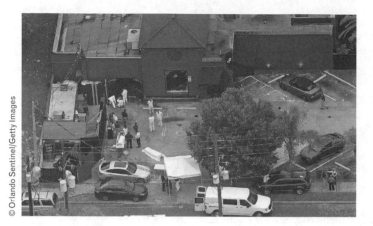

People who survive severely traumatic events, such as the nightclub shooting in Orlando in June 2016, are at risk of developing PTSD.

study found that following the 2011 earthquake in Japan, more than half of the people living in one town—which was near the nuclear power plant and at risk of leaking radiation—showed some symptoms of PTSD (Kukihara, Yamawaki, Uchiyama, Arai, & Horikawa, 2014). Similarly, after the 9/11 terrorist attacks, higher rates of PTSD and psychological distress were reported by those who lived in close proximity to the attacks compared to those in other parts of the country (Schlenger et al., 2002). However, and as described in **Focus on Neuroscience**, even among people who all experience the same traumatic event, the risk of experiencing PTSD varies.

People with PTSD stay in a nearly constant state of physiological arousal so that they are able to respond quickly if this threat returns. This continual arousal exerts considerable wear and tear on the body, which in turn increases the risk of developing various health problems, including cardiovascular disease, stroke, respiratory symptoms, and cancer (Brudey et al., 2015; Chen et al., 2015; Kotov et al., 2015). For example, people with PTSD are at increased risk of experiencing heart failure, even after researchers take into account age, gender, BMI, and family history (Roy, Foraker, Girton, & Mansfield, 2015; Sumner et al., 2015). People with PTSD also experience higher levels of pain and disability (Outcalt et al., 2015).

The link between PTSD and serious health consequences is explained in part through the wear and tear this disorder causes on multiple body systems. For example, people with PTSD also engage in particular behaviors, such as smoking and excessive alcohol use, that harm health (Dennis et al., 2014). People with PTSD are also more likely to engage in disordered eating behaviors, such as vomiting, laxative use, fasting, and overexercise (Mitchell, Porter, Boyko, & Field, 2016).

FOCUS ON NEUROSCIENCE

How the Brain Responds to a Terrorist Attack

Researchers in one study examined the effects of experiencing stress—a terrorist attack—on brain activity (McLaughlin, Busso, Duys, Green, Alves, Way, & Sheridan, 2014). As part of a study on childhood trauma, a research team conducted brain scans on adolescents living in the Boston area to assess how they responded to both negative and positive images. Then, one month following the April 2013 bombing at the Boston Marathon, researchers asked these adolescents to complete online surveys assessing their experience of PTSD, such as having difficulty concentrating and continuing to think about the bombing even when they tried not to.

Findings revealed that adolescents whose brain scans at the first testing session—prior to the bombing—showed greater activation in their amygdala (a part of the brain that processes emotions) to negative images, such as people feeling sad, fighting, or threatening someone, were at greater risk of developing PTSD at the time of the second testing. These findings suggest that people whose brains react more to negative images in general are at greater risk of developing PTSD following stressful life experiences. They may also explain why some people but not others develop PTSD even after exposure to the same circumstances.

Memory and Cognition

Stress may have a substantial impact on memory and cognition. People who are under high stress may have trouble concentrating or focusing on a particular task because other thoughts continue to come into their minds (Lyubomirsky & Nolen-Hoeksema, 1995; Sarason, Sarason, Keefe, Hayes, & Shearin, 1986). Have you ever misread a question on an exam and gotten the answer wrong, even though you knew the right answer? For example, as you take an exam that is not going well, you may start thinking, "Everyone else seems to be nearly finished," or "If I don't do well on this test, I will get a C in this course," which in turn increases stress and makes it even harder for you to focus. Long-term stress leads to the loss of neurons in the hippocampus, which in turn impairs memory (Sapolsky, 1992). This finding helps explain with high rates of work stress correspond to worse scores on a memory test (Rutledge et al., 2009).

Even ongoing types of environmental stressors, such as loud noise, can lead to cognitive problems. One study examined reading and memory skills in children ages 8 to 12 who lived near a noisy airport (Hygge, Evans, & Bullinger, 2002). After the airport was shut down, the children's reading and memory scores improved, whereas children who lived near the new airport showed a decline in scores on these measures.

Behavioral Choices

As described in the prior section, stress impacts virtually every biological system in the body, which in turn has major implications for physical health. But stress also impacts health indirectly by influencing people's behavior. Here's a simple example: many college students find that they seem to always get sick during or right after exam week. In this case, what factors might lead to the link between stress and illness? Many college students report engaging in generally poor health practices during exam week, such as eating junk food, drinking large amounts of coffee and other caffeinated beverages, getting less sleep, and reducing (or completely stopping) exercise. Thus, one explanation for the sickness that always seems to follow exams is that people who are experiencing stress often engage in behaviors that impact health.

Considerable research reveals that people who are experiencing high levels of stress are less likely to engage in health-promoting behaviors, such as exercising and getting adequate amounts of sleep, and are more likely to engage in health-impairing behaviors, such as eating less-nutritious foods and smoking cigarettes (Conway, Vickers, Ward, & Rahe, 1981; Jackson, Knight, & Rafferty, 2010; Ng & Jeffery, 2003). As shown in Figure 4.8, people who are experiencing chronic stress, meaning stress that lasts more than a month, are particularly likely to engage in behaviors that harm their health. Similarly, people who experience higher levels of stress report poorer eating habits, including eating more high-fat and high-sugar foods, eating fewer main meals and vegetables, and engaging in more emotional eating, meaning eating in response to a bad mood (Diggins, Woods-Giscombe, & Waters, 2015; O'Connor, Jones, Conner, McMillan, & Ferguson, 2008). Not surprisingly given these eating habits, stress is also linked with weight gain (Block, He, Zaslavsky, Ding, & Ayanian, 2009; Hannerz, Albertsen, Nielsen, Tüchsen, & Burr, 2004; Michels et al., 2015). These findings suggest that the association between stress and illness may be moderated in part by unhealthy behaviors.

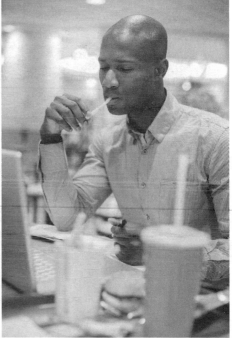

© iStockphoto.com/NicolasMcComber

Think about your own behavior during final exams. Do you engage in health-promoting behaviors or those that can hurt your health?

People who are experiencing stress also tend to get less sleep, which in turn is associated with negative health outcomes (Cohen, Doyle, Alper, Janicki-Deverts, & Turner, 2009; Zunhammer, Eichhammer, & Busch, 2014). For example, one study examined immune cell activity in a group of healthy men who were kept awake between 3 and 7 a.m. (Irwin et al., 1994). As predicted, this type of sleep deprivation led to decreases in immune cell activity that returned only after the men had a good night's sleep. Although this study examined the negative consequences of deliberately disrupting sleep, naturalistic studies reveal similar findings. Children and adolescents who experience more stressful life events also report having lower sleep quality, including feeling drowsy during the day, having more trouble falling asleep, and waking up in the middle of the night (Ly, McGrath, & Gouin, 2015). Unfortunately, this lower quality of sleep is associated with increases in cortisol level, indicating that experiencing stress leads to physiological changes at least in part due to the effect on sleep quality.

This link between psychological states, health behaviors, and health outcomes is particularly hazardous for people who are clinically depressed. Researchers in one study examined the association between depression and likelihood of experiencing a cardiovascular event, such as a stroke or heart attack, in men with coronary heart disease (Whooley et al., 2008). Depressed people were 31% more likely to experience a cardiovascular event than nondepressed people, even after controlling for disease state and other risk factors. However, when researchers controlled for level of physical activity, the association between depression and likelihood of experiencing a cardiovascular event disappeared. In sum, depression has an indirect, not direct, effect on the experience of cardiovascular events; depressed people are less likely to exercise than nondepressed people, which in turn increases the risk of a heart problem.

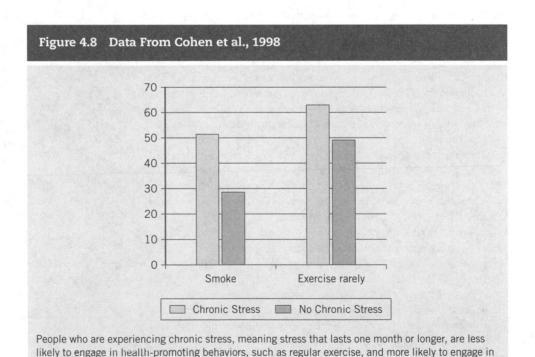

Figure 4.8   Data From Cohen et al., 1998

People who are experiencing chronic stress, meaning stress that lasts one month or longer, are less likely to engage in health-promoting behaviors, such as regular exercise, and more likely to engage in harmful behaviors, such as smoking. These behaviors, in turn, increase the likelihood of getting sick.

Source: Cohen, Frank, Doyle, Skoner, Rabin, & Gwaltney (1998).

Table 4.4 Summary of Additional Effects of Stress

Type of Effect	Example
Psychological well-being	Anxiety, depression
Posttraumatic stress disorder (PTSD)	Disruptive memories, flashbacks, and nightmares; severe anxiety
Memory and cognition	Impaired memory, lower scores on cognitive tests
Behavior	Poor eating habits, more substance abuse, less sleep, negative interpersonal behavior

Finally, stress can lead to negative interpersonal behavior. After the devastating Hurricane Andrew hit south Florida in 1992, destroying and damaging homes, reports of domestic violence increased dramatically (Polusny & Follette, 1995). Sexual drive is also affected by stress; women are less likely to ovulate, and men are more likely to have difficulty achieving and maintaining an erection (Sapolsky, 1994).

Table 4.5 Information YOU Can Use

- Given all the hazards of stress on psychological and physical well-being, one of the best ways you can promote good health is to avoid stress whenever possible. So, think about the impact of your choices—the environment in which you live, your job, your relationships—on the amount of stress you experience, and try to make choices that reduce the amount of stress in your life.

- Everyone experiences some stress, but people vary considerable in how they appraise or think about particular events. You have a choice about how to interpret and experience particular events in your life, so, whenever possible, appraise events you experience as exciting challenges and not distressing stressors.

- Many of the negative effects of stress on health occur at least in part because people fail to take care of themselves during periods of stress. Thus, during times of stress, take care of yourself—eat healthy foods, get enough sleep, maintain your exercise routine, and avoid adopting bad habits such as smoking and alcohol use.

SUMMARY

Sources of Stress

- Personal relationships are a major source of stress. Relationships can cause conflict, and more serious family issues, such as an illness or divorce, are especially stressful. Even positive relationships cause stress.

- Work pressures can create considerable stress. Such stress is particularly intense for people with jobs involving saving people's lives and for those who have little control over their work lives.

- People experience stress from environmental pressures, such as noise, crowding, and pollution, as well as shorter-term environmental factors, such as the political climate. Living in poverty is especially stressful, in part because it creates many additional stressors.

- Major cataclysmic events, such as natural disasters, terrorist attacks, and mass shootings, clearly cause considerable stress. Even watching media coverage of terrorist attacks can lead to stress.

- Pressures within ourselves, such as when we are torn between two different goals, is another factor that can cause stress. This type of stress includes approach-approach conflict, approach-avoidance conflict, and avoidance-avoidance conflict.

Measuring Stress

- Many researchers use self-report inventories, in which people list the number of major life events they have experienced in a given period of time. However, these measures don't take into account the subjective experience of an event or whether it is positive or negative and may exclude some ongoing stressful events. Other researchers measure stress in terms of daily hassles or small uplifting events. However, these measures also have some limitations, including the correlation between major and minor life stresses, the inclusion of specific health-related behaviors in such measures, and people's own degree of perceived stress.

- Researchers can also use physiological measures to assess stress. These can include measures of physiological arousal, including heart rate, blood pressure, respiration, and changes in the skin's resistance to electrical current (galvanic skin response, or GSR). They can also include biochemical measures, which assess the presence of particular hormones, such as norepinephrine, epinephrine, and cortisol. However, physiological measures have some limitations; the use of such measures can in and of themselves be stressful, their data is influenced by factors other than stress, and they tend to be expensive and time-consuming to use and interpret.

Models of the Stress Response

- According to the Cannon's fight-or-flight response model, when a person is threatened, the immediate response is to either fight off the stressor or escape from it. This leads to stimulation of the sympathetic nervous and endocrine systems, which causes a dramatic rise in epinephrine (adrenaline) and norepinephrine (noradrenaline). The increase in these hormone levels leads to physiological responses that prepare someone to either fight off a threat or run from it.

- According to the General Adaptation Syndrome (GAS), stress first leads to the alarm stage, in which the body mobilizes to fight off a threat. Next, there is the resistance stage, which occurs when the body continues trying to respond to the threat. Finally, when the threat continues for a long time, occurs repeatedly, or is very severe, the exhaustion stage may set in.

- More recent research has led to revisions of these models. First, different types of stressors are associated with different types of physiological reactions. The duration of the stressor also influences the physiological response. People may also vary in how they respond to stress.

- According to the transactional, or relational, model, the meaning a particular event has for a person predicts its experience. First, people engage in primary appraisal in which they interpret the situation and what it will mean for them. They then engage in secondary appraisal in which they assess the resources available for coping with the situation.

- Finally, the term *eustress* describes the benefits associated with stress. Moderate levels of stress lead to small amounts of arousal, providing extra energy, and can help people perform at their best. Moreover, individuals who experience some adverse life events may develop increased resilience, which in turn leads to greater physical and psychological well-being.

Physical Consequences

- The nervous system, which includes the central nervous system (the brain and spinal cord) as well as the peripheral nervous system, controls the body's overall reaction to stress. The peripheral nervous system includes the somatic nervous system and the autonomic nervous system, which in turn consists of the sympathetic and parasympathetic divisions. The sympathetic division mobilizes the body to react in the face of a threat; the parasympathetic division demobilizes the body to conserve energy.

- The endocrine system releases hormones into the bloodstream. During times of stress, the sympathetic nervous system activates the sympathetic adrenomedullary (SAM) system, which initiates the fight-or-flight response to stress, and the hypothalamic-pituitary-adrenal (HPA) axis, which puts into motion a slower neuroendocrine response to stress.

- The primary function of the cardiovascular system is for the heart to generate the force necessary to pump blood to transport oxygen to and remove carbon dioxide from each cell in the body. Prolonged periods of high blood pressure cause a buildup of fatty acids and glucose on blood vessel walls, which forces the heart to work even harder to pump blood. Over time, this can lead to considerable damage to the heart and arteries and contribute to both minor and major health problems.

- The immune system provides three levels of protection. Initially, the skin protects the body from bacteria and viruses. The immune system also works to eliminate foreign materials that contact or enter the body. The body's third line of defense consists of specialized white blood cells called lymphocytes, including B cells and T cells. Stress has a number of negative effects on the immune system.

- The field of psychoneuroimmunology examines the complex connection between psychosocial factors, such as stress, and the nervous, cardiovascular, endocrine, and immune systems.

Additional Effects of Stress

- Stress can lead to a variety of negative emotions, such as fear, anxiety, and sadness. Ongoing, or chronic, stress, is particularly likely to lead to negative psychological consequences. Moreover, depression is directly linked with poorer overall health; it increases the risk of developing serious health problems, including heart disease and stroke.

- Posttraumatic stress disorder (PTSD) is caused by exposure to some type of extreme stressor, such as war, a natural disaster, or physical assault. Symptoms of PTSD include reliving the event through memories, flashbacks, and nightmares; avoiding any reminders of the event; and having severe anxiety. PTSD is more likely among those who are more affected by a particular event. People with PTSD stay in a near constant state of physiological arousal so that they are able to respond quickly if this threat returns. This continual arousal exerts considerable wear and tear on the body, which in turn increases the risk of developing various health problems.

- Stress causes problems with memory and cognition. People who are under high stress may have trouble concentrating or focusing because other thoughts continue to come into their minds. Even ongoing types of environmental stressors, such as loud noise, can lead to cognitive problems.

- Stress also impacts health indirectly by influencing people's behavior. People who are experiencing high levels of stress are less likely to engage in health-promoting behaviors and are more likely to engage in health-impairing behaviors. Finally, stress can lead to negative interpersonal behavior, including domestic violence and sexual problems.

5

MANAGING STRESS

Learning Objectives

5.1 Compare how different coping styles approach managing stress

5.2 Examine how social support influences the experience of stress and predicts health outcomes

5.3 Describe how religion and spirituality influence health as well as various explanations for this association

5.4 Explain the impact of personality on the experience and management of stress

5.5 Summarize different strategies for reducing stress

What You'll Learn

5.1 Why people with good neighbors are less likely to experience a heart attack

5.2 Why attending religious services may extend your life

5.3 Why happy people are less likely to develop a cold

5.4 How meditation can help prevent cardiovascular disease

5.5 Why spending time in nature reduces anxiety, depression, and stress

Preview

In the last chapter, you learned about the various factors that can cause stress, and the substantial impact of stress on psychological and physical health. But here's the good news: **stress management**, meaning behavioral and cognitive strategies for reducing reactions to stress, can help people improve the quality—and quantity—of their lives. This chapter will describe the role of coping strategies, personality, social support, and religious and spiritual beliefs in helping people manage the ongoing challenges of daily life.

127

THE IMPACT OF COPING STYLES

LO 5.1

Compare how different coping styles approach managing stress

As described by Richard Lazarus and Susan Folkman (1984), **coping** refers to an individual's efforts to manage the stressful demands of a specific situation, such as working to solve a problem, finding a new way to look at the situation, or distracting oneself from the problem. In this section, you'll learn about two distinct approaches people use to manage stressful life experiences.

Problem-Focused Coping

One common strategy for managing challenging situations is trying to confront and change the stressor. This is called **problem-focused coping** and is often used when something constructive can be done to help solve the problem, or at least make the situation better (Folkman & Lazarus, 1980; Folkman, Lazarus, Dunkel Schetter, DeLongis, & Gruen, 1986). Problem-focused coping can include a number of different approaches, such as seeking assistance from others, taking direct action, and planning (see Table 5.1; Carver, Scheier, & Weintraub, 1989; Folkman & Lazarus, 1980). For example, a college student who is feeling stress due to the pressure of balancing academic work with athletic commitments could remove the stressor by dropping a class, manage the stressor by structuring specific times for studying each day, or relieve stress by sharing these feelings with a friend.

Is tackling a problem directly beneficial in terms of health? Yes: most research suggests that people who use problem-focused coping show better adjustment, probably because this type of coping helps people effectively eliminate problems (Dunkel Schetter, Feinstein, Taylor, & Falke, 1992; Penley, Tomaka, & Wiebe, 2002). For example, while students who procrastinate experience less stress than other students early in the semester, by the end of the semester

Table 5.1 Sample Items Testing Coping Styles
These questions are answered on a scale of 1 to 4, with 1 meaning "I usually don't do this at all" and 4 meaning "I usually do this a lot."
Active Coping
I concentrate my efforts on doing something about it.
I take direct action to get around the problem.
Planning
I try to come up with a strategy about what to do.
I make a plan of action.
Suppression of Competing Activities
I put aside other activities in order to concentrate on this.
I keep myself from getting distracted by other thoughts or activities.
Restraint Coping
I force myself to wait for the right time to do something.
I hold off doing anything about it until the situation permits.

Seeking Social Support for Instrumental Reasons

I ask people who have had similar experiences what they did.

I try to get advice from someone about what to do.

Seeking Social Support for Emotional Reasons

I talk to someone about how I feel.

I try to get emotional support from friends or relatives.

Positive Reinterpretation and Growth

I look for something good in what is happening.

I learn something from the experience.

Acceptance

I learn to live with it.

I accept that this has happened and that it can't be changed.

Turning to Religion

I seek God's help.

I try to find comfort in my religion.

Focus on and Venting of Emotion

I get upset and let my emotions out.

I let my feelings out.

Denial

I refuse to believe that it has happened.

I pretend that it hasn't really happened.

Behavioral Disengagement

I give up the attempt to get what I want.

I just give up trying to reach my goal.

Mental Disengagement

I turn to work or other substitute activities to take my mind off things.

I sleep more than usual.

Alcohol/Drug Disengagement

I drink alcohol or take drugs, in order to think about it less.

This scale assesses 14 different strategies people sometimes use to cope with problems.

Source: Carver, Schierer, & Weintraub (1989).

(when procrastinating is finally catching up with them), they experience greater stress and have more symptoms of illness (Tice & Baumeister, 1997). Students who directly handle their problems by keeping up with regular course reading and assignments thereby avoid the considerable stress faced at the end of the semester by those who have ignored these responsibilities. Similarly, law students who use active coping to manage the stress of taking the bar exam show lower levels of anxiety (Iida, Gleason, Green-Rapaport, Bolger, & Shrout, 2017).

Emotion-Focused Coping

In some cases, however, the stress can't simply be removed or eliminated, meaning that problem-focused coping doesn't really work. In these cases, changing how you think about the stress can be helpful in reducing its negative effects, a strategy called **emotion-focused coping** (Folkman & Lazarus, 1980; Lazarus & Folkman, 1984). This type of coping can involve either **approach (vigilant) coping**, meaning changing how one thinks about the problem or venting about the problem to others, or **avoidance (minimizing) coping**, meaning denying or avoiding the problem. For example, someone who has a fight with a close friend could discuss these feelings with another person to try to make sense of the sadness or simply try to put it out of his mind as a way of avoiding feeling sad. (We will talk specifically about the role of social support, a type of approach coping, later in this chapter.)

Approach-Focused Coping

Some forms of approach-focused coping, such as changing how one thinks about a problem, can help reduce the negative effects of stress (Lazarus & Folkman, 1984). For example, writing about emotional experiences, which is one form of approach-focused coping, leads to considerable benefits for both psychological and physical health (Langens & Schuler, 2007; Low, Stanton, & Danoff-Burg, 2006; Pennebaker & Beall, 1986; Smyth, 1998). In one study, early-stage breast cancer patients were randomly assigned to write over four sessions about one of three topics: their deepest thoughts and feelings regarding breast cancer, their positive thoughts and feelings regarding their experience with breast cancer, or facts about their breast cancer experience. (Stanton, Danoff-Burg, Sworowski, et al., 2002). Data at the three-month follow-up revealed that compared to those who only wrote about the facts of their illness, women who wrote about their intimate thoughts and feelings regarding the diagnosis reported significantly fewer physical symptoms, and women who wrote about either their most intimate thoughts or positive thoughts has fewer medical appointments for cancer-related morbidities. This work indicates that simply having people write about traumatic emotional experiences improves immune system functioning and can have clinically significant effects on health. Other research reveals similar positive health effects of writing about traumatic events for people with a number of different chronic illnesses (Petrie, Fontanilla, Thomas, Booth, & Pennebaker, 2004; Smyth, Stone, Hurewitz, & Kaell, 1999). However, and as described in **Focus on Diversity**, the benefits of writing about one's problems may not be seen in all cultures.

The use of *positive reappraisal*, meaning finding some beneficial aspects of even negative events, is another type of approach-focused coping that benefits health. For example, HIV-positive men who see some positive aspects of their diagnosis, such as shifting their values and priorities, show a slower rate of progression of the disease and survive for longer periods of time (Thompson, Nanni, & Levine, 1994). These results suggest that responding in a positive way to stressful events may be associated with better immune response, which in turn leads to better physical well-being.

A specific type of positive reappraisal that can reduce stress, and in turn lead to better health, is having a sense of humor. Specifically, people who use humor to manage stressful life events, including coping with chronic illness and terrorist disasters, show reduced distress and fewer physical symptoms (Fritz, Russek, & Dillon, 2017). The use of humor is associated with improved physiological responses to stress, including lower blood pressure and improved immune system functioning (Lefcourt, Davidson-Katz, & Kueneman, 1990; Lefcourt, Davidson, Prkachin, & Mills, 1997). Humor may help people cope with stressors at least in part by distracting them from their problems. For example, one study found that patients who joked and laughed prior to dental surgery experienced less anxiety during the procedure (Trice & Price-Greathouse, 1986). As Dan Shapiro, a clinical psychologist and author, says, "We all have a choice as to how to respond to stressful situations. Take losing one's luggage. We can respond with humor: 'Has my luggage gone somewhere interesting? Is it having a good time?' or we can take it as a calamity" (Brody, 2001).

Avoidance Coping

Another form of emotion-focused coping is avoidance coping, such as denying or avoiding thinking about a problem to take your mind off it (Roth & Cohen, 1986; Suls & Fletcher, 1985). Although avoiding problems can be adaptive for short-term stressors, such as a blind date or job interview, in the case of longer-term and more severe stresses, avoidance coping can have negative consequences (Carver et al., 1993; Classen, Koopman, Angell, & Spiegel, 1996; Penley, Tomaka, & Wiebe, 2002). For example, women who have breast cancer and rely on avoidance coping prior to their surgery show higher levels of negative affect after their surgery than those who use other coping strategies (Stanton & Snider, 1993). In this case, emotion-focused

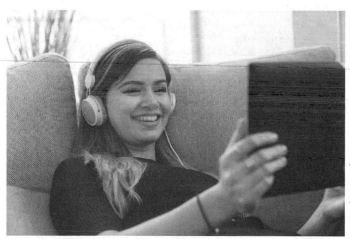

Finding some humor in a stressful situation is literally good for your health.

© iStockphoto.com/JGalione

strategies such as wishful thinking (e.g., "hoped a miracle would happen") are detrimental, perhaps because their use interferes with effective cognitive processing and problem solving directed toward those decisions. Avoiding thinking about a traumatic event also prevents individuals from understanding and ultimately coming to terms with the experience (Pennebaker, 1989; Wegner, 1994). The use of denial or distraction can also lead people to delay seeking medical care in response to various health symptoms, which can have serious consequences (as discussed in *Chapter 13: Managing Health Care*).

Moreover, deliberately trying to avoid thinking about negative events is very difficult and thus requires considerable effort (Pennebaker, 1989). Have you ever tried to *not* think about something (an ex-boyfriend, a particularly gruesome scene from a movie, a failed test) and then found that thoughts about this "forbidden" topic dominate your mind? Research by Dan Wegner and his colleagues (1990) reveals that constantly exerting effort to avoid thinking about something upsetting leads to chronic physiological arousal, which can lead to decreases in immune cell activity as well as higher blood pressure and heart rate (Pennebaker, Hughes, & O'Heeron, 1987; Petrie, Booth, & Pennebaker, 1998).

Conclusions

In sum, most research now suggests that both problem-focused and emotion-focused coping can be effective, as long as they are used to cope with specific types of problems. Specifically, while problem-focused coping is very effective in the case of stressors that you can change by actively confronting them, in cases in which you have no opportunity for improving the situation, the use of problem-focused coping may lead to feelings of frustration and disappointment (Roth & Cohen, 1986). On the other hand, while emotion-focused coping can be detrimental if you simply refuse to try to fix a manageable problem, this approach may be very effective when there is little that can be done to change a negative situation (Terry & Hynes, 1998). For example, you may need to use problem-focused coping when trying to constructively resolve a conflict with your dating partner but must use emotion-focused coping if your efforts to solve the problem fail and the relationship ultimately ends. People who cope with events using the "right" type of strategy therefore experience fewer symptoms of anxiety and depression (Forsythe & Compas, 1987; Terry & Hynes, 1998). Because different types of situations call for different types of coping, individuals who are comfortable using a number of different coping styles have a higher likelihood of minimizing their stress in a variety of challenging situations.

THE POWER OF SOCIAL SUPPORT

LO 5.2

Examine how social support influences the experience of stress and predicts health outcomes

Many people rely on support from family members and friends, especially during difficult times. And as you'll learn in this section, social support plays a very important role in helping people manage the small and large stresses in daily life. Social support also has a substantial impact on both psychological and physical well-being.

Types of Social Support

Although the term **social support** describes general help that people may receive, we can actually receive very different types of support (Cohen, 1988; House, 1981; House & Kahn, 1985). For example, college students may receive financial support from their parents or guardians, emotional support from their friends, and academic support from professors. You can use **Table 5.2: Test Yourself** to measure the different types of support you receive.

Table 5.2 Test Yourself: What Types of Social Support Do You Receive?

Please rate whether each of the following items is true or false.

1. If I had to go out of town for a few weeks, someone I know would look after my home, such as watering the plants or taking care of the pets.

2. If I were sick and needed someone to drive me to the doctor, I would have trouble finding someone.

3. If I were sick, I would have trouble finding someone to help me with my daily chores.

4. If I needed help moving, I would be able to find someone to help me.

5. If I needed a place to stay for a week because of an emergency, such as the water or electricity being out in my home, I could easily find someone who would put me up.

6. There is at least one person I know whose advice I really trust.

7. There is no one I know who will tell me honestly how I am handling my problems.

8. When I need suggestions about how to deal with a personal problem, there is someone I can turn to.

9. There isn't anyone I feel comfortable talking to about intimate personal problems.

10. There is no one I trust to give me good advice about money matters.

11. I am usually invited to do things with others.

12. When I feel lonely, there are several people I could talk to.

13. I regularly meet or talk with my friends or members of my family.

14. I often feel left out by my circle of friends.

15. There are several different people I enjoy spending time with.

Give yourself one point for each of the following items answered true: 1, 4, 5, 6, 8, 11, 12, 13, 15, and one point for each of the following items answered false: 2, 3, 7, 9, 10, 14. Then, sum up your scores on items 1 to 5 to assess tangible support, items 6 to 10 to assess appraisal support, and items 11 to 15 to assess belongingness support.

Source: Cohen, Mermelstein, Kamarck, & Hoberman (1985).

Emotional support describes the expression of caring, concern, and empathy for a person as well as the provision of comfort, reassurance, and love to that person. Most people who are confronted with stressful life events want to be able to talk about these events with others, and having a "listening ear" can be very valuable. One study of cancer patients found that more than 90% saw emotional support as one of the most valuable types of support (Dunkel Schetter, 1984; Dunkel Schetter & Wortman, 1982). Similarly, college students may need emotional support to cope with the stress of a relationship breakup, a poor exam grade, or the divorce of their parents.

Belongingness support is similar to emotional support in that it too includes a focus on being able to talk to others, but this type of support refers primarily to the availability of social companionship (Cohen et al., 1985). People are interested in having others with whom they can engage in social activities, such as going out to dinner, seeing a movie, and attending a party. People who are unemployed—and hence lose one valuable type of social integration—particularly benefit from having belongingness support, and they experience more psychological symptoms when they do not have this type of support (Cutrona & Russell, 1990).

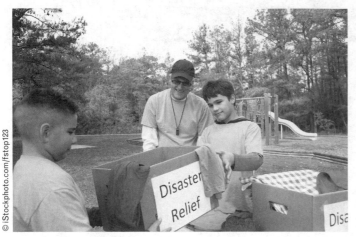

Instrumental, or tangible, support is particularly valuable for victims of natural disasters, who often need considerable assistance in restoring and/or rebuilding their homes, belongings, and community.

Instrumental, or *tangible*, *support* refers to the provision of concrete assistance, such as financial aid, material resources, or needed services. For example, you may need instrumental support from your parents to pay for textbooks and from your friends to help carry your belongings when you move to a new apartment. Victims of natural disasters, such as hurricanes, floods, and earthquakes, are particularly in need of tangible support (Kaniasty & Norris, 1995; Norris & Kaniasty, 1996).

Informational, or *appraisal*, *support* refers to advice and guidance about how to cope with a particular problem. For example, you may depend on your professors for this type of support when you are trying to find a summer internship and depend on your friends for such support when choosing classes to take. Victims of natural disasters, who need advice about how to organize cleanup efforts and arrange to receive government aid, also benefit from this type of support.

People also benefit from receiving *esteem*, or *validational*, *support*, meaning the affirmation of self-worth. This type of support gives a person feedback that he or she is valued and respected by others. One study on long-term recovery from heart surgery found that patients who believed they received considerable esteem support from their spouses had the highest levels of emotional well-being and were the least likely to experience disruption of their everyday lives (e.g., problems with social interaction, recreational activities, sleep, walking) or symptoms of heart trouble even as long as one year after surgery (King, Reis, Porter, & Norsen, 1993).

Although this section has described the different types of social support that can be provided, all of these types are not interchangeable. According to the **matching hypothesis**, individuals benefit from receiving the type of social support that fits their particular problem (Cohen & Wills, 1985; Cutrona & Russell, 1990). Specifically, in the case of controllable events, meaning those that can be solved or fixed, people benefit most from receiving practical types of support. For example, instrumental support is associated with better psychological and physical well-being for new parents, who are struggling with caring for an infant and may therefore appreciate offers of food, childcare, or housecleaning. On the other hand, in the case of uncontrollable events, such as the loss of a spouse, practical types of support will not be as effective because they will not help people solve or eliminate the stressor. Emotional support should therefore be more valuable in these cases. In support of this view, breast cancer patients benefit from having emotional support but not from instrumental support (Helgeson & Cohen, 1996). This research all points to the importance of receiving the "right type" of support for a given problem.

Moreover, the type of social support people find most useful may vary based on their culture. For example, Asians and Asian Americans benefit more from implicit social support, meaning support that is provided simply through the awareness of one's connection to a broader social network, whereas European Americans benefit more from explicit support, meaning support that is provided through a direct request for assistance (Taylor, Welch, Kim, & Sherman, 2007). People may particularly benefit from social support that is in line with culturally valued norms. One study of Latina women with arthritis revealed a strong reliance on family members, and especially daughters, for support, whereas people from more individualistic cultures may rely more on friends (Abraído-Lanza & Revenson, 1996). Similarly, social support buffers the role of perceived stress on mental and physical health among Mexican Americans but not among members of other racial groups (Shavitt et al., 2016).

In sum, while social support in general is valuable, the benefit of such support varies as a function of culture.

Benefits of Social Support

Having greater social support is associated with a variety of positive health outcomes. In fact, social support may play as large a role in predicting physical health as eating healthy foods and engaging in regular exercise (Yang, Boen, Gerken, Li, Schorpp, & Harris, 2016). The effects of having high-quality relationships may even be quite long-lasting; one recent longitudinal study revealed that having close friendships during the teenage years is associated with better physical health in adulthood, even when researchers take into account factors such as income, BMI, and drug use (Allen, Uchino, & Hafen, 2015). This section will describe the impact of social support on various aspects of health, including preventing illness, coping with illness, recovering from surgery, and, most important, predicting life expectancy. Next, it will describe the value of receiving diverse types of support as well as the benefits of giving social support.

Preventing Illness

People with high-quality social support are less likely to experience both minor and major health problems. For example, college students who have more and higher-quality social interactions have fewer health problems and visits to the campus infirmary (Reis, Wheeler, Kernis, Spiegel, & Nezlek, 1985). People who are gay, lesbian, or bisexual and feel accepted by others are more likely to come out, which in turn predicts experiencing fewer physical symptoms (e.g., stomach pain, headaches; Legate, Ryan, & Rogge, 2017). Higher levels of social support also seem to protect people against more serious health problems. People with poor social relationships are more likely to develop coronary heart disease and to have a stroke (Berkman, 1985; Blumenthal et al., 1987; Valtorta, Kanaan, Gilbody, Ronzi, & Hanratty, 2016). Similarly, men who receive low levels of social support are twice as likely to have high levels of prostate-specific antigen (PSA), a marker of prostate cancer, as those with high levels of support (Stone, Mezzacappa, Donatone, & Gonder, 1999).

What explains the link between more social support and better health? One possibility is that support changes physiological reactions in the body (Kennedy, Kiecolt-Glaser, & Glaser, 1990; Uchino, Cacioppo, & Kiecolt-Glaser, 1996; Uchino, Uno, & Holt-Lunstad, 1999). In line with this view, people with higher levels of social support have lower heart rates and blood pressure (Bland, Krogh, Winkelstein, & Trevisan, 1991; Linden, Chambers, Maurice, & Lenz, 1993; Undén, Orth-Gomér, & Elofsson, 1991; Whisman, 2010). For example, college students who complete various stressful arithmetic tasks in the presence of a friend have a lower heart rate than those who complete these tasks alone (Kamarck, Manuck, & Jennings, 1990).

People with higher levels of social support also have more effective immune systems and hence are better able to fight off major and minor illnesses (Jaremka et al., 2013; Jemmott & Locke, 1984; Jemmott & Magliore, 1988; Uchino et al., 1996). For example, lesbian, gay, and bisexual young adults who receive higher levels of family support show a reduced cortisol response to stressors (Burton, Hatzenbuehler, & Bonanno, 2014). Individuals who have a larger social network are even more resistant to the common cold (Cohen, Doyle, Skoner, Rabin, & Gwaltney, 1997; Cohen & Herbert, 1996).

Coping With Illness

People with high levels of social support recover more quickly from illnesses when they do get sick. For example, those with greater social support recover more rapidly from kidney disease (Dimond, 1979), leukemia (Magni, Silvestro, Tamiello, Zanesco, & Carl, 1988), and stroke (Robertson & Suinn, 1968). They are also better able to cope with serious illnesses, including cancer, diabetes, and HIV (Gremore et al., 2011; Manne, Ostroff, Winkel, Grana, & Fox, 2005). For example, HIV-positive men who are satisfied with the social support they have received are less likely to be depressed one year later and show higher levels of T cell counts (a marker of immune system strength) as long as five years later (Hays, Turner, & Coates, 1992; Theorell et al., 1995).

Recovering From Surgery

Not surprisingly, social support helps people cope with the major stressor of surgery. Among individuals who are undergoing surgery, those who receive higher levels of social support experience less pain, use less pain medication, show a faster recovery time from surgery, and are less likely to have to return to the hospital for complications post-surgery (Helgeson, 1991; Kulik & Mahler, 1989). One study found that people with high levels of social support showed less anxiety, received lower doses of narcotics, and were released from the hospital 1.42 days faster than those with lower levels of support (Krohne & Slangen, 2005). For pregnant women, greater social support is associated with fewer complications during delivery, less use of anesthetics, and a shorter overall labor (Kennell, Klaus, McGrath, Robertson, & Hinckley, 1991; Sosa, Kennell, Klaus, Robertson, & Urrutia, 1980).

Life Expectancy

Most important, greater social support is associated with lower rates of mortality (Giles, Glonek, Luszcz, & Andrews, 2005; Kaplan et al., 1988; Welin et al., 1985). The first published study on the link between social support and mortality was conducted by Berkman and Syme (1979), who collected data on social support and physical health from a representative sample of nearly 7,000 men and women living in Alameda County, California, in 1965. Researchers then collected mortality data from 1965 to 1974 to examine death rates as a function of social ties. At every age, people who lacked social ties were two to three times more likely to die during this period than those with social ties, and greater social support reduced the risk of each of the separate causes of death, including heart disease, cancer, and circulatory disease. This study therefore provides compelling evidence about the importance of social relationships.

Other research supports this finding that greater social support is associated with increased longevity. In one study, researchers examined the effects of social ties, meaning connections to a broader social network, on rates of both mortality and on coronary heart disease in 28,369 male health professionals (Eng, Rimm, Fitzmaurice, & Kawachi, 2002). Over a 10-year follow-up, the risk of mortality for men with fewer social ties was significantly higher than that in more socially integrated men, even after controlling for age, occupation, health behaviors, general physical condition, coronary risk factors, and dietary habits. For example, men with a moderately low number of social ties were more than twice as likely to die from accidents and suicides than men with the highest number of social connections. Other research has shown similar findings with women (House, Robbins, & Metzner, 1982). These findings help explain why married people live longer than unmarried people (Liu, 2009), why people who are married live longer following a stroke than those who are unmarried (Dupre & Lopes, 2016), and why twice as many single people die from coronary heart disease as married people (Schwarzer & Leppin, 1992).

The association between social support and life expectancy is found even in people who are critically ill (Berkman, Leo-Summers, & Horowitz, 1992; Ruberman, Weinblatt, Goldberg, & Chaudhary, 1984). One study of over 1,000 heart disease patients found that those with greater social support, as defined by having a spouse or close confidant, had lower rates of mortality (Williams et al., 1992). Eighty-two percent of those who were married or had a close confidant lived for at least five years, compared to only 50% of those without such support. Similarly, people who have cancer survive longer if they have extensive social support, either from friends and family members or through a support group (Helgeson, Cohen, & Fritz, 1998; Spiegel & Kato, 1996). One study of breast cancer patients, for example, found that women who participated in a support group lived for an average of 36.6 months following the intervention versus 18.9 months for those in the control group (Spiegel, Kraemer, Bloom, & Gottheil, 1989). However, other research has not replicated these findings (Goodwin et al., 2001). (You'll learn more about the role of social support in helping people cope with chronic illness in *Chapter 10: Understanding and Managing Chronic Illness*.)

The Value of Diverse Types of Support

Although most of the research on the link between social support and health has examined the importance of such support from a spouse or close friend, support in general is what is important, not support from a particular person. One study of over 5,000 American adults over four years found that people who felt more connected to their neighbors—including feeling like they were a part of their neighborhood, that the neighbors were friendly, and that they had neighbors who would help them if they got into trouble—were less likely to experience a heart attack (Kim, Hawes, & Smith, 2014). In fact, even when the researchers took into account other factors (such as sociodemographic, behavioral, biological, and psychosocial factors), every increase in feelings of neighborhood cohesion—which was measured on a seven-point scale—was associated with a 17% reduction in risk of experiencing a heart attack.

What You'll Learn
5.1

As pet lovers will not be surprised to learn, even social support from our pets can reduce feelings of stress and thereby lead to better psychological and physical well-being (McConnell, Brown, Shoda, Stayton, & Martin, 2011). In line with this view, pet owners who take a math test in the presence of their pet experience lower heart rates and blood pressure reactivity than those whose pets are not present (Allen, Blasovich, & Mendes, 2002). People with pets have fewer doctor visits: those who had experienced many stressful events and did not have a pet had an average of 10.37 doctor visits during the year compared to 8.38 for pet owners (Siegel, 1990). Interestingly, the effect between pet ownership and doctor visits was true only for those who owned a dog; having a cat or a bird did not seem to produce the same beneficial effects. As shown in Figure 5.1, having a dog is even linked with an increased likelihood of survival after experiencing a heart attack.

The Value of Giving Social Support

Interestingly, giving social support may also lead to better health. One study that followed older couples over five years revealed that people who reported providing no instrumental or emotional support to others were more than twice as likely to die over the next five years as those who gave such support (to friends, spouses, relatives, neighbors) (Brown, Nesse, Vinokur, & Smith, 2003). This effect remained even when researchers considered other factors, such as age, health, and income, suggesting that giving support may in fact be good for your health. **Research in Action** describes how giving support to other people may help buffer the negative effects of daily life stress.

The Downside of Social Support

This section has, understandably, focused on the numerous ways in which social support may lead to better health. In some cases, however, social support can have negative implications for psychological and physical well-being. People sometimes receive social support that is intended to be helpful but is actually detrimental in terms of health (Dakof & Taylor, 1990;

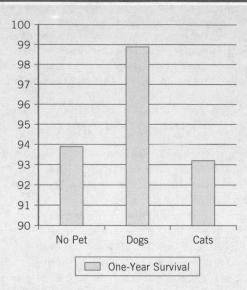

Figure 5.1 Data From Friedmann and Thomas, 1995

One year after experiencing a heart attack, people who owned at least one dog were significantly more likely to be alive than those who had no pet or owned a cat. Can you think of some explanations for why owning a dog seemed to be better for your health than owning a cat?

Source: Data from Friedmann & Thomas (1995).

Thoits, Hohmann, Harvey, & Fletcher, 2000; Wortman & Lehman, 1985). For example, if you are depressed about a recent relationship breakup, friends may encourage you to "drown your sorrows" by drinking alcohol, which obviously is not a great strategy for enhancing your health. Similarly, people can give unwanted advice, discourage open discussion of the problem, or push for a too-rapid recovery following an illness or negative event (Dakof & Taylor, 1990; Dunkel Schetter & Wortman, 1982). In fact, people who experience more problematic, or undermining, social support are at greater risk of experiencing coronary heart disease (Davis & Swan, 1999). Similarly, although in general people who are married show better health outcomes than those who are unmarried, the quality of the marriage also matters; patients who undergo heart surgery and are high in marital satisfaction are three times as likely to be alive 15 years later as those in low-satisfaction marriages (King & Reis, 2012). These findings indicate that it isn't just the presence of social relationships that helps promote good health, but rather the quality of these relationships. As described in ***Chapter 6: Injury and Injury Prevention***, physical, sexual, and/or emotional violence from an intimate partner can cause both minor and major injuries.

Explaining the Social Support–Health Link

Although research consistently indicates a strong link between social support and health, the precise mechanism leading to this association is less clear. Specifically, some researchers believe that social support is beneficial primarily when people are feeling tremendous stress, whereas others believe that support is generally useful across all daily life situations. Let's examine these two hypotheses.

RESEARCH IN ACTION

Why Giving Support Is a Good Idea

Although this section has focused on the benefits of receiving social support, some recent research shows that giving social support—to friends, acquaintances, and even strangers—can reduce the negative impact of stress on mental health. In one study, researchers asked people to report their feelings and experiences in daily life every day for two weeks (Raposa, Laws, & Ansell, 2016). This report included any stressful life events they had experienced as well as whether they had engaged in any type of helping behavior (e.g., holding a door open for someone, helping someone with homework). Their findings revealed that people who had given more help to others reported higher levels of positive emotions and better overall mental health. The benefits of providing such help were particularly strong on days in which people experienced the most stress; in fact, those who reported not helping much in a given day had more negative emotions in response to experiencing high daily stress, whereas those who reported more helping had no such increases following high stress. Additional support for the value of giving social support is found in research showing that giving support activates parts of the brain that process reward and not in parts of the brain that process stress (Inagaki et al., 2016). In sum, giving social support to other people may be another effective way of coping with stress.

Buffering Hypothesis

As described in ***Chapter 4: Understanding Stress***, as a person experiences repeated stressors and their accompanying physiological reactions, his or her body may experience a state of *allostatic load*, which leads to great susceptibility to illness and disease. According to the **buffering hypothesis**, social support provides a buffer from such daily life stress, which in turn protects people from the negative health-related consequences of stress, such as increases in blood pressure, cortisol, and depression (Wills, 1985) (see Figure 5.2). For example, when one spouse is particularly busy at work, the other spouse may do more housework and "pick up the slack" to reduce his or her partner's responsibilities and thereby reduce the spouse's experience of stress. Similarly, although adolescents show more negative mood and physical symptoms on days in which they experience more stress, those who feel supported by their parents show fewer negative effects of stress (Lippold, Davis, McHale, Buxton, & Almeida, 2016).

Considerable research provides support for the buffering hypothesis by showing that the benefits of social support are greatest for people who are experiencing high levels of stress, including people who have a chronic disease (Baek, Tanenbaum, & Gonzalez, 2014; Hays et al., 1992), are experiencing natural disasters (Fleming, Baum, Gisriel, & Gatchel, 1982; Kaniasty & Norris, 1993), or have low income (Shankar, McMunn, Demakakos, Hamer, & Steptoe, 2017). For example, having a supportive spouse buffers the negative effects of socioeconomic stress on blood pressure, thereby reducing the risk for cardiovascular disease (Cundiff, Birmingham, Uchino, & Smith, 2016).

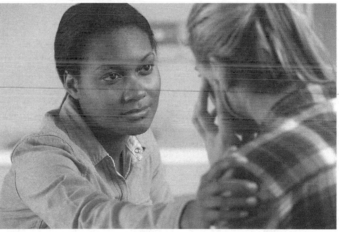

© iStockphoto.com/monkeybusinessimages

Emotional support, such as listening, comforting, and providing reassurance, is particularly valuable during times of high stress.

Figure 5.2   Models of the Buffering and Direct Effects Hypotheses

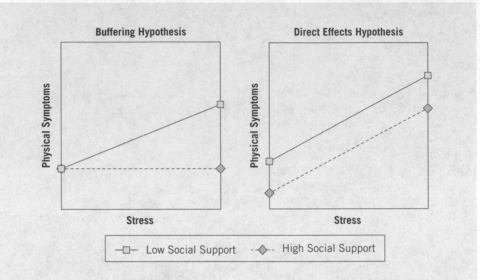

The buffering hypothesis suggests that social support is particularly beneficial to health during times of stress, whereas the direct effects hypothesis suggests that social support is always beneficial.

Source: Created by Catherine A. Sanderson.

Similarly, for low-income Mexican American women, higher levels of economic stress predict higher cortisol levels, but only if they receive low levels of family support (Jewell, Luecken, Gress-Smith, Crnic, & Gonzales, 2015).

One explanation for how social support may buffer people from stress is that those with high levels of social support think about difficult situations in a more positive way. Because they know that others will provide help to them during times of need, they perceive potentially stressful events as less impactful. For example, a person who receives little support from a spouse may see the loss of employment as a very negative event posing substantial problems for the family, whereas someone who receives high levels of support from a spouse could interpret the loss of a job as a somewhat negative event, but also as an opportunity to investigate a new career path; the loss of a job might then be perceived as less stressful. In line with this view, women with breast cancer who receive high levels of social support show lower levels of stress and higher levels of posttraumatic growth (meaning they are able to find some benefit in their experience) and subjective well-being (McDonough, Sabiston, & Wrosch, 2014).

Higher levels of social support may also help people cope more effectively with potentially stressful events. People who have support from friends and family may have more resources to cope with the stressful events and may therefore see these events as less problematic. If your car breaks down and you can't get to work, having a friend who will drive you or loan you a car could substantially reduce your concern about this car trouble. In line with this view, people who receive more social support following a natural disaster show lower levels of psychological distress, including symptoms of depression and PTSD, later on, in part because the presence of such support reduces the experience of stress (Chan, Lowe, Weber, & Rhodes, 2015; Paul et al., 2015). Similarly, although in general men who experience many stressful life events have greater mortality over the next decade, this effect is actually found only for those who have received low levels of emotional support; apparently, receiving high levels of emotional support buffers these men from the negative health consequences of stressful life events (Rosengren, Orth-Comer, Wedel, & Wilhelmsen, 1993).

Having high levels of social support may help people adopt healthier behaviors. For example, people with high levels of social support are better able to stop smoking because the presence of this support reduces their stress during quit attempts (Bandiera, Atem, Ma, Businelle, & Kendzor, 2016). Smokers with greater social support are also less likely to relapse after quitting smoking, presumably because this support helps buffer the effect of difficult withdrawal symptoms (Creswell, Cheng, & Levine, 2015).

The positive effects of supportive relationships are quite long-lasting. For example, college students who report having had difficult childhoods—meaning a lack of warmth from their parents and/or caregivers—show higher levels of cortisol on days in which they experience more stressful events (Miller & Chen, 2010). In contrast, for students who had more positive childhood environments, lower levels of cortisol were found on days in which they experienced more stress. This finding suggests that having a supportive childhood environment has lasting benefits in terms of individuals' ability to manage stress in later life.

Direct Effects Hypothesis

Although the buffering hypothesis suggests that social support benefits health only during times of high stress, other researchers believe that social support benefits health regardless of level of stress (Wills, 1985). According to this perspective, individuals benefit from having social support during times of low stress as well as high stress. This **direct effects hypothesis** posits that having high levels of social support is always advantageous to health. For example, you may be helped by having emotional support from your friends when you are under a lot of stress at exam time, but you may also be helped from having this support during low-stress times.

In line with this hypothesis, people with good social relationships consistently show better health-related behavior, regardless of level of stress (Stroebe & Stroebe, 1996). People with more social support consume fewer alcoholic drinks, are less likely to smoke and engage in risky sexual behavior, and are more likely to wear a seat belt (Barrera, Chassin, & Rogosch, 1993; Businelle et al., 2010; Cohen & Lemay, 2007; Darbes & Lewis, 2005). Individuals with high levels of social support are also more likely to use health care services (Wallston, Alagna, DeVellis, & DeVellis, 1983), adhere to medical regimens (Christensen et al., 1992; Gonzalez et al., 2004; Wallston et al., 1983), self-manage chronic conditions (Brody, Kogan, Murry, Chen, & Brown, 2008), and follow recommended cancer screenings (Messina et al., 2004). One meta-analysis revealed that across different types of medical regimens, patients with cohesive families are 1.74 times more likely to adhere, whereas those from families in conflict are 1.53 times less likely to adhere (DiMatteo, 2004).

As described previously, people with high levels of social support also show important physiological changes within their bodies. For example, people who report receiving more social support from family, friends, and spouses are less likely to show markers of inflammation, which is associated with the development of many serious health conditions, including cardiovascular disease, diabetes, dementia, and arthritis (Yang, Schorpp, & Harris, 2014). High levels of social support are also associated with changes in part of the brain that are associated with social and emotional processing, suggesting that receiving support helps people more effectively manage their feelings in the face of stressful life experiences (Sherman, Cheng, Fingerman, & Schnyer, 2015).

Conclusions

Although this section has described two competing models describing the social support–health link, some research provides support for both explanations. For example, researchers in one study measured levels of stress, social support, companionship, and physical symptoms in over 1,000 California residents (Rook, 1987). This study distinguished between *social support*, defined as having people to talk to about personal issues, help with household tasks, and consult when making important decisions, and *social companionship*, defined as having people with whom to eat meals, visit, and engage in recreational activities. The findings indicate that social support assisted people in times of stress (in line with the buffering hypothesis), whereas social companionship led to positive well-being regardless of stress levels (in line with the direct effects hypothesis). This work suggests that researchers must distinguish between practical types of support, such as direct help with problem solving and assistance with tasks, which may be particularly beneficial to health when people are experiencing stress, and companionate support, such as listening to people's problems and providing emotional support, which may be beneficial to health in general.

THE INFLUENCE OF RELIGION AND SPIRITUALITY

LO 5.3

Describe how religion and spirituality influence health as well as various explanations for this association

Religion plays a very important role in the lives of many people. A large-scale survey of Americans conducted in 2014 revealed that 89% of people say they believe in God and 77% describe themselves as affiliated with some type of formal religion (Pew Research Center, 2015). About half of all Americans engage regularly in some type of religious activity, such as praying daily (55%) or attending services at least monthly (50%). Although some people distinguish between religiosity—a formal link to religious organizations—and spirituality—a personal orientation toward religious beliefs—most people see these two concepts as quite similar. This section will examine the link between religious and spiritual beliefs and health and then offer several explanations for this association.

The Religion/Spirituality–Health Link

People who are involved in religion experience better psychological health (Bergin, Masters, & Richards, 1987; Koenig, McCullough, & Larson, 2001; McFadden, 1995; Nicholson, Rose, & Bobak, 2010). For example, among people who are caregivers for

FOCUS ON NEUROSCIENCE

How Religious and Spiritual Beliefs Change the Brain

To examine how having religious and spiritual beliefs helps protect against depression, researchers recruited adults who were either at high or low risk of developing depression based on their family history (Miller et al., 2013). Participants were placed in an MRI machine to test their brain structure and activity and asked how important their religious or spiritual beliefs were to them. The findings indicated that people who placed a higher importance on such beliefs also had a greater thickness in the brain cortex, which is the same part of the brain that shows thinning in people who are at high risk of depression. Thus, people with religious or spiritual beliefs may protect themselves from the natural cortical thinning that occurs in those at risk of developing depression. In other words, holding such beliefs may counteract the thinning that would otherwise be expected, particularly among those with a family history of depression.

people with Alzheimer's disease or cancer (a potentially very stressful situation), those who have strong religious beliefs are less likely to experience depression (Rabins, Fitting, Eastham, & Zabora, 1990). As described in **Focus on Neuroscience**, holding religious or spiritual beliefs seems to change the brain in ways that protect against depression.

Moreover, religious involvement, such as attending religious services and holding strong religious beliefs, is associated with better health, including lower levels of cancer, heart disease, stroke, and suicide (Levin, 1994; McCullough, Hoyt, Larson, Koenig, & Thoresen, 2000). People with stronger religious beliefs also have fewer complications and shorter hospital stays following heart surgery (Contrada et al., 2004). This general finding about the link between religious beliefs and good health holds for all different types of religious and spiritual beliefs. For example, Jewish Americans of every denomination who participate actively in their faith report significantly better health than Jews who are secular or nonpracticing (Levin, 2015).

What You'll Learn
5.2

Most important, people who have strong religious faith have a longer life expectancy (George, Ellison, & Larson, 2002; Lutgendorf, Russell, Ullrich, Harris, & Wallace, 2004; McCullough et al., 2000). In one study, researchers examined data from over 74,000 women, who answered questionnaires about their diet, lifestyle, and health every two years and about their religious service attendance every four years (Li, Stampfer, Williams, & VanderWeele, 2016). Compared with women who never attended religious services, those who attended more than once per week had 33% lower mortality risk during the 16-year study period and lived an average of five months longer, even when researchers took into account a variety of other factors, such as diet, physical activity, alcohol consumption, smoking status, body mass index, social integration, depression, race, and ethnicity. Those who attended weekly had a 26% lower risk and those who attended less than once a week had a 13% lower risk, and this behavior lowered their risk of both cardiovascular mortality (27%) and cancer mortality (21%). Similarly, open heart surgery patients who experienced strength and comfort from their religious beliefs were less likely to die in the six months following surgery (Oxman, Freeman, & Manheimer, 1995). These findings provide powerful evidence for the link between religiosity and longevity.

Although religiosity and spirituality are generally associated with good health, they also can have some drawbacks (Koenig et al., 2001). Some religions, such as Jehovah's Witnesses and Christian Scientists, forbid some types of medical care, including blood transfusions and immunizations. For example, Jehovah's Witnesses believe that there is no distinction in God's eyes between having a blood transfusion and drinking someone else's blood, and therefore anyone who receives a transfusion will be "turned away" from eternal salvation. People with strong religious beliefs may also delay seeking medical care or refuse lifesaving medications and procedures because they believe prayer and other religious methods of managing illnesses will lead to positive outcomes. In line with this view, one study demonstrated that one reason why more Black women die from breast cancer than White women is because some of their cultural beliefs lead them to delay seeking medical care (Lannin et al., 1998). For example, Black women are much more likely than White women to believe that "if a person prays about cancer, God will heal it without medical treatments." In sum, religious beliefs seem to have a beneficial effect on health only when these beliefs are used in conjunction with standard medical care, not as a replacement for such care, and in conjunction with other coping mechanisms.

Explaining the Religion/Spirituality–Health Link

What leads to this association between religious and/or spiritual beliefs and greater physical health (Koenig et al., 2001; Plante & Sherman, 2001; Seybold & Hill, 2001)? One explanation is that many religions directly encourage healthy behaviors, such as abstaining from smoking, alcohol/drug use, and risky sexual behaviors, which in turn leads to greater physical well-being (Gorsuch, 1995). The Mormon, Muslim, and Southern Baptist religions, for example, forbid the use of alcohol. In turn, one recent study revealed that the association between church attendance and better physical health is at least partially a function of the lower rates of substance abuse seen in those who attend church regularly (Koenig & Vaillant, 2009). Women who regularly attend religious services are also more likely to get regular mammograms and Pap smears and to perform breast self-exam (Benjamins, 2006). However, many of these studies control for—meaning they take into account—people's other health behaviors and still find an association between religion and health.

Another possibility is that substantial social support is provided within many religious communities, which in turn leads to greater health. People who are religious may belong to a church, temple, or other organization that brings them together on a regular basis with others who share their general views. One study found that 41% of community members reported they would use their clergy for help with personal problems (Pergament, 1997). In line with the view about the importance of social support, frequency of attendance at religious services is positively associated with health, whereas frequency of prayer is negatively associated with health (Nicholson et al., 2010). Religious groups may therefore serve as a type of self-help group and may benefit health in similar ways to other such groups, such as Alcoholics Anonymous.

A third possibility is that religion gives people a sense of meaning, which may in and of itself have beneficial effects on health (Emmons, 2005; Silberman, 2005). In one study, researchers examined changes in spirituality/religiousness following diagnosis of HIV and disease progression (as measured by T cells and level of HIV in the blood every six months) over four years (Ironson, Stuetzle, & Fletcher, 2006). People who reported an increase in spirituality/religiousness after the diagnosis had significantly higher levels of T cells over the four-year period, and these results held true even after controlling for other measures (including church attendance, initial disease status, use of medication, age, gender, race, education, health behaviors, depression, hopelessness, optimism, coping strategies, and social support). In sum, these findings suggest that an increase in spirituality/religiousness, a type of emotion-focused coping, after HIV diagnosis predicts slower disease progression.

Religious commitment may also lead people to rely on more adaptive coping mechanisms (Ai, Park, Huang, Rodgers, & Tice, 2007; Pargament, 1997). Many people use religion as a way of coping with potentially stressful events, including medical problems, accidents, and problems with loved ones (see Table 5.3; Pargament, 1997). For example, one study of

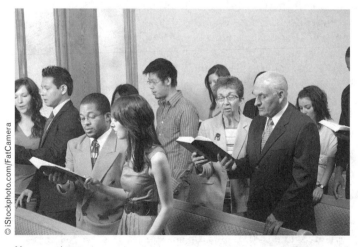

© iStockphoto.com/FatCamera

Many people report praying as a way of coping with stressful life events.

parents who had lost a baby to sudden infant death syndrome found that parents who felt that religion was important to them engaged in more cognitive processing about the experience, which in turn led to greater well-being later on (McIntosh, Silver, & Wortman, 1993). Similarly, among patients undergoing a heart procedure, those who were higher in religiosity were more likely to use positive religious coping—such as seeking spiritual support and God's love and care—which in turn was associated with less distress (Ai et al., 2007). Finally, people who have strong spiritual beliefs may benefit in terms of health because their religion provides some type of meaning for even seemingly senseless tragedies. Seeing the benefits of a negative experience gives people a chance to confront and cope with thoughts and feelings about the trauma but with a focus on its positive aspects, which in turn can lead to greater psychological and physical well-being.

Table 5.3 The Use of Religion to Cope With Traumatic Events

- "After the flight attendant explained emergency landing procedures, we were left with our thoughts. That's when I began praying. I closed my eyes and thought, "Dear Lord, I pray that you'll guide the pilot's hands." I also thought that if God wanted to take my life, that it was OK with me. I was full of peace. Here I was sitting on the edge of eternity. I wasn't facing the end of my life."

- "The plane smelled like a house after a fire. I was exhilarated to be alive but deeply grieved when I could see and smell death. It was like being at the doorstep of hell. I pulled my Bible out of my bag. That's all I wanted."

- "I did what I needed to do to prepare to die. My thought at the time was that I wanted to be reborn into a family where I would be able to hear the teachings of Buddha. I'd done a lot of Buddhist meditation in my life, and this trained me to become one-pointed in my awareness. I was totally focused on the brace position."

These quotes are from survivors of United Flight 232, which made a crash landing in a field in Iowa on its way from Denver to Chicago on July 19, 1989. As you can see, many passengers thought about their religious beliefs during this traumatic event.

Source: Created by Catherine A. Sanderson using data from Pargament K. I. (1997). *The psychology of religion and coping: Theory, research, practice.* New York, NY: Guilford.

Although most people see religiosity and spirituality as quite similar, recent research suggests that religion and spirituality influence health in distinct ways (Aldwin, Park, Jeong, & Nath, 2014). Specifically, religious beliefs and attendance seems to help people manage health-related behaviors, such as by lowering smoking rates and reducing alcohol consumption. Spirituality, on the other hand, seems to influence how people regulate their feelings, which in turn can have beneficial effects on such outcomes as blood pressure, cardiac responsiveness, and immune system functioning.

THE ROLE OF PERSONALITY

LO 5.4

Explain the impact of personality on the experience and management of stress

As soon as you meet someone for the first time, you notice what the person is like. Is she or he friendly, outgoing, and energetic, or is the person anxious, withdrawn, and fearful? If I ask you to describe your closest friends or your siblings, you can probably list a number of these types of personality traits, meaning basic characteristics of the person that are relatively stable across situations and over time. But why do people differ so much in terms of their personalities, and where do these traits come from? According to personality psychologists, at least some personality traits are strongly influenced by heredity (Eysenck, 1967; Izard, Libero, Putnam, & Haynes, 1993). This is why identical twins who are raised apart often show very clear similarities in their personalities, whereas children who are raised together but have no genes in common (e.g., adopted children) may show little or no resemblance in terms of personality to other members of their family. These traits are formed by people's experiences in the world, not just their biology; hence, our personalities reflect the environment in which we were raised. This section first examines how four personality factors are associated with psychological and physical well-being: positive states, conscientiousness, internal locus of control/hardiness, and negative states. Then, you'll learn different explanations for the link between personality and health.

Positive States

As described in *Chapter 1: Introduction*, a growing trend in psychology is to focus on positive emotions, such as happiness, joy, enthusiasm, and contentment (Seligman & Csikszentmihalyi, 2000). These **positive states** include extraversion (feelings of energy and sociability), positive affect (Costa & McCrae, 1980, 1992; Eysenck, 1967), and **optimism** (the expectation that good things will happen in the future and bad things will not (Peterson, 2000; Scheier & Carver, 1993; Snyder et al., 1996). Table 5.4, for example, illustrates how researchers might assess people's overall level of optimism.

Considerable research reveals that people who are high in positive emotions experience better psychological well-being (Costa & McCrae, 1980; Scheier & Carver, 1987). For example, women who are optimistic show lower levels of distress following breast cancer diagnosis (Carver et al., 1993), HIV-positive men who are optimistic are less worried about developing AIDS (Taylor et al., 1992), and people who are optimistic are less depressed following unsuccessful attempts at in vitro fertilization (Litt, Tennen, Affleck, & Klock, 1992). Researchers in one study examined how students, faculty, and staff coped with a school shooting (Vieselmeyer, Holguin, & Mezulis, 2017). People who were high on **resilience**, a character strength that allows an individual to grow and even thrive in the face of adversity, and **gratitude**, a tendency to appreciate the positive aspects of one's life, showed lower levels of posttraumatic stress, suggesting that they were better able to cope with a severely upsetting event.

What You'll Learn
5.3

People with generally positive mood states also experience better physical well-being: they have lower rates of both major and minor illnesses, including asthma, sore throats, flu, arthritis, ulcers, hypertension, diabetes, and even strokes and coronary heart disease (Friedman & Booth-Kewley, 1987a; Pressman & Cohen, 2005). For example, researchers in one study exposed people to a cold virus (using nasal drops) and then examined whether personality traits, including positive affect, protected people from becoming sick (Cohen, Alper, Doyle, Treanor, & Turner, 2006). As predicted, participants who were higher on positive affect were less likely to develop cold symptoms as assessed through either self-reported symptoms or mucus production. This association remained even when researchers considered other variables that could help explain susceptibility to colds, including age, sex, education, race, body mass, and overall health. Thus, this research provides powerful evidence that our moods may influence our likelihood of becoming sick.

Table 5.4   Sample Items From the Optimism Scale

1. In uncertain times, I usually expect the best.

2. If something can go wrong for me, it will.

3. I always look on the bright side of things.

4. I'm always optimistic about my future.

5. I hardly ever expect things to go my way.

6. Things never work out the way I want them to.

7. I'm a believer in the idea that "every cloud had a silver lining."

8. I rarely count on good things happening to me.

Items 2, 5, 6, and 8 are reverse-scored so that lower scores indicate greater optimism.

Source: Scheier & Carver (1985).

The benefits of positive mood states on physical well-being are found even among people with more serious illnesses. For example, following surgery for coronary heart disease, optimists recover more quickly, report lower pain intensity, and are less likely to be rehospitalized (Fitzgerald, Tennen, Affleck, & Pransky, 1993; Ronaldson, Poole, Kidd, Leigh, Jahangiri, & Steptoe, 2014; Scheier et al., 1989, 1999). Most important, people who are higher in positive states show longer life expectancy (Levy, Lee, Bagley, & Lippman, 1988; Reed, Kemeny, Taylor, Wang, & Visscher, 1994; Terracciano, Lockenhoff, Zonderman, Ferrucci, & Costa, 2008). In fact, researchers in one recent study found that compared to people who were the least optimistic, those who were most optimistic were less likely to die of cancer, heart disease, or stroke during the six-year study follow-up (Kim et al., 2017). The benefits of optimism remained even when researchers took into account other factors associated with life expectancy, such as high cholesterol, smoking, and exercise. People who explain events in an optimistic way are also less likely to die from accidental or violent causes than those without this beneficial explanatory style (Peterson, Seligman, Yurko, Martin, & Friedman, 1988).

However, and contrary to the impression you might get from folklore and popular psychology, you cannot heal yourself from serious disease simply by having a positive mind-set. Although some research suggests that positive affect is associated with longer survival in people who are HIV-positive and those with breast cancer (Levy et al., 1988; Moskowitz, 2003), most research finds no association between positive affect and longevity in patients with serious illness, presumably because emotions are likely to have no impact on survival for those who are quite far along in their illness progression.

Moreover, optimism can also have costs. Specifically, people who are unrealistically optimistic about their risk of various health problems may fail to protect themselves adequately from such problems (Weinstein, 1984, 1987). In fact, some research suggests that optimists have a higher mortality rate, perhaps because they are more careless about their health (Friedman et al., 1993; Martin et al., 2002). This is a case in which optimists' views that "it won't happen to me" can lead to risky health-related behavior, which in turn can have serious consequences. Thus, it may be that while optimism in general is good for health, too much optimism can be bad.

Conscientiousness

Conscientious people are hardworking, motivated, and persistent (McCrae & Costa, 1987). They show high levels of self-restraint (e.g., may write a term paper even when they'd rather be watching reality television) and focus intensely on their goals (e.g., may carefully choose summer internships that help them achieve their career ambitions). On the other hand, people who are low in conscientiousness are easygoing and somewhat disorganized; for example, they may have trouble deciding on a career path and meeting deadlines.

Considerable research indicates that conscientiousness is associated with better physical health (Kern & Friedman, 2008; Martin, Friedman, & Schwartz, 2007; Terracciano et al., 2008). One meta-analysis revealed that conscientiousness is negatively related to all risky health-related behaviors, including tobacco use, drugs, risky sex, violence, risky driving, and alcohol use, and positively associated with all health-promoting behaviors, including a healthy diet and exercise (Bogg & Roberts, 2004). Similarly, **Focus on Development** describes the powerful association between childhood personality traits and health-related behavior later on. As you'll learn in *Chapter 13: Managing Health Care*, conscientiousness is also associated with improved immune function in people living with HIV, perhaps in part because conscientious people are more likely to adhere to medical regimens and use active coping styles (O'Cleirigh, Ironson, Weiss, & Costa, 2007). Finally, and as you might expect, given their greater frequency of health-promoting behavior, conscientious people also live longer. In fact, for both men and women, those in the top 25% of conscientiousness are less likely to die at a given age than those who are in the bottom 25% of conscientiousness (Martin, Friedman, & Schwartz, 2007).

FOCUS ON DEVELOPMENT

Why Conscientious Kids Become Thin Adults

Researchers in one longitudinal study examined teachers' assessments of over 2,000 elementary school children's personality traits (including conscientiousness, extraversion, agreeableness, openness/intellect, and emotional stability) (Hampson, Edmonds, Goldberg, Dubanoski, & Hillier, 2013; Hampson, Goldberg, Vogt, & Dubanoski, 2006). For example, teachers were asked to indicate how a particular child ranked in terms of conscientiousness (e.g., *organized*, *dependable*, *self-disciplined*) compared to his or her peers. Forty years later, researchers contacted these now-grown children and examined their rates of health-related behaviors. Findings indicated that childhood personality traits were associated with health later on, including all four health outcomes: smoking, alcohol use, body mass index, and overall health. Findings revealed that children rated by their teachers as more conscientious had better global health status as adults, including lower rates of obesity, cholesterol, and risk for cardiovascular disease. This association was found even when researchers took into account other factors, such as ethnicity, socioeconomic status, gender, and other personality traits. These findings indicate that children who are conscientious—meaning organized, disciplined, and dependable—tend to adopt healthier habits as adults, which reduces their risk of disease and injury. In turn, children who are truthful, reliable, and hardworking live on average about two years longer than those who are described as impulsive and lacking in self-control (Friedman et al., 1993).

Internal Locus of Control/Hardiness

People vary considerably on the extent to which they believe they have control, or mastery, over their lives (Rotter, 1966). People who have a strong internal locus of control believe that their decisions and behaviors impact their outcomes, whereas those with an external locus of control believe they have little control over events and experiences in their lives (Abramson, Metalsky, & Alloy, 1989; Peterson, 2000; Peterson, Seligman, Yurko, Martin, & Friedman, 1998). For example, students who have an internal locus of control could explain a bad grade on an exam as being due to not enough studying, whereas those with an external locus of control might explain such a grade based on the trickiness of the test. Similarly, a person most likely to stay healthy in the face of stress shows high hardiness, meaning a commitment to goals and activities, a sense of control over what happens to him or her, and a view of stressful events as challenging rather than threatening (Kobasa, Maddi, & Kahn, 1982). Such individuals are committed to their work and their families and believe that what they do is important and under their own control. In fact, demanding situations can lead hardy people to perform particularly well. Table 5.5 provides some examples of perspectives of those high versus low in hardiness.

As discussed in *Chapter 4: Understanding Stress*, having a sense of control over events in one's life is an important predictor of health. Thus, not surprisingly, people who are hardy and those with an internal locus of control experience better psychological well-being (Florian, Mikulincer, & Taubman, 1995; Peterson, Seligman, & Vaillant, 1988). For example, people who believe they have control suffer less depression in response to major illnesses, such as kidney failure, coronary heart disease, and cancer (Helgeson, 1992; Marks, Richardson, Graham, & Levine, 1986; Taylor, Lichtman, & Wood, 1984). Similarly, cancer patients who have greater perceptions of control (over their illness, interpersonal relationships, and symptoms) are less depressed than those who have low perceived control (Thompson, Sobolew-Shubin, Galbraith, Schwankovsky, & Cruzen, 1993).

Feelings of control are also associated with improved physical well-being and longer life expectancy. One study examined levels of mastery—meaning a sense that you can

Table 5.5   Quotes From People Who Are High or Low in Hardiness

High Hardiness

- "I realize that setbacks are a part of the game. I've had 'em, I have them now, and I've got plenty more ahead of me. Seeing this—the big picture—puts it all in perspective, no matter how bad things get."

- "I had a sense of peace inside that assured me that this loss would pass just as all of life passes. . . . At the funeral I knelt in front of him and the same peace came over me. The next day I was out back chopping wood, just as three generations of family had done on this land before me."

- "The key to dealing with loss is not obvious. One must take the problem, the void, the loneliness, the sorrow, and put it on the back of your neck and use it as a driving force. Don't let such problems sit out there in front of you, blocking your vision. . . . Use hardships in a positive way."

Low Hardiness

- "I was certain I would die on the table . . . never wake up. . . . I felt sure it was the end. Then I woke up with a colostomy and figured I have to stay inside the house the rest of my life. Now I'm afraid to go back to the doctor's and keep putting off my checkups."

- "I was apprehensive all the time—he was sick for years and each day that I got out of bed, I was thinking that he was going to die. It was always in the back of my mind, always. Another fear I have is of falling. Therefore, I never go anywhere for fear I'll fall in a strange place."

- "I have arthritis and every day I feel stiffer than the day before. Simple jobs around the house look so big to me and I feel fatigued oftentimes before I begin them. Sometimes I stay in bed for much longer than I should and get up feeling worse. I worry too much. . . . Life has never been a rose garden."

These quotes illustrate differences in how people who are high in hardiness think about the potentially stressful events of their lives compared to those low in hardiness.

Source. Colerick (1985).

control your outcomes—in over 20,000 patients, and then health records over the next six years (Surtees, Wainwright, Luben, Khaw, & Day, 2006). Patients who were high in a sense of mastery showed lower rates of mortality from all causes, including cardiovascular disease and cancer. Similarly, researchers in one study examined quotes from baseball players that appeared in newspaper articles describing why the team won or lost (Peterson & Seligman, 1987). Men who gave internal, stable, and global explanations for bad events lived a shorter life, as did those who offered external, unstable, and specific explanations for good events. Having a perception of control may be particularly important for helping people cope—and thereby stay healthy—during times of high stress. For example, business executives who were low in hardiness and had experienced many stressful life events report experiencing high levels of illness; those who were high in hardiness remained healthy even when they experienced many stressful life events (Kobasa et al., 1982).

Negative States

Although thus far we've focused on personality factors that can lead to beneficial types of health-related behavior, other personality factors are associated with poor psychological and physical health. This section will describe the link between neuroticism (negative affect), Type A behavior, and hostility/disagreeableness and health.

Neuroticism (Negative Affect)

Neuroticism, or **negative affect**, is a broad personality dimension that refers to the tendency of some people to experience negative emotions, such as distress, anxiety, nervousness, fear, shame, anger, and guilt, often (Watson & Clark, 1984). Although everyone experiences these feelings at times, people who are high in negative affect are in a "bad mood" quite frequently. They are likely to worry about upcoming events, dwell on failures and shortcomings, and have a less favorable view of themselves and others.

People who are high in neuroticism describe experiencing a greater number of physical symptoms and illness, including cardiovascular problems, digestive problems, pain, and fatigue (Affleck, Tennen, Urrows, & Higgins, 1992; Costa & McCrae, 1987; Vassen, Røysamb, Nielsen, & Czajkowski, 2017). For example, college students who experience high levels of negative affect report more physical complaints, such as headaches, diarrhea, and sore throat (Watson, 1988; Watson & Pennebaker, 1989). Although cross-sectional research—meaning studies that rely on reports of personality and symptoms at the same point in time—can't determine whether neuroticism causes physical problems or whether physical symptoms cause negative feelings (or a third variable predicts both neuroticism and illness), longitudinal studies do reveal that people who are higher in negative affect at one time are more likely to report experiencing a variety of physical symptoms, including fatigue, dizziness, sleep disturbance, and energy loss, over time (Leventhal, Hansell, Diefenbach, Leventhal, & Glass, 1996).

Careful readers will note that much of the research described thus far shows merely that neuroticism is associated with *complaining* more about physical symptoms as opposed to actually *experiencing* more physical symptoms. However, research using more objective measures of health also shows such associations (Lahey, 2009; Wilson, Krueger, Gu, Bienias, Mendes de Leon, & Evans, 2005). People who are high in neuroticism are more likely to have a variety of health problems, including ulcers, chronic fatigue syndrome, headaches, nausea, asthma, arthritis, and coronary heart disease (Charles, Gatz, Kato, & Pedersen, 2008; Suls & Bunde, 2005; Watson, 1988; Watson & Pennebaker, 1989). Neuroticism is also associated with longevity. A longitudinal study of over 5,000 adults found that neuroticism is associated with greater mortality from cardiovascular disease, even after controlling for age, sex, and other risk factors (such as smoking and alcohol use) (Shipley, Weiss, Der, Taylor, & Deary, 2007). Similarly, cancer patients who are high on neuroticism have a 150% higher death rate than those who are low on neuroticism (Nakaya et al., 2006).

Type A Behavior

The **Type A behavior** pattern is characterized by three features (Friedman & Booth-Kewley, 1987b; Matthews, 1988). First, Type A people experience high levels of time urgency—they are irritated by and impatient with time delays and constantly try to do more than one thing at a time. If you walk and talk fast, interrupt slow speakers (or finish their sentences), race through yellow lights, and hate waiting in line, you may have a tendency toward Type A behavior. Second, Type As have a strong competitive drive and are focused on doing better than other people in all sorts of situations (work and play). For example, Type As engage in competitive leisure activities more than Type Bs—they may prefer playing tennis (in which there is a clear winner and loser) to doing aerobics (Kelly & Houston, 1985). Finally, Type As are quick to experience anger and may lash out at others in frustration.

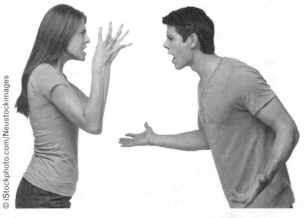

© iStockphoto.com/Neustockimages

People with certain personality traits, such as Type A behavior pattern and hostility, become angry with little provocation, which may lead to negative health outcomes.

As you can probably imagine, the type of behavioral tendencies Type A people show are linked with worse health (Friedman & Rosenman, 1974). For example, Type As report experiencing more minor illnesses, such as coughs, allergies, headaches, and asthma attacks, as well as more gastrointestinal problems, such as ulcers, indigestion, and nausea, than Type Bs (people without such behavioral tendencies) (Suls & Marco, 1990; Woods & Burns, 1984; Woods, Morgan, Day, Jefferson, & Harris, 1984). People with Type A behavior are also more likely to experience major health problems, including hypertension and heart attacks (Rosenman & Friedman, 1961; Suinn, 1975).

Although researchers often refer to "Type A behavior" as representing a single type of behavior, Type A behavior actually has three distinct types: impatience/speed, job involvement, and hard-driving. Moreover, the link between hostility and coronary heart disease is quite strong; the link between other components of Type A behavior and health is much weaker. In fact, some research suggests that people who are labeled Type A are simply expressive, efficient, and ambitious people who are coping well with their personal and professional lives and are not at increased risk of experiencing health problems (Friedman, Hall, & Harris, 1985). In contrast, and as we discuss next, "real Type As," namely, those who are tense, repressed, and hostile, are the ones most likely to experience physical problems.

Hostility/Disagreeableness

People who are high in **hostility/disagreeableness** have more negative moods and fewer positive moods (Cook & Medley, 1954; Smith, Pope, Sanders, Allred, & O'Keefe, 1988). But this personality trait focuses specifically on people's expectations about and interactions within their interpersonal relationships. People who are hostile or disagreeable believe that others are motivated by selfish concerns and expect that other people will deliberately try to hurt them (Miller, Smith, Turner, Guijarro, & Hallet, 1996) (see Table 5.6). In turn, because of their general mistrust and cynicism about other people's motivations, hostile people don't hesitate to express these feelings—they are often uncooperative, rude, argumentative, condescending, and aggressive.

Table 5.6 Sample Items From the Hostility-Guilt Inventory

1. Once in a while I cannot control my urge to harm others.
2. I can't help being a little rude to people I don't like.
3. When someone makes a rule I don't like I am tempted to break it.
4. Other people always seem to get the breaks.
5. I commonly wonder what hidden reason another person may have for doing something nice for me.
6. I can't help getting into arguments when people disagree with me.
7. Unless someone asks me in a nice way, I won't do what that person wants.
8. My motto is "Never trust strangers."
9. Whoever insults me or my family is asking for a fight.
10. If somebody annoys me, I am apt to tell him what I think of him.

This scale assesses a person's general level of hostility, including feelings of antagonism, cynicism, and aggression.

Source: Buss & Durkee (1957).

Hostility is associated with poorer health, including higher rates of hypertension and coronary heart disease as well as shorter life expectancy (Barefoot, Dodge, Peterson, Dahlstrom, & Williams, 1989; Jorgensen, Johnson, Kolodziej, & Schreer, 1996; Miller et al., 1996). One prospective study assessed hostility in 200 healthy women and then followed these women over 10 years (Matthews, Owens, Kuller, Sutton-Tyrrell, & Jansen-McWilliams, 1998). Even after controlling for variables such as smoking, women who had higher hostility scores in the earlier testing were more likely to show symptoms of cardiovascular disease 10 years later. Similarly, men who were high in hostility during young adulthood were five times more likely to develop coronary heart disease by the 30-year follow-up than those who were low in hostility (Barefoot, Dahlstrom, & Williams, 1983). They were also nearly seven times as likely to have died before the time of the follow-up. Although this study does not indicate why men who are hostile die at younger ages than those who are not hostile, it clearly suggests that hostility matters.

Explaining the Personality–Health Link

Thus far, we have examined the link between many different personality variables and psychological and physical well-being. However, we have not discussed the factors that may lead to this association. Do positive states directly enhance health, perhaps by improving our health-related behaviors, coping styles, or availability of social support? Alternatively, or perhaps additionally, are the health benefits of positive states good for our health because they influence how our bodies respond physiologically to stress, thus preventing harmful processes that lead to disease? This section describes several possible pathways that may account for the association between personality and health (see Figure 5.3).

Stress

First, individuals' personalities may influence how much stress they experience—or how much stress they perceive they are experiencing (Hemenover & Dienstbier, 1996). As described by Barbara Fredrickson's **broaden-and-build theory**, positive emotions broaden people's attention and cognition, which in turn leads to increases in physical, intellectual, social, and psychological resources (Fredrickson, 2001; Fredrickson & Joiner, 2002). People who are high in positive emotions may reappraise stressful situations in a less threatening way, which is a pretty good mechanism for reducing the negative physiological effects of particular challenges (Davis, Nolen-Hoeksema, & Larson, 1998; Florian et al., 1995; Hemenover, 2001). In line with this view, people who experience negative life events and are low in **grit**, a trait measuring passion and motivation to achieve a longer-term goal, report more thoughts about suicide, whereas those who are high in grit do not, suggesting people who are high on grit are better able to cope with such events (Blalock, Young, & Kleiman, 2015). Similarly, and as shown in Figure 5.4, police officers who dealt with traumatic events during Hurricane Katrina—such as recovering bodies, preventing looting, and rescuing people—were less likely to develop PTSD if they were high in positive states (life satisfaction, resilience, gratitude) (McCanlies, Mnatsakanova, Andrew, Burchfiel, & Violanti, 2014).

On the other hand, people who are high in negative emotions are likely to create additional stress in their lives. People with such personality traits anticipate that others will act aggressively toward them and thus may behave antagonistically first, which in turn elicits the aggressive behavior they expected (Smith, 1992). For example, people who are high in hostility or negative affect experience more frequent and severe daily hassles and major life events and report more conflict in their jobs, marriages, and families (Ormel & Wohlfarth, 1991; Smith et al., 1988). Similarly, when playing games, Type As view their opponents as more competitive and hard-driving than Type Bs do, and not surprisingly, they elicit more

Figure 5.3 Model Explaining the Personality–Health Link

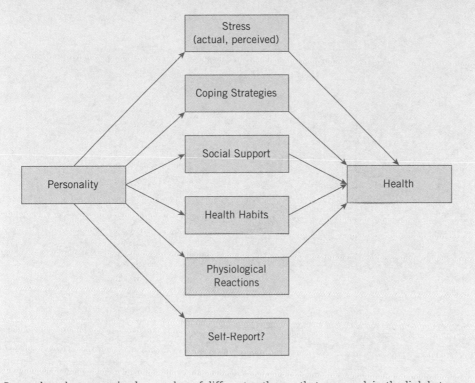

Researchers have examined a number of different pathways that may explain the link between personality and health.

Source: Created by Catherine A. Sanderson.

competitive and aggressive responses from others (Ortega & Pipal, 1984; Rhodewalt, Hayes, Chemers, & Wysocki, 1984; Sorensen et al., 1987).

Physiological Mechanisms

Personality may also influence health through its impact on physiological mechanisms. For example, individuals who are high in positive states show faster cardiovascular recovery following stress (Tugade & Frederickson, 2004). They also show lower cortisol increases and higher levels of T cells, even in the face of stressors (Segerstrom, Taylor, Kemeny, & Fahey, 1998; Taylor et al., 2008). For example, researchers in one study measured levels of optimism in women with ovarian cancer before starting chemotherapy (de Moor et al., 2006). Women with higher levels of optimism at the start of chemotherapy showed a greater decline in a marker of cancer at the end of chemotherapy. Similarly, people who have a greater sense of purpose in life experience fewer physiological effects of stress, even after controlling for other aspects of psychological well-being associated with such biological reactions (Zilioli, Slatcher, Ong, & Gruenewald, 2015).

In contrast, people who are high on negative states not only experience higher levels of stress but also show greater physiological reactions to stress, including cardiovascular response and immune functioning (Scheier & Carver, 1987). Think about what happens to your body

Figure 5.4 Data From McCanlies et al., 2014

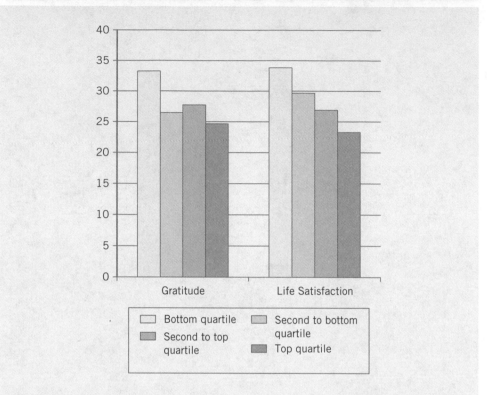

Police officers who were high in life satisfaction or gratitude were less likely to develop PTSD after dealing with the traumatic events following Hurricane Katrina than those who were lower on such measures. This study provides some evidence for the power of personality traits to buffer one from negative life experiences.

Source: Data from McCanlies, Mnatsakanova, Andrew, Burchfiel, & Violanti (2014).

when you yell at someone—your heart rate probably increases, and, although you may not be aware of it, so does your blood pressure. People who regularly experience this higher level of physiological arousal may be at greater risk of developing cardiovascular problems because they exert so much wear and tear on their blood vessels and heart (Siegman, Anderson, Herbst, Boyle, & Wilkinson, 1992). In turn, people who are hostile—and constantly on guard against slights from others—have consistently higher heart rates and blood pressure than those who are low in hostility, show more rapid cardiovascular reactions to stressful situations, and take longer for their bodies to return to normal functioning following a stressful interaction (Smith, 1992; Suarez, Kuhn, Schanberg, Williams, & Zimmermann, 1998). Similarly, when people who are Type A feel threatened or challenged, they show greater changes in heart rate, blood pressure, and adrenaline levels than Type Bs (Contrada, 1989; Lyness, 1993). Not surprisingly, these increased reactions to stress lead to wear and tear on the heart over time.

Coping Strategies

Another explanation for the personality–health link is that personality traits influence the use of different coping strategies, which in turn impacts health. People who are high in positive emotions tend to use more adaptive and functional strategies for coping with problems and are less likely to use destructive coping strategies (Carver et al., 1993; Drach-Zahavy & Somech, 2002; Gloria & Steinhardt, 2014; McCrae & Costa, 1986; Williams, Wiebe, & Smith, 1992). For example, optimists recover from surgery faster than pessimists, in part because they sought out as much information as possible about what to expect and how best to cope with recovery, whereas pessimists tend to dwell on negative aspects of the experience or block out thoughts about the recovery process (Scheier et al., 1989). Similarly, people who are high on **self-compassion**, meaning a tendency to treat oneself with kindness and compassion, tend to construe negative events in less dire terms than people low in self-compassion (Allen & Leary, 2010). They also show less internalization and self-blame, which in turn reduces the experience of stress. In contrast, people who are high in neuroticism and have an external locus of control tend to rely on maladaptive coping strategies (Hewitt & Flett, 1996).

Social Support

Personality factors may also influence how much social support a person has (Lepore, 1995; Smith, 1992). In line with this view, Xu and Roberts (2010) examined positive feelings in a sample of over 6,000 adults and then evaluated death rates over the next 28 years. Although positive feelings predicted lowered risk of all causes of mortality, this association was largely caused by social networks, meaning that people with high levels of positive emotions tend to have larger social support networks, which in turn leads to better health. In contrast, people who are hostile, neurotic, and pessimistic may experience high levels of interpersonal conflict (in part because they treat others in an antagonistic way) and have difficulty both seeking and accepting social support (Houston & Vavak, 1991; Sarason, Sarason, & Shearin, 1986; Smith, 1992). For example, people who are low in hostility experience less stress when they have a friend with them while they give a difficult speech, whereas people who are high in hostility do not show any benefit from the presence of such support (Lepore, 1995).

Health Habits

As you can probably imagine, personality factors may influence individuals' health habits. People who are high in conscientiousness, optimism, and extraversion and those with have an internal locus of control are more likely to engage in health-promoting behaviors, including taking vitamins, engaging in regular exercise and healthy eating, avoiding cigarette smoking and drugs, engaging in safer sexual behaviors, and safe driving (Korotkov, 2008; Scheier & Carver, 1992; Trobst, Herbst, Masters, & Costa, 2002). In contrast, people who are high in neuroticism, hostility, and Type A behavior are more likely to smoke, abuse alcohol, eat less healthy foods, engage in unsafe sex, avoid exercise, sleep less, and drink caffeine (Costa & McCrae, 1987; Folsom et al., 1985; Leiker & Hailey, 1988; Miller et al., 1996). For example, people who are high in neuroticism engage in fewer health-promoting behaviors and more risk-taking behavior when driving (Booth-Kewley & Vickers, 1994). This type of careless behavior may explain why people who have pessimistic explanatory styles have higher rates of death from accidents and violence but not from cancer or cardiovascular disease (Peterson et al., 1998). Personality can even predict health-related behavior over time: children who are higher in hostility in first grade are more likely to smoke cigarettes, drink alcohol, and use marijuana during high school (Hampson, Tildesley, Andrews, Luyckx, & Mroczek, 2010), and children who are high in negative affect are more likely to be obese as adults (Pulkki-Råback, Elovainio, Kivimäki, Raitakari, & Keltikangas-Järvinen, 2005).

Personality factors may also influence people's behavior following an illness, such as whether they adhere to a recommended medical regimen or follow diet and exercise advice (Gonzalez et al., 2004; Wiebe & Christensen, 1997). For example, cardiac patients who are optimistic are more likely to take vitamins, eat low-fat foods, enroll in a rehabilitation program, successfully reduce their weight, follow a recommended diet, and start exercising

(Scheier et al., 1989; Shepperd, Maroto, & Pbert, 1996). Similarly, conscientious people, who have the self-control to overcome potential barriers (e.g., fear) and to complete difficult, aversive, and stressful tasks (e.g., getting a mammogram, having an HIV test) tend to follow health care advice, whereas those who are low in conscientiousness simply abandon medical regimens that are distasteful in some way (Christensen & Smith, 1995; Schwartz et al., 1999). In contrast, hostile people and those with Type A behavior patterns may even react against doctors' orders to exert their independence (Lee et al., 1992; Rhodewalt & Smith, 1991).

Self-Report

Finally, the link between personality and health could be a function of self-report—in other words, personality traits may influence how focused people are on their physical health, and hence how likely they are to notice various aches, pains, and symptoms (and not just how many symptoms they notice). Those who are high in negative affect, for example, may interpret relatively minor and normal symptoms as more painful and problematic than people with low negative affect (Watson, 1988; Watson & Pennebaker, 1989). To test this possibility, research has included physiological tests of health, such as immune system functioning, cardiovascular fitness, and measures of cholesterol levels (Costa & McCrae, 1987). This work generally suggests that there is little association between personality traits and actual physical measures of health. For example, researchers in one study asked people about their cold symptoms (e.g., runny nose, congestion) and also gathered more objective data (e.g., mucus output) (Cohen et al., 1995). Although people who were high in negative affect complained more about various health problems (e.g., headaches, chest pains, stomachaches), there was no evidence that they actually experienced more health problems (e.g., elevated blood pressure, serum lipids). Similarly, people who are high in negative affect complain of all kinds of physical problems and symptoms but do not actually show evidence of increased health problems or earlier mortality—there is no evidence from biological tests that they experience more problems, visit the doctor more often, take medicine more often, or miss school/work more often.

Conclusions

In sum, although the model suggests that each pathway between personality and health is separate and distinct from all others, clearly these pathways could be, and probably often are, interrelated. Personality factors are likely to influence the type of coping strategy used, which in turn influences the amount of stress experienced. Similarly, the amount of social support a person receives may impact the amount of stress he or she experiences, the coping strategies used, and even the person's health habits, any or all of which could in turn influence health. Moreover, the findings on the link between personality and health are entirely correlational, meaning it is impossible to determine the factors that explain these associations. In other words, while evidence certainly shows that particular personality traits—such as agreeableness, conscientiousness, and neuroticism—are linked with health, we know less about how much such traits matter and why (Strickhouser, Zell, & Krizan, 2017). Finally, and perhaps most important, these findings suggest that our own interpretation of and reaction to stressful life events can influence health outcomes. Thus, make an effort to adopt a positive outlook and be conscientious in your health habits, regardless of your natural tendencies.

STRATEGIES FOR REDUCING STRESS

LO 5.5

Summarize different strategies for reducing stress

Throughout this chapter, you've learned how various personal and situational factors help people manage stress. This final section describes specific strategies that help people reduce their feelings of stress and thereby experience better health.

Relaxation

Another approach to managing stress is to change one's physiological responses to stress, which in turn can reduce its harmful effects on physical health. The *relaxation response* is a coordinated set of physiological changes that support rest and restoration and are characterized by greater activation of the parasympathetic nervous system, leading to a lower heart rate, blood pressure, and breathing rate. There are many strategies for activating the relaxation response, including imagery, hypnosis, meditation, yoga, and progressive muscle relaxation.

In the **progressive muscle relaxation** technique for managing stress, people focus on consciously tensing and then releasing each part of their body (hands, shoulders, legs, etc.) one at a time (Jacobson, 1938). This helps patients learn to distinguish states of tension from states of relaxation, thereby helping them learn how to calm themselves down in virtually any stressful situation. Progressive muscle relaxation can also be paired with *systematic desensitization*, an approach that helps people build up tolerance to a particular stressful object or event. In this technique, the person is asked to describe the specific causes of his or her anxiety and then to create a hierarchy of different stimuli associated with that anxiety. As shown in Table 5.7, these fears are ranked such that relatively low-anxiety-causing stimuli fall at the bottom of the hierarchy and higher-anxiety-provoking stimuli sit at the top of the hierarchy. The therapist then asks the patient to focus on the least-anxiety-provoking image while encouraging the person to relax. Whenever the patient experiences anxiety, the therapist asks him or her to focus on a less-stressful stimulus. Gradually, as the patient is able to think about a low-level stimulus without feeling anxiety, the therapist continues to higher-level (more anxiety-provoking) stimuli; this process, over time, enables people to build up their tolerance to the stressful situation.

The technique of *biofeedback* also helps people distinguish between states of tension and relaxation, but with a particular focus on how these psychological states influence their physiological reactions. Patients are attached to a monitor that shows their physiological response (heart rate, muscle tension, sweat), and they are able to learn how their thoughts and feelings influence their physiological reactions. Biofeedback is an effective way to help people

Table 5.7 Sample Desensitization Hierarchy for Coping With Fear of Injected Shots
1. You are reading a magazine and there is a photograph of someone getting a shot.
2. You are watching a television show or movie in which someone gets a shot.
3. You receive a letter from your college stating that before you return in the fall you must have a tetanus vaccine.
4. You call the health center to make an appointment for your vaccination.
5. You leave your room on the morning of your appointment.
6. You park at the health center.
7. You sit in the line to receive your shot.
8. Your name is called by the nurse.
9. You sit in the room as the nurse wipes your arm with alcohol.
10. You watch the nurse approach with the needle.

Source: Created by Catherine A. Sanderson.

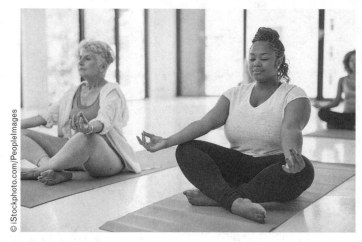

Meditation, and other strategies for relaxation, can have beneficial effects on health.

What You'll Learn
5.4

learn strategies for decreasing stress as well as the impact of stress on their physical reactions.

All of these relaxation techniques can reduce the negative effects of stress on psychological and physical health. For example, high school students who learn progressive muscle relaxation during their regular health class show a decrease in blood pressure (Ewart et al., 1987); women with breast cancer who receive relaxation training report reduced levels of depression (Gudenkauf et al., 2015); and patients who are trained in *meditation* show reductions in neck pain (Jeitler et al., 2015). Using such techniques can also lead to long-term health benefits. One study with teenagers who had high blood pressure found that those who meditated twice a day—for just 15 minutes each time—had a lower risk of developing cardiovascular disease than those who simply received education about how to lower blood pressure and the risk for cardiovascular disease (Barnes, Kapuku, & Treiber, 2012). Training patients with severe coronary heart disease in relaxation techniques, such as meditation, can even lead to a reversal in the amount of arteriosclerosis present (Ornish et al., 1998).

Mindfulness

It feels good to relax, and it's easy to understand how relaxation—a kind of escape from real or imagined stressors—might undo the physiological and psychological symptoms of stress. The benefits are perhaps more surprising, though, when we consider the effects of simply paying attention to our thoughts, or **mindfulness**. As shown in Table 5.8, mindfulness can be described as a state of concentrated awareness of what is happening in the present moment (Brown & Ryan, 2003). It consists of simply paying attention to ongoing events and experiences, and thereby avoiding letting one's mind become preoccupied with other thoughts or concerns. So, while talking with a friend, you would focus intensely on this interaction and not allow yourself to think about what you will do later on or how stressful your day has been. Various approaches for increasing mindfulness include meditation, breathing practices, body awareness, yoga, and tai chi.

Considerable research demonstrates that mindfulness can have beneficial effects on stress, depression, and anxiety in both healthy people and those with serious health conditions (Gu, Strauss, Bond, & Cavanagh, 2015; Khoury, Sharma, Rush, & Fournier, 2015). Mindfulness training leads to decreases in stress and anxiety in pregnant women (Guardino, Dunkel Schetter, Bower, Lu, & Smalley, 2014); lower levels of pain, fatigue, depression, and PTSD symptoms in veterans (Banks, Newman, & Saleem, 2015; Kearney et al., 2016; Stephenson, Simpson, Martinez, & Kearney, 2017); and improved psychological functioning among breast cancer survivors (Huang, He, Wang, & Zhou, 2016). Even online mindfulness-based interventions have a small but significant beneficial impact on depression, anxiety, and well-being (Spijkerman, Pots, & Bohlmeijer, 2016).

Most important, mindfulness can improve physical health. For example, breast cancer survivors who received training in mindfulness-based stress reduction showed a reduction in fear of recurrence as well as improved physical functioning (Lengacher et al., 2014). Mindfulness-based stress reduction interventions also decrease fatigue and increase immune function response in cancer patients (Johns, Brown, Beck-Coon, Monahan, Tong, & Kroenke, 2015; Witek-Janusek et al., 2008), reduce stress and injury in student-athletes

Table 5.8 Mindfulness Scale

The following statements are about your everyday experience. Using a 1–6 scale, please indicate how frequently or infrequently you currently have each experience (1 = almost always to 6 = almost never).

1. I find it difficult to stay focused on what's happening in the present.

2. I tend to walk quickly to get where I'm going without paying attention to what I experience along the way.

3. It seems I am "running on automatic," without much awareness of what I'm doing.

4. I rush through activities without being really attentive to them.

5. I do jobs or tasks automatically, without being aware of what I'm doing.

6. I find myself listening to someone with one ear, doing something else at the same time.

7. I drive places on "automatic pilot" and then wonder why I went there.

8. I find myself doing things without paying attention.

This scale measures mindfulness, meaning how able you are to show concentrated awareness of and attention to ongoing events.

Source: Brown & Ryan (2003).

(Petterson & Olson, 2016), and decrease pain in patients with migraines or back pain (Braden et al., 2016; Feuille & Pargament, 2015).

Mindfulness may help reduce the negative effects of stress on health by giving people specific strategies they can use to manage stress. For example, researchers in one study randomly assigned members of a surgical intensive care unit—meaning people who experience high levels of work-related stress—to receive an eight-week mindfulness-based intervention (which included yoga, meditation, and mindfulness) or a no-treatment control (Duchemin, Steinberg, Marks, Vanover, & Klatt, 2015). This intervention led to decreases in nervous system activation and risk of burnout, indicating that while stress levels of the job didn't change, people's ability to manage that stress improved in important ways.

Exercise

Another technique for coping with stressful events is exercise. Exercise improves mood and reduces anxiety and depression (McCann & Holmes, 1984). Exercise may also lead to reductions in symptoms of PTSD and depression in people with PTSD (Rosenbaum et al., 2015). Most important, because exercise reduces the effect of stress on cardiovascular and psychoneuroendocrine responses (including heart rate, blood pressure, and cortisol), people who engage in regular exercise experience fewer negative physiological effects of stress than people who do not (Forcier et al., 2006; Zschucke, Renneberg, Dimeo, Wüstenberg, & Ströhle, 2015).

In turn, and not surprisingly, people who exercise more frequently report fewer illnesses (Roth, Wiebe, Fillingim, & Shay, 1989). One study examined the associations between physical fitness, stress, and number of visits to the campus health center (Brown, 1991). Students who were high in stress and low in physical fitness made the most visits, whereas those who were high in stress but also high in fitness made as few visits as those under low stress. So, the next time you are feeling blue, think about going for a jog—or a brisk walk, if even the thought of jogging is stressful!

Spending Time in Nature

What You'll Learn
5.5

One of the easiest ways to reduce stress is to simply spend time outside. In fact, spending time in nature is associated with lower levels of depression and blood pressure and higher levels of energy and personal well-being (Ryan et al., 2010; Shanahan et al., 2016). People who regularly spend time in nature—including city parks and private gardens—report lower rates of stress and stress-related illnesses (Grahn & Stigsdotter, 2003) as well as better overall physical and mental health and fewer health-related complaints (De Vries, Verheij, Groenewegen, & Spreeuwenberg, 2003).

To examine the benefits of nature on health, researchers in one study combined mental health data from a statewide survey and satellite data showing how much vegetation was present in various neighborhoods (Beyer et al., 2014). Their findings were remarkable: across all income levels, people who lived in a neighborhood with less than 10% tree canopy were much more likely to report depression, stress, and anxiety. In other words, a poor person living in a forest area was more likely to be happy than a wealthy person living on a treeless block in a fancy neighborhood. These findings suggest that simply planting trees, grass, and flowers is a relatively easy way of reducing stress.

What is it about spending time in nature that leads to such dramatic benefits? Researchers believe that exposure to nature basically switches the body from the "fight-or-flight" response (as you learned about in *Chapter 4: Understanding Stress*) to a "rest-and-digest" model (Kuo, 2015; Li, 2010). This switch allows the body to divert resources toward the immune system, which in turn leads to important long-term health advantages.

Therapy

The strategies described in this section can all help people reduce the normal stresses of daily life. But for some people—and in some situations—additional support is needed. People who are facing intense and lasting stress may find therapy with a trained professional an essential part of coping. Many models of therapy, such as cognitive behavioral therapy, use some of the same principles described in this chapter to help people change their thoughts about stress as well as their behavioral responses to stress. Drug therapy, including anti-anxiety and antidepressant medication, may also be useful in treating severe psychological distress.

Table 5.9   Information YOU Can Use
• Think about how you choose to cope with stressful events in your life, and make sure you are using effective strategies for managing the particular situation you are in. For situations you can fix, problem-focused coping is probably the best bet, but for situations that are not solvable, emotion-focused coping can be most effective.
• Because everyone experiences some stress, it is essential that you figure out how best to cope with that stress. Think about what approaches help you manage stress, such as exercising, relaxing, social support, laughing, or religious beliefs, and try to adopt one or more of those strategies when you are experiencing stress.
• Your outlook—including your personality, beliefs, and mood—influences your physical well-being, so try to maintain positive states, including extraversion and positive affect, whenever possible. In other words, focus on seeing the glass as half full instead of half empty!

- People who are conscientious live longer, in part because they show amazing self-control and thus have the ability to focus on long-term goals over short-term gratification. In turn, conscientiousness is associated with better health-related behavior, including healthy eating, exercise, and adherence to medical recommendations. So, the next time you are faced with short-term temptations, try to focus on the longer-term consequences of such a choice . . . and exercise self-restraint yourself.

- Try to form larger social networks, since having more people to rely on increases the likelihood of having a particular type of support available when you need it. This might be a particularly important strategy to use when you are in new environments (e.g., starting college, moving to a new city), which may be stressful and in which you may not already have many sources of support. You should also try to maintain closer contact with old friends.

- Consider getting a pet . . . and preferably a dog. Research reveals that pet owners experience better psychological and physical well-being.

- If you have religious and spiritual beliefs, embrace the health-related benefits of such a perspective by attending religious services, praying, and/or appreciating your connection to something meaningful and bigger than yourself. All of these beliefs and behaviors are linked with positive health outcomes.

SUMMARY

The Impact of Coping Styles

- One common strategy for managing challenging situations is trying to confront and change the stressor. This is called problem-focused coping and is often used when something constructive can be done to help solve the problem or at least make the situation better. Problem-focused coping can include seeking assistance from others, taking direct action, and planning. Most research suggests that people who use problem-focused coping show better adjustment.

- Another coping strategy is changing how you think about the stress, which is called emotion-focused coping. This type of coping can involve either approach (vigilant) coping, meaning changing how one thinks about the problem or venting about the problem to others, or avoidance (minimizing) coping, meaning denying or avoiding the problem. Some forms of approach-focused coping, such as positive reappraisal and having a sense of humor, lead to health benefits. Avoidance coping can have negative consequences in the case of longer-term and more severe stresses.

- Both problem-focused and emotion-focused coping can be effective, as long as they are used to cope with specific types of problems. Individuals who are comfortable using a number of different coping styles have a higher likelihood of minimizing their stress in a variety of challenging situations.

The Power of Social Support

- Many people rely on different types of social support from others. These include emotional support, belongingness support, instrumental (or tangible) support, informational (or appraisal) support, and esteem (or validational) support.

- According to the matching hypothesis, individuals benefit from receiving the type of social support that fits their particular problem. However, culture influences the type of social support people find most beneficial.

- Having greater social support is associated with a variety of positive health outcomes. People with high-quality social support are less likely to experience both minor and major health problems, recover more quickly from illnesses when they do get sick, and cope better with surgery. Most important, greater social support is associated with increased longevity, even in people who are critically ill.

- Support in general is what is important, not support from a particular person. Even social support from our pets can reduce feelings of stress, as can giving social support to others. However, social support can also have negative implications for psychological and physical well-being.

- According to the buffering hypothesis, social support provides a buffer from daily life stress and thus is particularly beneficial during times of high stress. In contrast, the direct effects hypothesis posits that having high levels of social support is always advantageous to health, regardless of level of stress.

The Influence of Religion and Spirituality

- Many people find that religiosity—meaning a formal link to religious organizations—and spirituality—meaning a personal orientation toward religious beliefs—are helpful in managing stress and improving health outcomes. People who are involved in religion experience better psychological health, better physical health, and even a longer life expectancy. However, religiosity and spirituality can have some negative health-related consequences, such as avoiding or delaying medical treatment

- There are many different explanations for the link between religious and/or spiritual beliefs and greater physical health. One explanation is that many religions directly encourage healthy behaviors, such as abstaining from smoking, alcohol/drug use, and risky sexual behaviors, which in turn leads to greater physical well-being. Another possibility is that substantial social support is provided within many religious communities, which in turn leads to greater health. A third possibility is that religion gives people a sense of meaning, which may in and of itself have beneficial effects on health. Religious commitment may also lead people to rely on more adaptive coping mechanisms for managing stressful events.

The Role of Personality

- People who are high on positive states experience better psychological well-being, better physical well-being, and greater life expectancy. However, people cannot heal themselves simply by having a positive mind-set, and some positive states may lead to negative health-related outcomes.

- Conscientious people experience better physical health, perhaps in part because they engage in more health-promoting behavior.

- People who have a strong internal locus of control experience better psychological and physical health, as do those who are high in hardiness. Both of these traits are associated with better psychological and physical well-being.

- Other personality factors are associated with poor psychological and physical health. These include neuroticism (negative affect), Type A behavior, and hostility/disagreeableness.

- There are several explanations for the link between personality and health. First, individuals' personalities may influence how much stress they experience—or perceive they are experiencing. Personality may also influence health through its impact on physiological mechanisms, such as cardiovascular recovery and immune functioning. Another explanation is that personality factors influence the use of different coping strategies, the amount of social support a person receives, and/or her or his health habits. Finally, the link between personality and health could be a function of self-report, meaning how focused people are on their physical health.

Strategies for Reducing Stress

- One strategy for managing stress is relaxation, which can include imagery, hypnosis, meditation, or yoga. In the progressive muscle relaxation technique, people focus on consciously tensing and then releasing each part of their body, one at a time. The technique of biofeedback helps people learn how psychological states influence their physiological reactions.

- The technique of mindfulness, meaning a state of concentrated awareness in terms of what is happening in the present moment, is another form of managing stress. It consists of simply paying attention to ongoing events and experiences and thereby avoiding letting one's mind become preoccupied with other thoughts or concerns.

- Another technique for coping with stressful events is exercise, which reduces anxiety and depression as well as the negative physiological effects of stress.

People who exercise more frequently also report fewer illnesses.

- Spending time in nature is associated with lower levels of depression and stress as well as lower blood pressure and fewer stress-related illnesses. Exposure to nature helps the body relax, which in turn leads to important long-term health advantages.

- People who are facing intense and lasting stress may find therapy with a trained professional an essential part of coping. Many models of therapy help people change their thoughts about stress as well as their behavioral responses to stress. Drug therapy may also be useful in treating severe psychological distress.

6

INJURY AND INJURY PREVENTION

Learning Objectives

6.1 Describe different types and consequences of injuries

6.2 Compare the risk of injury across the lifespan

6.3 Summarize the causes of and risk factors for unintentional injuries

6.4 Summarize the causes of and risk factors for intentional injuries

6.5 Describe strategies for preventing injuries

What You'll Learn

6.1 How concussions can lead to lasting consequences

6.2 Why conscientious people may be riskier drivers

6.3 Why publicizing mass killings can have deadly consequences

6.4 Why paid parental leave reduces child abuse

6.5 How texting bans save lives

Preview

One of the major goals of health psychology is to prevent the development of health problems, which is a much easier and cheaper way of increasing life expectancy and life quality than treating established medical problems. Preventing injuries—which cause over 26 million visits to an emergency room each year in the United States—can therefore have a substantial impact on both the quality and length of people's lives (Centers for Disease Control and Prevention, 2016b). In turn, one of the goals of Healthy People 2020 is to prevent unintentional injuries and violence and reduce their consequences. In this chapter, you'll learn about different types of injuries and their causes, their frequency across the lifespan, and strategies for preventing injuries.

UNDERSTANDING INJURY

Describe different types and consequences of injuries

One of the challenges of understanding the substantial impact of injuries is that we often misunderstand how behavioral choices can cause various types of injuries. This section will examine different types of injuries as well as their consequences.

Types of Injury

Although injuries in general cause numerous fatalities and continuing problems, different types of injuries are caused by different factors. Specifically, psychologists divide injuries into two distinct types: unintentional injuries and intentional injuries.

Unintentional injuries are often described as "accidents" because the person who experienced the injury did not mean for it to happen. However, the leading cause of death in every age group between age 1 and 44 is unintentional injury (Centers for Disease Control and Prevention, 2016e). Many unintentional injuries are caused by car accidents, fires, drowning, falls, and poisoning. This type of injury could include someone developing a sprained neck following a car crash, becoming paralyzed after falling from a balcony, or dying from an accidental drug overdose.

Although unintentional injuries are often called "accidents," many of these injuries could be prevented (as you'll learn later in the chapter). For example, in the United States about 90 people a day die from car accidents (Centers for Disease Control and Prevention, 2016f). Because many of these accidents—or at least the deaths caused by them—could be prevented through behavioral choices, such as wearing a seat belt, obeying the speed limit, and refusing to drive while intoxicated, this is a compelling example of the role that individuals' behavior plays in influencing physical health.

Other types of injuries are described as **intentional injuries**, meaning the person who caused the injury meant for it to happen. Intentional injuries are caused by violent behavior. This type of injury includes self-directed behavior, such as suicide and nonsuicidal self-injury, in which a person deliberately attempts to harm himself or herself. Physical assaults and homicides, in which a person deliberately injures one or more people, are also considered intentional injuries.

Consequences of Injuries

Nearly 200,000 Americans die from injuries each year, and for people ages 1 to 44, injuries are the leading cause of death (Heron, 2016). In fact, in the first half of life, more Americans die from injuries—such as motor vehicle crashes, falls, or homicides—than from any other cause, including cancer, HIV, or heart disease.

Many additional people experience nonfatal injuries. The leading causes of nonfatal injuries are falling, being struck by or against someone or something (such as walking into a wall or colliding with another player during a game), and overexertion (such as carrying a too heavy box or performing a repetitive movement) (Centers for Disease Control and Prevention, 2017v). Over 80 million Americans each year seek medical treatment at a doctor's office or hospital for an injury, and 2.5 million people are hospitalized due to injuries. In some cases, nonfatal injuries may lead to lasting problems that lead to lasting disability, such as in the case of spinal cord and brain injuries.

What You'll Learn 6.1

You've undoubtedly heard about the growing concern about the lasting effects of head injuries experienced by athletes. Approximately 20% of high school athletes experience a concussion at some point, which is probably a low estimate since athletes may fail to report concussion symptoms (Kroshus, Garnett, Hawrilenko, Baugh, & Calzo, 2015). Side effects of concussions include headaches, dizziness, confusion, tiredness, and irritability, as well as problems with memory (Bergman et al., 2013). Moreover, head injuries can cause lasting deficits in cognitive abilities, including problems with processing information and performing executive functions (meaning the ability to initiate actions, monitor and change behavior, and plan future behavior; Crawford, Knight, & Alsop, 2007; Howell, Osternig, Van Donkelaar, Mayr, & Chou, 2013; McAllister et al., 2012). Any type of repetitive head contact, such as that sustained during tackling in football or hockey or headers in soccer, can cause brain damage, even if the contact does not cause a concussion or result at the time in clear signs of injury.

People who suffer multiple concussions may experience severe neurological damage, including chronic traumatic encephalopathy (CTE), which is linked with dementia and even suicide. One recent study published in the *Journal of the American Medical Association* examined signs of CTE in the brains of former National Football League (NFL) players (Mez et al., 2017). Of the 111 brains examined, 110 showed signs of CTE. In contrast, a comparison group of brains from former high school and college football players revealed somewhat lower rates of CTE, suggesting that more years playing football increases the risk of developing such severe damage. Although this study used a nonrandom sample of athletes, since families with concerns about players' long-term damage may be more likely to have donated their brains following their death, its findings are in line with those from other studies suggesting that repeated head injuries can lead to long-term brain damage. Such findings have led some players to retire in the prime of their careers, giving up lucrative salaries, to protect themselves from future consequences.

Injuries exert a huge cost on society, not only in terms of physical health and life expectancy but also in terms of financial costs. The total cost of injuries in the United States in 2013 was $671 billion (Centers for Disease Control and Prevention, 2016b). The costs associated with fatal injuries were $214 billion, while nonfatal injuries accounted for over $457 billion. These costs included both direct costs of medical treatment and indirect costs due to lost work productivity.

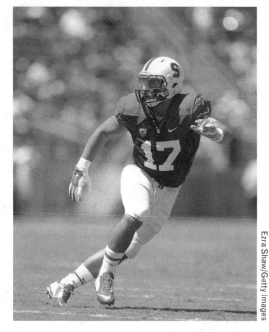

Ezra Shaw/Getty Images

A. J. Tarpley played one year in the NFL before retiring at the age of 23 due to concerns about the long-term effects of concussion.

RISK OF INJURY ACROSS THE LIFESPAN

Although overall injuries are the fourth leading causes of death (following heart disease, cancer, and respiratory disease), the risk of injury, as well as death caused by injury, varies considerably across the lifespan (Heron, 2016) (see Table 6.1). This section will examine the risk of injury by age, including infancy and childhood, adolescence and young adulthood, and adulthood and older adulthood.

LO 6.2

Compare the risk of injury across the lifespan

Infancy and Childhood

Although infants in the first year of life face a higher likelihood of death than older children (often due to complications associated with premature birth), childhood in general is a time of relatively low mortality. However, and as shown in Figure 6.1, the leading cause of death for children from ages 1 to 14 is unintentional injury, and the fourth leading cause of death, following cancer and heart disease, is homicide (Heron, 2016).

Table 6.1   Leading Causes of Death by Age

- Birth to Age 1: Congenital anomalies, premature birth, SIDS
- Ages 1 to 4 years: Injuries, congenital anomalies, homicide
- Ages 5 to 9 years: Injuries, cancer, congenital anomalies
- Ages 10 to 14 years: Injuries, cancer, suicide
- Ages 15 to 24 years: Injuries, suicide, homicide
- Ages 25 to 34 years: Injuries, suicide, homicide
- Ages 35 to 44 years: Injuries, cancer, heart disease
- Ages 45 to 54 years: Cancer, heart disease, injuries
- Ages 55 to 64 years: Cancer, heart disease, injuries
- Ages 65 years and over: Heart disease, cancer, respiratory disease

Although heart disease, cancer, and respiratory diseases are overall the leading causes of death, more people ages 1 to 44 years die from injuries than any other cause.

Source: National Center for Health Statistics (2017).

The specific types of unintentional injuries that lead to death vary considerably by age (Heron, 2016) (see Table 6.2). For infants younger than 1, suffocation causes the vast majority of injury deaths. For children ages 1 to 4, the leading causes of injury-related death are drowning and car accidents. For children ages 5 to 9, injury-related deaths are most commonly caused by car accidents, drowning, and fire/burns. For children ages 10 to 14, most injury-related deaths have historically been caused by car accidents; however, suicide is now the leading cause of injury-related death in children ages 10 to 14. This change is due in part to substantial decreases in the prevalence of fatal car accidents but also reflects an increase in rates of youth suicide.

Figure 6.1   Leading Causes of Death for Children Ages 1 to 14

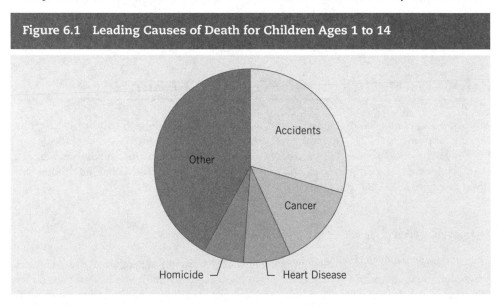

Source: Created by Catherine A. Sanderson, based on data from Heron, M. (2016). Deaths: Leading causes for 2014. *National Vital Statistics Reports, 65*(5), 1–96.

Table 6.2	Leading Causes of Injuries Leading to Death in Children

- Younger than 1: Unintentional suffocation, homicide, car accident
- Ages 1 to 4: Drowning, car accident, homicide
- Ages 5 to 9: Car accident, drowning, fire/burns
- Ages 10 to 14: Suicide, car accident, homicide

Although the types of injuries leading to death vary considerably by age, injuries are the leading cause of death in children ages 1 to 14.

Source: Kochanek, Murphy, Xu, & Tejada-Vera (2016).

Children also experience many nonfatal injuries. The leading cause of nonfatal injury in children of all ages is falling, such as falling down stairs, out of a window, or out of a bed. Falls from playground equipment are also relatively common during childhood. Other sources of injury during childhood include being struck by or against something (such as running into an opening door), stings and bites (from insects, animals, other children), and, for children ages 10 to 14, overexertion (such as from pushing too hard during sports practice). As described in **Focus on Development**, early sport specialization contributes to injuries in children, which can have lasting consequences.

Adolescence and Young Adulthood

Injury is also one of the leading causes of deaths for adolescents and young adults (ages 15 to 24) (Heron, 2016). As shown in Figure 6.2, over 40% of deaths in people in this age group are caused by accidents, and the second and third leading causes of death in this age group are suicides and homicides. In sum, 73% of deaths to adolescents and young adults are caused by either unintentional or intentional injuries.

FOCUS ON DEVELOPMENT

The Hazards of Early Sport Specialization

As you may have heard, there is a growing trend among youth athletes toward sport specialization, meaning focusing on excelling at a single sport instead of playing a variety of different sports. Unfortunately, evidence now suggests that this choice may increase athletes' risk of experiencing an injury. For example, researchers in one study of high school athletes found that those who specialized in a single sport, or trained in one sport for more than eight months out of the year, were more likely to report a history of knee or hip injuries (Bell et al., 2016). Moreover, athletes who specialize in an individual sport, such as gymnastics or tennis, are at higher risk for experiencing overuse injuries than those who play team sports. Kids who play individual sports usually start training at a younger age and spend more hours a week training, which both may increase their risk of developing an overuse injury. These findings suggest that parents and coaches should encourage young athletes to pursue a range of different types of sports and other activities and to limit the amount of time they spend training to avoid lasting injuries (Pasulka, Jayanthi, McCann, Dugas, & LaBella, 2017).

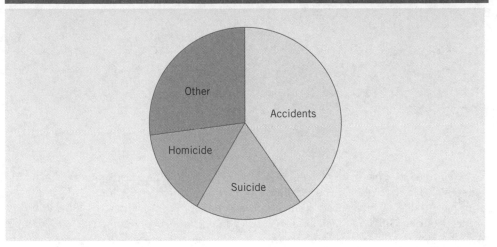

Figure 6.2 Leading Causes of Deaths for Adolescents and Young Adults (Ages 15–24)

Source: Created by Catherine A. Sanderson, based on data from https://www.cdc.gov/nchs/data/hus/hus16.pdf#019.

The leading cause of unintentional injuries leading to death in people age 15 to 24 is car accidents (Heron, 2016). Many of these accidents are a result of unsafe driving, including speeding, driving under the influence of alcohol, and driving while distracted (e.g., talking on a cell phone, texting). (You'll learn more about why car accidents are so prevalent for this age group in the next section.) Unintentional poisoning, meaning overdoses, also causes an increasing number of unintentional deaths in this age group.

Adolescents and young adults also experience nonfatal injuries. The leading causes of such injuries during this age period are being struck by or against something, falling, and motor vehicle accidents. Some of the same factors that contribute to fatal injuries, such as alcohol use and unsafe driving, also contribute to nonfatal injuries.

Adulthood and Older Adulthood

As shown in Figure 6.3, injuries cause about 20% of all deaths in adulthood. However, the impact of injuries on fatalities changes dramatically with age. Unintentional injuries are the leading cause of death in adults ages 25 to 44 but only the third leading cause of death in adults ages 45 to 64, following cancer and heart disease (Heron, 2016). In older adults, meaning those 65 and older, unintentional injuries cause only 2.5% of all deaths; chronic diseases cause most of the deaths for people in this age group.

The specific causes of injury-related deaths vary some with age (Heron, 2016). For adults ages 25 to 64, poisoning, meaning drug overdose, is the leading cause of injury-related death, followed by car accident. For those ages 25 to 34, homicide is the third leading cause of injury-related death, whereas for those ages 35 to 64, suicide is the third leading cause of injury-related death. However, the leading causes of injury-related deaths are quite different for adults ages 65 and higher. The vast majority of injury-related deaths in older adulthood are caused by falls; car accidents and suicide are the second and third leading causes of injury-related deaths, respectively.

Although throughout adulthood, falls are the leading cause of nonfatal injury, falls are especially common in older adults (Bergen, Stevens, & Burns, 2016). Risk factors for experiencing

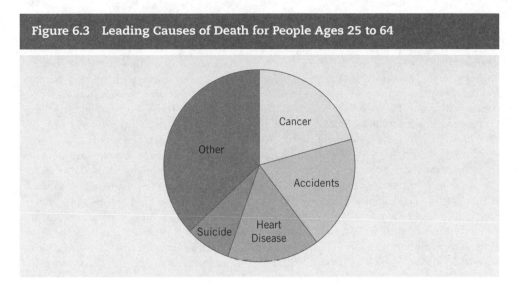

Figure 6.3   Leading Causes of Death for People Ages 25 to 64

Source: Data from Heron (2016).

falls including poor vision, lack of physical activity (which causes impairments in balance as well as loss of muscle tone), side effects of medications, and other chronic diseases, such as arthritis and Alzheimer's disease; many of these factors are more prevalent with age. Falls can lead to serious problems, including head injuries and broken bones. The other two major causes of nonfatal injuries in adulthood are being struck by something or someone and overexertion.

UNDERSTANDING UNINTENTIONAL INJURY

As described in the prior section, unintentional injuries are a leading cause of death through-out the lifespan and can also result in nonfatal injuries with sometimes serious and lasting consequences. In this section, you'll learn about the most common causes of such deaths as well as risk factors contributing to such injuries.

LO 6.3

Summarize the causes of and risk factors for unintentional injuries

Common Causes of Unintentional Injury

Although for many years, car accidents were the leading cause of injury-related death in the United States, more people now die from drug overdoses than in car accidents. This section examines the three leading causes of death from unintentional injuries: poisoning, car accidents, and falls.

Poisoning

Poison describes any substance that can be harmful to your health if too much of that substance is taken into your body via any mechanism (e.g., eaten, inhaled, injected, or absorbed through the skin). The most common type of poisoning in adults is the use of illegal drugs, such as cocaine or heroin, or the use of prescription drugs, such as opiates. In children, poisoning often occurs when someone accidentally consumes a drug, such as when a toddler mistakes a medication for candy. Poisoning can even happen unintentionally and without a person's awareness. For example, carbon monoxide poisoning can be caused by poorly vented gas furnaces and appliances, gas generators, and the indoor use of charcoal grills or portable stoves.

Poisoning is the leading cause of unintentional injury–related death in the United States (Heron, 2016). The majority of these deaths involve the use of an opioid. Although some of these deaths are caused by the use of illicit drugs, such as heroin, an increasing number are caused by the use of prescription opioids, such as oxycodone, methadone, and hydrocodone (as shown in Figure 6.4). In fact, 91 Americans die every day from an opioid overdose. Moreover, almost 2 million Americans abuse prescription opioids each year, and every day over 1,000 people are treated in emergency rooms for misusing prescription opioids.

Prescription opioids have been used for years to treat moderate to severe pain and hence are often prescribed for patients who need assistance in managing the pain caused by surgery, a severe injury, or a serious health condition, such as cancer. However, many people are now using opioids to manage the pain associated with less serious chronic types of pain, such as back pain or osteoarthritis. Many of these people may initially intend to use opioids for only a short period of time but then find themselves addicted and hence unable to stop. (This process of addiction is described in more detail in *Chapter 7: Substance Use and Abuse*.) Moreover, many people who become addicted to prescription opioid drugs then start using heroin, which is cheaper and more readily available.

Although anyone can become addicted to, and overdose on, both prescription and illicit drugs, certain people are at greater risk than others. The number of deaths caused by prescription opioid deaths is highest among those ages 25 to 54 years, and higher in men than in women (Centers for Disease Control and Prevention, 2017r). Prescription drug overdose rates are also higher among non-Hispanic Whites and American Indians/Alaskan Natives than

Figure 6.4 Increases in Overdose Deaths Over Time

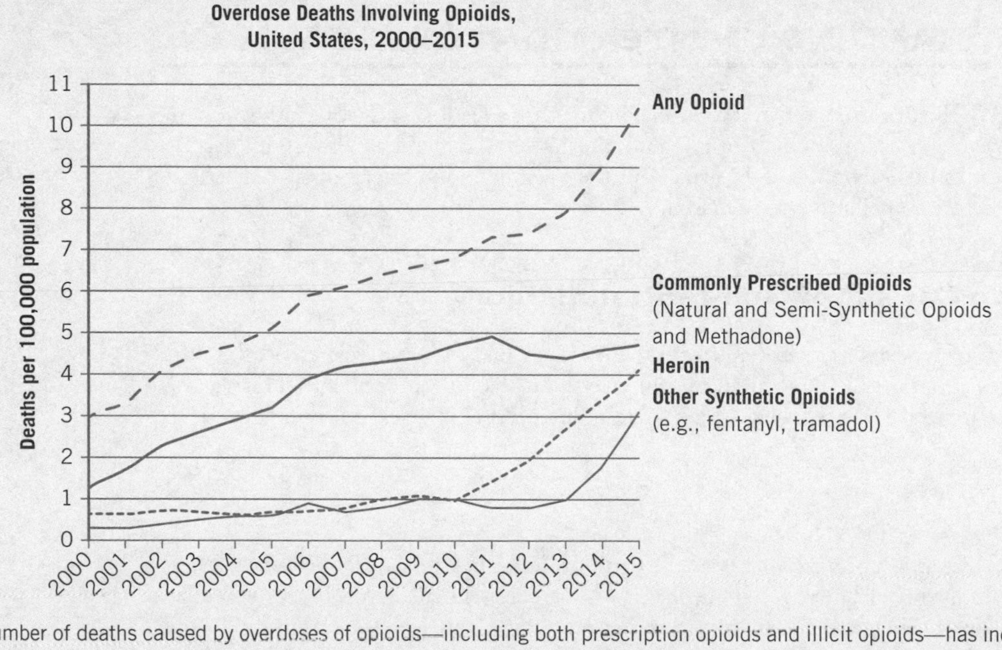

The number of deaths caused by overdoses of opioids—including both prescription opioids and illicit opioids—has increased substantially in recent years. Moreover, these numbers are probably an underestimate, since in about 20% of drug overdose deaths, a specific drug is not listed on the death certificate.

Source: Centers for Disease Control and Prevention (2017), https://www.cdc.gov/drugoverdose/data/analysis.html.

among non-Hispanic Blacks and Hispanics. Heroin use is more common in men than in women, although rates of use among women are rapidly increasing. Heroin use is most common among White people ages 18 to 25 with relatively low income.

Although relatively few deaths in children are caused by poisoning—because they do not abuse drugs as frequently as older people—an estimated 60,000 children visit emergency rooms each year due to medication poisonings (Safe Kids Worldwide, 2017). Very young children (ages 1 and 2) are most at risk for experiencing poisoning. The most common causes of poisoning among young children are cosmetics and personal care products, household cleaning products, and pain relievers. In many cases, children simply ingest something they've seen a parent, sibling, or grandparent take, which can include prescription drugs as well as over-the-counter drugs, nutritional supplements, or vitamins. One recent study found that rates of children seen at a hospital or poison control center for marijuana exposure increased substantially following state legalization (Wang et al., 2016).

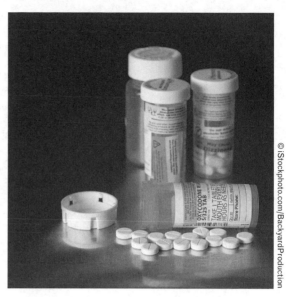

Drug overdose deaths have increased substantially over the last 20 years and show no signs of decreasing. In fact, estimates are that approximately 64,000 people died from drug overdoses in 2016, the largest number of such deaths ever recorded (Centers for Disease Control and Prevention, 2017s).

Car Accidents

Car accidents are the largest cause of unintentional injury deaths in people ages 5 to 24 (Heron, 2016). Each year in the United States alone, more than 32,000 people are killed and another 2 million are injured from car accidents. Car accidents also cause other types of lasting but not fatal injuries. For example, car accidents are the leading cause of spinal cord injuries (O'Connor, 2002). Car accidents can also lead to relatively minor injuries, such as fractures, sprains/strains, internal bleeding, and bruising.

Many of these deaths are caused by behavioral choices. For example, one in three deaths from car accidents involves a drunk driver, and nearly one in three deaths involves speeding (Centers for Disease Control and Prevention, 2016f). Deaths from car accidents also result from people not wearing seat belts and not having children in properly installed car seats and booster seats. One study analyzing data from over 18,000 children (ages 14 and younger) who were involved in a fatal crash found that 20% were unrestrained or inappropriately restrained, suggesting that increasing children restraint use would be an effective strategy for reducing unintentional injuries (Wolf et al., 2017).

Distracted driving also contributes to a substantial number of car crashes each year. Every day in the United States, nine people are killed and over 1,000 people are injured from crashes resulting from a distracted driver (National Center for Statistics and Analysis, 2017). Distraction can be visual, such as when you take your eyes off the road, but can also be manual, when you take your hands off the steering wheel, or cognitive, meaning you take your mind off driving. Although talking on a cell phone and texting while driving are two common types of activities that can lead to distraction, other distractions that can impair driving include eating or drinking, applying makeup, and adjusting the radio. Researchers in one study using a driving simulator found that people texting made as many driving errors—such as speeding, straying from their lane position, and delayed reaction time—as those with a blood alcohol concentration of .07 (Leung, Croft, Jackson, Howard, & McKenzie, 2012).

Falls

The third leading cause of unintentional injury–related death in the United States is falls (Heron, 2016). Moreover, nonfatal falls cause many serious injuries, such as broken bones and head injuries. Over 800,000 people are hospitalized for a fall-related injury, such as hip fracture or brain injury, each year. More than 95% of hip fractures are caused by falling, and falls are the most common cause of traumatic brain injury.

Not surprisingly, age has a substantially impact on the likelihood of being injured or dying in a fall (Heron, 2016). Falls are the leading cause of nonfatal injuries for all children ages 0 to 19, with approximately 8,000 children every day—and nearly 2.8 million children a year—being treated in an emergency room for a fall-related injury. For very young children, many of these injuries are caused by falls from cribs, playpens, and bassinets, whereas in older children, fall-related injuries are often a result of playground accidents (Tinsworth & McDonald, 2001; Yeh, Rochette, McKenzie, & Smith, 2011).

Falls are also a very common cause of injury, and are the leading cause of injury-related deaths, in older adults, as described earlier in this chapter (Heron, 2016). Approximately 2.8 million people ages 65 and older are treated in the emergency room each year for injuries resulting from a fall, and over 300,000 older people are hospitalized for a hip fracture each year. Many of these falls are caused by hazards in the home, such as broken or uneven steps, throw rugs, or clutter. Simple changes in the environment can therefore dramatically reduce the risk of falls.

Risk Factors for Unintentional Injury

Although unintentional injuries, and even deaths, are often seen as "accidents" that are simply a part of daily life, the reality is that many of these injuries are caused by specific predictable (and thus preventable) causes. These include personality traits, substance abuse, social influence, and poverty.

Personality Traits

As you might predict, people vary considerably in their overall likelihood of engaging in risky behavior that leads to injury. For example, people with angry, impulsive personality traits are more likely to engage in aggressive driving behavior, such as swearing at or threatening to hurt another driver (Stephens & Sullman, 2015). These people become irate easily, such as by slow drivers and traffic disruptions. This type of driving behavior, in turn, increases their likelihood of being involved in a car accident (Wickens, Mann, Ialomiteanu, & Stoduto, 2016). People who are high on sensation-seeking and impulsivity also show riskier driving behavior, which increases the likelihood of accidents (Dahlen, Martin, Ragan, & Kuhlman, 2005; Schwebel, Severson, Ball, & Rizzo, 2006).

Particular personality traits may also lead people to be more susceptible to the influence of media violence. For example, although people who watch a lot of television are at greater risk overall of experiencing an injury, this association is especially strong for people who are high in hostility (Fabio et al., 2015). In fact, for people who are high in hostility, watching more television is associated with a 40% greater likelihood of being hospitalized due to an injury five years later. Researchers believe people who are high in hostility are more likely to imitate risky behaviors they see on television, experience higher levels of physiological arousal from observing media violence, and may become desensitized to violent behavior after repeated exposure. All of these factors lead to an increase in risky, and violent, behaviors, which increases the likelihood of injury.

In contrast, other personality traits predict a lower likelihood of injury. As you may remember for *Chapter 5: Managing Stress*, people who are conscientious are less likely to engage in all types of risky health-related behaviors, including substance abuse, violence, and risky driving (Bogg & Roberts, 2004; Schwebel, Severson, Ball, & Rizzo, 2006). For example, one study of 103 male military personnel found that conscientiousness was associated with safer driving behavior, such as following the speed limit and obeying driving rules (Booth-Kewley & Vickers, 1994). Similarly, a study of teenage drivers found that conscientiousness predicted lower rates of risky driving (such as rapid starting, hard breaking, and sharp turns), which in turn led to fewer crashes and near crashes (Ehsani et al., 2015).

What You'll Learn
6.2

However, conscientiousness is not always linked with safer driving. Researchers in one recent study examined the association between personality traits and distracted driving in two groups of drivers: teenagers (ages 16 to 19) and older adults (ages 65 to 85) (Parr et al., 2016). Participants completed measures assessing personality as well as their frequency of engaging in distracted driving behaviors, such as talking on their cell phones and sending text messages. Among teenage drivers, higher levels of conscientiousness were associated with an increase in both texting and using a cell phone while driving. Although you might expect that people higher in conscientiousness would be more cautious, these drivers may feel a need to diligently respond to others, which in turn leads to such risky behavior. However, conscientiousness was not associated with distracted driving in older adults, demonstrating that personality traits may predict risky behavior in different ways across the lifespan.

Substance Abuse

Substance use is another behavioral choice that increases the likelihood of many different types of injury. As you'll learn more about in *Chapter 7: Substance Use and Abuse*, the physiological effects of alcohol impair people's ability to process information and consider the long-term consequences of their behavior (Gable, Mechin, & Neal, 2016; Sevincer & Oettingen, 2014; Steele & Josephs, 1990). Alcohol use also directly impacts people's ability to drive safely in a number of ways, including by reducing muscle coordination and impairing vision and perception.

These physiological effects of alcohol, not surprisingly, contribute to numerous types of injuries. Nearly 10,000 Americans are killed in alcohol-related driving accidents, which accounts for nearly one third (31%) of all traffic-related deaths in the United States and 28 people every single day (Centers for Disease Control and Prevention, 2016f). Alcohol also increases the risk of experiencing other types of unintentional injuries, such as falls, drownings, and burns. For example, one study examining hospital admissions found that nearly half of all people admitted for pedestrian and near-drowning injuries had consumed alcohol (Miller & Spicer, 2012).

Not surprisingly, substance abuse also increases the risk of both using and overdosing on opioids. People who are addicted to alcohol are twice as likely to be addicted to heroin, and people who are addicted to prescription opioids are 40 times as likely to be addicted to heroin (Centers for Disease Control and Prevention, 2017w). Moreover, using heroin along with alcohol or other drugs substantially increases the likelihood of overdosing.

Social Influence

Social factors exert a strong influence on the likelihood of injury, and are a particularly strong influence during adolescence. For example, although the presence of friends has no impact on adults' driving behavior, adolescents who are driving with friends engage in more risky driving than they do when alone (Gardner & Steinberg, 2005). Moreover, adolescents who believe their friends are watching them engage in riskier behavior than when they are alone (Chein, Albert, O'Brien, Uckert, & Steinberg, 2011). These findings about the impact of friends on teenage drivers has led many states to restrict newly licensed teenagers from driving with peers unless an adult is also in the car.

Not surprisingly, riskier driving increases the risk of car accidents. For example, researchers in one study analyzed factors contributing to serious car crashes by teenage drivers (Curry, Mirman, Kallan, Winston, & Durbin, 2012). Both male and female drivers with peer

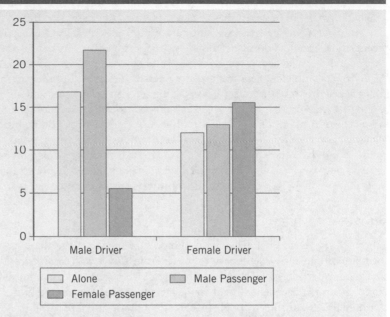

Figure 6.5 Data From Simons-Morton, Lerner, and Singer, 2005

Alone Male Passenger
Female Passenger

Male teenage drivers show riskier driving behavior—including speeding and following too closely—in general than do female teenage drivers, but are particularly likely to do so with a male passenger and are particularly safe when driving with a female passenger. In contrast, female teenage drivers show little difference in driving behavior as a function of whether they are driving alone or with a male or female passenger.

Source: Data from Simons-Morton, Lerner, & Singer (2005).

passengers were more likely to be distracted just before a crash than when teens were driving alone. Specifically, 71% of males and 47% of females reported they were distracted by something inside the vehicle (e.g., texting, eating, looking at other passengers) before they crashed. Moreover, males with passengers were nearly six times as likely to perform an illegal maneuver (such as running a stop sign or doing an illegal U-turn) and twice as likely to drive aggressively (such as speeding or tailgating) as those driving alone. As shown in Figure 6.5, male teenage drivers are especially likely to drive aggressively in the presence of other males.

Encouragingly, parents can play a valuable role in decreasing risky behavior that is linked to injuries. For example, teenagers who report having close relationships with their parents are less likely to engage in substance abuse, which in turn reduces the risk of unintentional injuries (Kuntsche, van der Vorst, & Engels, 2009; Schofield, Conger, & Robins, 2015). Parent monitoring of teenagers' behavior also reduces the risk of substance abuse (Borawski, Ievers-Landis, Lovegreen, & Trapl, 2003; Lac & Crano, 2009). Moreover, and as described in **Focus on Neuroscience**, a mother's presence in a car activates particular parts of the brain that regulate behavior, which in turn leads teenagers to make safer driving choices.

Poverty

One consistent finding is that people who are living in poverty are at greater risk of experiencing an injury. Specifically, compared with children from higher socioeconomic backgrounds, children living in poverty are more likely to experience recreation or play injuries and are more likely to die from fires, falls, and drownings (Birken & MacArthur, 2004). Studies in both Philadelphia and Boston reveal that children living in lower-income neighborhoods are more than twice as likely to die in a house fire than children living in higher income neighborhoods (Shai & Lupinacci, 2003; Wise, Kotelchuck, Wilson, & Mills, 1985).

One explanation for this link between socioeconomic status and risk of injury is that people living in poverty experience less safe physical environments. For example, children living in poverty are less likely to live in homes with working smoke alarms and safe hot-water temperatures, which increases their risk of experiencing fire and scalding burns (Gielen et al., 2012; Warda, Tenenbein, & Moffatt, 1999). Similarly, a study in New York City found that playgrounds in low-income areas had more maintenance-related hazards, such as rusty play equipment and inadequate fall surfaces, than playgrounds in high-income areas (Suecoff, Avner, Chou, & Crain, 1999).

Another explanation is that the link between poverty and risk of injury is explained by a lack of family resources (Schwebel & Gaines, 2007). For example, families living in poverty often lack money to provide safer environments, such as by buying car seats or installing smoke detectors. Children living in poverty also spend more time unsupervised, which substantially increases their risk of injury. In line with this view, parents with low-paying jobs that make paying for childcare difficult are more likely to leave children at home alone.

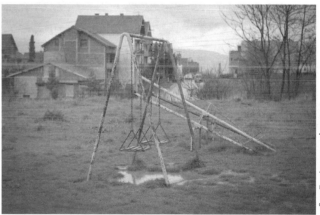

Children living in poverty are significantly more likely to experience an unintentional injury, in part because they often live in less safe environments.

©iStockphoto.com/ZN_images

Parents living in poverty also tend to have less education compared to families with greater financial resources, which is linked with an increased risk of childhood injuries (Schwebel & Gaines, 2007). In line with this view, children who are born to mothers younger than age 20 and with less than a high school education are at significantly greater risk of dying due to injuries than children born to mothers older than 30 and those with a college education (Scholer, Hickson, & Ray, 1999; Scholer, Mitchell, & Ray, 1997).

Families living in poverty are also likely to experience more stressful life events, which in turn may increase the risk of injury. Parents who are experiencing stress may be distracted and thus less able to provide careful supervision of children. In line with this view, among low-income mothers with a child under the age of five, experiencing more stressful life events is associated with a higher rate of injury (Vaughan, Anderson, Agran, & Winn, 2004). In fact, the presence of stressful life events is a more important predictor of the rate of injury than physical factors related to the home environment, such as the presence of childproof locks on cabinets, the presence of stairs, and the presence of broken locks and doors.

Finally, people living in poverty are more likely to use drugs, which in turn increases the risk of addiction and overdose (Adelman & Taylor, 2003; Jones, Logan, Gladden, & Bohm, 2015). Although the specific link between poverty and drug use is unclear, one possibility is that people living in poverty use drugs as a way of coping with the stresses of their daily lives. Another explanation is that parents living in difficult financial circumstances are less able to provide supervision, which increases the likelihood that children will start using drugs. People living in poverty also typically have less ability to access services to treat drug addiction.

UNDERSTANDING INTENTIONAL INJURY

LO 6.4

Summarize the causes of and risk factors for intentional injuries

Intentional injury is caused by deliberate violent behavior that is intended to inflict harm. This section describes the most common causes of and risk factors for experiencing intentional injuries.

Common Causes of Intentional Injury

Many deaths, and even more injuries, are caused each year by violent behavior. This includes behavior that is intended to harm oneself, such as cutting or suicide, or others, such as homicide or sexual assault. As you'll learn in this section, intentional injuries can be caused by strangers as well as by family members.

Suicide

Suicide is the 10th overall leading cause of death in the United States, with more than 42,000 suicides occurring each year (Heron, 2016). Suicides cause many more deaths each year than homicides or HIV/AIDS; on an average day, 121 people die by suicide in the United States. As shown in Figure 6.6, nearly half of all suicides are committed by guns. Moreover, many more people attempt suicide or consider attempting suicide.

Although rates of death by suicide have increased steadily over the last 20 years, the risk of suicide varies considerably by age. As you learned earlier in this chapter, suicide is one of the leading causes of deaths for adolescents and young adults. Suicide rates are particularly high in lesbian, gay, and bisexual teenagers. One study of nearly 30,000 high school students revealed that lesbian, gay, and bisexual (LGB) students were more than five times as likely to have made a suicide attempt in the previous 12 months as heterosexual students (21.5% versus 4.2%) (Hatzenbuehler, 2011). Students living in gay-supportive environments, however, were less likely to make an attempt than those living in less supportive environments, suggesting that bullying and discrimination may contribute to the increased risk of suicide among LGB teenagers. Rejection by family members is particularly impactful in terms of suicide risk; lesbian, gay, and bisexual young adults who reported higher levels of family rejection during their teenage years were more than eight times as likely to report a suicide attempt than those experiencing no or low levels of rejection (Ryan, Huebner, Diaz, & Sanchez, 2009).

Figure 6.6 Suicide Deaths by Method Used

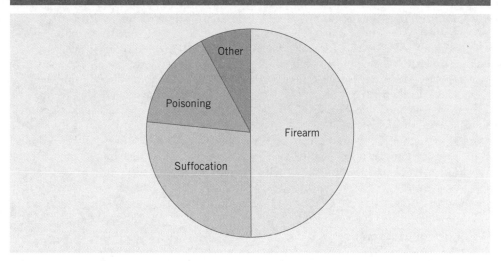

Source: Created by Catherine A. Sanderson, based on data from https://www.cdc.gov/nchs/fastats/suicide.htm.

Older adults are also increasingly at risk of death by suicide. Rates of suicide are increasing rapidly in middle-age men (ages 45 to 64), with White men being particularly at risk of dying by suicide (Curtin, Warner, & Hedegaard, 2016; Hu, Wilcox, Wissow, & Baker, 2008). One factor that is thought to contribute to these high rates is economic pressure, which middle-age men may feel acutely as they try to provide for their families. In support of this view, rates of mortality in this age group are higher than expected among men without a college degree and in poorer states (Alabama, West Virginia, Mississippi) (Case & Deaton, 2015; Squires & Blumenthal, 2016). Men may also be less willing than women to seek help for depression and hence be less likely to get support from family members, friends, or a therapist.

The risk of suicide varies substantially by gender. Women attempt suicide approximately three times more often than men (American Foundation for Suicide Prevention, 2017). However, more men than women die from suicide; men are four times as likely to die from suicide as women. This gender difference is caused at least in part by the differences in methods used—men tend to use "more effective" methods, such as firearms and hanging, whereas women are more likely to use "less effective" methods, such as poisoning (Fine, Rousculp, Tomasek, & Horn, 1999). Firearms are the most commonly used method of suicide among males (56.9%), whereas poisoning is the most common method of suicide for females (34.8%) (Heron, 2016).

The risk of suicide also varies substantially by race/ethnicity. In 2015, the rate of suicide was highest among American Indians and Alaska Natives, followed by Whites. Lower rates of suicide are found among Latinos, Asians, and Blacks (Heron, 2016). Similarly, the percentages of adults age 18 or older having suicidal thoughts in the last year is higher among American Indians/Alaskan Natives (4.8%) and Whites (4.1%) than among Latinos (3.6%), Asians (3.3%), and Blacks (2.9%).

Nonsuicidal Self-Injury

Self-directed violence also includes **nonsuicidal self-injury**, meaning the deliberate, self-inflicted destruction of body tissue resulting in immediate damage, without suicidal intent and for purposes not culturally sanctioned (Sieman & Hollander, 2001). This type of injury includes cutting, scratching, and burning the skin in an attempt to harm oneself. Approximately 383,000 people in the United States are treated at an emergency room each year for self-inflicted injuries (Centers for Disease Control and Prevention, 2017u).

Nonsuicidal self-injury is sadly quite prevalent in both the high school and college populations. A study of high school students found that 15% reported engaging in self-harming, with such behavior being more common in girls than in boys (Laye-Gindhu & Schonert-Reichl, 2005). Moreover, over half of girls (53%) and 28% of boys reported having thought about harming themselves in some way. Such behavior is often triggered by feelings of depression, loneliness, and negative feelings about the self (e.g., anger, dislike, inadequacy). Similarly, a study of students at eight universities revealed that approximately 15.3% of students reported engaging in such behavior at some point (Whitlock et al., 2011). Women were more likely to self-injure because they were upset or with the hope that someone would notice them. Men were more likely to self-injure out of anger and following intoxication. Unfortunately, only 8.9% of students reported disclosing such behavior to a mental health professional.

Homicide and Assault

Another leading cause of injury-related deaths is homicide, which is responsible for an estimated 15,809 deaths per year (Heron, 2016). In many cases, the person who commits the homicide is known to the victim. As shown in Figure 6.7, about 13% of homicides are committed by a family member, and another 29% are committed by someone known to the victim, such as a dating partner, friend, or acquaintance (Federal Bureau of Investigation, 2016). Over 70% of homicides are caused by guns.

The risk of homicide varies across the lifespan. Homicide is the third leading cause of death for people ages 10 to 24, the fourth leading cause for children ages 1 to 9, and the fifth leading cause for people ages 25 to 44 (Heron, 2016). It is not among the 10 leading causes for people age 45 and over. In addition, and as described in **Focus on Diversity**, there are substantial differences in the rate of homicide deaths as a function of both race and gender.

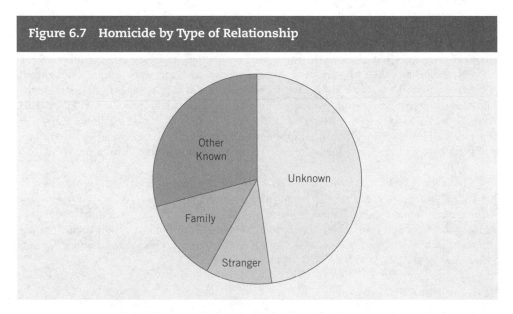

Figure 6.7   Homicide by Type of Relationship

Source: Created by Catherine A. Sanderson, based on data from https://ucr.fbi.gov/crime-in-the-u.s/2015/crime-in-the-u.s.-2015/offenses-known-to-law-enforcement/expanded-homicide.

Violent crimes also include assaults that are not fatal. In 2015, there were an estimated 764,449 aggravated assaults, meaning attacks intended to inflict severe bodily injury (FBI, 2016). Approximately 26% of these were committed with personal weapons, such as hands, fists, or feet; 24% used guns, 18% used knives or other cutting instruments, and other weapons were used in 31% of these assaults.

Teenagers and young adults are particularly at risk of experiencing an assault. Nearly 500,000 young people ages 10 to 24 are treated in emergency departments each year for injuries sustained due to violence-related assaults (Centers for Disease Control and Prevention, 2017y). Moreover, in a nationwide survey of high school students, about 6% reported not going to school on one or more days in the last 30 days because they felt unsafe at school or on their way to and from school.

Intimate Partner Violence (IPV)

Although we often think about violent behavior as occurring between strangers, violence occurs far too often between people in close relationships. **Intimate partner violence (IPV)** describes physical, sexual, or psychological aggression that is committed by a current or former romantic partner (Centers for Disease Control and Prevention, 2017n). IPV can include many different types of violence, including hitting, choking, stalking, or threats of physical violence. It may also include sexual assault. This type of violence can occur among heterosexual or same-sex couples.

Many people experience some type of violence from an intimate partner at some point in their lives. An estimated 27% of women and 11% of men in the United States report having experienced some type of sexual violence, physical violence, or stalking by an intimate partner (Smith et al., 2017). Moreover, a study of high school students revealed that 20% of female students and 10% of male students have experienced some form of physical or sexual violence from a dating partner in the last year (Vagi, Olsen, Basile, & Vivolo-Kantor, 2015). Such violence can cause minor or major injuries, such as bruises, broken bones, or traumatic brain injury. Each year, over 1,000 women and 200 men are murdered by a current or former intimate partner (U.S. Department of Justice, 2011).

Sexual violence on college campuses is a particular concern. Nearly 20% of female college students experience an attempted or completed sexual assault during their college years, with women being at particular risk during their first two years of college (Krebs, Lindquist, Warner, Fisher, & Martin, 2007). One recent study of nine colleges found that over 10% of women had experienced a completed sexual assault; most of these attacks were by men the women knew and trusted and often occurred while the women were incapacitated in some way, such as after drinking (Krebs et al., 2016). Although sexual assault is sometimes viewed as a concern only for women, men can also experience sexual assault. In fact, data from the study of nine colleges previously mentioned revealed that 3% of men reported experiencing sexual assault.

Child Abuse and Neglect

Child maltreatment describes four distinct types of behaviors: physical abuse, sexual abuse, emotional abuse, and neglect. Physical abuse includes punching, kicking, burning, or shaking a child and is typically what comes to people's minds when they think of child abuse. Sexual abuse may include sexual contact between an adult and a child but could also include exposing one's own genitals to a child or taking sexually explicit photos of a child. Emotional abuse describes rejecting, ignoring, or belittling the child or failing to give appropriate affection. The majority of child abuse cases—approximately 80%—involve neglect, which includes failing to give the child adequate food and clothing or leaving the child alone.

Child abuse and neglect are far too prevalent in the United States. An estimated 683,000 children are the victims of abuse and neglect, and about 1,670 children die from abuse or neglect each year (Heron, 2016). Moreover, these estimates are probably low, since many cases may not be reported. Consequences of child abuse include impaired cognitive and social skills, lower language development, blindness, and cerebral palsy (due to head trauma). Sadly, most of this abuse and neglect is caused by parents.

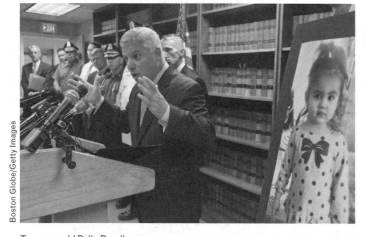

Two-year-old Bella Bond's body was found inside a plastic garbage bag on the shore of Deer Island in Boston, Massachusetts, in June 2015. Her mother and mother's boyfriend were arrested and charged with her murder.

Sexual Violence

Sexual violence, meaning sexual activity when consent is not obtained or given, is a significant problem in the United States. Although sexual violence can happen to anyone, most victims are female, and most such violence is committed by a male the victim knows. One national survey revealed that 18.3% of women, and 1.4% of men, reported experiencing rape at some point in their lives (Black et al., 2011). In addition, over 5% of both men and women report having experienced some type of sexual violence (other than rape), such as sexual coercion or unwanted sexual contact, in the last year.

Risk Factors for Intentional Injury

A number of factors influence a person's risk for experiencing different types of violence. These include individual differences, substance abuse, social influence, poverty, and access to firearms.

Individual Differences

Many people who attempt suicide are suffering from a serious psychological disorder, such as major depressive disorder or bipolar disorder. In fact, estimates are that over 90% of the people who commit suicide have a psychological disorder (Cavanagh, Carson, Sharpe, & Lawrie, 2003). Many of these people have clinical depression, in which they feel an overwhelming sense of hopelessness and despair, have difficulty engaging in basic life tasks (e.g., working, studying, spending time with friends), and do not see their lives as improving in the future. **Table 6.3: Test Yourself** assesses a person's overall sense of hopelessness about her or his current and future lives, which is a risk factor for suicide (Ellis & Rufino, 2015). (If you, or someone you know, scores high on this measure, please seek help by talking to someone you trust or calling the National Suicide Prevention Lifeline at 1-800-273-8255.)

People who are high on impulsivity are more likely to commit violence against themselves as well as others (O'Connor & Nock, 2014). People who are impulsive do not think through the consequences of their actions and thus are more likely to act on a whim. In turn, people who are impulsive may react to feeling bad about themselves in some way by engaging in self-harm. In line with this view, girls with attention-deficit hyperactivity disorder (ADHD), and in particular those who are high on impulsivity, are three to four times more likely to attempt suicide and two to three times more likely to commit self-injury than those who do not have ADHD (Hinshaw et al., 2012). Similarly, people who are impulsive, and thus have difficulty with self-control, are more likely to engage in acts of aggression and violence (Bushman et al., 2016; Loeber & Farrington, 1998). One large-scale study found that men convicted of violent crimes had significantly lower scores on self-control, the inverse of impulsivity, than did those not convicted of violent crimes (Caspi et al., 1994).

People who are high on perfectionism, meaning an unrelenting self-pressure to be perfect, are also at increased risk of committing or attempting suicide (Blatt, 1995; Flett, Hewitt, & Heisel, 2014; O'Connor & Nock, 2014). According to the perfectionism social disconnection model, people who feel that others require them to be perfect, or themselves have an

---

Table 6.3 Test Yourself: Are You at Risk of Harming Yourself?

Please rate the following statements on a scale of 1 to 5 (*1 = strongly disagree to 5 = strongly agree*).

1. The world would be better off without me.
2. Suicide is the only way to solve my problems.
3. I can't cope with my problems any longer.
4. There is nothing redeeming about me.
5. I don't deserve to live another moment.
6. I can't stand this pain anymore.
7. I've never been successful at anything.
8. I am completely unworthy of love.
9. It is impossible to describe how badly I feel.
10. I can't tolerate being this upset any longer.

This scale measures feelings of pervasive hopelessness and helplessness, which predict suicidal intention. Higher scores indicate greater degrees of suicidal intent.

Source: Ellis & Rufino (2015).

excessive need to appear as perfect to others, experience a lack of social connection to others, and this feeling of aloneness can result in suicidal ideation and attempts (Hewitt, Flett, Sherry, & Caelian, 2006). In support of this model, college students who think about committing suicide have more perfectionistic tendencies than those without such thoughts (Hamilton & Schweitzer, 2000).

These consistent findings about the link between perfectionism and suicidal intent indicate that environments that place a high value on appearing perfect may lead to unintended, and dangerous, consequences. In line with this view, interviews with both high school students and their parents in a community in which at least 19 high school students, or recent graduates, had committed suicide over the last 15 years revealed an environment with intense pressure to succeed—both academically and athletically—which left teenagers feeling unable to admit to failure or to needing help (Mueller & Abrutyn, 2016). One teenage described her friend, who had committed suicide, as follows:

> Like, she likely felt that she was a failure. And so, I think it's definitely tied to her thoughts about her own place in the stupid high school drama that we all grew up in, and her ability to survive—in a very basic sense—the culture of what she was dealing with. So, yeah. I think she probably felt like a failure. (pp. 888–889)

Substance Abuse

As described previously, substance use causes a number of physiological effects that impair people's ability to process information and consider the long-term consequences of their behavior. Moreover, substance use may also reduce people's normal inhibitions against engaging in violent behavior (Bushman, 1997; Weafer & Fillmore, 2012). These factors may all increase a person's risk of experiencing intentional injuries, including self-directed and interpersonal violence.

People with substance abuse disorders are at greater risk of committing suicide (Arsenault-Lapierre, Kim, & Turecki, 2004; Nordentoft, Mortensen, & Pedersen, 2011). In fact, people who abuse alcohol and/or drugs are six times as likely to attempt suicide as people who do not engage in substance abuse (Wilcox, Conner, & Caine, 2004). People who engage in substance abuse often also have other risk factors for suicide, such as depression or financial problems. Substance abuse is also more common in people who are generally impulsive, which may also contribute to a greater tendency to engage in impulsive behavior, including self-harm. Given the link between substance abuse and suicide, researchers in one study examined the link between restrictive alcohol policy and rates of suicide (Xuan et al., 2016). As predicted, states with more restrictive policies have lower rates of suicide, presumably because alcohol is less readily available.

People who engage in substance abuse are also at greater risk of engaging in violent behavior toward other people, including intimate partner violence and child abuse and neglect (Berger, 2005; Laslett, Room, Dietze, & Ferris, 2012). For example, male college students are more likely to commit acts of physical, psychological, or sexual aggression toward their female partners after drinking (Shorey, Stuart, McNulty, & Moore, 2014). The ready availability of alcohol in a given community—meaning the number of places in which alcohol is sold—is also linked with greater intimate partner violence (McKinney, Caetano, Harris, & Ebama, 2009). Increases in alcohol availability in a given geographic area presumably lead to more drinking, which in turn leads to more interpersonal violence. Alcohol use is also associated with more severe types of IPV; those reporting severe IPV (e.g., having been hit, choked, or threatened with a knife or gun) were approximately twice as likely to report alcohol use compared to those who reported mild IPV (e.g., having had something thrown at them or having been pushed, shoved, or slapped) (McKinney, Caetano, Rodriguez, & Okoro, 2010).

Finally, alcohol use is linked with an increased risk of both homicide and assault (Bushman et al., 2016). Among all homicide victims, 39.9% had been drinking alcohol, and about two thirds of these had a blood alcohol concentration level greater than or equal to 0.08%, the legal limit for drunk driving (Naimi et al., 2016). Visits to the emergency room for violence-related injuries are higher when alcohol prices are lower, once again suggesting that raising alcohol prices decreases its use, which in turn decreases violent behavior (Page et al., 2016).

Social Influence

Considerable research points to the role of social influence in leading to intimate partner violence (Bushman et al., 2016). People who are exposed to domestic violence as children are at greater risk of committing intimate partner violence themselves as adults, perpetuating a cycle of abuse (Capaldi, Knoble, Shortt, & Kim, 2012). These children learn that violence is an acceptable way of resolving conflicts with romantic partners and thus are more likely to both commit such violence themselves and accept such treatment by their own romantic partners. In line with this view, a 20-year longitudinal study of over 500 families found that children who observed violence between their own parents were three times as likely to commit violence toward their own partners as adults (Ehrensaft et al., 2003).

Observing domestic violence in the home also increases the risk of engaging in self-directed violence (O'Connor & Nock, 2014). One study found that 17.3% of adults who had been exposed to chronic domestic violence between their parents during childhood had made a suicide attempt compared to only 2.3% of those who had not witnessed such violence (Fuller-Thomson, Baird, Dhrodia, & Brennenstuhl, 2016).

Social influence—from family members, peers, and the media—also increases the risk of suicide (O'Connor & Nock, 2014). Specifically, **suicide contagion** describes how the exposure to suicide or suicidal behaviors within one's family, one's peer group, or through the media can result in an increase in suicide attempts (Gould & Lake, 2013; Poijula, Wahlberg, & Dyregrov, 2001). Researchers believe that some people who hear about another's self-inflicted death decide to imitate them in the particular way in which they died. For example, in one high school, two students committed suicide within four days (Brent et al., 1989). In the next 18 days, an additional seven students attempted suicide and 23 others reported having thoughts about suicide. This tendency is particularly strong among adolescents, who tend to be more impressionable and easier to influence toward conformity. In line with this view, people who experience the sudden death of a friend or family member from suicide are 65% more likely to attempt suicide themselves than if the person died by natural causes (Pitman, Osborn, Rantell, & King, 2016).

Social contagion can even occur through suicides publicized in the mass media. For example, after a suicide of a famous figure is widely covered by the media, rates of suicide increase significantly (Phillips, 1982; Phillips & Carstensen, 1986). This type of conformity occurs even if the suicide occurs on a television show—more suicide attempts occur in the weeks following a television movie about suicide or a suicide in a soap opera than in the weeks preceding (Gould & Shaffer, 1986).

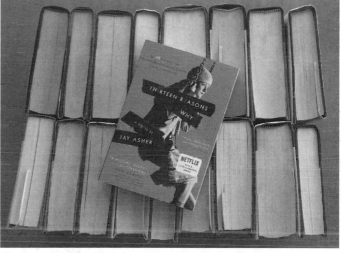

AP Photo/Ross D. Franklin

In the spring of 2017, the National Association of School Psychologists issued a warning that vulnerable teenagers should not watch the Netflix series *Thirteen Reasons Why*, which focuses on a teenage girl who commits suicide. Research on suicide contagion suggests that exposure to such a program increases the likelihood that at-risk teenagers will attempt to harm themselves.

Researchers in one study examined whether media reports of high-profile homicides, such as mass killings and school shootings, increase the likelihood of similar acts occurring later on (Towers, Gomez-Lievano, Khan, Mubayi, & Castillo-Chavez, 2015). First, they gathered data on all mass killings (meaning those that killed four or more people) that occurred in the United States as well as all shootings that occurred in a school. Next, they examined whether these violent incidents predicted an increased likelihood for similar events to be carried out in the near future. Sadly, their findings revealed that both mass killings and school shootings increase the likelihood of similar acts in the next 13 days. Researchers believe that these acts may inspire already at-risk people to act on their intentions to commit violence.

Social contagion also helps predict other-directed violence. A large-scale study of gun violence in Chicago demonstrated that more than 60% of gun violence occurs within people directly connected through social networks (Green, Horel, & Papachristos, 2017). Specifically, if one member of a social network—defined as someone a person was arrested with for the same offense—is shot, it increases the likelihood of others in the social network being shot over the next 125 days.

Poverty

As described previously, people living in poverty are more likely to experience unintentional injuries; unfortunately, poverty is also a risk factor for experiencing intentional injuries, including assault, homicide, and even suicide (Bushman et al., 2016; Krueger, Bond, Rogers, & Hummer, 2004; Loeber et al., 2005; Luo, Florence, Quispe-Agnoli, Ouyang, & Crosby, 2011). In fact, people living in households at or below the federal poverty level experience more than twice as many nonfatal violent behaviors—such as assault, robbery, and rape—as people living in wealthier households; Harrell, Langton, Berzofsky, Couzens, & Smiley-McDonald, 2014). One study of a specific neighborhood in Boston with high poverty and high crime rates, coupled with low social trust, accounted for 10% of the city's homicides annually even though it only contained 2% of the city's population (Harding, 2010). Gun violence is particularly common in high-poverty areas. People living in predominantly poor urban neighborhoods are more likely to experience a gunshot wound injury, and 83% of gun homicides among teenagers occur in populations with high poverty levels (Males, 2015; Zebib, Stoler, & Zakrison, 2017).

Children living in poverty are also at more risk of experiencing neglect and abuse. Children living in poverty are far more likely to experience abusive head trauma, or shaken baby syndrome, which is the third leading cause of head injuries in young children and can lead to permanent disability and even death (Boop, Axente, Weatherford, & Klimo, 2016). They are also three times as likely to die from child abuse as those living in communities with low rates of poverty (Farrell et al., 2017). One explanation for this link between poverty and intentional violence is that families living in poverty experience higher levels of stress, which in turn may lead to more violent behavior in the home. In line with this view, rates of domestic violence are higher during major economic recessions (Schneider, Harknett, & McLanahan, 2016). Researchers believe that men who feel anxious and out of control over their jobs and financial security respond by exerting control/abuse over their romantic partners. Another explanation for the increased risk of experiencing violent behavior in high-poverty communities is the ready availability of guns, as will be discussed in the next section (Bushman et al., 2016).

Researchers in one study examined whether paid parental leave—which could reduce the stress of parenting an infant—reduced rates of child abuse (Klevens, Luo, Xu, Peterson, & Latzman, 2016). Deliberately inflicted head trauma—often caused by shaking the baby—is a leading cause of fatal child abuse and is most likely to occur when infants are between 9 and 20 weeks (a period in which crying is frequent). In this study, researchers compared rates of hospital admissions for abusive head injury in California, which introduced 12 weeks of paid family leave in 2004, to that in other states without this policy. Even after taking into account other factors linked with child abuse, such as unemployment and low educational attainment, instituting paid parental leave was associated with a decrease in admissions for head trauma for children under age two. In contrast, other states without this policy experienced an increase in such admissions during this same period. This is one example of how laws can substantially reduce the rate of injuries, as you'll learn more about in the final section of this chapter.

Access to Firearms

Another factor that contributes to both self-directed and other-directed violence is access to firearms (O'Donnell, 1995). As described previously, guns are used in nearly 50% of suicides and two thirds of homicides (Heron, 2016). People living in a house where a firearm is kept are almost five times as likely to die by suicide than people living in gun-free homes (Bailey et al., 1997; Kellerman, Rivara, & Rushford, 1992; Kellerman et al., 1993; Resnick et al., 1997). Having a gun available also increases the likelihood that a suicide attempt will be successful; suicide attempts with a gun are 140 times more likely to lead to death than those using any other method (Bostwick, Pabbati, Geske, & McKean, 2016). As shown in Figure 6.8, many of the states with the highest rates of suicides are those with the most ready access to guns.

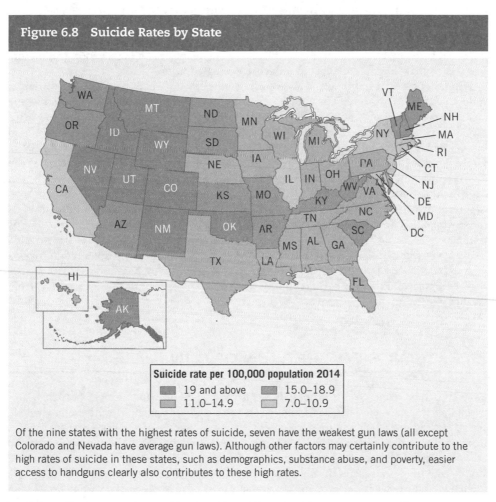

Figure 6.8 Suicide Rates by State

Suicide rate per 100,000 population 2014
- 19 and above
- 15.0–18.9
- 11.0–14.9
- 7.0–10.9

Of the nine states with the highest rates of suicide, seven have the weakest gun laws (all except Colorado and Nevada have average gun laws). Although other factors may certainly contribute to the high rates of suicide in these states, such as demographics, substance abuse, and poverty, easier access to handguns clearly also contributes to these high rates.

Source: https://www.economist.com/blogs/graphicdetail/2016/04/daily-chart-20. Reprinted with the permission of Economist Newspaper Group.

This research examined the association between rates of household firearm ownership and suicide across the 50 states (Miller, Lippmann, Azrael, & Hemenway, 2007). The researchers used state-level survey data assessing household firearm ownership, mental illness, and alcohol/illicit substance use and dependence to examine the relationship between owning a gun and rates of firearm, nonfirearm, and overall suicide. The researchers took into account poverty, unemployment, mental illness, and drug and alcohol dependence and abuse. The findings revealed that residents of all ages and both sexes are more likely to die from both firearm suicides and overall suicides when they live in communities in which more households contain firearms. Interestingly, there was no association between rates of firearm ownership and rates of suicides not caused by firearms. This finding suggests that firearm ownership levels are strongly associated with higher rates of suicide at least in part because the readily availability of guns in a community increases the rate of successfully completed suicide.

Conclusions

Although this section has described various distinct risk factors for experiencing intentional injury, in reality many of these risk factors are correlated. For example, families living in poverty are more likely to engage in both child abuse and substance abuse, making it difficult to tell which of these factors is most strongly predictive of violent behavior (Bushman et al., 2016). Relatedly, people who are high on perfectionistic tendencies may be particularly impacted by living in communities that place a strong emphasis on high achievement; these two factors may therefore interact to influence suicidal ideation.

In other cases, it is difficult to determine whether the link between particular variables reflects nature or nurture. The finding that children and teenagers who experience the death of a parent to suicide are three times as likely to commit suicide themselves and twice as likely to be hospitalized for depression as those with living parents may be explained by social influence, and in particular modeling of parents' self-harm (Wilcox et al., 2010). However, this increased risk of suicide for children whose parents committed suicide may also be caused by genetics; in other words, perhaps a genetic predisposition to depression explains this link. Similarly, among people in one study who had attempted suicide, 46% reported growing up with one or both parents who abused alcohol, compared to 21% of those who didn't attempt suicide (Alonzo, Thompson, Stohl, & Hasin, 2014). Although this finding suggests that family alcohol abuse may increase the risk of suicide, it is also possible that a genetic link explains both parents' substance abuse (which may be an attempt to cope with depression) and people's own self-harm. In sum, this section has described risk factors that are associated with intentional injury but not the precise way in which such factors predict injury.

STRATEGIES FOR PREVENTING INJURIES

Given the tremendous costs in terms of life expectancy, disability, and financial burden, health psychologists have focused on developing strategies for preventing injuries. These can include **active strategies**, which require people to engage in some type of action to prevent injuries from occurring or to decrease the harm resulting from such injuries. Wearing a helmet while bicycling, driving at a safe speed, and keeping windows locked are all examples of active strategies. Other approaches to injury prevention are passive—they do not require people to change their behavior or take any action but rather change people's environment. These **passive strategies** are often particularly effective in preventing injuries because they do not require continuing effort. Requiring all cars to have air bags, placing wood chips underneath playground equipment, and installing smoke detectors are all examples of passive strategies. This section will describe three distinct approaches to injury prevention: providing education, creating legislation, and changing communities.

Providing Education

In some cases, people are simply not aware of how their behavior may increase the risk of injuries. Interestingly, mothers are less likely to take steps to prevent falls than to prevent other types of injuries, such as burns, drowning, and poisoning, perhaps due to a mistaken belief that fall injuries aren't particularly serious (Morrongiello & Kiriakou, 2004). Providing such education is therefore a relatively simple strategy for preventing injuries. For example, providing clinicians and staff members working with elderly people in home case, outpatient rehabilitation, or senior centers with information on preventing serious fall-related injuries led to a 9% lower rate of serious fall-related injuries and an 11% lower rate of use of medical services for fall-related injuries (Tinetti et al., 2008). Similarly, a Seattle campaign to promote helmet use employed widespread educational messages to raise parents' awareness about the importance of helmet use, provided a subsidy to reduce the cost of purchasing helmets, and recruited prominent sports figures from the Seattle Seahawks, the Seattle Mariners, and the University of Washington Huskies football team to describe how helmets are just a standard part of the sports uniform (Bergman, Rivara, Richards, & Rogers, 1990; Rivara et al., 1994). Helmet use increased from 5% to 23% following this campaign.

Skills Training

One of the clearest examples of the benefits of providing skills training is seen in preventing drowning deaths. Over 3,500 people drown from non-boating-related incidents each year in the United States, meaning about 10 deaths a day, and this is the leading cause of injury-related death among children ages 1 to 4 and the second leading cause of death among children ages 5 to 9 (Heron, 2016). Moreover, for every child who dies from drowning, five receive emergency department care for nonfatal submersion injuries, which can cause brain damage that results in long-term disabilities ranging from memory problems and learning disabilities to the permanent loss of basic functioning (i.e., permanent vegetative state). Black children and teenagers are more than five times as likely to drown as their White peers, largely because Black children are less likely to receive swimming lessons (Gilchrist & Parker, 2014). Although swimming instruction alone isn't adequate to prevent drowning, especially for very young children, learning basic water safety skills can help reduce its risk.

Education and skills training can also help reduce the risk of intentional injuries. For example, school-based programs that teach students about the problem of violence and its prevention as well as skills intended to reduce aggressive or violent behavior (e.g., emotional self-awareness, self-esteem, positive social skills, social problem solving, conflict resolution, teamwork) lead to lower rates of violent and aggressive behavior (Hahn et al., 2007). Skills training can also be useful in reducing the risk of violent behavior in the college population. For example, to test the effectiveness of an education program on sexual assault, first-year college women either were given brochures providing information on sexual assault (the control group) or completed a four-session program, which included information on how to assess risk from acquaintances as well as training in physical and verbal strategies for use in defending against sexual assault (Senn et al., 2015). As shown in Figure 6.9, women who received this program were less likely to experience either attempted or completed rape. Women who received this program also reported lower levels of nonconsensual sexual contact.

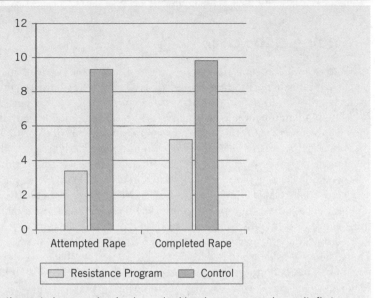

Figure 6.9   Data From Senn et al., 2015

Compared to women in the control group, who simply received brochures on sexual assault, first-year college women who received specific training in assessing their risk of experiencing sexual violence and training in effective verbal and physical skills to defend against such violence reported lower rates of both attempted and completed rape.

Source: Data from Senn, Eliasziw, Barata, Thurston, Newby-Clark, Radtke, & Hobden (2015).

Given the substantial risk of deaths by suicide among young people, suicide prevention programs are another potentially effective strategy for reducing this type of behavior. After completing a school-based program that describes the warning signs of suicide, risk factors for suicide and depression, and steps to take if they or a friend feel suicidal, high school students are less likely to report they have considered suicide or have attempted suicide three months later (King, Strunk, & Sorter, 2011). For example, researchers in one study randomly assigned 2,100 high school students to participate in either a suicide intervention program, called Signs of Suicide, or a control condition (Aseltine & DeMartino, 2004). This program teaches adolescents that suicide is directly related to depression, which is a treatable mental illness, and describes the signs of depression for adolescents to recognize in themselves and others. Follow-up data three months later revealed that adolescents who participated in this program showed increases in knowledge and attitudes about depression and suicide and reported significantly lower rates of suicide attempts. Similarly, educating doctors about the signs of, and effective treatments for, depression can help prevention rates for completed suicides as well as suicide attempts (Mann et al., 2005).

Mass Media Approaches

Mass media campaigns can be a relatively cost-effective strategy for providing education about strategies for reducing both intentional and unintentional injuries. Several states, including Colorado, Kentucky, and New York, have implemented community-based programs to increase booster seat use among children ages four to eight, including community awareness campaigns and school-based programs, public service announcements, billboards, and booster seat distribution events and car seat checkpoints. Distracted-driving programs in both California and Delaware that featured the phrase *Phone in One Hand. Ticket in the Other*, coupled with an increase in high-visibility police enforcement of distracted-driving laws, led to substantial decreases in handheld cell phone use in both states (Chaudhary, Connolly, Tison, Solomon, & Elliott, 2015).

Mass media campaigns have also been used to help educate people about the risks of suicide. One large-scale campaign in California, which included television and Internet advertising as well as billboards, was designed to increase awareness of the signs of suicide and give people information on how to help someone at risk of harming herself or himself (Ramchand, Roth, Acosta, & Eberhart, 2015). Researchers estimate that more than half of all California adults have been exposed to this campaign, and that people who have seen this message are more confident in knowing how to respond to someone in need of help.

Creating Legislation

Even when people are aware of the behaviors they should take to reduce the risk of injury, they do not always engage in safer behavior. The data showing that texting while driving increases the risk of car crashes, for example, is well known, and yet many people continue to engage in this behavior. Creating state or federal laws requiring or forbidding particular behaviors is therefore often necessary to increase people's motivation to change their behavior (Dannenberg, Gielen, Beilenson, Wilson, & Joffe, 1993; Heishman, Kozlowski, & Henningfield, 1997; Jacobson, Wasserman, & Anderson, 1997; Kaplan, Orleans, Perkins, & Pierce, 1995).

Motor Vehicle Laws

Because motor vehicle–related injuries are one of the leading causes of death, many laws attempt to reduce the risk of such injuries. These include laws that mandate particular speed limits, require seat belt use and the use of car seats for infants and children, and forbid driving while holding a phone. For example, many states require children to sit in car seats or booster seats while in the car and do not allow children under the age of 12 to ride in the front seat (Durbin, Chen, Smith, Elliott, & Winston, 2005). Similarly, given the concerns about driving accidents caused by "driving while calling," some communities have now banned the use of handheld cell phones as well as texting while driving. Estimates are that requiring seat belts in New York State alone saved an estimated 220 lives in the first six months of the program and prevented over 7,000 injuries (Latimer & Lave, 1987).

Researchers in one study examined the impact of laws banning texting while driving on crash-related deaths (Ferdinand et al., 2014). Specifically, this study compared rates of deaths caused by car accidents between states without any texting-while-driving ban, states that allow officers to give a ticket only if the driver is pulled over for another offense (such as running a red light or speeding), and states that allow officers to stop a driver for texting while driving even if the office doesn't have another reason for stopping the vehicle. The findings indicated that states that allow police officers to give people a ticket simply for texting—with no other reason—experienced a 3% reduction in fatal car accidents, meaning an average of 19 deaths per year prevented, compared to states that don't have such laws. These laws have been particularly effective in preventing deaths among young drivers, meaning those ages 15 to 21, who are presumably the least experienced drivers yet at the most risk of texting while driving; states experienced an 11% reduction in deaths of young drivers after instituting such a law.

Many laws about alcohol use, such as those preventing the sale and possession of alcohol by people under age 21, are designed to prevent drunk driving by teenagers. State laws regarding the possession and purchase of alcohol lead to an estimated 11.2% reduction in drunk driving (Fell, Fisher, Voas, Blackman, & Tippetts, 2008). Moreover, making it illegal to

What You'll Learn
6.5

use a false identification to purchase alcohol leads to fewer fatal crashes involving alcohol use in drivers under age 21.

Gun Control

Given the overwhelming link between the availability of guns and rates of homicide, laws restricting access to guns are a particularly effective way of reducing intentional injuries. Countries that pass laws restricting the ability to purchase and own guns show reductions in gun violence, including injuries, homicides, and suicides (Santaella-Tenorio, Cerdá, Villaveces, & Galea, 2016). Similarly, state laws requiring comprehensive background checks prior to purchasing a gun lead to reductions in both homicides and suicides (Sen & Panjamapirom, 2012). The laws that are most effective in reducing such deaths are those restricting people with restraining orders, mental illness, or fugitive status from purchasing a gun. In fact, estimates are that implementing three laws—background checks for all gun purchases, background checks to buy ammunition, and required identification of firearms through the bullets they fire—would lead to a substantial decrease in gun deaths (Kalesan, Mobily, Keiser, Fagan, & Galea, 2016).

Laws that restrict who can purchase a gun are particularly effective at reducing intimate partner violence. Specifically, states that adopt policies restricting people who have been convicted of engaging in domestic violence or have a restraining order due to domestic violence from acquiring a gun and violent acts show a 7% reduction in intimate partner homicide (Vigdor & Mercy, 2006). Cities that adopt similar laws show even greater declines—an average of 19%—in homicides committed by an intimate partner (Zeoli & Webster, 2010).

Laws that require people to get a license to own a gun may help reduce suicides in part because such requirements lead to a delay between wanting to buy a gun and being able to successfully purchase one. Suicidal ideation is often a result of a momentary impulse, which can pass over time; decreasing people's ability to immediately act on suicidal intentions is therefore extremely helpful, especially since suicide attempts using a gun are usually fatal (O'Connor & Nock, 2014). For example, one study found that a law in Connecticut requiring people to pass a background check before getting a license to buy a handgun led to a 15.4% reduction in suicide rates; similarly, Missouri's repeal of a law requiring a license to buy a handgun led to a 16.1% increase in suicide rates (Crifasi, Meyers, Vernick, & Webster, 2015).

Fire Prevention

Laws can also be used to prevent fire deaths, which cause over 3,000 deaths and over 15,000 injuries a year (Heron, 2016). Two thirds of deaths caused by home fires are a result of smoking that accidentally leads to fires on beds or upholstered furniture. Although many of these deaths could be prevented by smoke detectors, 60% of the deaths caused by fire occur in homes without working smoke detectors. Twenty percent of the deaths caused by fire occur as a result of home heating equipment, such as portable space heaters. In all of these cases, laws requiring working smoke detectors and/or sprinklers, or forbidding the use of portable space heaters, could prevent many fire-related injuries and deaths.

Helmet Use

Although wearing a helmet while biking is a very important strategy for reducing serious injuries, people are often reluctant to wear them. However, more than 1,300 people die each year from injuries sustained while riding a bicycle, often because of collisions with cars, and 90% of those people might have lived if they had worn a helmet (Sacks, Holmgreen, Smith, & Sosin, 1991). Helmet use also reduces the number of injuries to the face, head, and brain (Thompson, Nunn, Thompson, & Rivara, 1996; Thompson, Rivara, & Thompson, 1996).

The use of a helmet is particularly important for motorcycle riders. After a Michigan state law requiring helmets was repealed, fewer motorcyclists involved in crashes were wearing a helmet and trauma centers reported a 14% increase in head injuries seen in motorcyclists (Carter et al., 2017). Moreover, the type of head injuries also changed; the proportion with only a mild concussion fell 17% whereas the proportion with a skull fracture increased 38%. Similarly, head injury deaths increased by 66% following repeal of a Pennsylvania law requiring helmets for motorcycle riders (Mertz & Weiss, 2008). This study points out the truth in a common emergency room expression: "What do you call motorcycle riders without helmets? Organ donors."

Changing Communities

Community-based efforts, which focus on changing the physical environment and/or social norms, can help reduce both intentional and unintentional rates of injury (Klassen, MacKay, Moher, Walker, & Jones, 2000). These approaches are designed to reach multiple people within the same geographic area, such as a school, neighborhood, or city.

Modifying the Physical Environment

Changes to the environment can lead to dramatic reductions in unintentional injuries. One large-scale program in New York City made safety changes to dangerous intersections to create safer environments for children to walk or bike to school (Muennig, Epstein, Li, & DiMaggio, 2014). These changes included installing speed bumps, creating designated biking lanes, and changing the timing of lights to give pedestrians more time to cross the street. Even simple changes in a community, such as changing the start time for high schools, can lead to dramatic reductions in injuries, as described in **Research in Action**.

Changes to the physical environment can also help reduce intentional injuries. For example, researchers in one recent study examined the outdoor conditions in which teenagers

RESEARCH IN ACTION

Why Later School Start Times Can Save Lives

Considerable research has shown that teenagers often get too little sleep, at least in part because a biological shift in circadian rhythms that occurs with puberty means they just don't feel tired until later at night, compared to adults (Carskadon, Wolfson, Acebo, Tzischinsky, & Seifer, 1998). Unfortunately, many high schools start before 8 a.m., meaning teenagers often arrive at school—and, even more important, may drive to school—feeling sleepy. To examine the effects of school start time on accidents, researchers compared rates of crashes in two different counties in Virginia; one had a high school start time of 8:45 a.m. and the other had a start time of 7:20 a.m. (Vorona et al.,

2014). Although there were no differences in rates of crashes among adult drivers in the two counties, the weekday crash rate for teenage drivers was about 29% higher in the county in which high school classes began at 7:20 a.m. than in the adjacent county in which high school classes started at 8:45 a.m. Moreover, further analyses evaluating the causes and types of crashes found that the county with the early school start time had a significantly higher rate of run-off-road crashes, which is a common feature of drowsy-driving accidents. These findings suggest that simply delaying school start times can reduce the rate of injuries, and presumably deaths, in teenage drivers.

were killed compared to neighborhoods in which fewer teenagers died (Culyba et al., 2016). As you can probably predict, neighborhoods in which teenagers were killed were much more likely to show neglected conditions, such as vacant lots, poor lighting, and fewer parks. These findings suggest that modifying certain aspects of the community may help reduce youth violence in urban areas. In line with this view, fixing abandoned buildings, such as replacing broken windows and doors and cleaning the facade, in urban areas leads to substantial decreases in gun assaults in the surrounding areas (Kondo, Keene, Hohl, MacDonald, & Branas, 2015). Similarly, creating green space on vacant lots, which are often found in low-income areas, makes neighborhood residents feel safer and may even reduce assaults (Garvin, Cannuscio, & Branas, 2013). Although the precise mechanisms that explain this association aren't clear, researchers believe vacant lots overgrown with vegetation and trash may make it easier for people to hide illegal guns and engage in other types of illegal activities, such as drug use. Transforming these lots into green spaces by planting grass and trees and removing trash may make it more difficult for people to engage in such activities, which in turn reduces rates of crime and violence.

Changing the physical environment also helps reduce rates of self-directed violence. For example, installing barriers and safety nets in so-called suicide hot spots (in which many people attempt suicide) can reduce deaths in these locations by as much as 90% (Pirkis et al., 2015). One large-scale study compared rates of suicide before and after the

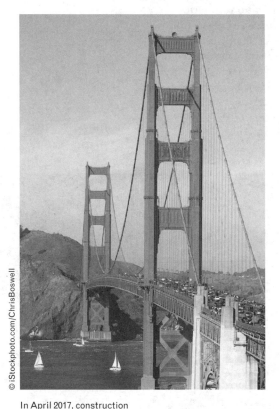

In April 2017, construction started on a stainless-steel net under the Golden Gate Bridge in an attempt to prevent the frequent suicide attempts that take place on this bridge each year.

institution of various suicide-prevention measures—such as placing signs and crisis telephones, increasing suicide patrols, and adding safety nets—at known hot spots, such as bridges and tall buildings, around the world. Deaths dropped from an average of 5.8 suicides each year before these measures were added to an average of 2.4 deaths per year afterward. Although initially public health researchers feared that people with suicidal intent would simply choose other means by which to harm themselves, installing barriers on hot spot locations does not seem to lead to increases in suicides in other places or by other means (e.g., Law, Sveticic, & De Leo, 2014).

Community-based efforts that change the physical environment as well as provide education on injury prevention are particularly effective. For example, the Safe Kids/Healthy Neighborhood Injury Prevention Program in Harlem, New York, targeted numerous aspects of the community, including renovating playgrounds, involving children in safe and fun activities (e.g., dance, arts, sports), offering classes on injury and violence prevention, and providing safety equipment (e.g., bicycle helmets) (Davidson et al., 1994). Rates of injuries declined 44% following the intervention, demonstrating the power of community-based efforts in improving physical health.

Changing the physical environment can also help reduce unintentional injuries in the home. Falls in the home can be prevented through installing grab bars in bathrooms, using window locks and stair gates, and adding brighter outdoor lighting on stairs. Changing the physical environment is especially important for families with a pool, since many drownings of young children occur in home swimming pools (Centers for Disease Control and Prevention, 2016h). In fact, using a four-sided fence to completely enclose a pool compared to three-sided property-line fencing (in which children can still gain access to the pool from inside a house) leads to an 83% reduction in the risk of childhood drowning (Thompson & Rivara, 2000).

Modifying Social Norms

Other programs have focused on changing norms in a given community. One of the most successful programs to reduce gang-related violence in inner cities was started in Boston in 1995 (Braga, Kennedy, Waring, & Piehl, 2001). This program, called Operation Ceasefire, was coordinated by police officers, community groups, and researchers to both reduce the availability of guns in the community and to strongly incentivize gang members to avoid carrying guns. Gang members were warned of serious penalties for carrying guns, such as two-year prison sentences for simply carrying a weapon, coupled with increased police presence in the community. However, gang members were also given appealing alternatives to crime as a job, such as free access to job placement and counseling. This program led to a 63% reduction in monthly youth homicides as well as a 44% decrease in the monthly number of youth gun assaults. These findings provide powerful evidence that broad community efforts can successfully reduce interpersonal violence, even in very at-risk communities.

Communitywide programs designed to prevent violence and homicides in inner cities have also been effective in other communities. For example, the Trauma Response Team, a program started in Syracuse, New York, involves collaboration between the police department, hospitals, and community members to respond to shootings in high-crime neighborhoods (Jennings-Bey et al., 2015). This team responds immediately after a shooting to try to deescalate violence that could occur in retaliation. First, the team provides support—at the scene of the crime and at the hospital—to family members and friends of the victim. Second, the team focuses on where subsequent feuds between rival gangs could happen and sets up hot dog grill stands at those locations. These efforts have led to a 20% reduction in gang-related homicides. Similar programs that connect community members, hospital workers, and police officers have led to reductions in violence in other communities, including New Orleans (McVey et al., 2014), Baltimore (Webster, Whitehill, Vernick, & Curriero, 2013), and Chicago (Skogan, Hartnett, Bump, & Dubois, 2008).

Other communitywide programs have been implemented to reduce suicides. For example, after the town of Somerville, Massachusetts, experienced a number of teenage deaths due to both suicide and unintentional opiate overdoses, a broad effort was implemented in an attempt to prevent further deaths (Hacker, Collins, Gross-Young, Almeida, & Burke, 2008). This effort included raising awareness about the dangers of substance abuse, increasing the availability of mental health services, developing additional recreational opportunities for teenagers, and enhancing awareness of risk factors for both suicide and substance abuse. Following the implementation of these efforts, rates of suicides as well as hospitalizations for both self-injury and drug overdose declined, suggesting that broad-scale community efforts can be quite effective.

Table 6.4 Information YOU Can Use

- Protect yourself from car accidents, which is the leading cause of injury-related death for adolescents and young adults. Make sure to wear a seat belt, obey the speed limit, and turn off your phone before driving. Most important, don't ever drive after drinking or be a passenger in a car with a driver who has consumed alcohol.

- Given the link between owning a firearm and both homicides and suicides, don't have a gun in your house.

- Suicide is a common cause of death for adolescents and young adults, and thus suicidal thoughts need to be taken very seriously. If you or someone you know is having thoughts about killing themselves, talk to an adult you trust—a teacher, parent, doctor, or religious leader—immediately.

(Continued)

Table 6.4   (Continued)

- Drownings in both pools and natural bodies of water are common causes of death and injury, so make sure to protect yourself. Learn how to swim and obey all water-safety guidelines, including wearing a life jacket at all times when on a boat and avoiding swimming after alcohol use.

- Fires at home cause many injuries and deaths each year but are highly preventable. Try not to smoke inside your home, and if you do smoke in your home, never smoke in bed or leave burning cigarettes unattended. Make sure to install smoke alarms and test them monthly.

SUMMARY

Understanding Injury

- Unintentional injuries refer to injuries in which the person who caused the injury did not mean for it to happen. Many unintentional injuries are caused by car accidents, fires, drowning, falls, and poisoning. Other types of injuries are described as intentional injuries, meaning the person who caused the injury meant for it to happen. Intentional injuries are caused by violent behavior, such as suicide, homicide, or sexual assault.

- For people ages 1 to 44, injuries are the leading cause of death, and many additional people experience nonfatal injuries. Injuries exert a huge cost on society, not only in terms of physical health and life expectancy but also in terms of financial costs, including both the direct costs of medical treatment and indirect costs due to lost work productivity.

Risk of Injury Across the Lifespan

- Childhood in general is a time of relatively low mortality. However, the leading cause of death for children from ages 1 to 14 is unintentional injury, and the fourth leading cause of death, following cancer and heart disease, is homicide. The leading causes of injury-related deaths during childhood vary by age but include suffocation, drowning, car accidents, fire/burns, and, for older children, suicide and homicide. Children may also experience nonfatal injuries, which can have lasting consequences.

- Injury is also one of the leading causes of death for adolescents and young adults (ages 15 to 24); 73% of all deaths in adolescents and young adults are caused by some type of injury. The leading causes of death for people in this age group are accidents, suicides, and

homicides. The leading causes of unintentional injuries are car accidents and poisoning.

- Injuries cause about 20% of all deaths in adulthood, but the impact of injuries on fatalities changes dramatically with age. Unintentional injuries are the leading cause of death in adults ages 25 to 44 and the third leading cause of death in adults ages 45 to 64 but cause very few deaths in those 65 and older. The leading causes of death for adults are poisoning, car accidents, homicides, suicides, and, for older adults, falls.

Understanding Unintentional Injury

- The three leading causes of death caused by unintentional injuries are poisoning, car accidents, and falls. Poisoning is the leading cause of unintentional injury–related death in the United States. The most common type of poisoning in adults is the use of illegal drugs, such as cocaine or heroin, or the use of prescription drugs, such as opiates. In children, poisoning often occurs when someone accidentally consumes a drug. Poisoning can also cause nonfatal injuries. Car accidents are the largest cause of unintentional injury deaths in people ages 5 to 24 and cause other types of lasting but not fatal injuries. Many of these deaths are caused by behavioral choices, such as drinking and driving, speeding, distracted driving, failing to wear a seat belt, and not having children in properly installed car seats and booster seats. The third leading cause of unintentional injury–related death in the United States is falls. Nonfatal falls cause many serious injuries, such as broken bones and head injuries. Falls are the leading cause of nonfatal injuries for all children ages 0 to 19 and are the leading cause of injury-related deaths in older adults.

- Many of these injuries are caused by specific predictable (and thus preventable) causes. People with particular personality traits, including hostility, sensation-seeking, and impulsivity, show riskier behaviors, which increases the likelihood of accidents. Other personality traits, such as conscientiousness, generally—but not always—predict safer behavior, and thus a lower likelihood of injury. Substance use is another behavioral choice that increases the likelihood of many different types of injury. The physiological effects of alcohol impair people's ability to process information and consider the long-term consequences of their behavior, reduce muscle coordination, and interfere with vision and perception. Social factors exert a strong influence on the likelihood of injury and are a particularly strong influence during adolescence. Parents can play a valuable role in decreasing risky behavior that is linked to injuries. Although people who are living in poverty are at greater risk of experiencing an injury, the mechanisms explaining this relationship are not clear. Possible explanations include exposure to less safe physical environments, a lack of family resources to provide safety features and adequate supervision, lower levels of maternal education, more stressful life events, and increased rates of substance abuse.

Understanding Intentional Injury

- Many deaths, and even more injuries, are caused each year by violent behavior. Suicide is the 10th overall leading cause of death in the United States, and many more people attempt suicide or consider attempting suicide. Self-directed violence also includes nonsuicidal self-injury, such as cutting, scratching, or burning the skin in an attempt to harm oneself. Intentional injuries and deaths can also be caused by other-directed violence, such as homicide, assault, or sexual violence. Although we often think about violent behavior as occurring between strangers, violence occurs far too often between people in close relationships. This includes intimate partner violence as well as child abuse and neglect.

- A number of factors influence a person's risk for experiencing different types of violence. Individual-difference factors that are linked with violent behavior include psychological disorder (e.g., major depressive disorder or bipolar disorder), impulsivity, and perfectionism. Substance abuse is linked with an increased likelihood of committing all types of violent behavior, including suicide, homicide, assault, intimate partner violence, and child abuse and neglect. Considerable research points to the role of social influence in leading to both self-directed and other-directed violence. Suicide contagion describes how exposure to suicide or suicidal behaviors within one's family, one's peer group, or through the media can result in an increase in suicide attempts. Social contagion also helps predict other-directed violence. People living in poverty are at increased risk of experiencing intentional injuries, including assault, homicide, and child abuse and neglect. Finally, another factor that contributes to both self-directed and other-directed violence is access to firearms. However, many of these factors are interrelated, and it is difficult to disentangle the precise risks associated with each.

Strategies for Preventing Injuries

- Providing education about strategies for reducing the risk of injury is a relatively simple approach that can be quite effective. Teaching people about their risk of injury, coupled with skills to reduce their risk of injury, can help prevent both unintentional and intentional injuries. Mass media campaigns can be a relatively cost-effective strategy for providing such education.

- Creating state or federal laws requiring or forbidding particular behaviors is often necessary to increase people's motivation to change their behavior. The adoption of such laws has led to reductions in deaths caused by car accidents, guns, fires, and bicycle/motorcycle accidents.

- Community-based efforts, which focus on changing the physical environment and/or social norms, can help reduce both intentional and unintentional rates of injury. Changes to the environment can lead to dramatic reductions in injury rates, including reducing rates of pedestrian and car accidents as well as homicides, assaults, and suicides. Similarly, programs that focus on changing norms in a given community have led to reductions in homicides, assaults, and suicides.

7

SUBSTANCE USE AND ABUSE

Learning Objectives

7.1 Describe the power of nicotine and the consequences of tobacco use

7.2 Explain factors that contribute to smoking

7.3 Describe what alcohol abuse is and its consequences

7.4 Summarize various explanations for alcohol abuse

7.5 Describe different types of drugs and their consequences

7.6 Compare different strategies for reducing substance abuse

What You'll Learn

7.1 How social media images can increase smoking in teenagers

7.2 How alcohol advertisements influence drinking

7.3 How citywide smoking bans help smokers quit

7.4 Why increasing taxes on cigarettes leads to lower rates of alcohol use

7.5 How becoming more mindful can reduce substance abuse relapse

Preview

Smoking and alcohol use are two of the most common health-compromising behaviors, and often they are used in combination (Sher, Gotham, Erickson, & Wood, 1996; Shiffman et al., 1994). These two behaviors also lead to many of the major health problems, as well as causes of death, in the United States today, including cancer, coronary heart disease, accidents/unintentional injuries, and even homicides and suicides. In this chapter, you'll learn about the very

(Continued)

serious health consequences of smoking cigarettes and excessive alcohol use and the factors that lead people to engage in these behaviors. Next, you'll learn about the prevalence and consequences of other types of illicit drug use. Finally, and perhaps most important, this chapter will end with a description of strategies for preventing and treating substance abuse. Given how common these behaviors are in young adults, perhaps you'll even learn something that may extend the quality and quantity of your life.

UNDERSTANDING SMOKING

LO 7.1

Describe the power of nicotine and the consequences of tobacco use

Estimates suggest that 36.5 million people in the United States smoke, meaning 15.1% of American adults, including a somewhat higher percentage of men than women (16.7% versus 13.6%) (Centers for Disease Control and Prevention, 2017d). (Although views about smoking are pretty negative in the United States, smoking is seen less negatively in other parts of the world, in which rates of smoking are even higher; you'll learn more about the global problems associated with smoking in *Chapter 14: Conclusions and Future Directions*.) Both Whites (16.6%) and Blacks (16.7%) are more likely to smoke than Latinos (10.1%), who in turn are more likely to smoke than Asian Americans (7%). Smoking is particularly high among Native Americans (21.9%). Smoking is more common in people who have lower levels of education: 34.1% of adults with a general education development (GED) degree smoke, compared to only 3.6% of those with a graduate degree. Smoking is also correlated with income: 26.1% of adults who live below the poverty line smoke, compared to only 13.9% of those who live at or above it. Finally, rates of smoking vary considerably by state (see Figure 7.1). In this section, you'll learn about the power of nicotine, a chemical found in all tobacco products, and the consequences of tobacco use.

The Power of Nicotine

Every day in the United States, more than 3,000 teenagers smoke their first cigarette, and over 2,000 become daily cigarette smokers. Although smoking by teenagers has declined over the last few years, many teenagers and young adults are now using other forms of tobacco, including e-cigarettes, vapes, and hookahs. In fact, a recent report by the United States surgeon general found that e-cigarettes are the most commonly used form of tobacco by teenagers (U.S. Department of Health and Human Services, 2016). These newer forms of tobacco use involve either inhaling a small amount of nicotine in liquid form directly (in the case of e-cigarettes) or through water vapor in the air (in the case of hookahs or vapes). Moreover, and as described in **Focus on Development**, both e-cigarettes and vapes often include tobacco mixed with other flavors, such as honey, candy, or chocolate, which can increase their appeal to children.

Understanding Addiction

Addiction refers to the condition in which a person has a physical and psychological dependence on a given substance, such as cigarettes, alcohol, or caffeine (my own personal addiction). Addiction is caused by repeatedly consuming a particular substance, which over time leads the body to adjust to the presence of that substance and to incorporate it into the "normal" functioning of the body's tissues. In the case of cigarettes, and other forms of tobacco use, people

Figure 7.1 Smoking Rates by State

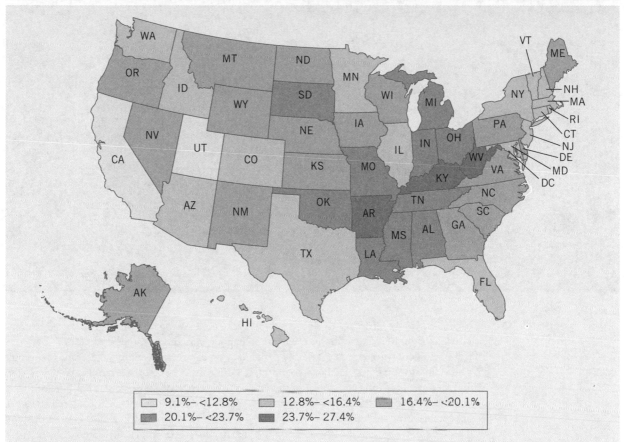

Legend:
- 9.1%–<12.8%
- 12.8%–<16.4%
- 16.4%–<20.1%
- 20.1%–<23.7%
- 23.7%–27.4%

Smoking rates vary considerably by region of the country, with smoking rates being highest in the Midwest and lowest in the West. What factors do you think explain these differences?

Source: Retrieved from the Centers for Disease Control and Prevention (2017), https://www.cdc.gov/tobacco/data_statistics/fact_sheets/adult_data/cig_smoking/index.htm.

experience various physiological reactions, such as increasing alertness, blood pressure, and heart rate, caused by the nicotine in these substances. However, these effects are maintained only while there is nicotine in the bloodstream—when it fades over time, these effects are gone.

Addiction also leads to two other physiological effects. First, people who are dependent on a given substance develop **tolerance**, in which their bodies no longer respond at the same level to a particular dose but rather need larger and larger doses to experience the same effects. Virtually all smokers start by smoking just a few cigarettes a day, but as the body builds up a tolerance to nicotine, they need more and more cigarettes to get the same positive effects. They also experience unpleasant **withdrawal** symptoms, such as irritability, difficulty concentrating, fatigue, nausea, and weight gain, when they discontinue using the substance, which makes quitting really hard (Hughes & Hatsukami, 1986).

Most adolescents don't understand how quickly addiction can happen and believe they can smoke cigarettes occasionally, or even regularly, for a few years and then easily quit. A study with over 25,000 high school students found that most teenage smokers report smoking because they enjoy it (58.6%) and because it relaxes them (53.7%) (Borderías, Duarte,

Escario, & Molina, 2015). Only 25% of these adolescents recognize they are addicted to cigarettes. Unfortunately, addiction to tobacco can happen very quickly; one study found that 86% of the adolescent smokers are physically dependent on cigarettes, which makes it more difficult to quit (Christophi, Pampaka, Paisi, Ioannou, & Difranza, 2016). Although most teenagers who smoke believe that quitting would be fairly easy, only 16% of adolescents had quit smoking when they were contacted again four years later (Zhu, Sun, Billings, Choi, & Malarcher, 1999).

Smoking, including the desire to smoke as well as the ease with which people become addicted to nicotine, may be at least partially based in genetics (Pomerleau, Collins, Shiffman, & Pomerleau, 1993). Research indicates that about 60% of smoking behavior may be inherited—for example, twin studies indicate that identical twins are much more likely to be similar in their smoking behavior than fraternal twins (Heath & Madden, 1995). Moreover, genetic factors contribute not only to whether a person smokes but also influence the age at which smoking begins, the number of cigarettes smoked per day, and the persistence and intensity of smoking (Heath & Martin, 1993). Heredity may also influence how pleasant or unpleasant someone finds tobacco. Yet another explanation for how genetic factors lead to smoking is that they cause personality traits (e.g., rebelliousness) that then lead to smoking. (You'll learn more about the link between personality and smoking later in this chapter.)

The Challenge of Quitting

Although an estimated 68% of adult smokers in the United States want to quit and 55% report having quit smoking for at least a day in an attempt to stop smoking, smoking is a very difficult habit to break (Babb, Malarcher, Schauer, Asman, & Jamal, 2017). In fact, most people who successfully quit have made 30 or more quit attempts before they are successful (Chaiton et al., 2016). Even people who are highly motivated to quit smoking have great trouble stopping; 40% of people who have had a laryngectomy (which is typically performed to treat throat cancer) continue to smoke, as do more than 50% of those who have experienced a heart attack or surgery resulting from lung cancer (Stolerman & Jarvis, 1995).

What predicts successful quitting? People who smoke less than a pack a day (i.e., have less nicotine dependence), have fewer smoking friends, have less stress, have higher levels of education and are employed, perceive the negative effects of smoking, and have intrinsic motivation and more positive expectations about quitting are more successful in quitting (Hertel et al., 2008; Shiffman et al., 1996). Having support from others, including family, friends, and coworkers, is also helpful (Cohen & Lichtenstein, 1990; Scholz et al., 2016). Not surprisingly, individuals who are higher in self-efficacy for both quitting smoking and maintaining smoking cessation are more successful in quitting (Baldwin et al., 2006; Van Zundert, Ferguson, Shiffman, & Engels, 2010).

On the other hand, other factors are linked with more difficulty in successfully quitting. People who are more concerned about gaining weight following smoking cessation are, not surprisingly, less likely to successfully quit: one study found that women who were not concerned about gaining weight had a quit rate of 21% compared to 13.1% for those who were extremely concerned about gaining weight (Jeffery, Hennrikus, Lando, Murray, & Liu, 2000). People who continue to drink alcohol also have more difficulty quitting, perhaps in part because alcohol use is often linked with smoking, and thus triggers cravings (Koçak et al., 2015).

Consequences of Tobacco Use

Smoking is the leading cause of preventable mortality in the United States, causing an estimated 480,000 deaths per year in the United States alone (Centers for Disease Control and Prevention, 2017d). In fact, more people die as a result of cigarette smoking than as a result of car accidents, HIV, guns, illegal drug use, and alcohol use combined. Smoking causes an estimated 90% of all lung cancer deaths; smokers are 25 times more likely to develop lung cancer than nonsmokers. Smoking is also linked with other types of cancer, including cancer of the bladder, colon, liver, kidney, stomach, pancreas, and esophagus. Smoking can also lead to a range of other major illnesses, such as coronary heart disease, stroke, emphysema, bronchitis, and diabetes. Smoking by pregnant women increases the risk of miscarriages, lower birth weights, and other health complications (Grunberg, Brown, & Klein, 1997). Moreover, even people who are light smokers experience very serious health consequences; compared to never smokers, people who smoke between one and 10 cigarettes a day are more than six times as likely to die from respiratory diseases and about one and a half times as likely to die from cardiovascular disease (Inoue-Choi et al., 2017).

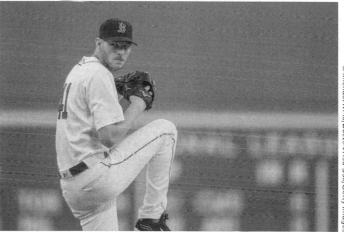

Chicago White Sox pitcher Chris Sale began chewing tobacco in 2007, at age 18. But in June 2014, he quit and hasn't chewed tobacco since. What led to his decision? He quit the day that Major League Baseball Hall of Famer Tony Gwynn died from oral cancer.

Although the health hazards of cigarette smoking are clear, other forms of tobacco, such as chewing tobacco, e-cigarettes, and vapes, are also associated with negative consequences. An estimated 10% of male high school students use smokeless tobacco (Centers for Disease Control and Prevention, 2016g). The use of smokeless tobacco is most common in White boys, especially those who are involved in organized athletics, probably because of the frequent role modeling of this behavior among professional athletes (Tomar & Giovino, 1998). Although the risk associated with smokeless tobacco is not as great as that associated with smoking, chewing tobacco is associated with oral cancer as well as cardiovascular disease. For example, men who chew tobacco have twice the risk of dying from coronary heart disease as those who do not (Bolinder, Alfredsson, Englund, & deFaire, 1994; Winn et al., 1981).

What causes the numerous health consequences of smoking? First, nicotine constricts blood vessels and increases heart rate, cardiac output, and blood pressure, so the heart becomes overworked. Cigarette smoke contains high levels of carbon monoxide, which reduces the amount of oxygen in the blood and thereby leads to arteriosclerosis (hardening of the arteries). Again, this increased buildup of plaque in the arteries forces the heart to work harder to pump blood. Also, tars, small particles of residue in smoke, contain carcinogens, or cancer-causing agents, that lead to abnormal growth of cells in the mouth, throat, and lungs. Moreover, as smoke repeatedly passes through the bronchial tubes, it disrupts the ability of the cilia (fine, hairlike structures that line the bronchial tubes) to effectively clear the lungs of foreign particles. The carcinogens therefore have consistent contact with the bronchial tubes, which is how smoking substantially increases the risk of lung cancer.

FACTORS CONTRIBUTING TO SMOKING

LO 7.2

Explain factors that contribute to smoking

Most people are aware of the very serious, and even life-threatening, consequences of smoking. So, what leads people to start smoking? This section describes the role of various psychosocial factors contributing to smoking.

Social Learning

First, teenagers may smoke as a way of trying out a new identity. Although teenagers may hold some negative views about smokers, such as that they are unhealthy, foolish, and not so good at schoolwork, smokers are also viewed as tough, cool, rebellious, mature, socially precocious, and more interested in the opposite sex (Aloise-Young, Hennigan, & Graham, 1996; Dinh, Sarason, Peterson, & Onstad, 1995). (Not coincidentally, advertisements for cigarettes often promote smokers as having precisely these qualities.) These perceptions about smokers can lead other adolescents to consider smoking themselves to try to seem glamorous, older, or more mature. Adolescents who see themselves as tough, liking to be with a group, consumers of alcohol, and interested in the opposite sex are especially likely to think about starting to smoke (Chassin, Presson, Sherman, Corty, & Olshavsky, 1981). For example, one study with fifth- and seventh-graders found that those who saw smokers in a positive way—meaning viewing them as cool, good at sports, independent, and good-looking—were more likely to start smoking later (Dinh et al., 1995). In fact, the more positive an adolescent's view of smokers, the more likely he/she is to smoke.

Social factors, including modeling and peer pressure, may contribute to smoking. Most first smoking occurs in the presence of a peer, and adolescents who smoke typically have friends who smoke (Mercken, Candel, Willems, & de Vries, 2009; Mittelmark et al., 1987; Otten, van Lier, & Engels, 2011). One study of over 50,000 middle and high school students revealed that the largest association of current smoking was the number of friends who smoked (Evans, Powers, Hersey, & Renaud, 2006). Having more than three friends who smoke is a particularly strong predictor, perhaps because such teenagers come to see more benefits of smoking over time (Morrell, Song, & Halpern-Felsher, 2010; Wills, Resko, Ainette, & Mendoza, 2004). In fact, having friends who smoke is a stronger predictor of adolescent smoking than having a family member who smokes. Having friends who smoke can also encourage smoking simply by providing more access to cigarettes. One study of middle and high school students found that nonsmokers receive an average of 0.16 offers of cigarettes per week as compared to 4.22 offers for smokers (Ary & Biglan, 1988). Similarly, and as described in **Focus on Diversity**, acculturation (meaning the adoption of beliefs and behaviors of another culture) to United States culture may lead immigrants to start smoking.

FOCUS ON DIVERSITY

How Acculturation Impacts Smoking in Latinos

Latinos have lower rates of smoking than Whites or Blacks, perhaps because Latino cultural values and practices emphasize the importance of engaging in health-promoting behaviors. However, these generally healthier practices may decline with acculturation as Latinos adopt the riskier health-related behaviors of United States culture, including smoking. In line with this view, higher levels of acculturation are linked with higher rates of smoking (Abraído-Lanza, Chao, & Flórez, 2005). Specifically, Latinos who have lived in the United States for a longer period of time are more likely to smoke than those who have spent less time in the United States. These effects are particularly strong for women; more acculturated women are twice as likely to smoke as less acculturated women. Other research finds that first-generation Latinos are less likely to smoke than third-generation Latinos, who presumably have adapted more to American culture (Echeverría, Gundersen, Manderski, & Delnevo, 2015). Similarly, young Latino adults who speak only or mostly English at home—indicating greater acculturation to American culture—report more acceptance of smoking than those who speak only or mostly Spanish at home. These findings suggest that adapting to American culture may be bad for immigrants' health.

Researchers in one study surveyed 1,500 tenth graders at a Los Angeles high school about their friendship networks, online social media activities, and rates of risky smoking and alcohol use (Huang et al., 2014). Although there was no association between the size of friendship networks and risky behaviors, teenagers whose friends posted images of their own partying and drinking on social media were more likely to report smoking and drinking themselves. The effects of having friends post images of such behavior was particularly strong for teenagers whose close friends did not drink.

Parents' attitudes and behaviors also influence whether teenagers smoke (Chassin, Presson, Todd, Rose, & Sherman, 1998; Villanti, Boulay, & Juon, 2011). Among those with a family history of smoking, 26.6% become adult smokers as compared to 12.5% of those whose parents did not smoke (Chassin, Presson, Rose & Sherman, 1996). Parents who started smoking earlier and smoke high amounts and have smoked over time are especially likely to have kids who smoke (Chassin et al., 2008). On the other hand, parents who monitor behavior, have expectations for not smoking, and both discuss and punish smoking are less likely to have kids who smoke—in part because they may restrict access to friends who smoke (Simons-Morton, Chen, Abroms, & Haynie, 2004). In turn, children who see their parents as strongly antismoking are seven times less likely to smoke than those who see their parents as not strongly against smoking (Murray, Johnson, Luepker, & Mittelmark, 1984).

What You'll Learn
7.1

Media Influence

The media—including seeing actors, athletes, and rock stars smoke as well as seeing smoking in movies—also contributes to smoking, in part by portraying smoking as glamorous and cool (Dalton et al., 2003; Grunberg et al., 1997; Heatherton & Sargent, 2009; Sargent, Tanski, & Gibson, 2007). Teenagers who watch more smoking in movies are more likely to report having tried a cigarette, even after taking into account other factors that predict smoking, including age, race, personality, and parent smoking (Sargent et al., 2005). Specifically, only 2% of adolescents who had seen the least amount of smoking reported having tried a cigarette compared to 22% of those who had seen smoking the most. Sadly, the presentation of smoking occurs even in films targeted to very young children. One study even found that tobacco use (including cigarettes, cigars, and pipes) was portrayed in 56% of G-rated animated children's films, including *Bambi*, *Lady and the Tramp*, and *The Lion King* (Goldstein, Sobel, & Newman, 1999).

Exposure to smoking in movies increases teenagers' likelihood of smoking in several ways. First, after exposure to smoking in movies, teenagers see smokers as higher in social status and develop greater intentions to smoke (Pechmann & Shih, 1999). Viewing movies with smoking also leads teenagers to have positive expectancies about smoking, and to identify with smokers (Tickle, Hull, Sargent, Dalton, & Heatherton, 2006; Wills, Sargent, Stoolmiller, Gibbons, & Gerrard, 2008). In turn, compared to adolescents whose favorite stars didn't smoke in a movie (or smoked only once), adolescents whose favorite stars smoked in a movie two or more times were much more likely to have positive attitudes toward smoking and report being more likely to smoke in the future themselves (Tickle, Sargent, Dalton, Beach, & Heatheron, 2001). Finally, viewing movies with smoking leads teenagers to have more friends who smoke, which in turn increases the accessibility of cigarettes and pressure to smoke (Wills et al., 2007).

Personality

Teenagers who smoke have distinct types of personalities (Burt, Dinh, Peterson, & Sarason, 2000; Windle & Windle, 2001). Specifically, they are higher in novelty-seeking and rebelliousness and lower in achievement motivation (Audrain-McGovern et al., 2006; Brook et al., 2008; Otten, Bricker, Liu, Comstock, & Peterson, 2011). Smoking is also associated with other risk-taking behaviors, such as alcohol and drug use, sexual activity with multiple partners, and deviant behaviors (e.g., vandalism, running away from home, graffiti) (Costello, Dierker, Jones, & Rose, 2008; Emmons, Wechsler, Dowdall, & Abraham, 1998). Although adolescents who smoke may be less academically oriented and less involved in school sports, they are not antisocial—in fact, adolescents who smoke tend to be extraverted and spend considerable time socializing with friends (Stein, Newcomb, & Bentler, 1996).

As you might predict, teenagers who smoke are lower in self-control. Children who were rated by their teachers as low in self-control at ages 10 and 11 were more likely to start smoking later on (Daly, Egan, Quigley, Delaney, & Baumeister, 2016). They also smoked more cigarettes and had more difficulty quitting. This association between lack of self-control and likelihood of smoking remained even after researchers took into account other factors that predict smoking, such as parental smoking, socioeconomic status, and intelligence.

Another individual difference factor that may prompt smoking in girls is a concern about weight. In line with this view, high school girls who are trying to lose weight and who have symptoms of eating disorders are more likely to smoke than those without such concerns (French, Perry, Leon, & Fulkerson, 1994). Advertising campaigns that link smoking with thinness in women reinforce this link. For example, college women who smoke experience greater urges to smoke after seeing images of thin women than after seeing neutral images, suggesting that experiencing weight concerns may prompt the desire to smoke (Lopez, Drobes, Thompson, & Brandon, 2008). In sum, it's not an accident that one of the best-selling brands for women is Virginia Slims (Grunberg, Winders, & Wewers, 1991).

Positive Reinforcement

Although smoking is clearly an addiction, the precise processes that lead to nicotine addiction are unclear. This section describes the three different types of theories to explain it: nicotine-based models, affect-based models, and combined models.

Nicotine-Based Models

According to the **nicotine fixed-effect model**, nicotine stimulates reward-inducing centers in the nervous system (Leventhal & Cleary, 1980). Nicotine increases the levels of neuroregulators, such as dopamine, norepinephrine, and opioids, which in turn lead to better memory and concentration and reduced feelings of anxiety and tension. Nicotine has a number of reinforcing physiological effects, including speeding up the heart and relaxing the skeletal muscles. These physiological effects lead to simultaneous mental alertness and physical relaxation. These positive effects are reinforcing, so people are motivated to continue smoking in order to experience these physiological benefits. This model is very simple—it basically proposes that smoking feels good, so people are motivated to continue the behavior.

The **nicotine regulation model** extends the fixed-effect model by predicting that smoking is rewarding only when the level of nicotine is above a certain "set point" in the body (Leventhal & Cleary, 1980). In other words, individuals need to smoke enough cigarettes to maintain a certain amount of nicotine in the bloodstream or they do not experience the physiological effects of smoking. To test this model, researchers provided smokers with either low- or high-nicotine cigarettes and then counted how many cigarettes the smokers consumed during a two-week period (Schachter, 1977). Heavy smokers liked the high-nicotine cigarettes much more than the low-nicotine cigarettes, and they also smoked more of the low-nicotine cigarettes than the high-nicotine ones. Moreover, many of the heavy smokers who were (unknowingly) given low-nicotine cigarettes reported feeling especially irritable and anxious. This finding suggests that the amount of nicotine does matter, at least for heavy smokers.

However, both of these nicotine-based models have limitations. First, because nicotine disappears from the blood a few days after smoking ceases, quitting should not be that difficult. But ex-smokers often continue to crave cigarettes even after they have not smoked for some time. Second, these models ignore environmental pressures that can prompt smoking, such as stress and anxiety. Finally, even heavy smokers do not smoke enough to compensate for the decline in nicotine resulting from tolerance, and although nicotine-replacement methods (e.g., the patch, nicotine gum) ease some withdrawal symptoms, they do not end smokers' cravings for cigarettes.

Affect-Regulation Model

Tomkins's **affect-regulation model** proposes that people smoke to attain positive affect or to reduce negative affect (Tomkins, 1966, 1968). Many smokers report that smoking enhances the pleasure of other events, such as eating a meal or having sex (as movies so often portray). Smokers also smoke to reduce negative affect, such as anger, guilt, or fear; these negative emotions increase smokers' urge to smoke as well as the number of cigarettes smoked (Ameringer, Chou, & Leventhal, 2015). Similarly, people who are depressed are more likely to smoke and have more difficulty quitting (Cooper, Borland, Mckee, Yong, & Dugué, 2016; McCaffery, Papandonatos, Stanton, Lloyd-Richardson, & Niaura, 2008; Zawertailo, Voci, & Selby, 2015). As shown in Figure 7.2, for people who are high in social phobia, smoking reduces social anxiety.

Support for the affect-regulation model is also found in research showing a link between stress and smoking. For example, compared to people who are experiencing low stress, smokers who are experiencing high stress smoke more cigarettes and take more puffs (Schachter, 1977). As described in *Chapter 4: Understanding Stress*, one explanation for the link between poorer health outcomes, as well as increased rates of smoking, in people with lower incomes is the ongoing experience of greater stress (Businelle et al., 2010). Similarly, nonsmoking adolescents whose parents experience a job loss are 87% more likely to try smoking in the next

Figure 7.2   Data From Dahne et al., 2015

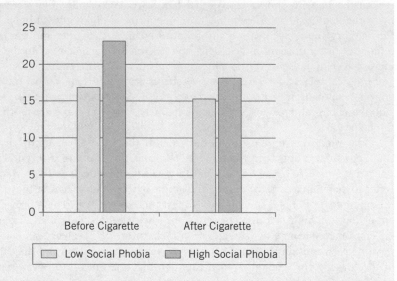

After experiencing a social stress, people who are high in social phobia experience more negative feelings than those low in social phobia. However, smoking a cigarette leads to a substantial reduction in negative feelings for those high in social phobia, whereas smoking has no significant impact on negative feelings for those low in social phobia. These findings suggest that smoking may be used to reduce social anxiety for those high in social phobia.

Source: Data from Dahne, Hise, Brenner, Lejuez, & MacPherson (2015).

year than those whose parents don't experience this loss, suggesting that stress in the home may lead to smoking (Unger, Hamilton, & Sussman, 2004).

Although some people may smoke occasionally to manage negative affect, over time they may become addicted to cigarettes if they come to rely on smoking as their only effective strategy for coping with unpleasant emotions. In line with this view, one large national health study found that smokers who were depressed were 40% less likely to quit than those who were not depressed (Anda et al., 1990). The first time I taught health psychology, one of my students came to me during the final exam with a very important question—she was feeling very nervous and wanted permission to go outside and smoke a cigarette to calm herself down! (Although I reluctantly agreed to her request, I had to wonder what she had really learned in the course about the dangers of smoking.)

Combined Models

According to the **multiple regulation model**, the combination of physiological and psychological factors leads to addiction. This model predicts that smoking is initially used to regulate emotions (in line with Tomkins's model), but over time how smokers feel becomes linked with how much nicotine they have in their blood (Leventhal & Cleary, 1980). For example, an individual who is anxious may initially smoke a cigarette to feel more comfortable (the act of holding something in his or her hand, the feeling of fitting in with others, etc.). In this case, external stresses (e.g., taking a difficult exam, attending a party) lead to the desire to smoke. Over time, however, the repeated pairing of smoking and reduction in anxiety becomes linked. At this point, low levels of nicotine in the blood trigger feelings of anxiety (and a craving for cigarettes), even if the person is not in a stressful situation. So, people learn to smoke as a way of reducing the negative feelings that result from a drop in nicotine levels. Because smoking can be used both to reduce arousal (and thereby reduce stress) and create arousal (and thereby increase stimulation), nicotine can easily become paired with positive as well as negative states.

The **biobehavioral model** also suggests that both psychological and physiological factors lead people to continue to smoke over time (Pomerleau & Pomerleau, 1989). This model proposes that nicotine has a number of physiological effects that make people feel good (e.g., improves memory and concentration, reduces anxiety and tension), which leads people to readily become dependent on smoking. Smokers then become dependent (both physically and psychologically) on using nicotine to experience these positive effects. In fact, smokers who are trying to quit often return to smoking precisely because they find it difficult to concentrate and relax without having a cigarette (and, most important, the nicotine that it provides).

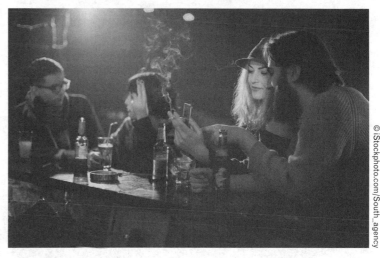

Many people initially smoke to regulate their moods in some way; however, over time the level of nicotine in the body and mood become integrally linked such that simply a drop in nicotine in the blood can trigger a negative mood, which in turn motivates smoking.

UNDERSTANDING ALCOHOL USE AND ABUSE

LO 7.3

Describe what alcohol abuse is and its consequences

Most adults drink alcohol at least occasionally—70.1% of Americans ages 18 and over have had a drink in the last year, and 56% have had a drink in the last month (Substance Abuse and Mental Health Services Administration, 2016). Rates of alcohol use also vary as a function of gender, ethnicity, and education. As you might guess, men are more likely than women to drink: 61.3% of men report having a drink in the past year compared to 51.1% of women. Drinking is more common among Whites (60.9% have drank within the last month) than among Hispanic or Latinos (47.5%), Blacks (48.3%), and Asian Americans (42.9%). Interestingly, although smoking is more common among people with lower levels of education, the reverse is true in terms of alcohol use. Sixty-nine percent of college graduates drink alcohol on a regular basis, compared to only 35% of those with less than a high school education. And even though alcohol use is illegal for those under age 21, large-scale national surveys reveal that 33% of high school students have drunk some alcohol in the past 30 days (Kann et al., 2016). In this section, you'll learn about how alcohol abuse is defined as well as its consequences.

Defining Alcohol Abuse

Although many people drink moderate amounts of alcohol, other people engage in excessive alcohol use. Excessive alcohol use includes *heavy drinking*, meaning consuming four or more drinks on one day for women and five or more drinks on one day for men, and *binge drinking*, meaning drinking large enough quantities of alcohol to bring a person's blood alcohol concentration to .08 (which typically happen when someone drinks four or five drinks within a two-hour period; see Table 7.1). As you might expect, men are more likely to engage in heavy drinking and binge drinking than women (Clarke, Norris, & Schiller, 2017). For example, 31.6% of men compared to only 18.9% of women report having had at least one heavy drinking day in the past year. Heavy drinking is also more common in White people (31.2% report heavy drinking at least once in the past year) than in Blacks (15.4%) and Latinos (22.1%). Heavy drinking is more common in younger people; over 30% of people ages 18 to 44 report having had at least one heavy drinking day in the last month, compared to only about 22% of those ages 45 to 64 and 8% of those 65 and older.

Alcohol use, at least in some people, can lead to serious problems. **Alcohol use disorder (AUD)** is a medical condition that is characterized by both alcohol abuse and dependence and occurs when drinking causes a person distress or harm (American Psychiatric Association, 2013). Table 7.2 describes the 11 symptoms of AUD, which is rated in severity based on the number of symptoms. People with two to three of these symptoms are classified as having a mild AUD, people with four to five symptoms have a moderate AUD, and people with six or more symptoms have a severe AUD.

Table 7.1   How to Calculate Your Estimated Blood Alcohol Content

Body Weight	1	2	3	4	5	6	7	8	9	10	11	12
100 lb.	.038	.075	.113	.150	.188	.225	.263	.300	.338	.375	.413	.450
110 lb.	.034	.066	.103	.137	.172	.207	.241	.275	.309	.344	.379	.412
120 lb.	.031	.063	.094	.125	.156	.188	.219	.250	.281	.313	.344	.375
130 lb.	.029	.058	.087	.116	.145	.174	.203	.232	.261	.290	.320	.348
140 lb.	.027	.054	.080	.107	.134	.161	.188	.214	.241	.268	.295	.321
150 lb.	.025	.050	.075	.100	.125	.151	.176	.201	.226	.261	.276	.301
160 lb.	.023	.047	.070	.094	.117	.141	.164	.188	.211	.234	.258	.281
170 lb.	.022	.045	.066	.088	.110	.132	.155	.178	.200	.221	.244	.265
180 lb.	.021	.042	.063	.083	.104	.125	.146	.167	.188	.208	.228	.250
190 lb.	.020	.040	.059	.079	.099	.119	.138	.158	.179	.198	.217	.237
200 lb.	.019	.038	.056	.075	.094	.113	.131	.150	.169	.188	.206	.225
210 lb.	.018	.036	.053	.071	.090	.107	.125	.143	.161	.179	.197	.215
220 lb.	.017	.034	.051	.068	.085	.102	.119	.136	.153	.170	.188	.205
230 lb.	.016	.032	.049	.065	.081	.098	.115	.130	.147	.163	.180	.196
240 lb.	.016	.031	.047	.063	.078	.094	.109	.125	.141	.156	.172	.188

To estimate the percentage of alcohol in your blood based on the number of drinks you've had in relation to your body weight:

1. Count your drinks (1 drink *equals* 1 ounce of 100-proof liquor, one 5-ounce glass of table wine, or one 12-ounce bottle of regular beer).

2. Use the chart to find the number of drinks opposite your body weight, and then find the percentage of blood alcohol listed.

3. Subtract from this number the percentage of alcohol "burned up" during the time elapsed since your first drink. This figure is 0.015% per hour. (Example: 180-lb. man has 8 drinks in 4 hours equals 0.167% minus (0.015 × 4) = 0.107%.

Source: Reprinted from the California Department of Motor Vehicles, https://www.dmv.ca.gov/portal/dmv/detail/pubs/hdbk/actions_drink.

Table 7.2 The Eleven Symptoms of Alcohol Use Disorder

1. Alcohol is often taken in larger amounts or over a longer period than was intended.

2. There is a persistent desire or unsuccessful efforts to cut down or control alcohol use.

3. A great deal of time is spent in activities necessary to obtain alcohol, use alcohol, or recover from its effects.

4. Craving, or a strong desire or urge to use alcohol.

5. Recurrent alcohol use resulting in a failure to fulfill major role obligations at work, school, or home.

6. Continued alcohol use despite having persistent or recurrent social or interpersonal problems caused or exacerbated by the effects of alcohol.

7. Important social, occupational, or recreational activities are given up or reduced because of alcohol use.

8. Recurrent alcohol use in situations in which it is physically hazardous.

9. Alcohol use is continued despite knowledge of having a persistent or recurrent physical or psychological problem that is likely to have been caused or exacerbated by alcohol.

10. Tolerance, as defined by either of the following:

    (a) A need for markedly increased amounts of alcohol to achieve intoxication or desired effect

    (b) A markedly diminished effect with continued use of the same amount of alcohol.

11. Withdrawal, as manifested by either of the following:

    (a) The characteristic withdrawal syndrome for alcohol (refer to criteria A and B of the criteria set for alcohol withdrawal)

    (b) Alcohol (or a closely related substance, such as a benzodiazepine) is taken to relieve or avoid withdrawal symptoms.

Source: Data from the National Institute of Alcohol Abuse and Alcoholism, https://pubs.niaaa.nih.gov/publications/dsmfactsheet/dsmfact.pdf.

Although there are many different approaches to treating alcohol abuse, more than 50% of people drop out of treatment; even among those who continue, fewer than half of these remain successful over the long term (Stark, 1992). Typically, those who are older, have a higher socioeconomic status, have stable employment and social relationships, and have little or no history of other types of substance abuse are successful in stopping their alcohol abuse. You will learn about strategies for treating alcohol abuse later in this chapter.

Consequences of Alcohol Use

Alcohol use has a number of negative health consequences. The best known is liver damage caused when fat accumulates in the liver and blocks blood flow, which can eventually lead to cirrhosis, a buildup of scar tissue in the liver (Eckardt et al., 1981). Not surprisingly, excessive drinking can lead to structural changes in the brain that cause impairments in cognitive, behavioral, and emotional functioning (Crews & Vetreno, 2016; Delin & Lee, 1992; Du et al., 2014; Sawyer et al., 2016; Sutherland, Sheedy, & Kril, 2014). For example, consuming large amounts of alcohol activates neurons that lead people to

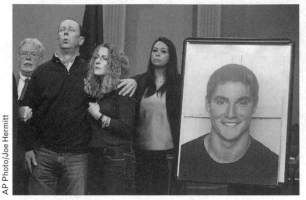

On February 4, 2017, 19-year-old Timothy Piazza died as a result of traumatic brain injury, which resulted from several falls (including down a flight of stairs). These injuries occurred following a night of heavy drinking during fraternity initiation at Penn State University. Eight members of the fraternity have been charged with involuntary manslaughter.

crave alcohol, and to then work to accomplish this goal (such as reaching for another bottle of tequila) (Wang et al., 2015). One of the most serious consequences of excessive alcohol use is the development of Wernicke-Korsakoff syndrome; symptoms include severe memory problems, disorientation, and drowsiness (Parsons, 1977). Heavy drinking can also lead to the development of some types of cancer, including cancer of the liver, esophagus, or larynx (Levy, 1985).

Excessive alcohol use by pregnant women has a number of negative effects on the growing fetus (Larroque et al., 1995). *Fetal alcohol syndrome*, which is caused by insufficient protein in the mother's diet, can be caused by excessive drinking during pregnancy and may result in significant problems for the fetus, including mental retardation, growth problems, and nervous system problems.

Alcohol use can also lead indirectly to a number of other health problems. Excessive alcohol use contributes to an estimated 88,000 deaths in the United States each year, and one in ten deaths among adults ages 20 to 64 (Centers for Disease Control and Prevention, 2016c). Nearly 11,000 people in the United States die in motor vehicle crashes that involve an alcohol-impaired driver each year, which accounts for nearly one third of all motor-vehicle related deaths (Department of Transportation, 2015). Alcohol use is also associated with higher rates of homicides, suicides, sexually transmitted diseases, falls, and burns.

Explaining the Alcohol–Consequences Link

Why does alcohol use lead to so many risky behaviors with potentially detrimental health consequence, such as unsafe sex, drunk driving, and injuries? First, the physiological effects of alcohol lead to impaired information processing and reduced self-awareness (Sayette, 1999). In turn, alcohol use reduces the association between attitudes and behavior, so people are more likely to engage in extreme or excessive behaviors that are not in line with their actual beliefs (Steele & Josephs, 1990). Sometimes such uninhibited behavior might simply make you feel silly—imagine dancing on a table wearing a lampshade, for example. But in other cases, alcohol use can lead to more problematic behavior, such as increased aggression. For example, people who consume alcohol and then rate the intentionality of various behaviors (e.g., "she cut him off in traffic") see such acts as more intentional than those who are sober (Begue, Bushman, Giancola, Subra, & Rosset, 2010).

Alcohol use also leads to a state called **alcohol myopia**, in which individuals are unable to engage in the complex cognitive processing required to consider the long-term consequences of their behavior, and instead base decisions primarily on the most salient and immediate cues (Gable, Mechin, & Neal, 2016; Sevincer & Oettingen, 2014; Steele & Josephs, 1990). For example, people who are sober may recognize that engaging in unprotected sex could have substantial long-term consequences (e.g., unintended pregnancy, transmission of STD/AIDS) and therefore refuse to have sex without a condom, whereas those who are intoxicated may act based entirely on the immediate situation (e.g., their desire to engage in sex) and may ignore the more distant consequences of this decision (Gordon, Carey, & Carey, 1997; MacDonald, Zanna, & Fong, 1995; Murphy, Monahan, & Miller, 1998; Vanable et al., 2004).

Alcohol myopia theory also proposes that people who are intoxicated experience *drunken self-inflation*, meaning they see themselves in an idealized way (Banaji & Steele, 1989; Steele & Josephs, 1990). This drunken self-inflation unfortunately also leads people to experience *drunken invincibility*, a feeling that one is invulnerable to the dangers he or she might normally experience. This is why even people who know that driving while intoxicated is not a good idea may believe—after a few drinks—they are able to drive "even better" when drunk. For example, heavy drinkers view the potential negative consequences of drinking, such as being arrested for driving under the influence and doing embarrassing things, as much less serious than do light drinkers (Hansen, Raynor, & Wolkenstein, 1991). Unfortunately, college students who are unrealistically optimistic about the likelihood they will experience problems due to alcohol use are more likely to experience negative events, including missing classes, getting injured, and getting in trouble with security or local police, over the next two years (Dillard, Midboe, & Klein, 2009).

Benefits of Moderate Alcohol Use

Although I've focused thus far on all the negative consequences of alcohol abuse, there is some evidence that alcohol use in moderation can actually have some benefits. Most research suggests that the link between alcohol use and health is a U-shaped curve—people who drink light to moderate amounts of alcohol have better health than those who drink heavily (not surprising) and those who do not drink at all (very surprising) (Fuchs et al., 1995). For example, one study followed more than 2,000 people over a 10-year period and divided participants into four groups based on their drinking habits—nondrinkers, light drinkers (two or fewer drinks per day), moderate drinkers (three to five drinks per day), and heavy drinkers (six or more drinks per day; Klatsky, Friedman, & Siegelaub, 1981). Nondrinkers and moderate drinkers had a similar death rate; heavy drinkers had the highest death rate, and light drinkers had the lowest death rate (nearly half the rate of the heavy drinkers).

Researchers have proposed a number of explanations for these health benefits of moderate drinking. One possibility is that alcohol increases the rate of high-density lipoprotein cholesterol (HDLC), which in turn helps protect people from heart disease (Gaziano et al., 1993; Linn et al., 1993). Moderate alcohol use can also lead to other benefits, including increased bone density (Felson, Zhang, Hannan, Kannel, & Kiel, 1995), protection from heart attacks and blood clots (Ridker, Vaughan, Stampfer, Glynn, & Hennekens, 1994), and lower rates of depression (Lipton, 1994).

However, the data on the link between moderate drinking and positive health outcomes are difficult to interpret, largely because these studies may show correlation, not causation (Stockwell et al., 2016). People who drink moderately versus those who don't may differ in other ways, such as behavior and genetics, which may better explain the link between moderate drinking and positive health outcomes.

EXPLANATIONS FOR ALCOHOL ABUSE

Many researchers believe that people learn to abuse alcohol the same way that they learn other behaviors: by reinforcement and modeling (Maisto, Carey, & Bradizza, 1999). This section describes explanations for alcohol abuse, including tension-reduction theory, social learning theory, personality, and biological/genetic.

LO 7.4

Summarize various explanations for alcohol abuse

Tension-Reduction Theory

According to **tension-reduction theory**, people drink alcohol to cope with or regulate negative moods, including feelings of tension, anxiety, and nervousness (Cooper, Russell, Skinner, Frone, & Mudar, 1992; Greeley & Oei, 1999; McCaul, Hutton, Stephens, Xu, & Wand, 2017; Swendsen et al., 2000). Specifically, a person who is feeling nervous or anxious may reduce the unpleasant tension by drinking alcohol, which then reinforces his or her drinking behavior. In line with this theory, people who have experienced more negative interpersonal events, such as conflicts with family and friends, report more frequent alcohol use (Carney, Armeli, Tennen, Affleck, & O'Neil, 2000), and people drink more on days in which they experience more negative mood (Dvorak, Pearson, & Day, 2014). Data from a large cross-cultural study revealed that people who worked longer hours were more likely to engage in risky drinking (Virtanen et al., 2015). Specifically, compared to those who worked a standard 35- to 40-hour work week, those who worked 49 to 54 hours were 13% more likely to engage in risky drinking, and those who worked more than 55 hours per week were 12% more likely to engage in risky drinking, suggesting that people may use alcohol to cope with job-related stress.

Although tension-reduction theory was one of the first theories describing the link between psychological factors and alcohol use, overall research provides only mixed support for its usefulness in predicting drinking (Greeley & Oei, 1999). First, most evidence suggests that some people do indeed consume alcohol to reduce tension, but many others do not. This reliance on alcohol to cope with negative events is particularly likely for men and for those who have fewer other coping skills (Cooper et al., 1992). This theory also ignores the often powerful role of people's expectations about the consequences of alcohol use, which, at least in some cases, may have a greater impact on behavior than actual alcohol use. Finally, this theory focuses only on the use of alcohol to cope with negative events (e.g., tension, stress) and thereby fails to explain the use of alcohol to celebrate positive events; people often report drinking to enhance or intensify positive emotions as well as drinking more on days with positive interpersonal events, such as being complimented and feeling cared for (Carney et al., 2000; Mohr et al., 2001).

Social Learning Theory

According to Bandura's **social learning theory** (1969), and as described in *Chapter 3: Theories of Health Behavior*, children learn attitudes and behaviors by watching others, including their parents, siblings, and peers (Maisto et al., 1999). So, children learn about the use of alcohol when they see people relaxing with a cocktail after a long day at the office, celebrating with a champagne toast at a wedding, and drinking beer while socializing at a party. Not surprisingly, children who have parents with lenient attitudes toward alcohol, and who experience alcohol-related problems, are more likely to engage in excessive drinking and to experience such problems themselves (Mares, van der Vorst, Engels, & Lchtwarck-Aschoff, 2011). Although in many cases children are raised by their biological parents, making it difficult to disentangle the effects of nature and nurture, adoption studies show that people drink more when they are raised by people who engage in excessive drinking (McGue, 1999). For example, 48% of adopted males raised in families with an alcoholic parent develop alcoholism, as compared to only 24.5% of those raised in families without such role models.

What You'll Learn
7.2

Moreover, even if children don't directly observe these models for alcohol use in their daily lives, television and movies provide numerous examples of the link between fun and drinking (Gibbons et al., 2010; Grube & Wallack, 1994). Alcohol use is frequently portrayed even in films marketed to children, including G-rated animated films such as *Pinocchio*, *Pocahontas*, and *Beauty and the Beast* (Goldstein et al., 1999). Exposure to drinking in movies is associated with more alcohol consumption later on, in part because exposure to alcohol use in the media leads to increases in the favorability of the adolescents' drinker prototypes, their willingness to drink, and their tendency to affiliate with friends who drink.

Advertisements for alcohol—including on television and the radio, in magazines, and on billboards—also model alcohol use norms, and can lead to increased intentions to drink as well as alcohol consumption (Collins, Ellickson, McCaffrey, & Hambarsoomians, 2007; Grube & Wallack, 1994). Such advertisements, not accidentally, typically show young, attractive people drinking in appealing settings (at parties, on the beach, etc.) and having a very good time—they don't show senior citizens drinking while they play shuffleboard. Researchers in one study examined whether advertisements of specific brands of alcohol in national magazines and on television predicted consumption of these brands by underage drinkers (Siegel et al., 2015). As predicted, teenagers were five times more likely to consume brands that were advertised on national television and 36% more likely to consume brands that were advertised in national magazines, compared to brands that don't advertise in the media. These findings held true even after researchers took into account other factors that could influence consumption, such as affordability, and thus provide powerful evidence of the impact of alcohol advertisement on underage consumption.

Watching people drink, both in real life and in the media, also creates norms that alcohol use is appropriate and desirable. People drink more when they are part of a group than when alone, especially when they are with people who are drinking heavily (Maisto et al., 1999). They also drink more when they have friends who drink heavily. In line with this view, adolescents who participate in after-school activities, such as clubs and sports, with peers who drink are more likely to drink themselves (Fujimoto & Valente, 2013). Interestingly, the mere belief that other people are drinking heavily can lead people to drink more—even if this belief is wrong. A number of studies have demonstrated that college students often believe that there is too much alcohol use on campus but believe other students like the amount of alcohol use. Moreover, the mere perception of a "heavy-drinking norm" can lead students to have more positive attitudes about alcohol and even to drink more (Baer & Carney, 1993; Baer, Stacy, & Larimer, 1991; Gibbons et al., 2010; Marks, Graham, & Hansen, 1992; Prentice & Miller, 1993).

Social learning theory also describes how observing people's behavior creates expectations about the consequences of that behavior. In turn, children as young as preschool and elementary school age have expectations about the effects of alcohol based on parental modeling as well as the portrayal of alcohol use in the media. Although these expectations are initially negative (e.g., they see alcohol as having unpleasant consequences), they get increasingly positive as children mature (Cooper, Frone, Russell, & Mudar, 1995; Goldman, Del Boca, & Darkes, 1999; Maisto et al., 1999). As shown in **Table 7.3: Test Yourself**, these expectations include the belief that alcohol use enhances social situations and interpersonal encounters in various ways, including by increasing social expressiveness (e.g., "makes me more friendly") as well as "sexual prowess" (Goldman et al., 1999). Not surprisingly, people who have more positive expectations about alcohol are more likely to drink (Corbin, Iwamoto, & Fromme, 2011; Sher et al., 1996; Smith, Goldman, Greenbaum, & Christiansen, 1995; Stacy, Newcomb, & Bentler, 1991). For example, college students who report experiencing positive consequences from drinking—such as better sex, making people laugh, or standing up for a friend—report more frequent binge drinking (Zaso et al., 2016).

Personality

Many studies have examined whether certain personality traits, including neuroticism/negative affect, impulsivity/disinhibition, and extraversion/sociability, are associated with alcohol-related problems (Sher, Trull, Bartholow, & Vieth, 1999). Support for the link between personality traits and such problems is primarily found in correlational studies. For example, alcoholism is associated with high rates of anxiety (Kessler et al., 1997; Kushner, 1996), antisocial and borderline personality disorder (Regier et al., 1990), and extraversion. However, many of these studies suffer from a major flaw: they examined people at a single point in time; hence, they simply can't determine whether personality traits lead to alcohol abuse, whether alcohol abuse over time leads to changes in personality traits, or whether a third variable leads to personality traits as well as alcohol abuse.

Table 7.3 Test Yourself: Why Do You Drink?

Please rate the following statements in terms of how frequently each of these reasons motivates you to drink alcoholic beverages (1 = never/almost never to 4 = always/almost always).

1. As a way to celebrate

2. Because it is what most of your friends do when you get together

3. To be sociable

4. Because it is customary on special occasions

5. Because it makes a social gathering more enjoyable

6. To relax

7. To forget your worries

8. Because you feel more self-confident or sure of yourself

9. Because it helps when you feel depressed or nervous

10. To cheer up when you're in a bad mood

11. Because you like the feeling

12. Because it's exciting

13. To get high

14. Because it's fun

15. Because it makes you feel good

The first five items describe social motives, the next five items describe coping motives, and the last five items describe enhancement motives. If you drink, why do you do it?

Source: Cooper et al. (1992).

Although relatively little research has examined the link between personality traits and alcohol-related problems over time, several longitudinal studies do indicate that personality traits can predict future alcohol abuse (Bates & Labouvie, 1995; Chassin, Presson, Rose, & Sherman, 1996; Zucker & Gomberg, 1986). For example, adolescents who at age 18 had lower scores on harm avoidance (e.g., choosing to avoid danger, preference for safe activities) and control (measures of cautiousness and rationality) were more likely to engage in alcohol abuse at age 21 (Caspi et al., 1997). Similarly, several studies suggest that high extraversion scores are associated with alcohol problems later on, especially in women (Kilbey, Downey, & Breslau, 1998; Prescott, Neale, Corey, & Kendler, 1997). But even longitudinal studies do not tell us whether a third variable is involved. As described in the next section, biological and genetic factors may in fact influence both personality and alcoholism.

Biological/Genetic Factors

A number of researchers have examined whether certain people are born with some type of predisposition for alcohol abuse (Enoch et al., 2016; McGue, 1999). Because studies involving children born and raised with their biological parents do not allow researchers to distinguish whether alcohol problems are the reflection of genetic factors or environmental factors, researchers usually conduct twin studies (in which they compare rates of alcohol abuse in identical twins—who share all their genes—as compared to fraternal twins—who share half their genes) or adoption studies (in which they compare rates of alcohol abuse in children's biological parents and adoptive parents), which reveal a genetic influence in the development of drinking problems (Schuckit, 1985). For example, if one member of a same-sex twin pair is an alcoholic, the risk of the other twin being alcoholic is twice as great if the twin is identical as opposed to fraternal. Similarly, adopted children with an alcoholic biological parent are four times more likely to become problem drinkers than other adoptees. A series of studies indicates that people with a particular gene are more likely to become alcoholics than those without this gene, although not everyone with this gene develops alcoholism—about 45% of alcoholics have this gene, as compared to only 26% of nonalcoholics (Cloninger, 1991). Having this gene does not mean that a person will definitely become an alcoholic, but it increases the likelihood.

Genes may influence the risk of developing problems with alcoholism in numerous ways, including sensitivity to alcohol, response to alcohol, and risk of developing dependence (Kumsar & Dilbaz, 2015; Manzardo, Mcguire, & Butler, 2015; Thompson & Kenna, 2015). One explanation for how a genetic predisposition may lead someone to have problems with alcohol is that this gene reduces sensitivity to the effects of alcohol (McGue, 1999; Newlin & Thomson, 1990; Schuckit & Smith, 1996). For example, after consuming a set amount of alcohol, high-risk people report feeling less drunk and show less impairment on various tasks than low-risk people, which then leads to overdrinking. People with a family history of alcoholism may also find alcohol more rewarding and less anxiety provoking than those without this predisposition (Newlin & Thomson, 1990). In other words, genetic factors may lead people to experience more positive effects of alcohol use and fewer negative consequences. People with a genetic predisposition to alcohol use disorders also show differences in brain function and structure, including changes in the amygdala, hippocampus, and thalamus (Alvanzo et al., 2015; Cohen-Gilbert, Sneider et al., 2015; Cservenka, 2016; Cservenka, Alarcón, Jones, & Nagel, 2015; Dager et al., 2015). These differences may cause deficits in controlling inhibitions as well as processing rewarding and emotional experiences, which all contribute to an increased risk of developing problems with alcohol.

Finally, genetic factors may influence personality, which in turn leads to alcohol abuse (McGue, 1999). As described previously, alcoholics differ from nonalcoholics in a number of ways, including impulsivity, sensation-seeking, extraversion, and neuroticism (Sher et al., 1999; Yarosh et al., 2014). For example, teenagers with particular variations in one gene—linked with impulsivity—are more likely to engage in binge drinking (Peña-Oliver et al., 2016). Future research is clearly needed to disentangle these complex relationships.

UNDERSTANDING DRUG USE

LO 7.5

Describe different types of drugs and their consequences

Although tobacco and alcohol are the most commonly used drugs in our society, an estimated 10% of Americans report having used some other type of illicit drug in the last month (Centers for Disease Control and Prevention, 2017m). In this section, you'll learn about different types of drugs as well as the very serious consequences of their use.

Types of Drugs

All drugs alter our mental processes in some way, such as by changing our conscious awareness, mood, and/or perception. Drugs are divided into four distinct categories based on the physiological effects they create in the body. Keep in mind that each of these categories includes drugs that are legal, such as caffeine and codeine, and drugs that are illegal, such as heroin and cocaine. However, legal drugs may be misused in various ways, including being used in illegal quantities, consumed in illegal ways, or taken by someone who does not have a prescription for their use. As shown in Figure 7.3, over 20% of young adults (ages 18 to 25) report having used some type of illicit drug in the last month, with marijuana being by far the most commonly used (Substance Abuse and Mental Health Services Administration, 2014).

Depressants, or sedatives, act on the central nervous system to slow down normal bodily activity, including in the brain, heart, and muscles. In turn, their use causes decreases in arousal and anxiety and increases in relaxation and drowsiness. Alcohol is a legal depressant, as are prescription drugs used to treat anxiety, such as Valium and Xanax, and sleep disorders.

Narcotics, or opiates, are designed to mimic the body's normal process of managing pain by binding to opioid receptors in the brain, spinal cord, and other parts of the body. This process in turn reduces feelings of pain and produces a feeling of pleasure or euphoria. Narcotics include illegal drugs, such as heroin, as well as drugs legally available with a prescription, such as morphine, codeine, and oxycontin. Although narcotics may be used safely for a brief period of time to treat severe pain, legal use can, over time, lead to misuse, including taking the drug in a larger amount than is recommended and taking the drug without a prescription. As you'll

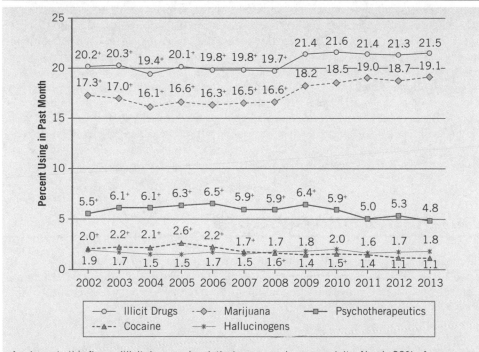

Figure 7.3   Prevalence of Illicit Drug Use in the Past Month by Young Adults in the United States

As shown in this figure, illicit drug use is relatively common in young adults. Nearly 20% of young adults report having used marijuana in the last month, although fewer than 5% report having used psychotherapeutics (stimulants, sedatives, tranquilizers, pain relievers), hallucinogens, or cocaine.

Source: Substance Abuse and Mental Health Services Administration (2014).

learn in the next section, opiate addiction is a growing problem in the United States and is associated with extremely serious consequences.

Stimulants are designed to create physiological arousal, which leads to increases in energy and alertness and reductions in fatigue. For example, many people use a widely available stimulant, coffee, to start their day. These drugs stimulate the central nervous system by raising levels of the neurotransmitter dopamine in the brain, which causes increases in heart rate, blood pressure, and body temperature. Illegal stimulants include cocaine, amphetamines, and crystal meth.

Stimulants are also used legally to treat attention-deficit hyperactivity disorder (ADHD). Adderall, for example, is a prescription stimulant used to help people with ADHD pay attention and maintain concentration. However, Adderall, and other drugs used to treat attention-related problems, may be used illegally, meaning by people without a prescription and/or in larger than recommended quantities. One study revealed that over 60% of college students had been offered a prescription stimulant, and 31% had actually used such a stimulant without a prescription (Garnier-Dykstra, Caldeira, Vincent, O'Grady, & Arria, 2012). Interestingly, and as described in **Research in Action**, college students often don't see the illegality of using such stimulants, in addition to their potential for leading to longer-term health problems, as particularly problematic.

Hallucinogens, or psychedelics, distort perception in some way, meaning people see and hear things that are not really there. Hallucinations work, at least in part, by temporarily disrupting the functioning of neurotransmitters in the body, which can create feelings of relaxation, euphoria, and heightened sensations. These drugs include marijuana (the most commonly used illicit drug), LSD, mescaline, psilocybin (found in certain types of mushrooms), and PCP. Each of these different hallucinogens includes different chemicals, which in turn influence the body in distinct ways. For example, the effects of marijuana are due to a chemical called tetrahydrocannabinol (THC), which affects parts of the brain that control pleasure, memory, thinking, concentration, sensory and time perception, and movement.

Although this section has divided drugs into four distinct categories, these divisions are not necessarily so clear. At very low levels, alcohol is a stimulant, increasing energy, whereas with increased consumption, alcohol is a depressant, relaxing the body and brain. Similarly, the drug MDMA (3,4-methylenedioxy-methamphetamine), often known as Molly or Ecstasy,

RESEARCH IN ACTION

Is Using Drugs to Get Ahead Cheating? It Depends!

Researchers in one recent study examined whether college students viewed using drugs to get ahead differently depending on how these drugs were used (Dodge, Williams, Marzell, & Turrisi, 2012). Approximately 1,200 first-year college students read a questionnaire describing drug use in two scenarios. One student ("Bill") was a sprinter for his college track team who didn't have adequate time to train and therefore used steroids to perform better in his championship meet (which he then won). The other scenario described "Jeff," who didn't have adequate time to study for exams and therefore used a stimulant (Adderall) to help him focus while studying (and he ended up doing better than expected). Although each of these students used a drug, participants rated the steroid user as more of a cheater than the stimulant user. Moreover, students who were athletes, as well as those who had previously used prescription drugs illegally themselves, were especially likely to see Bill, the steroid user, as engaging in worse behavior than Jeff, the stimulant user. These findings indicate that students view the use of performance-enhancing drugs in an academic setting as less serious than the use of such drugs in an athletic setting.

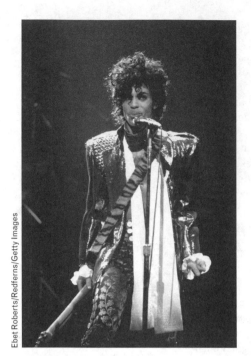

On April 21, 2016, singer Prince died of an accidental overdose of fentanyl, an opioid drug.

is similar to both a stimulant and a hallucinogen; it increases energy and positive emotions but also leads to distortions in sensations and time.

Consequences of Drug Use

All drugs contain chemicals that change the way cells in the brain send, receive, and process information. For example, opiates cause cells in the brain to release abnormally large amounts of dopamine, a neurotransmitter that leads to very positive feelings. When a person continues to use opiates, her or his body reduces its own production of this chemical, which leads the person to continue to take even more of the drug in order to experience the same positive feeling (this is the process of *tolerance*, as described earlier in this chapter). This process over time leads to addiction.

Although drugs vary considerably in the specific effects they have on the body, they all alter the body's normal physiological processes and can have serious, and lasting, side effects. These effects can include impairments in learning, judgment, memory, and decision making. In turn, college students who abuse sedatives—such as Xanax, Valium, or Ambien—are more likely to report experiencing both regret following sex and sexual assault (Parks, Frone, Muraven, & Boyd, 2017). Although the perpetrator is always responsible for any acts of sexual assault, people who are under the influence of drugs may be less able to recognize the danger they are facing and/or successfully fight off an assault. Illegal drugs can also have undesirable physical side effects, such as nausea, constipation, vomiting, and convulsions.

Most important, the use of illegal drugs can also lead to serious, even life-threatening, effects. For example, narcotics and depressants both slow breathing and heart rate, which can lead someone to become unconscious and even die. As described in ***Chapter 6: Injury and Injury Prevention***, drug overdose is the number-one cause of injury-related death in the United States; an estimated 91 Americans die every day from an opiate overdose (Centers for Disease Control and Prevention, 2017x).

Unfortunately, the growing trend toward legalizing marijuana use may lead to increases in its use and abuse, especially by teenagers. Researchers in one study compared high school students' beliefs about the harmfulness of marijuana as well as their use of the drug in the past month in states that had legalized recreational marijuana use versus those that had not (Cerdá et al., 2017). Their findings revealed that perceived harmfulness was decreased in states that had legalized marijuana more than in those that had not. Not surprisingly, its use was also increased in these states. These findings suggest that beliefs about marijuana and the prevalence of its use may change further as more states move toward legalizing this drug in some way.

STRATEGIES FOR REDUCING SUBSTANCE ABUSE

LO 7.6

Compare different strategies for reducing substance abuse

Given the substantial consequences of all forms of substances on health, public health researchers have focused considerable effort on reducing the prevalence of tobacco use, alcohol abuse, and illegal drug use. Such approaches include preventing people from initiating these behaviors, treating these addictions in current users, and helping former users avoid relapse.

Preventing Substance Abuse

Because most people who engage in substance abuse start at an early age, efforts to prevent such problems must target adolescents before they begin such behaviors; these are primary prevention strategies (Flay et al., 1987). The initial efforts to prevent such behaviors in teenagers focused on their severe long-term negative effects, such as dying of lung cancer (in the case of cigarette use). One of the most famous, and widely used, approaches to preventing drug use was Project DARE (Drug Abuse Resistance Education), which began in the early 1980s as a partnership between schools and police officers. This program was designed to teach students about the hazards of drug use and encourage them to resist social pressures to engage in substance abuse. Unfortunately, multiple studies have revealed that this program is ineffective, in part because it doesn't teach strategies needed to refuse drugs or opportunities to develop such skills (Ennett, Tobler, Ringwalt, & Flewelling, 1994; West & O'Neal, 2004).

This approach is basically unsuccessful for several reasons. First, many teenagers who begin to engage in such behavior are already aware of these dangers—but perceive them as not personally relevant, in part because teenagers usually intend to quit before they experience the longer-term consequences. Second, even those who believe they are at risk of various health consequences may perceive the shorter-term benefits of engaging in such behavior (e.g., looking "mature," feeling relaxed, fitting in) as more important than the distant, long-term consequences. More recent substance abuse prevention programs have therefore focused on alternative strategies, including social influence and life skills–training programs, mass media campaigns, and legal approaches.

Social Influence Programs

Social influence programs include a number of components designed to make them effective in keeping adolescents away from smoking (Flay et al., 1987). First, these programs inform teenagers of the immediate physiological and social consequences of engaging in substance use, such as the financial cost of smoking, rejection by potential dating partners who don't like the smell of smoke, and having stained teeth and bad breath. In fact, emphasizing minor but short-term consequences is more effective in changing attitudes toward smoking than emphasizing the serious long-term health consequences (Pechmann, 1997)! These programs also appeal to adolescents' desire for independence by pointing out the manipulative nature of cigarette ads. The underlying message is that people who buy cigarettes are giving in to advertising slogans, whereas those who refuse to smoke are independent and self-reliant (very appealing traits to most teenagers). Third, because peers play a major role in the initiation and maintenance of smoking, these programs often emphasize that many adolescents are against drug use. Adolescents tend to overestimate the number of others who are engaging in risky behaviors, and they believe that others have more favorable perceptions of the behaviors and those who engage in them (Graham, Marks, & Hansen, 1991; Marks, Graham, & Hansen, 1992). Finally, social influence programs are typically presented by desirable role models, namely, slightly older students (e.g., high school students leading groups for junior high school students). These peer leaders demonstrate strategies for resisting peer pressure to engage in substance abuse and allow participants to role-play various situations to practice their responses.

Encouragingly, some research suggests that social influence programs may reduce the rate of adolescent smoking. One study with sixth-grade students revealed that those who received a social influence program were significantly less likely to try cigarettes by the end of eighth grade than those who did not receive such a program (47% versus 60%, respectively) (Best et al., 1984). Moreover, this program was even effective in helping students who were already smoking occasionally—at the two-year follow-up, 63% of those who received this program had quit smoking as compared to only 28% of those who did not receive this program. Social influence programs should ideally start early, before students have started to engage in substance abuse, but also continue during middle school/junior high and high school.

Social influence programs may also try to change people's perceptions about how common drinking is among their peers. As described earlier, the perception that most other people drink heavily can lead to increased alcohol abuse, even if this perception is wrong. In one study, "high-risk" first-year students (those who were already heavy drinkers) met individually with a psychologist who gave them personal feedback, including how much more they drank than most students, the health consequences of heavy alcohol use, and environmental risk factors for heavy drinking, such as belonging to a sorority or fraternity and having heavy-drinking friends (Marlatt et al., 1998). Although these heavy-drinking students continued to experience more alcohol-related problems than the average college student, two years later only 11% of those who received this feedback were judged alcohol-dependent as compared to 27% of heavy drinkers who did not receive this type of feedback.

Life Skills–Training Approaches

Life skills–training approaches are based on the assumption that adolescents who lack self-esteem and self-confidence may turn to drugs both as a way of feeling better about themselves and because they lack the skills necessary to stand up to peer pressure (Flay, 1987). These programs may include some of the same components as social influence programs, such as information about the negative short-term consequences of such behaviors and the impact of manipulative media messages, but they also provide adolescents with general assistance in enhancing self-esteem and social competence, techniques for resisting persuasive appeals, and skills for verbal and nonverbal communication. One study demonstrated that seventh-grade students in New York who received 15 sessions of life-skills training over four to six weeks were less likely to report smoking than those who did not receive such training, even as much as one year later (10% versus 22%, respectively) (Botvin, Baker, Renick, Filazzola, & Botvin, 1984).

Even college students may benefit from training in assertiveness skills. For example, one study assigned college students who had been identified as problem drinkers to either a skills-training group, an information-only group, or a no-treatment group (Kivlahan, Marlatt, Fromme, Coppel, & Williams, 1990). Those in the skills-training group received information about strategies for drinking moderately as well as training in relaxation and assertiveness skills. They were specifically given the goal of drinking just to get their blood alcohol content (BAC) to 0.055 and were given information about how to set drinking limits to reach (but not exceed) this level. In contrast, those in the information-only condition received information about the effects of alcohol, the alcohol industry, and alcoholism. Findings at the one-year follow-up indicated that those in the skills-training condition reported having had only 7.6 drinks in the past month, as compared to 16.8 drinks for those in the information-only condition (and 15.4 drinks for those in the control condition).

Mass Media Approaches

A number of mass media approaches, including television, magazine, and billboard ads, have been used to try to prevent substance abuse, often by portraying the negative effects of engaging in such behavior. Many ads designing to prevent drunk driving, for example, emphasize tragic outcomes that result from driving while intoxicated. Media approaches are also commonly used to prevent teenage smoking, and can be quite effective both for preventing teenagers from initiating smoking and for reducing rates of smoking in light (not yet addicted) smokers. Rates of teenage smoking were found to be lower in communities exposed to a smoking prevention ad campaign, which included describing the short-term costs of smoking (e.g., smelly breath and clothes), demonstrating how to refuse offers of cigarettes, and emphasizing that most teenagers did not smoke (Flynn et al., 1992). For example, two years after the advertising campaign, 9.3% of high school students in communities without such ads reported smoking, compared to 5% of those in communities that received them. These lower rates of smoking remained as long as six years later, indicating that including media anti-smoking ads can be a very important tool in preventing teenage smoking.

The first national anti-smoking campaign, called the "truth" campaign, created edgy television, radio, and print ads that focused on exposing the tobacco industry's deceptive marketing techniques that try to lure in teenage smokers. Following this campaign, smoking prevalence among students decreased from 25.3% to 18.0% between 1999 and 2002 (Farrelly, Davis, Haviland, Messeri, & Healton, 2005). Estimates are that 22% of this decline was attributed to this campaign. Similarly, one survey of 16,000 12- to 17-year-olds both before and after the "truth" media campaign revealed that those in markets with high levels of exposure to this campaign had more negative beliefs about tobacco industry practices and more negative attitudes about the tobacco industry (Hershey et al., 2005). In turn, they were less likely to be receptive to such advertising and had lower intentions to smoke.

In February 2014, the Food and Drug Administration (FDA) launched its first national campaign to prevent teenage smoking. This campaign, called The Real Cost, focused on the cosmetic effects of smoking, the loss of control caused by addiction, and the dangerous mix of toxic chemicals found in cigarette smoke, and presented messages in a variety of outlets, including television, radio, on the Web, in social media, and on billboards. A national study conducted following the release of this campaign estimated that it led to a 30% decrease in smoking initiation by youths ages 11 to 18, thus preventing an estimated 350,000 people from acquiring this habit (Farrelly et al., 2017).

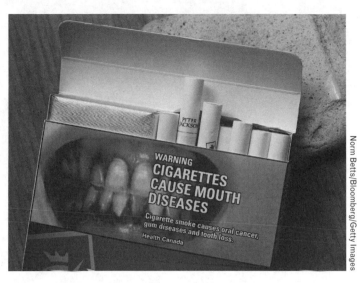
Norm Betts/Bloomberg/Getty Images

Although in 2009 the U.S. Congress approved a law requiring graphic warning labels on cigarette packages (a requirement in most other countries), tobacco companies have so far successfully sued to prevent such labels from appearing.

Government-Based Approaches

Large-scale legal approaches, such as banning the sale, advertising, and/or use of cigarettes, alcohol, and drugs, can help prevent substance abuse (Ashley & Rankin, 1988; Slater, Chaloupka, Wakefield, Johnston, & O'Malley, 2007). Laws prohibit advertisements for cigarettes and other tobacco products on television and place limits on alcohol advertising, including the hours in which such ads can appear on television and/or what they can portray.

One of the most obvious large-scale approaches to reducing substance use is the creation of laws that prohibit selling particular products to people under a certain age, such as 18 for cigarettes and 21 for alcohol. Other approaches include limiting the number of places where and the times in which alcohol can be bought. For example, in some states, alcohol is not sold on Sundays or in grocery and convenience stores. Unfortunately, these approaches are generally ineffective in decreasing substance use by teenagers. As you probably know, most college students are under 21, yet often they report having little trouble gaining access to alcohol. Similarly, teenagers may ask smokers of legal age to buy cigarettes for them.

However, bans restricting smoking in particular areas can be effective in preventing tobacco use. One study of 301 Massachusetts communities revealed that teenagers who lived in towns with a strong restaurant smoking regulation were less likely to become smokers

What You'll Learn
7.3

than those who lived in towns with weak regulations (Siegel, Albers, Cheng, Hamilton, & Biener, 2008). Specifically, although smoking regulations had no impact on the likelihood of a teenager trying smoking, these laws apparently impeded teenagers' progression from experimenting with cigarettes to becoming a regular smoker. Similarly, one recent national study examined rates of smoking in over 4,000 people ages 19 to 31 over eight years (Vuolo, Kadowaki, & Kelly, 2016). Participants in this study were interviewed every year, which allowed researchers to determine whether smoking bans in a particular city—such as laws forbidding smoking in workplaces, bars, and restaurants—led to changes in rates of smoking. During this period, smoking bans were widely implemented: 14.9% of people lived in a city with a smoking ban at the start of the study, whereas 58.7% lived in a city with a smoking ban eight years later. And these bans had a substantial impact on reducing smoking rates in men, with 19% of men living in a city without a ban reporting smoking in the last month compared to only 13% of those living in a city with a ban. The bans were particularly effective for leading men who were light smokers to quit and leading men to never start smoking at all; they unfortunately didn't lead men who were heavy smokers (smoking more than a pack a day) to quit, presumably because these men were truly addicted to cigarettes. Surprisingly, smoking rates didn't differ for women, with 11% of women reporting smoking in the last month, regardless of where they lived.

Other large-scale approaches, such as raising cigarette prices, can also help prevent smoking. One recent study found that even a $1 increase in the price of a package of cigarettes resulted in a 7% reduction in rates of heavy smoking (defined as at least 10 cigarettes per day) (Mayne et al., 2017). Moreover, among heavy smokers, such an increase led to a 35% reduction in the average number of cigarettes smoked.

Treating Substance Abuse

The very first step in treating people with alcohol use disorders or drug addiction is **detoxification**, in which the person withdraws completely from the drug they are abusing. This process takes about a month and can include severe symptoms, such as intense anxiety, tremors, and hallucinations (Miller & Hester, 1980). Detoxification may take place in a hospital or rehabilitation center with the use of medication when the symptoms of withdrawal are particularly severe, but it can sometimes take place in an outpatient setting. In fact, recent research suggests that outpatient—or community—detoxification may lead to better outcomes (and is less expensive) (Nadkarni et al., 2016).

But detoxification is only the first step in treating addiction. Recovering from addiction is a long process, and a number of different approaches may be used, either alone or in combination, to help people avoid returning to destructive patterns of behavior. Although some people are able to stop substance abuse on their own, many people do need assistance in making such a behavior change (Prochaska & Benowitz, 2016; Sobell, Cunningham, & Sobell, 1996). This section will describe a variety of approaches used to treat addiction, including pharmacological approaches, aversive strategies, cognitive-behavioral therapies, and self-help programs.

Pharmacological Approaches

Because one of the major problems of quitting smoking is the experience of nicotine withdrawal symptoms, United States Public Health Service guidelines suggest that all smokers be offered some type of drug treatment to help manage these symptoms (Fiore et al., 2008). Different types of drugs work in distinct ways, including by reducing physical withdrawal symptoms and decreasing the rewarding effects of nicotine on the body, which in turn allows smokers to focus on behavioral and psychological strategies (Prochaska & Benowitz, 2016). Compared to placebo treatments, the use of such drugs doubles rates of successfully quitting smoking.

One of the most commonly used pharmacological treatments for quitting smoking is **nicotine-replacement therapy (NRT)** (Wetter et al., 1998). Some people use *nicotine-fading strategies*, such as reducing smoking by switching to low-nicotine cigarettes and then slowly weaning themselves off nicotine. One study found that 44% of those who gradually reduced the number of cigarettes they smoked were still abstaining one year later as opposed to only 22% of those who quit "cold turkey" (Cinciripini et al., 1995). Other people use *nicotine-replacement strategies*, such as gum and nicotine patches, which are effective in decreasing withdrawal symptoms and helping achieve short- and long-term success (Voci, Zawertailo, Hussain, & Selby, 2016; Zhang, Cohen, Bondy, & Selby, 2015).

Although nicotine-replacement strategies are the most commonly used medications to assist smokers in quitting, other drugs, such as varenicline and bupropion, may also be used to assist with managing the side effects of quitting. These approaches to quitting smoking are especially effective if used in combination with nicotine-replacement strategies (Chang et al., 2015; Tulloch, Pipe, Els, Clyde, & Reid, 2016). However, these drugs can have undesirable side effects, such as insomnia, nausea, constipation, and indigestion, and hence smokers may prefer to try other approaches before resorting to medication (Baker et al., 2016).

Medications can also be used to help treat the symptoms of both alcohol and opioid addiction. Three medications—disulfiram, acamprosate, and naltrexone—have been approved by the Food and Drug Administration (FDA) to treat alcohol use disorders (Winslow, Onysko, & Hebert, 2016). These drugs reduce the rewarding effects of alcohol, which in turn decreases cravings for alcohol and reduces the unpleasant symptoms of alcohol withdrawal, such as insomnia, anxiety, and restlessness. Other medications, such as methadone, buprenorphine, and naltrexone, are useful in treating opioid addiction. These drugs target the same areas in the brain as opioids and thereby reduce withdrawal symptoms and cravings.

Aversion Strategies

Aversion strategies are based on principles of classical conditioning—these approaches pair the use of a particular drug with some type of unpleasant stimulus, such as an electric shock, nausea, or unpleasant images (Miller & Hester, 1980). For example, every time a smoker takes a drag on the cigarette or an alcoholic takes a drink, he or she will receive a slightly painful electric shock or be told to think about vomit or excrement (Kamarck & Lichtenstein, 1985). After repeated pairings of a particular drug and some unpleasant outcome, people should begin to associate this drug with negative consequences, which will enable them to stop its use.

Aversion strategies can help people successfully change undesirable addictions. One study found that approximately 63% of people with a drinking problem who received this type of treatment remained abstinent one year later, although half of these then returned to drinking the second year (Wiens & Menustik, 1983). Aversion strategies also lead to significant increases in smoking cessation rates, especially for those with low levels of physical dependence on nicotine and for those who smoke for pleasure (Wetter et al., 1998; Zelman, Brandon, Jorenby, & Baker, 1992).

However, aversion strategies also have their limits. For example, one commonly used aversion-based strategy to treat people with alcohol use disorder works by giving people the drug Antabuse, which interferes with the breakdown of alcohol in the body and therefore leads to unpleasant physical reactions such as extreme nausea if the person drinks any alcohol. But people quickly learn that they can avoid these side effects by simply not taking the Antabuse.

Cognitive-Behavioral Approaches

Cognitive-behavioral programs focus on helping people become aware of their expectations about the benefits of using a particular drug as well as both the factors and situations that lead them to engage in substance abuse (Lang & Marlatt, 1982; Lichtenstein & Mermelstein, 1984; Sussman, Sun, & Dent, 2006). Once people understand the situations that lead them to want to engage in substance abuse, they can then start to avoid these situations (a technique called **stimulus control**). For example, people who are tempted to drink when they are with others who are drinking might avoid attending social events in which other people are drinking, at least initially. Similarly, reducing exposure to cues to smoking, such as removing the ashtrays in your home and only going to nonsmoking restaurants, can help smokers quit.

Because it is impossible to avoid all situations that prompt substance abuse, cognitive-behavioral strategies also involve teaching **response substitution**, meaning choosing another way to handle situations that lead someone to want to smoke (Lichtenstein & Mermelstein, 1984). Former smokers could, for example, decide to drink coffee or chew gum during stressful times. Because many people engage in substance use as a strategy for coping with anxiety, self-management approaches may also include training in stress management techniques, such as meditation and relaxation (Berkman, Dickenson, Falk, & Lieberman, 2011; Wetter et al., 1998). For example, instead of having a drink after a long day, people may learn to substitute other rewarding and positive behaviors, such as getting a massage, taking a long bath, or meditating. In this way, a negative addiction can be replaced by a positive addiction, or something else that the person enjoys.

Cognitive-behavioral programs also help people develop specific skills for handling tricky situations. Because interpersonal conflict is often a trigger for relapse, people need to learn new skills for coping with these situations. One recovered alcoholic reports, "I share my feelings and get out anything that's on my mind, including old issues. Before, I always hid my feelings behind masks, and I drank to get away from all the emotional baggage. Now I make sure it doesn't pile up" (Fletcher, 2001). People also need specific strategies for managing pressure to engage in substance abuse, such as offers of drinks and cigarettes by others. Telling friends that they will be the "designated driver" or that they are on medication that interacts with alcohol can be effective, for example, because it gives people an "acceptable out" for not drinking and thereby reduces peer pressure to drink (see Table 7.4).

Self-management strategies may also include setting clear and attainable goals so that people can experience quick feelings of success (Lichtenstein & Mermelstein, 1984; Petry, Martin, Cooney, & Kranzler, 2000; Sussman et al., 2006). The goals should also be reasonable—not smoking for a day can quickly (although not necessarily easily) be attained, whereas "never have another cigarette for the rest of my life" is not going to be quickly

---

Table 7.4   How Recovered Alcoholics Handle Pressure to Drink

1.   Just say no: "No thanks." "No, thank you."

2.   Simply say, "I don't drink"; "I no longer drink"; "Thanks, I don't drink."

3.   Explain that you have or had a drinking problem: "No, thanks. I'm a nonpracticing alcoholic"; "I had my quota years ago."

4.   Blame it on a health problem: "I have an allergy—drinking makes me break out in spots";

5.   "Drinking makes me sick."

6.   Ask the person to stop pushing: "Why is it so important to you that I drink?" "Because when I drink, I tend to take off my clothes and dance on the tables, and my husband doesn't like it."

These quotes are by people who have successfully overcome drinking problems.

accomplished. In fact, the slogan of Alcoholics Anonymous is "One day at a time." Providing some type of reward or incentive for reaching a desired goal is particularly effective at helping people maintain behavior change over time. Ex-smokers could, for example, plan to use the money they've saved on cigarettes to take a trip or buy new clothes. A specific type of reward-based approach, **contingency-contracting**, asks people to set up a contract that specifies the costs of relapsing. In this technique, smokers give some money to a friend (or therapist), with the understanding that if they are not smoking six months later, they get the money back. One Black woman who was trying to stop smoking gave her therapist $50 and told her that if she smoked, the money should be donated to the Ku Klux Klan!

Public Health Approaches

Other strategies for reducing substance abuse focus on large-scale public health approaches instead of changing individuals' behavior. For example, smoking is banned in particular situations, such as in the workplace, in schools, and on airplanes. Although these types of programs certainly help prevent the problems associated with passive smoking, smokers can just smoke more in other places to compensate. One study of the effects of a workplace ban on smoking found that although there was an initial decrease of levels of nicotine in the bloodstream of smoking employees one week after the ban was enacted, six weeks later nicotine levels were nearly back to baseline levels (Gomel, Oldenburg, Lemon, Owen, & Westbrook, 1993).

Other large-scale approaches, such as raising taxes on cigarettes and alcohol, thereby making the cost of engaging in such behaviors more expensive, can also help motivate people to change their behavior. In line with this view, more smokers reported quit attempts, and were successful in abstaining from cigarettes, after a tax increase in California raised cigarette prices (Reed, Anderson, Vaughn, & Burns, 2008). Similarly, one recent study found that an increase in Maryland's alcohol sales tax led to a 2.5% reduction in wine sales, a 3.2% reduction in beer sales, and a 5.1% reduction in liquor sales (Staras, Livingston, & Wagenaar, 2016). Increasing sales taxes on cigarettes also leads to reductions in alcohol consumption, presumably because smoking is often a trigger for drinking (Krauss, Cavazos-Rehg, Plunk, Bierut, & Grucza, 2014).

What You'll Learn
7.4

The use of graphic warning labels on cigarette packs, which are common in other countries but are not used in the United States, leads to both reduced intentions to smoke in the future and increases in intention to quit smoking (Blanton, Snyder, Strauts, & Larson, 2014; Cantrell et al., 2013; Pechmann & Reibling, 2006). To examine the effectiveness of graphic warnings on cigarette packages, researchers randomly assigned smokers to receive either text-only warnings or pictorial warnings on their cigarette packs for four weeks (Brewer et al., 2016). Smokers who received the pictorial warnings were more likely to attempt to quit smoking during the four-week trial than those who received the text-only warnings (40% versus 34%). Smokers who received the pictorial warnings were also more likely to report having successfully quit smoking, with 5.7% of those receiving such warnings having quit compared to 3.8% of those who received the standard warnings. The pictorial warnings also increased smokers' intentions to quit smoking, amount of thinking about the harms of smoking, and conversations about quitting. These findings provide powerful evidence that graphic warning labels can lead to reductions in smoking and literally save lives.

Self-Help Programs

Many substance abuse treatment programs encourage people to also participate in self-help groups both during and after formal treatment. Self-help programs can provide valuable social support during recovery and thereby help people maintain long-term changes in behavior. Self-help programs include Alcoholics Anonymous (AA), Narcotics Anonymous (NA), and Heroin Anonymous (HA).

Alcoholics Anonymous (AA) is the most widely known self-help program for alcohol abuse and is attended more often than any other alcohol program (Weisner, Greenfield, & Room, 1995). AA was started in the 1930s by people with drinking problems who found that sharing their problems and experiences with alcohol with others helped them remain sober. The process they used eventually evolved into 12 steps (see Table 7.5). People who are trying to stop drinking attend frequent meetings (daily, at least initially) in which members talk about their experiences with alcohol and their difficulty in quitting. The general AA philosophy is based on two principles. First, people who abuse alcohol are alcoholics and will remain that way for life, even if they never drink again. Second, consuming even a small amount of alcohol leads to an irresistible craving for more alcohol, and thus alcoholics must avoid all drinking.

Although it is difficult to systematically track AA's success rate given its anonymous nature, alcoholics who regularly attend AA meetings are more likely to maintain abstinence from alcohol as long as 18 months after beginning treatment (Humphreys, Blodgett, & Wagner, 2014; McCrady, Epstein, & Kahler, 2004). However, and as you learned in *Chapter 2: Research Methods*, people who choose to attend AA meetings may differ in some way from those who do not, which may explain such findings. But research using more rigorous methods—including randomized controlled trials (RCTs)—reveals that participation in AA is effective; specifically, alcoholics who were randomly assigned to receive treatment that strongly encouraged and supported AA participation showed higher rates of abstinence

Table 7.5 The 12 Steps of Alcoholics Anonymous

1. We admitted we were powerless over alcohol—that our lives had become unmanageable.

2. Came to believe that a power greater than ourselves could restore us to sanity.

3. Made a decision to turn our will and our lives over to the care of God as we understood Him.

4. Made a searching and fearless oral inventory of ourselves.

5. Admitted to God, to ourselves, and to another human being the exact nature of our wrongs.

6. Were entirely ready to have God remove all these defects of character.

7. Humbly asked Him to remove our shortcomings.

8. Made a list of all persons we had harmed and became willing to make amends to them all.

9. Made direct amends to such people whenever possible, except when to do so would injure them or others.

10. Continued to take personal inventory and, when we were wrong, promptly admitted it.

11. Sought through prayer and meditation to improve our conscious contact with God as we understand Him, praying only for knowledge of His will for us and the power to carry that out.

12. Having had a spiritual awakening as the result of these steps, we tried to carry this message to alcoholics and to practice these principles in all our affairs.

These 12 steps are the core of the Alcoholics Anonymous approach to drinking problems.

Source: Alcoholics Anonymous World Services (1977). The Twelve Steps and the Twelve Traditions are reprinted with permission of Alcoholics Anonymous World Services, Inc. ("A.A.W.S."). Permission to reprint the Twelve Steps and the Twelve Traditions does not mean that A.A.W.S. has reviewed or approved the contents of this publication, or that A.A. necessarily agrees with the views expressed herein. A.A. is a program of recovery from alcoholism only—use of the Twelve Steps and Twelve Traditions in connection with programs and activities which are patterned after A.A., but which address other problems, or in any other non-A.A., does not imply otherwise.

than those assigned to a control group (Walitzer, Dermen, & Barrick, 2009). As described in **Focus on Neuroscience**, for recovered alcoholics, simply saying the AA prayer may lead to changes in the brain that reduce the urge to drink.

Managing Relapse

Even when people seek medical treatment and attempt to follow recommendations, maintaining health behavior change over time is a major problem. Have you ever made a change in your health-related behavior, such as stopping smoking, starting exercising, or adopting a healthier diet, but then returned to your old—less healthy—habits after a few weeks or months (or sometimes even days)? This pattern of **relapse**, meaning returning to an unwanted behavior after beginning to change it, is very common. As shown in Figure 7.4, the relapse curves for alcohol use, smoking, and heroin use are very similar, with about two thirds of all relapses occurring in the first 90 days following treatment (Hunt, Barnett, & Branch, 1971; Ockene et al., 2000). This suggests that there is a common link to the process of relapse that may be similar across different types of addiction. This section examines the major theories of addiction and strategies used in relapse-prevention programs to help people successfully overcome addiction.

Theories of Addiction

The *moral or self-control theory* posits that people who engage in addictive behaviors, such as smoking, drinking, and gambling, have some type of moral weakness (Marlatt, 1985a). According to this theory, people who are lazy and undisciplined lack the "moral fiber" to stop engaging in these self-destructive behaviors. For example, the Temperance Movement during the 1940s and the ban of alcohol during Prohibition reflected this view, advocating that people must be protected from themselves. Moreover, because any problem with addiction is a result of a lack of personal impulse control or willpower, people who engage in these behaviors in excess deserve whatever negative consequences befall them. This model holds people

FOCUS ON NEUROSCIENCE

How Alcoholics Anonymous May Change Your Brain

One recent study provides strong evidence that the AA prayer may lead to changes in brain physiology, which in turn reduce alcohol cravings (Galanter, Josipovic, Dermatis, Weber, & Millard, 2016). Researchers recruited 20 long-term members of AA and placed them in an MRI machine. They were then shown pictures of either alcoholic drinks or people drinking alcohol to cue drinking behavior. These pictures were first shown after asking people to simply read neutral material from a newspaper, and then again after asking them to recite the AA prayer promoting abstinence. All participants reported some degree of alcohol craving after viewing the images and less craving after reciting the prayer. Moreover, MRI data demonstrated that praying led to increased activity in parts of the brain that control attention and emotion, indicating that these participants may be using the prayer to think and feel about these alcohol use triggers in different ways. These findings suggest that long-term members of AA have an ability to use the AA prayer to reduce the effects of alcohol triggers, which may help explain the effectiveness of this approach.

Figure 7.4 Relapse Curve

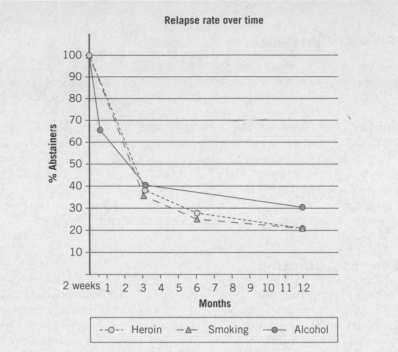

Relapse rate over time

The relapse curves for various addictions, including heroin use, smoking, and alcohol abuse, are very similar, suggesting that the relapse process across different issues shares some common points.

Source: Hunt, Barnett, & Branch (1971, p. 456).

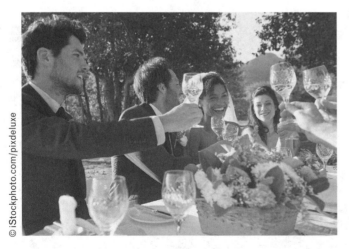

People who are trying to avoid alcohol use may, at least initially, try to avoid all settings in which alcohol is served in order to avoid temptation.

responsible for their own behavior and, thus, in one sense can be seen as empowering.

On the other hand, according to the **disease model**, addiction is caused primarily by internal physiological forces, such as cravings, urges, and compulsions; hence, the "addict" is unable to voluntarily control his or her behavior (Marlatt, 1985a). The disease model of addiction has an "all-or-nothing" view, which means that only lifelong abstinence is effective, and hence relapse is failure. Alcoholics Anonymous is based on this model and posits that the alcoholic is completely powerless over the disease and that alcoholism can never be cured, only controlled by completely abstaining from all alcohol use.

However, other approaches to treating addiction focus instead on reducing the negative consequences of substance abuse, not on eliminating such behavior entirely (Logan & Marlatt, 2010). Alcoholics could, for example, be taught to engage in moderate, or "controlled," drinking, and college students could learn to avoid binge drinking that can result in alcohol poisoning. Similarly, some smokers try to move to smokeless forms of tobacco, such as e-cigarettes or nicotine-replacement strategies, which reduces some of the negative effects of nicotine.

According to Bandura's *social learning theory*, people who engage in addictive behaviors have acquired these habits through learning, just like they learn other habits; hence, these behaviors can be examined and changed (Marlatt, 1985a). For example, people may learn to drink or smoke based on classical conditioning (the behavior of going to a pub leads to feeling relaxed, which leads to drinking, may turn into "Going to a pub leads to drinking"), operant conditioning ("I feel more confident when I drink"), observational learning or modeling ("Others I respect drink"), and cognitive factors ("Drinking helps me cope with stress"). This model focuses on understanding the determinants of the behavior and the consequences of the behavior. For example, many addictive behaviors are performed to reduce stress and, hence, represent maladaptive coping mechanisms.

Relapse-Prevention Programs

Relapse prevention programs teach people who are trying to make a long-term change in their behavior how to anticipate and cope with the very real problem of relapse (Marlatt, 1985b). These programs have two major goals: helping people identify high-risk situations, meaning those that are likely triggers of relapse, and helping people learn new ways to cope with these situations (see Table 7.6). In sum, relapse-prevention programs are like fire drills; people prepare for how they will act once a fire occurs so they can act this way easily and quickly when they are suddenly faced with a fire.

Triggers of Relapse

Many people who are trying to give up an addictive behavior find that one of the most common triggers of relapse is experiencing a particular emotional state associated with engaging in the behavior (Grilo, Shiffman, & Wing, 1989; Hodgins, el-Guebaly, & Armstrong, 1995). Negative emotional states (which account for 35% of relapses) are situations in which the individual is experiencing anger or frustration, depression, helplessness, or boredom and are likely to lead to the first lapse. Interpersonal conflict, with a spouse, friend, family member, or boss, is another common high-risk situation, and accounts for 16% of relapses. Finally, social pressure situations, which account for 20% of relapses, are those in which the individual is responding to the influence of another person or group of people exerting pressure to engage in the taboo behavior. This can be direct (e.g., "you should have some champagne; this is a

---

Table 7.6 What Would You Do?

- You've just picked up your car from the mechanic and the bill is twice as much as you expected it to be. As you drive home you find that the very thing you took the car in for is still not fixed. The car stalls in rush-hour traffic. You feel angry and frustrated; you crave a cigarette.

- You're at a party with friends. People are smoking and drinking. You're having a glass of wine and intense conversation. You always used to have a cigarette with your drink. It looks good.

- While waiting at the market checkout stand, you find yourself next to the cigarette stand and you notice that the market carries your old brand of cigarettes. Boy, do those cigarettes look good—you can almost taste one.

Ex-smokers are asked to read these situations and then quickly write down exactly what they would do as a way of testing how effective their coping strategy would be.

Source: Marlatt (1985a).

celebration") or indirect (e.g., all your friends are smoking while they play poker). Other high-risk states can include positive emotional states (using the drug to enhance positive feelings, making "special exceptions" for using a drug during times of celebration) and testing personal control (to see if one really is no longer addicted).

As described previously, triggers of relapse can also include particular locations, people, times of day, and life stressors (Marlatt & Gordon, 1980). Specific triggers, however, vary for different people. People with an alcohol addiction, for example, are very likely to relapse while in a bar or tavern—in one study 63% of the relapses occurred in this type of location. On the other hand, smokers are more likely to relapse at their homes (44%) or at work (19%). Relatively few people relapse in the morning, presumably because willpower is still high, but people often have particular times of day that are most difficult for them. Having a tough day (or week or month) can lead people to say, "I deserve a break," and hence trigger relapse (Brandon, Copeland, & Saper, 1995; Shiffman et al., 1996). The AA program uses the acronym HALT, which refers to avoiding being too hungry, angry, lonely, or tired, all of which are factors that can trigger a relapse (Fletcher, 2001).

Strategies for Preventing Relapse

First, individuals need to identify high-risk situations that may lead them to experience a craving for a particular substance (Marlatt, 1985b). As one recovered alcoholic described it, "Look for the common thread in your relapses. Break that thread" (Fletcher, 2001). After these high-risk situations have been identified, people can simply remove themselves from the situation. They could, for example, avoid going to bars or being in situations in which drinking is expected and could remove triggers for their behavior, such as ashtrays and wine glasses. One study with alcoholics found that training in cue exposure techniques, in which as part of therapy they were allowed to see and smell their preferred alcoholic beverage while imagining situational pressures to drink, led to much lower rates of drinking over time—only 44% of the patients who received this therapy were drinking at the six-month follow-up, as compared to 79% of those who received traditional therapy (Monti et al., 1993). People who participated in such training learned coping skills that they could apply in real-life situations later on, which in turn likely increased their self-efficacy for refusing alcohol in tempting situations.

Social support can help people maintain a new behavior (Black, Gleser, & Kooyers, 1990; McBride et al., 1998; Mermelstein, Cohen, Lichtenstein, Baer, & Kamarck, 1986). People who are trying to change their behavior should tell people they are close to as well as people they spend a lot of time with about their intentions. These other people can be asked to support the behavior change, such as by not smoking around them or offering them a drink with dinner and by expressing confidence in the person's ability to change the behavior (Cohen & Lichtenstein, 1990; Sorensen, Pechacek, & Pallonen, 1986). However, because relapse can be precipitated by a reaction against perceived imposition of rules or regulations governing the prohibited behavior, it is important that the person himself or herself makes the decision to change the behavior. For example, people can throw off this prohibition, particularly if they believe that others (family members, friends) are forcing them to abstain.

Therapists and support groups are most effective at maintaining behavior change when they continue their interaction with the patient over time, in part because such contact helps people maintain their self-efficacy for behavior change even in the face of great temptation and occasional lapses (Curry & McBride, 1994; Irvin, Bowers, Dunn, & Wang, 1999). For example, one study found that 14.7% of smokers who received a self-help quit kit had stopped smoking at a 12-month follow-up as compared to 19.8% of those who received the kit plus one telephone counseling session and 26.7% of those who received the kit plus up to six counseling sessions (Zhu et al., 1996). Similarly, and as shown in Figure 7.5, people who leave treatment for alcohol use disorder with a smartphone application that includes guided

Figure 7.5   Data From Gustafson et al., 2014

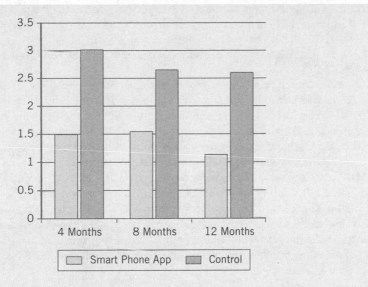

Patients who leave a residential treatment for alcohol use disorder with a smartphone application that supports recovery experience fewer risky drinking days (meaning drinking more than four drinks in one day for men or three drinks in one day for women) at all three time periods (four, eight, and twelve months) than patients who do not receive this added support.

Source: Data from Gustafson, McTavish, Chih, Atwood, Johnson, Boyle, ... Shah (2014).

relaxation and specific support if the person nears a high-risk location (such as a bar) experience fewer risky drinking days than people who do not receive this added support.

Another strategy for preventing relapse is helping people think about their old behaviors in new ways (Marlatt, 1985a). Relapse-prevention programs try to help people focus on the short-term versus the long-term consequences of engaging in the behavior (PIG, or the problem of immediate gratification). The immediate consequences of engaging in an addictive behavior may be particularly strong and positive (e.g., relaxation, feeling good, fitting in), whereas the long-term consequences may be less salient and largely negative (e.g., have trouble with work, develop serious health problems). So, people need to be trained to focus on the delayed effects of giving in to temptation. They also need to recognize that these responses arise and subside on their own (e.g., as opposed to thinking that these cravings will gain in intensity until they give in). Learning how to externalize and label their desires is one strategy for reducing the tendency to give in to the urge (e.g., "I am experiencing an urge to smoke" instead of "I really want a cigarette"). They may also need to be trained to reevaluate their expectancies for engaging in the behavior.

Finally, relapse-prevention strategies include preparing people to see a lapse in behavior as a single, isolated incidence as opposed to a disaster that can never be undone (Marlatt, 1985a). According to the *abstinence violation effect*, if people expect they will never give in to temptation, when and if they do have a lapse in behavior, they are likely to blame it on themselves, which could lead to a total relapse (Curry, Marlatt, & Gordon, 1987; Marlatt & Gordon, 1980). For example, if someone is trying to stop drinking but then has a glass of wine at a work dinner, he or she may feel guilty about that choice. But that person may then manage that guilt by drinking even more. People who are trying to change their behavior are therefore encouraged to commit to use only a single "dose" in the case of relapse, such as having one beer and not a six-pack, or one cigarette and not a pack. This limited type of relapse makes it easier to recover from a lapse. Relapse-prevention programs should therefore include exposure to some such high-risk settings to give people a chance to cope with such challenges in a controlled environment. If they face a temptation to engage in the addictive behavior, they should agree to wait at least 20 minutes before giving in. This will at least give them time to contemplate the behavior and not just act on the spur of the moment.

**What You'll Learn
7.5**

Some intriguing recent research suggests that increasing mindfulness, meaning a mental state characterized by awareness of and focus on one's present experience, can reduce the risk of relapse. For example, a mindfulness-based relapse-prevention (MBRP) program led to less alcohol and other drug use and fewer alcohol cravings, suggesting that building mindfulness practice into one's daily life could help with ongoing recovery (Grow, Collins, Harrop, & Marlatt, 2015). Researchers in one study compared the effectiveness of an MBRP program to a standard cognitive-behavioral relapse-prevention program (Bowen et al., 2014). Both programs included eight weeks of group sessions and a one-year follow-up. At the 12-month follow-up, people in the MBRP group reported fewer days of substance use and decreased heavy drinking compared with those who received the standard relapse-prevention program. These findings provide strong evidence that teaching mindfulness practices may help people manage the negative feelings and physiological cravings that can trigger relapse.

Table 7.7　Information YOU Can Use

- No one tries to become a smoker, but even a few cigarettes in high school and college can lead to a lifetime of addiction. So, try to resist even occasional smoking, since addiction can happen quickly. And although e-cigarettes are somewhat less harmful than traditional cigarettes, they still contain tobacco and can and do lead to addiction.

- Because many people smoke and/or drink to reduce tension, one of the best strategies for avoiding cigarettes and excessive alcohol use is to develop other strategies for relieving the stress that we all experience at times. Therefore, think about other things you can do when you are nervous about exams or sad after a relationship breakup: go for a run, watch a movie, or call a friend instead.

- One of the single largest causes of deaths in teenagers and young adults—which includes most of the readers of this textbook—is drinking and driving. So, please remember to never drink and drive yourself and never get in a car with a driver who has been drinking.

- Remember that drinking is not as prevalent as you might think it is: many college students believe that their peers drink far more than they actually do, in part because excessive drinking is likely to be more salient (and thus seem more prevalent) than not drinking or moderate drinking. So, don't be fooled by how much you think others are drinking; they aren't drinking as much as you think they are drinking (and they, too, often believe that there is too much drinking).

- Opiates are highly addictive and lead to very serious, even life-threatening, consequences. Avoid trying these drugs even once.

- When trying to make behavior changes, develop strategies to help you succeed. Identify high-risk situations and try to avoid them. Set clear and attainable goals and mark your progress toward achieving them. Learn strategies for coping with high-risk situations so that lapses, which will occur, don't turn into relapses.

Understanding Smoking

- Most smokers acquire the habit at a relatively young age and become addicted to the nicotine present in all types of tobacco use. Addiction is caused by repeatedly consuming a particular substance. People who are dependent on a given substance also develop tolerance, in which their bodies no longer respond at the same level to a particular dose, and experience unpleasant withdrawal symptoms when they discontinue using the substance. Smoking is a very difficult habit to break; both genetic/ biological and psychosocial factors influence people's likelihood of becoming addicted and ability to quit.

- Smoking is the leading cause of preventable mortality in the United States. Smoking causes an estimated 90% of all lung cancer deaths and is linked with many other types of cancer. Smokers are more likely to develop coronary heart disease and stroke as well as other major illnesses. Smoking also impacts fertility and pregnancy. Other forms of tobacco use, such as chewing tobacco and e-cigarettes, are also associated with negative consequences.

Factors Contributing to Smoking

- Social factors, including modeling and peer pressure, may lead teenagers to start smoking. They may also use smoking as a way of trying out a new identity, especially since smokers are seen as having particular qualities that are considered positive. Most first smoking occurs in the presence of a peer, and having friends who smoke increases the availability of cigarettes. Parents' attitudes and behaviors regarding smoking also influence whether teenagers smoke.

- The media contributes to smoking by portraying smoking as glamorous and cool. Teenagers who see more smoking in movies are more likely to start smoking themselves, in part because movies portray smokers as higher in social status and create positive expectancies about smoking.

- Teenagers who smoke have distinct personalities. They are higher in novelty-seeking and rebelliousness and lower in achievement motivation and self-control. Smoking is also associated with more tolerance for deviance and other risk-taking behaviors. Girls who are concerned about their weight may smoke as a strategy for weight loss.

- According to the nicotine fixed-effect model, nicotine stimulates reward-inducing centers in the nervous system, which leads to better memory and concentration and reduced feelings of anxiety and tension. The nicotine regulation model posits that smoking is rewarding only when the level of nicotine is above a certain "set point" in the body. Tomkins's affect-regulation model proposes that people smoke to attain positive affect or to avoid (or reduce) negative affect. According to the multiple regulation model, the combination of physiological and psychological factors leads to addiction; smoking is initially used to regulate emotions, but over time how smokers feel becomes linked with how much nicotine they have in their blood. The biobehavioral model suggests that nicotine leads to physiological effects that make people feel good, which lead smokers to become dependent on using nicotine to experience these positive effects.

Understanding Alcohol Use and Abuse

- Although many people drink moderate amounts of alcohol, other people engage in excessive alcohol use, including *heavy drinking* and *binge drinking*. Alcohol use disorder (AUD) is a medical condition characterized by both alcohol abuse and dependence and occurs when drinking causes a person distress or harm.

- Alcohol use leads to negative health consequences, including liver damage, structural changes in the brain, memory problems, and some types of cancer. Alcohol use by pregnant women has negative effects on the growing fetus. Alcohol use can also lead indirectly to other health problems, including motor vehicle accidents, homicides, suicides, sexually transmitted diseases, falls, and burns.

- Some evidence suggests that alcohol use in moderation can actually have some benefits. However, the data on the link between moderate drinking and positive health outcomes is difficult to interpret.

Explanations for Alcohol Abuse

- According to tension-reduction theory, people drink alcohol to cope with or regulate negative moods, including feelings of tension, anxiety, and nervousness. However, overall research provides only mixed support for its usefulness in predicting drinking.

- According to social learning theory, children learn attitudes and behaviors by watching others, including their parents, siblings, and peers. Television, movies, and advertisements also model alcohol use norms. Moreover, the mere belief that other people are drinking heavily can lead people to drink more—even if this belief is wrong. Observing people's alcohol use also creates positive expectations about the consequences of that behavior.

- Many studies have examined whether certain personality traits, including neuroticism/negative affect, impulsivity/disinhibition, and extraversion/sociability, are associated with alcohol-related problems. Although some support for the link between personality traits and such problems is found in correlational studies, these studies can't determine the association between traits and alcohol abuse. However, several longitudinal studies do indicate that personality traits can predict future alcohol abuse.

- Research using adoption and twin studies reveals a genetic influence in the development of drinking problems. Genes may influence the risk of developing problems with alcoholism in numerous ways, including sensitivity to alcohol, response to alcohol, and risk of developing dependence. Genetic factors may also influence personality, which in turn leads to alcohol abuse.

Understanding Drug Use

- All drugs alter mental processes in some way. Depressants, or sedatives, act on the central nervous system to slow down normal bodily activity, including in the brain, heart, and muscles. Narcotics, or opiates, mimic the body's normal process of managing pain by binding to opioid receptors, which reduces feelings of pain and produces a feeling of pleasure or euphoria. Stimulants create physiological arousal by activating the central nervous system, which causes increases in energy and alertness and reductions in fatigue. Hallucinogens, or psychedelics, distort perception in some way, meaning people see and hear things that are not really there. Hallucinations temporarily disrupt the functioning of neurotransmitters, which creates feelings of relaxation, euphoria, and heightened sensations.

- All drugs can have serious side effects, including impairments in learning, judgment, memory, and decision making. Drugs can also have undesirable physical side effects, such as nausea, constipation, vomiting, and convulsions. Most important, the use of certain drugs can lead to life-threatening effects.

Strategies for Reducing Substance Abuse

- Social influence programs inform teenagers of the short-term consequences of substance use, point out the manipulative nature of advertisements, and emphasize that many adolescents are against substance use. Life skills–training approaches provide teenagers with assistance in enhancing self-esteem and social competence, techniques for resisting persuasive appeals, and skills for verbal and nonverbal communication. Mass media approaches can help prevent substance abuse, as can public health approaches, such as banning the sale, advertising, and/or use of cigarettes, alcohol, and drugs, or raising taxes on such substances.

- The first step in treating people with substance abuse is detoxification, in which the person withdraws completely from the drug they are abusing. Various types of drug treatment can help reduce the rewarding effects of the substance and the unpleasant withdrawal symptoms and cravings. Aversion strategies work by pairing the use of a particular substance with some type of unpleasant stimulus. Cognitive-behavioral approaches help people become aware of their expectations about the benefits of using a particular drug as well as both the factors and situations that lead them to engage in substance abuse. They can then avoid these situations (stimulus control) and choose other strategies for handling such situations (response substitution). Public health approaches, such as banning use in particular situations, raising taxes, and requiring graphic warning labels, can reduce substance abuse. Self-help programs can provide valuable social support during recovery and help people maintain long-term behavior changes.

- The moral or self-control theory posits that people who engage in addictive behaviors have some type of moral weakness that leads them to engage in self-destructive behaviors. According to the disease model, addiction is caused by internal physiological forces, and hence the person is unable to voluntarily control his or her behavior. According to social learning theory, people who engage in addictive behaviors have acquired these habits through learning, just like they learn other habits; hence, these behaviors can be examined and changed. Relapse-prevention programs teach people how to anticipate and cope with barriers to maintaining long-term behavior change. Strategies for preventing relapse include identifying high-risk situations, receiving social support, learning to think about their old behaviors in new ways, and seeing a lapse in behavior as a single, isolated incidence.

8

OBESITY AND DISORDERED EATING

Learning Objectives

8.1 Describe the measurement and consequences of obesity, and the role of genetic factors in influencing weight

8.2 Summarize how psychosocial factors contribute to obesity

8.3 Compare different strategies for reducing obesity

8.4 Describe different types of eating disorders and the role of genetic factors in contributing to such disorders

8.5 Explain how psychosocial factors contribute to disordered eating

8.6 Compare different strategies for reducing disordered eating

What You'll Learn

8.1 How does a home team NFL loss impact snacking?

8.2 Why do most contestants on reality TV weight-loss shows regain their weight?

8.3 Does posting calories on menu items change ordering at Starbucks?

8.4 Can spending time on Facebook lead to disordered eating?

8.5 Why do some people overeat in response to stress?

Preview

Coverage of the "obesity epidemic" in the United States is widespread, including in newspapers, in magazines, online, and on television. Articles describe at length the health problems associated with obesity, and various strategies—exercise, drugs, surgery—to overcome it.

(Continued)

Yet these same media outlets regularly feature images of extremely thin women, and often muscular men, clearly suggesting that these body shapes represent the ideal. In this chapter, you'll learn about the complexities of predicting overweight and obesity as well as disordered eating, including their consequences, biological and psychosocial factors that contribute to their development, and strategies for both preventing and treating unhealthy eating.

UNDERSTANDING OBESITY

LO 8.1

Describe the measurement and consequences of obesity, and the role of genetic factors in influencing weight

Many Americans struggle to manage their weight. Over one third of American adults, and 17% of children and adolescence, are considered obese (Ogden, Carroll, Fryar, & Flegal, 2015). **Obesity** rates are particularly high among people of color; an estimated 48.1% of Black adults and 42.5% of Latino adults are obese, compared to 34.5% of White adults and only 11.7% of Asian American adults. Moreover, and as shown in Figure 8.1, the rate of obesity has climbed over the last 20 years, and is expected to continue to increase. This section describes how obesity is measured, its consequences, and the impact of genetic factors on weight.

Figure 8.1   Rates of Obesity Over Time

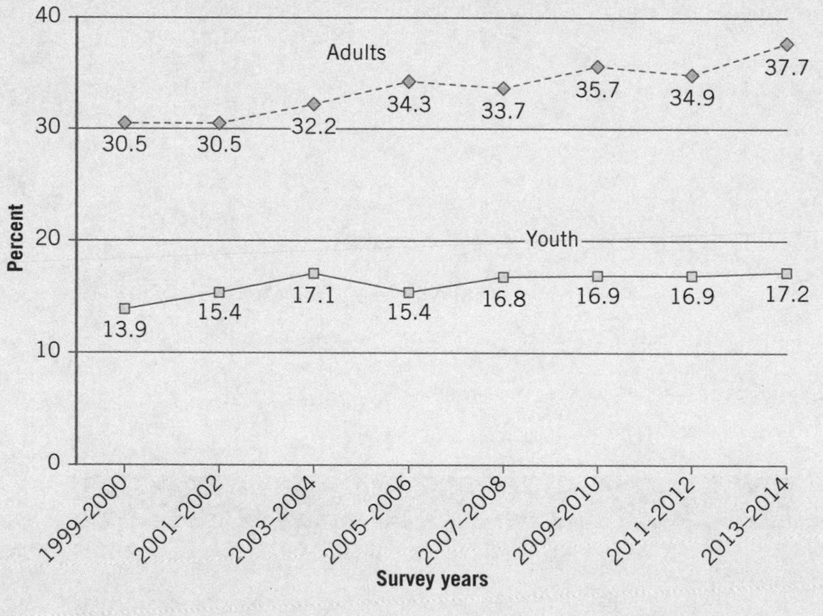

Rates of obesity have increased in both adults and youth (children, teenagers) over the last 20 years.

Source: Ogden et al. (2015).

Measuring Obesity

For many years, researchers relied on the use of tables that simply plotted normal weight ranges for people of various heights. Unfortunately, because muscle tissue and bones weigh more than fat, relying on only weight as a measure of obesity can cause some highly fit people, such as muscular athletes, to test as obese. A more accurate way to assess obesity is by calculating percentage of body fat, which can be tested by measuring a pinch of skin in several places on a person's body or (ideally) using a water immersion technique. However, because the pinch test is not particularly accurate and the water immersion method is time-consuming and expensive, body fat measures are not widely used to determine obesity.

The most common measure of obesity today is **body mass index (BMI)**, which is calculated by dividing a person's weight (in kilograms) by the person's height (in meters) and squaring the sum (see Table 8.1). A BMI between 19 and 24 is considered ideal; 25 to 29 is moderately **overweight** (about 15% to 30% over ideal weight); and people with indexes

Table 8.1   Body Mass Index (BMI) Calculation Table

BMI (kg/m²)	19	20	21	22	23	24	25	26	27	28	29	30	35	40
Height (in.)	Weight (lb.)													
58	91	96	100	105	110	115	119	124	129	134	138	143	167	191
59	94	99	104	109	114	119	124	128	133	138	143	148	173	198
60	97	102	107	112	118	123	128	133	138	143	148	153	179	204
61	100	106	111	116	122	127	132	137	143	148	153	158	185	211
62	104	109	115	120	126	131	136	142	147	153	158	164	191	218
63	107	113	118	124	130	135	141	146	152	158	163	169	197	225
64	110	116	122	128	134	140	145	151	157	163	169	174	204	232
65	114	120	126	132	138	144	150	156	162	168	174	180	210	240
66	118	124	130	136	142	148	155	161	167	173	179	186	216	247
67	121	127	134	140	146	153	159	166	172	178	185	191	223	255
68	125	131	138	144	151	158	164	171	177	184	190	197	230	262
69	128	135	142	149	155	162	169	176	182	189	196	203	236	270
70	132	139	146	153	160	167	174	181	188	195	202	207	243	278
71	136	143	150	157	165	172	179	186	193	200	208	215	250	286
72	140	147	154	162	169	177	184	191	199	206	213	221	258	294
73	144	151	159	166	174	182	189	197	204	212	219	227	265	302
74	148	155	163	171	179	186	194	202	210	218	225	233	272	311
75	152	160	168	176	184	192	200	208	216	224	232	240	279	319
76	156	164	172	180	189	197	205	213	221	230	238	246	287	328

Source: Bray & Gray (1988).

greater than 30 are considered obese (about 40% over ideal weight). Obesity, in turn, is divided into three distinct categories. People with a BMI of 30 to 35 are on the low end of obesity, those with a BMI of 35 to 40 have a moderate level, and those with a BMI of 40 or higher have "extreme" or "severe" obesity.

Although BMI is widely used as an easy test of obesity, this measure has some distinct limitations. Specifically, many people who are healthy may have a BMI indicating they are obese, and many people who are obese—as determined by their BMI—are actually healthy based on physiological data. For example, researchers in one study examined health data, including blood pressure and cholesterol, from over 40,000 adults (Tomiyama, Hunger, Nguyen-Cuu, & Wells, 2016). Their findings indicated that 47% of people classified as overweight, and 29% of those classified as obese, were healthy based on the physiological measures. On the other hand, 31% of people who were classified as normal weight were considered healthy based on physiological data. Thus, relying solely on BMI as a measure of health would classify an estimated 75 million American adults as unhealthy.

Consequences of Obesity

Regardless of how it is measured, obesity is associated with substantial consequences, including physical, psychological, and social.

Physical Consequences

Obesity is associated with a variety of negative physical consequences. People who are obese are at an increased risk of developing hypertension, kidney disease, gallbladder disease, diabetes, cardiovascular disease, and some types of cancer (Bray, 1992; Gallagher & LeRoith, 2015; Manson et al., 1990). In fact, being overweight or obese increases the risk of developing many different types of cancer, including breast, ovarian, colorectal, liver, and kidney (Lauby-Secretan et al., 2016). One of the most common health problems associated with obesity is *diabetes*, a chronic endocrine disorder in which the body is not able to produce or use the hormone insulin (as you'll learn more about in ***Chapter 10: Understanding and Managing Chronic Illness***). Type 2 diabetes (or non-insulin-dependent diabetes), which accounts for approximately 90% of diabetes cases, is most prevalent in older people and in those who are obese (Haffner, 1998). For example, 80% of people with Type 2 diabetes are obese, and a growing number of overweight children and adolescents are developing signs of diabetes (Sinha et al., 2002). Obesity in women is associated with infertility, miscarriage, and poor pregnancy outcomes (Talmor & Dunphy, 2015). Overweight and obese pregnant women are also at greater risk of premature death and cardiovascular disease, even when taking into account other variables, such as socioeconomic status, smoking, gestation at BMI measurement, preeclampsia, and low birth weight (Lee et al., 2015).

Most important, people who are overweight have higher rates of mortality, and are particularly at risk of dying from cardiovascular disease (Stevens et al., 1998; Yusuf et al., 2005). Being severely overweight is associated with even greater risks—very obese men and women (those with BMIs above 40) were twice as likely to die in a given period of time as those who were of normal weight (Bender, Trautner, Spraul, & Berger, 1998). In contrast, people with a BMI between 18.6 and 23.0 (for women) and 19.9 to 22.6 (for men) had the lowest rates of coronary heart disease, diabetes, and mortality (Lew, 1985).

Although this section has examined the negative physical effects of obesity, some research calls into question this association. First, the distribution of weight on a body may be a better predictor of health than simply the amount of weight (Wickelgren, 1998). People who have upper-body fat (e.g., "apples") are at a greater risk of experiencing major health problems, such as diabetes, hypertension, and cardiovascular disease, than those who have lower-body fat (e.g., "pears"). In fact, the weight accumulated around one's waist may be a better predictor of mortality than overall obesity (Folsom et al., 1993). One reason why having upper-body fat is associated with such negative health consequences is that fat cells in the abdomen are much larger than fat cells in the legs and butt; hence, abdominal fat cells are more likely to form fatty acids. In turn, high levels of fatty acids in the blood lead to higher levels of glucose in the blood as well as higher blood pressure. Second, obese people who are physically fit, and hence show normal levels of blood pressure and cholesterol, are at no greater risk of dying from cardiovascular disease or cancer than those who are of normal weight (Ortega et al., 2013). These findings suggest that fitness, not weight, is a better predictor of health outcomes.

Social and Psychological Consequences

Obese people also suffer negative social and psychological consequences. They tend to be rated as less likable, are at a disadvantage in dating people, get lower grades, earn less, and are generally the subject of negative social attitudes (Ryckman, Robbins, Kazcor, & Gold, 1989). Sadly, people who feel discriminated against due to their weight show increases in depression over time (Robinson, Sutin, & Daly, 2017).

One reason why there are such negative views about obese people is that obesity is often seen as something that is within a person's control—obese people are seen as slow, lazy, sloppy, and lacking in willpower (Ryckman et al., 1989; Thomas, Olds, Pettigrew, Randle, & Lewis, 2014). We often have the view that if they wanted to lose weight, they could just stop eating so much, so we blame obese people for their weight. But are obese people really different from others? No—the personality characteristics of obese and nonobese people are very similar (Poston et al., 1999).

The Role of Genetics

Genetic factors clearly play a role in obesity (Albuquerque, Manco, & Nóbrega, 2016; Albuquerque, Stice, Rodríguez-López, Manco, & Nóbrega, 2015). Obese people are more likely than nonobese people to have had obese parents and obese grandparents (Noble, 1997), and obese parents are more likely to have obese children. For example, about 7% of the children of normal-weight parents are obese, compared with 40% of the children in families with one obese parent and 80% in families with two obese parents (Mayer, 1980).

We cannot, however, attribute obesity solely to genetic factors based upon this correlation alone. After all, parents who are obese might tend to buy and cook mostly high-fat foods or encourage their children to overeat, which may point to an environmental cause of obesity. However, studies of adopted children provide some compelling evidence for the link between genetics and obesity. First, identical twins are very similar in terms of BMI regardless of whether they are raised together or apart, and identical twins are much more similar in BMI than are same-sex fraternal twins (Grilo & Pogue-Geile, 1991). Second, there is a much stronger relationship between the adopted children's and their biological parents' weight than there is between the children's weight and their adoptive parents' weight, and there is no significant correlation in weight between adopted siblings who are raised together (Grilo & Pogue-Geile, 1991). Genetic factors appear to predict about 40% to 70% of the variation in BMI (Comuzzie & Allison, 1998; Wardle, Carnell, Haworth, & Plomin, 2008).

Although research on the genetic factors predicting obesity is still relatively new, recent evidence suggests that genes may influence obesity in a variety of ways. This section examines how genes may influence food preferences and metabolism.

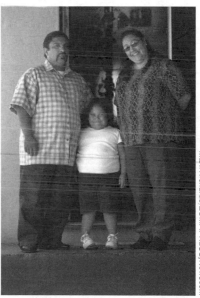

Although obese parents are more likely to have obese children, both genetic and environmental factors clearly contribute to this association!.

Mark Richards/ZUMAPRESS/Newscom

Genes Impact Food Preferences

Genes may influence how much—and even what—people want to eat. Research with mice demonstrates that a gene is responsible for directing the fat cells to release **leptin**, a hormone that decreases appetite and increases energy expenditure (Wang et al., 1999). In turn, when we lose weight (and lose fat cells), less leptin is released into our bloodstream, which may lead us to feel hungrier. Obese people might also have a genetic preference for energy-dense fat-containing foods, such as chocolate, ice cream, pastries, and whipped cream (Drewnowski, 1996). Because dietary fats are the most concentrated source of energy, people who are obese might be particularly sensitive to these foods.

Genes Impact Metabolism

Genes may also influence **metabolism**, the rate the body uses energy to carry out basic physiological processes, such as respiration, digestion, and blood pressure (Comuzzie & Allison, 1998). People who have a high metabolism are thought to use more energy to carry out these processes; hence, they burn off more calories. On the other hand, people with a lower metabolic rate gain more weight than people with higher metabolic rates, presumably because their bodies are not burning off as many calories (Ravussin et al., 1988). For example, when normal-weight people are asked to eat an extra 1,000 calories a day for eight weeks, some volunteers gain considerable amounts of weight (over 9 pounds), whereas others gain only small amounts (less than 1 pound) (Levine, Eberhardt, & Jensen, 1999). The biggest predictor of low levels of weight gain was the incidental physical activity (not intentional exercise) people engaged in as part of daily life, such as fidgeting, sitting up straight, and flexing their muscles. People may vary in how easily they engage in activities that burn fat.

According to **set-point theory**, each person's body has a certain weight that it strives to maintain, much like a thermostat device (Keesey, 1995). When you eat fewer calories, your metabolism slows to keep your weight at the same level. Because people's set points may vary based on heredity, some will be heavier and some will be lighter. One way it may work is that the set point is determined by the number of fat cells a person has (Leibel, Berry, & Hirsch, 1983). Although there is little or no difference in the number of fat cells between people of normal weight and those who are slightly overweight, people who are severely obese have many more fat cells. Another possibility is that the hypothalamus influences fat stores and/or levels of glucose or insulin in the blood, which in turn influence feelings of hunger and fullness. In line with this view, research with animals demonstrates that damage to a certain part of the hypothalamus can lead to a change in weight, perhaps by allowing a new set point to be established (Keesey & Powley, 1975).

Conclusions

Although genes do play some role in obesity, it is clear that they do not totally predict a person's weight. First, rates of obesity in the United States have increased dramatically in recent years, which means genetics can't explain it all (Hill & Peters, 1998; Katan, Grundy, & Willett, 1997). Second, people with the same genetic background who live in different parts of the world often have very different body weights (Hodge & Zimmet, 1994). For example, Japanese people who live in Japan are thinner than those who move to Hawaii, and Japanese people who live in Hawaii are thinner than those who move to the continental United States (Curb & Marcus, 1991). These differences in weight suggest that while genetics may play some role, cultural factors including diet and exercise also influence weight.

Even if genes do play some role in influencing weight, whether these genes are activated (an epigenetic effect) may depend on environment factors. For example, in-utero experiences, such as experiencing malnutrition or extreme stress, may activate genes that regulate appetite in ways that make weight gain more likely to occur (Burgio, Lopomo, & Migliore, 2014). These very early life experiences may also lead to changes in the hypothalamus, a part of the brain that regulates appetite. In line with this view, one study of 100,000 young men found that those whose mothers experienced the death of a close relative during or just before their pregnancy were significantly more likely to become overweight or obese as adults (Hohwü, Li, Olsen, Sørensen, & Obel, 2014). In fact, those whose mothers had lost their husbands—a particularly severe stressor—were at twice the risk of developing weight problems in adulthood.

Finally, explaining obesity as a function of genes may have negative consequences. Specifically, a belief that obese people have no control over their weight leads people to feel they have less control over their own weight (Dar-Nimrod, Cheung, Ruby, & Heine, 2014). In fact, simply reading a (fictitious) article suggesting that obesity is caused by genes leads people to later eat more cookies than reading an article suggesting obesity is caused by psychosocial factors! On the other hand, overweight people who read an article describing the role of environmental factors, such as the ready accessibility of junk food, in contributing to obesity show greater self-efficacy to lose weight (Pearl & Lebowitz, 2014). These findings point to the downside of overemphasizing the role of genes in predicting weight.

PSYCHOSOCIAL FACTORS CONTRIBUTING TO OBESITY

LO 8.2

Summarize how psychosocial factors contribute to obesity

Although genetic and biological factors do influence how much we eat, they aren't the whole story. There are probably many times you have eaten even when you have not been hungry, for instance. Maybe you eat when you are nervous; maybe you eat after you walk by a shop selling great-smelling cinnamon rolls in the mall; maybe you eat mindlessly while watching TV. All of these are examples of psychological factors that may lead to eating (and overeating). This section will examine various psychological factors that influence eating: the internal-external hypothesis, mood regulation, restraint theory, and sociocultural factors.

Internal-External Hypothesis

One of the earliest hypotheses explaining obesity was the **internal-external hypothesis**, which proposed that people often fail to listen to their internal cues for eating (namely, hunger), and instead pay attention to external cues, such as food taste, smell, and variety (Schachter, 1968). In line with this hypothesis, you've probably noticed that even when you are not hungry, tempting food smells and tastes can influence you to eat. We also eat more when we have a variety of different types of foods available (just think about a time you've overeaten at an all-you-can-eat buffet) (Rolls et al., 1981).

In support of Schachter's theory, obese people do eat more when foods taste particularly good (Kauffman, Herman, & Polivy, 1995). For example, when normal-weight people were placed on a hospital diet—meaning the only thing they could eat was a bland liquid diet shake—they basically took in the same number of calories as they did in normal life (Hashim & Van Itallie, 1965). In other words, they ate to maintain their weight, and presumably they relied on their internal cue of hunger to guide their eating. On the other hand, obese people consumed significantly fewer calories on this diet than they normally did, presumably because the external cues of eating were weak. These findings suggest that obese people show a close connection to the external circumstances of eating, whereas for normal-weight people, the close connection is between their physiological state—that is, their hunger—and the amount eaten.

More recent research, however, provides little support for the internal-external theory. First, even people of normal weight are not particularly good at interpreting internal signals for hunger, such as low blood sugar and stomach pains (Rodin, 1981). People are also not very good at surmising how many calories they have consumed or how many calories their bodies need to maintain weight. Second, people at varying weight levels, including those of average weight, can and do eat in response to external cues, such as the presence of food and whether other people are eating (Elliston, Ferguson, Schüz, & Schüz, 2017). For example, people vary in how appealing they find different types of snack foods, as well as how well they are able to control these desires (Nederkoorn, Houben, Hofmann, Roefs, & Jansen, 2010).

Restraint Theory

Restraint theory was developed in part to explain the mixed findings from research testing the internal-external theory. According to **restraint theory**, people are generally motivated to eat as a function of internal physiological signals that cue hunger (Herman & Polivy, 1984). However, when people are trying to lose weight—either because they are obese or because they are dieting—they deliberately ignore these internal signals and instead use cognitive rules to limit their caloric intake. For example, so-called restrained eaters might develop rules about eating only certain types of foods (e.g., celery, carrots, nonfat yogurt) and avoiding other types of foods (e.g., ice cream, brownies, meat).

This approach can be successful in helping people restrict their eating, but it can also backfire. Specifically, restrained eaters often develop an "all-or-nothing" mind-set about eating, which means that breaking the rules by eating small amounts of "forbidden food" can lead to overeating. For example, a person who is dieting but who gives in and eats a fattening first course at a dinner party may think, "Well, I've blown it now, so I may as well eat all I want." Similarly, while people who are high in restrained eating generally eat fewer calories than those who are not high in restraint, they eat substantially more than nonrestrained eaters if eating while walking—suggesting that "eating on the go" may distract restrained eaters from their goal (Ogden, Oikonomou, & Alemany, 2015). Similarly, when restrained eaters feel sad or stressed, they give up the cognitive rules and can then eat excessive amounts (Heatherton, Striepe, & Wittenberg, 1998).

However, other research suggests that restraint theory is not always a good predictor of eating behavior (Lowe, 1993). Specifically, people who are restrained eaters but are not at the moment actively trying to lose weight should overeat under various conditions (when they are sad, when they are stressed, etc.). On the other hand, people who are actively trying to diet may also develop rules to guide their eating, but these people should not engage in the same type of "all-or-nothing" eating that nondieting restrained eaters show. In support of this view, restrained nondieters eat more after they have first had a milkshake (because they have already blown their diet anyway), whereas restrained dieters eat significantly less after having a milk-shake (because they are actively trying to lose weight) (Lowe, Whitlow, & Bellwoar, 1991).

Mood Regulation

Considerable research indicates that people may eat to influence how they feel (a factor psychologists describe as *mood regulation*). For example, people eat when they experience negative affect (e.g., bored, angry, sad, stressed), presumably in an attempt to make themselves feel better (Elliston et al., 2017). As described in ***Chapter 4: Understanding Stress***, people who experience more stress eat more high-fat or high-sugar between-meal snacks, have less main meal and vegetable consumption, and show higher levels of emotional eating and hap-hazard planning of eating, which in turn can, not surprisingly, lead to weight gain (Hannerz, Albertsen, Nielsen, Tüchsen, & Burr, 2004; O'Connor, Jones, Conner, McMillan, & Ferguson, 2008; Sims et al., 2007). In line with this view, children who are exposed to serious stressors, such as poverty and family disruptions, are more likely to become obese during adolescence (Hernandez & Pressler, 2015).

To examine the impact of a pretty typical daily life stress on eating, researchers measured how professional football losses influence eating patterns in the team's home city (Cornil & Chandon, 2013). To test this question, data were collected on the total consumption of calories as well as the amount of saturated fats (e.g., pizza, cakes, cookies) consumed in cities (including those both with an NFL team and not). First, findings revealed there were no differences in calories or fats consumed on Sundays, regardless of whether the city had an NFL or not, and, for those with an NFL team, regardless of the game outcome. On Mondays, however, consumption of both calories and saturated fats increased in cities in which the home team lost and decreased in cities in which the home team won; there were no differences in rate of consumption for cities without an NFL team or for those in which the home team didn't play. Interestingly, the effect of game outcome on consumption was particularly strong in cities with the most devoted fans; saturated fat consumption increased by 28% in these cities following defeat (compared to 9% in the other cities) and decreased by 16% following victories (compared to 4% in the other cities).

Although the studies described thus far are correlational, and thus it is difficult to determine the precise way in which stress influences eating, experimental research yields similar findings. For example, people who are watching sad movies—such as the tragedy *Love Story*—eat substantially more popcorn than those who are watching a funny movie—such as the comedy *Sweet Home Alabama* (Garg, Wansink, & Inman, 2007). Bad moods are particularly likely to lead people to eat more "comfort foods" when they are trying to suppress such moods, indicating that people who aren't able to regulate their moods in an adaptive way show more signs of eating as a way of coping with bad emotions (Evers, Stok, & de Ridder, 2010).

There is rather mixed evidence, however, for the view that stress consistently leads to overeating (Rosengren et al., 2015). In fact, while some people seem to eat more when under stress, others eat less (Sproesser, Schupp, & Renner, 2014; Willenbring, Levine, & Morley, 1986). This tendency to eat more when stressed is more common among those who are obese and/or trying to lose weight (Baucom & Aiken, 1981; Friedman & Brownell, 1995). One study of female college students found that obese students ate nearly seven times as much during exam period as normal weight students, whereas there was virtually no difference in how much obese and nonobese students ate during less stressful periods of the semester (Slochower, Kaplan, & Mann, 1981). So, all of this research suggests that some people may indeed overeat when they are experiencing stress, but stress does not lead everyone to overeat. You can measure how much different emotions impact your eating by completing **Table 8.2: Test Yourself**.

What You'll Learn

8.1

Situational Factors

As you probably already know, situational factors influence not only how much we eat but also what we eat. These factors include social influences, the environment, and culture.

Social Influences

People eat more when they are with other people than when they are alone, and are particularly likely to eat more when eating with family and friends (de Castro, 1994; de Castro & de Castro, 1989; Feunekes, De Graaf, & Van Staveren, 1995; Lumeng & Hillman, 2007). Having other people around may lead to more eating in part because meals last longer. We may also be less sensitive to internal cues for hunger when we are with other people. For example, if you are eating alone, the amount you eat is influenced by how hungry you are (e.g., if you had a late or big lunch, you eat less for dinner), whereas if you are eating with other people, you eat the same amount regardless of when you have last had a meal.

Table 8.2 Test Yourself: Are You an Emotional Eater?

This scale measures the tendency to eat in response to different types of emotions. Rate how much each of the following emotions leads you to feel an urge to eat using a scale of 1 to 5 (1 = no desire to eat at all to 5 = an overwhelming urge to eat).

1. Angry
2. Discouraged
3. Jealous
4. Guilty
5. Nervous
6. Excited
7. Worried
8. Upset
9. Bored
10. Sad
11. Lonely
12. Blue

Add up your scores on items 1 to 4 (which assess anger/frustration), 5 to 8 (which assess anxiety), and items 9 to 12 (which assess depression).

Source: Arnow, Kenardy, & Agras (1995).

Obesity is also linked to particular social networks, meaning that people with social contacts who are obese are more likely to be obese themselves. One study of young adults found that those who were overweight and obese were more likely to have friends and romantic partners who were also considered overweight (Leahey, LaRose, Fava, & Wing, 2011). Moreover, data from a large social network study found that having friends or siblings who are obese increases one's own chances of becoming obese over time (Christakis & Fowler, 2007). Specifically, people's chances of becoming obese increased by 71% if they had a same-sex friend who became obese during that time, by 40% if they had a sibling who became obese, and by 37% if they had a spouse who became obese. (The link between obesity was not seen among neighbors or opposite-sex friends.) This research suggests that obesity may in fact be "contagious," perhaps indirectly, such as through the impact of obesity leading to changes in weight-related norms, and/or directly, such as through impacting food consumption.

Environmental Factors

As described in *Chapter 2: Research Methods*, a series of fascinating studies by Brian Wansink demonstrate that even subtle environmental factors, such as the size of the dish food is served on, influence how much we eat. For example, guests attending an ice cream party who are given a larger bowl serve themselves 31% more ice cream than those who are given a smaller bowl (Wansink, van Ittersum, & Painter, 2006). Similarly, people who serve themselves a snack mix of pretzels, nuts, and chips at a Super Bowl party take—and consume—56% more from large bowls than small ones (Wansink & Cheney, 2005). Even the brightness of a room can influence the types of food people eat (see Figure 8.2).

Figure 8.2   Data From Biswas et al., 2017

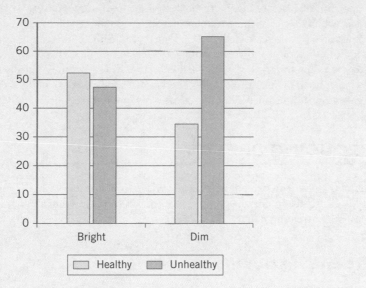

Even when dining at the same restaurant and ordering off the same menu, people who are seated in well-lit rooms are more likely to order healthy foods (such as grilled/baked fish, vegetables, or white meat) than those dining in dimly lit rooms, who are more likely to order unhealthy food (such as fried food or dessert). What explains this finding? Researchers posit that people feel more alert in bright rooms, which in turn increases their awareness of their food choices.

Source: Biswas, Szocs, Chacko, & Wansink (2017).

Cultural Factors

Cultural factors such as the availability and amount of food clearly contribute to obesity (Wadden, Brownell, & Foster, 2002). The United States has the highest rates of obesity in the world, but also a great abundance of fast-food restaurants featuring inexpensive and very fatty foods. Not surprisingly, people who live closer to fast-food restaurants have higher BMIs and eat fewer fruits and vegetables, presumably because less nutritious foods are much more readily available (Kruger, Greenberg, Murphy, Difazio, & Youra, 2014). Moreover, food is not simply readily available but is increasingly being served in larger amounts. Portions at both high-end and low-end restaurants (think "Super Size that") in the United States have become bigger over time, which encourages overeating (Hill & Peters, 1998). The original glass Coke bottles that were manufactured in the 1930s held 6½ ounces, whereas the current "single-size" plastic Coke bottle now holds 1 liter, which is five times as much.

These aspects of American culture—including the abundance of food and large portion sizes—help explain why immigrants who move to the United States increase in obesity over time (Goel, McCarthy, Phillips, & Wee, 2004). Specifically, although the prevalence of obesity was 16% among immigrants and 22% among U.S.-born individuals, only 8% of immigrants who had lived in the United States for less than a year were obese compared to 19% among those who had lived in the United States for at least 15 years. These findings suggest that exposure to American culture increases the risk of obesity.

Another factor contributing to obesity is a lack of access to affordable, nutritious foods, at least in certain communities. Specifically, the term *food desert* describes parts of the country in which people lack access to healthy foods—such as fruits, vegetables, and whole grains—because they do not live near a supermarket and do not have transportation to reach such a store (see Figure 8.3). People living in high-poverty areas, as well as areas with a large proportion of Black residents (regardless of income), are less likely to have access to healthy foods, which may contribute to their increased risk obesity, diabetes, and heart disease (Baker, Schootman, Barnidge, & Kelly, 2006). One recent study found that many neighborhood stores in a city sell little or no fresh fruits and vegetables, and that such stores often have higher prices than supermarkets that are further away (MacNell, Elliott, Hardison-Moody, & Bowen, 2017). In turn, people living in food deserts eat foods that are higher in fat, cholesterol, and sugars than those who live in other areas (De Choudhury, Sharma, & Kiciman, 2016).

REDUCING OBESITY

LO 8.3

Compare different strategies for reducing obesity

Given the physical, psychological, and social consequences of obesity, reducing rates of obesity is clearly an important goal. This section describes two distinct approaches: preventing obesity and treating obesity.

Preventing Obesity

Preventing obesity must begin in childhood because obese children are very likely to become obese adults (Kelsey, Zaepfel, Bjornstad, & Nadeau, 2014). Fat cells develop in childhood and

---

Figure 8.3 Food Deserts in the United States

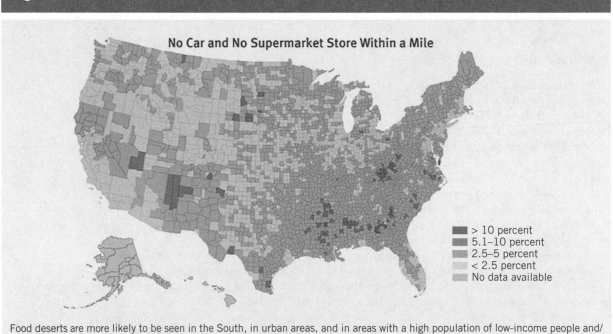

No Car and No Supermarket Store Within a Mile

> 10 percent
5.1–10 percent
2.5–5 percent
< 2.5 percent
No data available

Food deserts are more likely to be seen in the South, in urban areas, and in areas with a high population of low-income people and/or people of color.

Source: Data from U.S. Department of Agriculture and Centers for Disease Control and Prevention. Public Domain.

adolescence, and once they develop, they never disappear—they can get bigger or smaller, but they never disappear. One study examined the prevalence of adult obesity based on whether six-month-old infants were above or below the 75th percentile for weight (Charney et al., 1976). Only 8% of nonobese infants became obese adults as compared to 14% of obese infants (nearly double the rate). The risk of adult obesity is even greater for children who are obese at older ages. For example, 40% of obese seven-year-olds became overweight adults as compared to only 10% of nonobese seven-year-olds (Stark, Atkins, Wolff, & Douglas, 1981). This section describes effective strategies for preventing obesity.

Avoid Using Food as a Reward

Efforts to prevent obesity can be relatively simple, such as encouraging children to exercise and eat healthy foods and modeling healthy behavior, such as using fruits as dessert, eating healthy snacks, and exercising. However, parents should never use unhealthy food as a reward for good behavior even when it is really tempting to do so. One study of 427 parents of preschool children found that 56% reported promising children a special food, such as a dessert, for finishing their dinner and 48% reported promising children a special food for good behavior, such as cleaning their room (Stanek, Abbott, & Cramer, 1990). But what are the long-term effects of this approach? Children figure out very quickly that the "good foods" come after the "bad foods," and they in fact show an increased desire for "forbidden" foods.

Limit Television

Another important factor in preventing obesity is limiting television watching. First, watching television is a passive activity (particularly with the advent of the remote control). So, when children come home from school (or adults come home from work) and sit in front of the television, they aren't exercising. Studies with both adults (Ching et al., 1996) and children (Andersen, Crespo, Bartlett, Cheskin, & Pratt, 1998) have shown that people who watch a lot of television are more likely to be overweight than those who watch less television. Children from families in which the television is often on during meals also eat more salty snacks and sodas and less fruits, vegetables, and juices than those from families in which the television is rarely on (Coon, Goldberg, Rogers, & Tucker, 2001).

Watching television also exposes children to numerous advertisements for unhealthy foods, which in turn models bad eating habits (Story & Faulkner, 1990). The average child sees more than 20,000 TV commercials in a year, and the two most common types of ads are for toys and food. Moreover, in one study, 97.8% of the 5,000 television food-product advertisements viewed by children 2 to 11 years old were for foods high in fat, sugar, or sodium, and on average 46.1% of the total calories in these products came from sugar (Powell, Szczypka, Chaloupka, & Braunschweig, 2007). For example, 97.6% of cereal advertisements were for high-sugar cereals.

This constant exposure to television advertisements also leads children to develop stronger preferences for restaurants featuring unhealthy foods. More than half of 9- to 10-year-old children believe that Ronald McDonald knows what is good for children to eat (Horgen, Choate, & Brownell, 2001). Children also believe that food from McDonald's tastes better. Researchers in one study examined the effects of fast-food branding on children's taste preferences

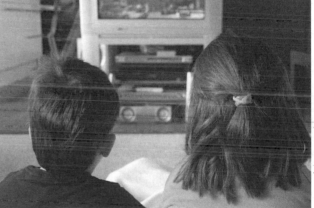

Children who watch considerable amounts of television are at increased risk of obesity, in part because they are exposed to many commercials for unhealthy foods and in part because they are less likely to participate in physical activity than children who watch less television.

(Robinson, Borzekowski, Matheson, & Kraemer, 2007). Sixty-three children tasted five pairs of identical foods and beverages in packaging from McDonald's and matched but unbranded packaging and were asked to indicate if they tasted the same or if one tasted better. Overall, children preferred the tastes of foods and drinks if they thought they were from McDonald's. Although children in general prefer the taste of food in a McDonald's package over food in a plain package, this preference is even stronger for children who live in homes with more television sets.

Encourage Physical Activity

Efforts to prevent weight can also focus on increasing the number of calories expended through exercise; in fact, increasing exercise is the single best predictor of long-term weight control (Wadden, 1993). Exercise helps with weight loss in a number of ways, including increasing metabolic rate (so calories are burned at a faster rate), increasing lean body mass (which requires more calories to maintain), and suppressing appetite. Engaging in regular exercise also leads to greater psychological and physical well-being; even moderate amounts of exercise can decrease anxiety and depression and reduce the risk of cardiovascular disease and diabetes (Helmrich, Ragland, Leung, & Paffenberger, 1991; Manson et al., 1992), lower blood pressure (Kokkinos et al., 1995), and protect against osteoporosis (Greendale, Barrett-Connor, Edelstein, Ingles, & Haile, 1995) as well as cancer (Meyerhardt et al., 2009; Wolin, Yan, Colditz, & Lee, 2009). Physical activity is even associated with longer life expectancy (Sun et al., 2010). Unfortunately, despite the numerous health benefits of exercise, only about half of all Americans meet the recommended guidelines for aerobic physical activity (meaning 150 minutes a week of moderate-intensity exercise or 75 minutes of vigorous physical activity) (Centers for Disease Control and Prevention, 2017g).

People who live in areas in which they can easily, and safely, walk are more likely to get adequate amounts of physical activity (Cunningham-Myrie et al., 2015; Jilcott Pitts et al., 2015). It is more difficult to maintain healthy exercise habits in neighborhoods without bicycle lanes and sidewalks, a lack of affordable exercise clubs, and fear of crime. Not surprisingly, people who live in walkable urban neighborhoods also show slower increases in rates of overweight, obesity, and diabetes than those living in less walkable ones, even when researchers take into account people's age, area income, and ethnicity (Creatore et al., 2016).

Get Enough Sleep

One of the easiest ways to prevent obesity is to get an adequate amount of sleep. Both sleep quantity and sleep quality influence levels of hormones that regulate appetite, meaning that sleep deprivation can increase feelings of hunger (Knutson, 2012). One recent meta-analysis revealed that people who are sleep-deprived consume about 385 additional calories the next day (Al Khatib, Harding, Darzi, & Pot, 2017). They also consume more fat, and less protein, which over time could lead to obesity. Moreover, and as described in **Focus on Development**, young children who stay up late at night are at greater risk of becoming obese adolescents.

Conclusions

Although preventing obesity is an important goal in terms of improving long-term health, parents need to be careful about the messages they send their children about weight and body image. In some cases, parents' concern about their children's weight can have unintended negative—and lasting—consequences. For example, children whose parents see them as overweight are more likely to develop concerns about their own weight and shape and to engage in unhealthy patterns of eating (such as binging and purging) (Allen, Byrne, & Crosby, 2014; Robinson & Sutin, 2017). They are also more likely to become overweight. Children whose parents see them as overweight gain more weight, perhaps because their parents' perceptions lead them to feel negatively about their bodies, which can cause stress and unhealthy eating habits, both of which lead to weight gain. Pediatricians therefore recommend that parents emphasize the importance of a healthy lifestyle and not achieving a particular weight (Golden, Schneider, Wood, Committee on Nutrition, Committee on Adolescence, & Section on Obesity, 2016).

Treating Obesity

It is no mystery that weight gain is at least partially a function of taking in more calories than the body burns off. Many people try to lose weight by making changes in their diet—in fact, as much as 25% to 30% of the adult American population is dieting at any one time (Bouchard, 1991). However, the amount of weight people lose on any of these diets tends to be small and temporary. These approaches don't focus on helping people make long-term changes in their dietary habits. It might be that eating only grapefruit for the rest of your life would allow you to maintain a very low body weight, but you would also suffer from various nutritional deficits. It is unrealistic to think that people could maintain health on some dieting approaches. This section describes various strategies that can effectively help people lose weight and maintain such weight loss over time.

Set Short-Term Goals

Setting short-term goals regarding exercise and eating is a great strategy for treating obesity and is more effective than setting longer-term goals (Bandura & Simon, 1977; Marcus et al., 2000; Wadden, 1993). For example, it is better to focus on cutting calories at each meal than on eliminating a certain number of calories each week or jogging three times a week. This type of short-term approach allows people to experience small successes in reaching their larger goals and thus can help them feel more confident in their ability to achieve their weight-loss goals. Setting specific realistic goals and working toward them helps motivation stay high and increases self-efficacy for following through on these behavior change intentions—which is particularly important since self-efficacy is one of the best predictors of whether someone engages in physical activity and adopts healthier eating habits (Anderson, Wojcik, Winett, & Williams, 2006; Fuemmeler et al., 2006; Kitzman-Ulrich, Wilson, Van Horn, & Lawman, 2010).

Similarly, the most effective techniques emphasize gradual weight loss (1 to 2 pounds a week), as opposed to more extreme approaches. The quick and extreme plans that are often featured on magazine covers just don't work—no one can safely lose 10 pounds in the week before spring break. In fact, one recent study examined whether 14 contestants who appeared on *The Biggest Loser* reality television program—and lost an average of 127 pounds during this show—were able to sustain their weight loss after the program ended (Fothergill et al., 2016). Unfortunately, six years later, contestants had regained an average of 90 pounds, in part because the very sudden and extreme weight loss led to a dramatic reduction in their metabolic rate, meaning their bodies simply burn calories more slowly, making weight loss more difficult to sustain.

Create Rewards

As you learned in *Chapter 3: Theories of Health Behavior*, operant-conditioning approaches, in which people receive some type of reward for adhering to a diet, losing weight, or sticking to an exercise program, can be very helpful (Jeffery, Wing, Thorson, & Burton, 1998; Wadden, 1993). For example, you could give yourself some type of reward for successfully meeting your weight-loss goals, such as a new pair of sunglasses or tickets to a concert you've been wanting to see. (Obviously, it's better to not use food as a reward to motivate yourself!) One study found that people who were given rewards (e.g., clothing, money, going to the movies) for engaging in regular exercise reported exercising an average of 2.29 times per week as compared to 1.36 for those who were not given such rewards (Noland, 1989). Operant-conditioning approaches may be especially useful for creating behavior change in children (Epstein, Paluch, Kilanowski, & Raynor, 2004).

Monitor Behavior

Monitoring exactly what, when, and where you eat can help you reduce calories (Wadden, 1993). People sometimes lack an understanding of precisely what they eat each day; therefore, they are confused when their dieting doesn't work. You may, for example, decrease the number of calories you eat at each meal, but if you consistently eat potato chips while you study or have a candy bar as a quick between-classes snack, you may not remember to count those calories. Also, people often overeat in social situations because they aren't even aware of how much they are eating. (Sadly, calories consumed while standing up still count.)

Once you have monitored the factors that lead to overeating, you can try to eliminate these triggers. Instead of stopping at Dunkin' Donuts for coffee and a doughnut on your way to class, you might try eating a bowl of cereal or fruit at home instead. If you eat while you watch TV, you might try eating when sitting at your dining room table with the TV off. Mindful eating is a particular type of self-monitoring that involves paying deliberate attention to what you are eating, including its taste, smell, texture, and so on. People who learn strategies for mindful eating make healthier food choices, which in turn can lead to weight loss (Hendrickson & Rasmussen, 2017). Even simple cues to how much you are eating can help people adopt healthier snacking habits. For example, people eat far fewer potato chips from a tube that contains chips dyed red interspersed at regular intervals that designate how many chips make up a single serving size than from a normal tube without such a visual cue (Geier, Wansink, & Rozin, 2012).

Self-monitoring is more effective if it includes regular prompts and reminders, such as mailings, signs, or phone calls, to keep people on track with the desired changes in their behavior (Anderson, Franckowiak, Snyder, Bartlett, & Fontaine, 1998; Eakin, Reeves, Winkler, Lawler, & Owen, 2010; Lombard, Lombard, & Winett, 1995; Marcus et al., 2000). For example, simply placing a sign saying, "Your heart needs exercise. Here's your chance" increases the number of people taking the stairs instead of the escalator (Brownell, Stunkard, & Albaum, 1980).

Similarly, obese dieters who received reminder calls to self-monitor their eating a couple of times a week didn't gain any weight during the diet-challenging eight-week holiday time (including the Thanksgiving to New Year's weeks), whereas those without these calls gained weight (Boutelle, Kirschenbaum, Baker, & Mitchell, 1999).

Make Small Changes

Other self-control approaches to weight loss focus on helping people make small changes in their behavior, or even in the way that they think about eating and weight loss (Wadden, 1993). Obese people might be encouraged to purchase healthy foods to snack on and to avoid keeping "problem foods" in the house; this way, if they overeat, they eat carrots as opposed to doughnuts. Similarly, people who are dieting may be advised to slow down their eating, perhaps by putting their fork down between each bite or chewing all of their food thoroughly. These methods focus on changing people's negative or unrealistic views about weight loss (e.g., "I will never be able to lose the weight"; "I should have lost the weight by now; this isn't working"). People who have struggled with obesity for some time may view their lack of weight-loss success as a sign of personal weakness and failure, which in turn can lead them to return to unhealthy eating patterns at the first sign of trouble.

People are also more likely to follow through on their intentions to change their eating and exercise habits when these behaviors can easily fit in with their daily lives and schedules. For example, people are more likely to continue exercising when they are exercising at home as opposed to in a health club (Perri, Martin, Leermakers, Sears, & Notelovitz, 1997). Although formal exercise classes can provide social support and motivation, exercising at home is cheaper and more convenient. Similarly, people who commit to engaging in several short bouts of exercise each day (four 10-minute bouts of exercise such as climbing the stairs or walking briskly outside) are more successful at maintaining this behavior than those who attempt to engage in one longer period of exercise such as a 40-minute exercise class (Jakicic, Winters, Lang, & Wing, 1999). Even simple lifestyle changes, such as using stairs rather than escalators, walking rather than driving to work, and parking farther away from store entrances, can be as effective as more organized exercise activities in weight reduction (Andersen et al., 1999; Dunn et al., 1999; Kujala, Kaprio, Sarna, & Koshenvuo, 1998; Wadden et al., 2002).

Get Social Support

Social influence techniques, such as exercising with a friend and participating in formal weight-loss groups, can often help people successfully make changes related to diet and exercise (Duncan & McAuley, 1993; Wadden, 1993; Wing & Jeffery, 1999). For example, one study with overweight adults found that participation in 20 weekly group sessions to encourage dieting and engaging in exercise led to a mean weight loss of 4.4 pounds, with 69% of participants losing at least that much weight (Hollis et al., 2008). Group approaches are especially effective in helping people lose weight because they provide social support as well as healthy competition. For example, rewarding people for the average weight loss in a group leads to greater success at maintaining weight loss over two years than rewarding people for only their own weight loss (Jeffery et al., 1984).

Informal support from family and friends also helps people adopt healthier eating and exercise habits (Anderson et al., 2006; Fuemmeler et al., 2006). For example, a study with adolescents found that having friends, parents, and siblings who support sport activities—and who watch such activities—is associated with more physical activity (Duncan, Duncan & Strycker, 2005). Believing your parents/peers care about your sports and come watch you play is associated with more physical activity. Interventions designed to decrease obesity in children are especially effective if parents are involved and supportive, including changing their own habits and/or assisting with cooking and providing healthier foods (Kitzmann et al., 2010).

Institute Societal Changes

Given the growing awareness of the health consequences of obesity, coupled with its increasing prevalence, a number of cities and states have implemented laws in an attempt to reduce obesity. These included laws requiring posting information on calories and nutrition in restaurants, restricting the sales of unhealthy foods in schools, and increasing taxes on unhealthy foods and drinks (Donaldson et al., 2015). As predicted, towns that increase the tax on sugar-sweetened beverages show reductions in their sales, coupled with increases in sales of other beverages, such as water and milk (Silver et al., 2017).

What You'll Learn 8.3

Researchers in one study examined the effects of posting calorie and nutrition information on purchases at Starbucks in New York City (Bollinger, Leslie, & Sorensen, 2011). Specifically, they compared the calories purchased per transaction and the amount spent before New York City passed a law requiring that such information be posted to assess its impact. As predicted, the number of calories purchased per transaction fell by about 6%, indicating that the law led to some changes in purchasing. Although there was basically no change in the beverage calories purchased, people chose lower-calorie food options following the posting of this information. However, there was no impact on the amount spent per transaction, indicating that posting of calorie information did not reduce sales (as companies often fear).

Utilize Drugs or Surgery

Four drugs have been approved by the United States Food and Drug Administration for use in treating obesity (Apovian et al., 2015; Kakkar & Dahiya, 2015). These drugs—lorcaserin (Belviq), phentermine/topiramate (Qsymia), naltrexone/bupropion (Contrave), and liraglutide (Saxenda)—are used only when other approaches have not been effective in reducing weight, and typically when the person is at risk of experiencing complications, such as diabetes and/or cardiovascular disease, as a result of the weight. Although these drugs can be effective in helping people lose weight, all drugs can have side effects and are thus used only after other approaches to treating obesity have failed.

Finally, in extreme cases, when obesity is a real threat to a person's health, surgical techniques can be used (Kral, 1992). One method is to wire shut a person's jaw for a certain amount of time so he or she can only drink fluids. Other surgical methods include stomach stapling (so that the person can eat only small amounts of food before feeling full) and removal of a portion of the small intestine (which prevents food from being absorbed into the body). Although these approaches often do lead to significant weight loss, they can have unpleasant side effects, including permanent diarrhea and long-term nutritional deficits. These methods are therefore used only in cases of severe obesity that have potentially life-threatening effects.

Conclusions

Obesity is an epidemic within the United States in part because environmental factors, such as the ready availability of cheap unhealthy foods and overall large portion sizes, encourage overeating. Moreover, losing weight, and maintaining that weight loss, is really hard. So, how can people lose weight and maintain that weight loss over time? A 10-year observational study of people who had lost at least 30 pounds, and managed to keep this weight off for at least a year, found that people who were successful showed consistent changes in their behavior (Thomas, Bond, Phelan, Hill, & Wing, 2014). Specifically, these people weighed themselves daily, engaged in regular physical activity, followed a low-fat diet, and avoided overeating. If you'd like to lose weight, try to adopt each of these strategies, and

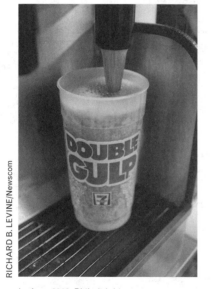

RICHARD B. LEVINE/Newscom

In June 2016, Philadelphia became the second city in the United States to increase taxes on sugar-added and artificially sweetened soft drinks, which research suggests will decrease their consumption. This tax will add 18 cents to the cost of a can of soda, $1.08 to a six-pack, and $1.02 to a 2-liter bottle.

remember that engaging in regular exercise—even if it doesn't result in weight loss—is good for psychological and physical well-being.

UNDERSTANDING DISORDERED EATING

LO 8.4

Describe different types of eating disorders and the role of genetic factors in contributing to such disorders

This section of the chapter is particularly difficult to write—and perhaps to read—because many students may feel personally impacted by some type of disordered eating. I remember attending summer camp one year when I was in high school and hearing a close friend talk about consuming over a gallon of ice cream and then vomiting it up. I remember watching a girl in high school jog around the school every day at lunchtime, getting thinner almost literally before my eyes. I remember staying overnight with a friend during college and seeing cookie crumbs beside the toilet. In this section, you'll learn about different types of eating disorders, psychosocial factors influencing their development, and strategies for both preventing and treating such disorders. But most important, keep in mind that disordered eating is a serious problem, and therefore it is really important to seek help if you or someone you know is engaging in these behaviors.

Types of Eating Disorders

Although all eating disorders involve some type of dysfunctional and unhealthy pattern of eating, the specific characteristics of various disorders differ substantially. This section describes the three most common types of disordered eating.

Anorexia Nervosa

Anorexia nervosa involves a drastic reduction in a person's food intake and an intentional loss of weight (maintaining a body weight 15% below one's normal weight based on height/weight tables, or a BMI of 17.5; American Psychiatric Association, 2013). This loss of weight eventually leads to amenorrhea, the absence of menstruation. People with anorexia nervosa are intensely focused on achieving and maintaining a very thin body size and have an excessive fear of gaining weight (see Table 8.3). They also overestimate their own body weight and thus see themselves as heavy even when they are actually quite thin (Hagman et al., 2015). Unfortunately, these dysfunctional body shape and size ideals lead them to engage in unhealthy patterns of eating and exercise. They typically eat only very small amounts of food (e.g., a Cheerio for breakfast, a bite of an apple for lunch, lettuce for supper) and may have a variety of eating rituals that they engage in as a way of avoiding eating (e.g., cutting food into very small portions, eating very slowly). People with anorexia may also engage in strenuous exercise in an effort to lose weight.

Anorexia is much more common in women than men and tends to be most prevalent in upper-middle-class and upper-class White women. Women who participate in weight-conscious activities, including ballet, gymnastics, and modeling, are at greatest risk of developing anorexia. Although the overall prevalence of anorexia nervosa in all women in the United States is approximately 1% (only 0.3% for men) (Hudson, Hiripi, Pope, & Kessler, 2007), some estimates suggest that 6% to 7% of women who attend professional schools for modeling and dance meet the criteria for having anorexia (Garner & Garfinkel, 1980).

Most important, anorexia can lead to very serious, in some cases life-threatening, problems; in fact, an estimated 4% of people with anorexia will die from this disease, which is the highest mortality rate among all psychiatric disorders (Crow et al., 2009; Kask et al., 2016). Anorexia can cause low blood pressure, heart damage, and cardiac arrhythmia, which in turn can lead to heart failure (Brownell & Fairburn, 1995; Comerci, 1990). Moreover, women who recover from anorexia still may suffer from long-term problems, including bone loss (because of undernutrition and amenorrhea) and infertility (Becker, Grinspoon, Klibanski, & Herzog, 1999).

Table 8.3   Diagnostic Criteria for Eating Disorders

Anorexia Nervosa

1. Restriction of energy intake relative to requirements, leading to a significantly low body weight in the context of age, sex, developmental trajectory, and physical health. Significantly low weight is defined as a weight that is less than minimally normal or, for children and adolescents, less than that minimally expected.

2. Intense fear of gaining weight or of becoming fat, or persistent behavior that interferes with weight gain, even though at a significantly low weight.

3. Disturbance in the way in which one's body weight or shape is experienced, undue influence of body weight or shape on self-evaluation, or persistent lack of recognition of the seriousness of the current low body weight.

Bulimia Nervosa

1. Recurrent episodes of binge eating. An episode of binge eating is characterized by both of the following:

   - Eating, in a discrete period of time (e.g., within any two-hour period), an amount of food that is definitely larger than most people would eat during a similar period of time and under similar circumstances.

   - A sense of lack of control over eating during the episode (e.g., a feeling that one cannot stop eating or control what or how much one is eating).

2. Recurrent inappropriate compensatory behavior to prevent weight gain, such as self-induced vomiting; misuse of laxatives, diuretics, enemas, or other medications; fasting; or excessive exercise.

3. The binge eating and inappropriate compensatory behaviors both occur, on average, at least once a week for three months.

4. Self-evaluation is unduly influenced by body shape and weight.

5. The disturbance does not occur exclusively during episodes of anorexia nervosa.

Binge Eating Disorder

1. Recurrent episodes of binge eating. An episode of binge eating is characterized by both of the following:

   - Eating, in a discrete period of time (e.g., within any 2-hour period), an amount of food that is definitely larger than what most people would eat in a similar period of time under similar circumstances.

   - A sense of lack of control over eating during the episode (e.g., a feeling that one cannot stop eating or control what or how much one is eating).

2. The binge-eating episodes are associated with three (or more) of the following:

   - Eating much more rapidly than normal.

   - Eating until feeling uncomfortably full.

   - Eating large amounts of food when not feeling physically hungry.

   - Eating alone because of feeling embarrassed by how much one is eating.

   - Feeling disgusted with oneself, depressed, or very guilty afterward.

3. Marked distress regarding binge eating is present.

4. The binge eating occurs, on average, at least once a week for 3 months.

5. The binge eating is not associated with the recurrent use of inappropriate compensatory behavior as in bulimia nervosa and does not occur exclusively during the course of bulimia nervosa or anorexia nervosa.

Source: Reprinted with permission from the *Diagnostic and Statistical Manual of Mental Disorders*, Fifth Edition (Copyright © 2013). American Psychiatric Association. All Rights Reserved.

Bulimia Nervosa

Bulimia nervosa is characterized by recurrent episodes of binge eating followed by purging (see Table 8.3; American Psychiatric Association, 2013). These episodes are typically triggered by some type of negative emotion, such as anxiety, tension, or even tiredness. During binges, bulimics rapidly consume enormous quantities of food. They typically select binge foods that are easy to swallow and vomit—fatty, sweet, high-energy foods. Bulimics then attempt to get rid of these calories, typically through vomiting or excessive exercise. This pattern of binge eating and purging occurs on a regular basis over some period of time. Bulimia is easier to hide than anorexia, in part because people with bulimia are typically normal weight. Although bulimia has a prevalence rate of approximately 1.5% in American women (0.5% in American men; Hudson et al., 2007), some surveys indicate that as many as 10% of women in college show symptoms of bulimia (Becker et al., 1999).

Bulimia can also cause a variety of medical problems, which are a result of the use of specific types of purging behaviors (e.g., vomiting and laxative use) (Comerci, 1990; Mehler, 2010; Mehler & Rylander, 2015). Frequent vomiting may cause tearing and bleeding in the esophagus, burning of the throat and mouth by stomach acids, and damage to tooth enamel. Frequent purging can also lead to deficiencies in various nutrients as well as anemia (an insufficient number of red blood cells), which both cause weakness and tiredness). An estimated 3.9% of people with bulimia die from this disorder, in part due to an increased rate of suicide (Crow et al., 2009). One study of over 10,000 adolescents and nearly 3,000 adults found that 53% of those with bulimia had thoughts about suicide (Crow, Swanson, Grange, Feig, & Merikangas, 2014).

Binge Eating Disorder

Although anorexia and bulimia are the most widely known disorders, the most common eating disorder is **binge eating disorder** (Hudson et al., 2007; Swanson, Crow, le Grange, Swendsen, & Merikangas, 2011). This disorder is characterized by repeatedly eating large quantities of food, often very quickly and to the point of discomfort, and feeling out of control during these episodes (see Table 8.3; American Psychiatric Association, 2013). People with binge eating disorder typically feel negative emotions, such as shame, distress and/or guilt, for their binge eating. An estimated 3.5% of females and 2% of males report having binge eating disorder at some point in their lives.

Not surprisingly, binge eating disorder often leads to obesity, and is prevalent in up to 30% of those seeking weight loss treatment. Binge eating can also lead to serious medical consequences. Consuming large quantities of food can cause damage to the stomach and intestines (Brownell & Fairburn, 1995) as well as hypoglycemia, which is a deficiency of sugar in the blood: following a binge of sweets, the pancreas releases excessive amounts of insulin, which drives down blood sugar levels and can leave a person feeling dizzy, tired, and depressed. Binge eating disorder may also cause disturbances to the metabolic system, which can lead to weight gain (Mitchell, 2015). Perhaps most important, more than a third of people with binge eating disorder have thoughts about suicide (Crow et al., 2014).

Subclinical Eating Disorders

Although relatively few people meet the diagnostic criteria for an eating disorder, many people, especially women, engage in some type of disordered eating. An estimated 4.4% of adolescents report having symptoms of disordered eating that do not reach clinical proportions (Swanson et al., 2011). Similarly, although relatively few people meet the diagnostic criteria for an eating disorder (only 2.9% of females and 0.01% of males), 11.5% of females and 1.8% of males ages 14 to 24 show at least some key symptoms of an eating disorder (Nagl et al., 2016). One study of college students found that 13.5% of women and 3.6% of men show some symptoms of disordered eating, such as losing substantial weight, believing they are fat when others describe them as too thin, and feeling that food dominates their life. And disordered eating occurs throughout the lifespan; an estimated 2 million adult women report using unhealthy strategies to lose weight, including fasting, vomiting, using diet pills, and taking laxatives (Biener & Heaton, 1995).

Common Features of Eating Disorders

Although the specific symptoms differ between those with anorexia, bulimia, and binge eating disorder, they also share some distinct similarities. First, people with eating disorders tend to overvalue the role of appearance and see themselves in very self-critical ways (Duarte, Ferreira, & Pinto-Gouveia, 2016). People with anorexia often believe that one must be attractive to be successful, and evaluate extremely thin women as more attractive and normal-weight women as less attractive, compared to women without anorexia (Hartmann et al., 2015; Horndasch et al., 2015). For example, one study of women with anorexia or bulimia found that when looking in a mirror, they spent more time looking at their most dissatisfying body parts than their more satisfying ones, whereas people without such a disorder show a more balanced looking pattern (Tuschen-Caffier et al., 2015).

Evidence also suggests that people with eating disorders may have difficulty understanding and regulating their emotions, and may engage in particular behaviors—such as bingeing, purging, and excessive food restriction—as a way of managing distressing emotions (Lavender et al., 2015). Specifically, people who experience stress show increases in negative affect, which in turn leads to disordered eating behaviors, including binge eating, and purging (Goldschmidt et al., 2014; Ivanova et al., 2015). In line with this view, people with binge eating disorder report a greater number of traumatic events—such as bereavement, accidents, and separation from a family member—in the six months preceding the start of their disorder than do people without this disorder, revealing more often three types of events: bereavement, separation from a family member, and accidents (Degortes et al., 2014). Lab-based research finds similar results; women who experience stress in a lab-based setting report increases in drive for thinness and bulimic symptoms (Sassaroli, Fiore, Mezzaluna, & Ruggiero, 2015).

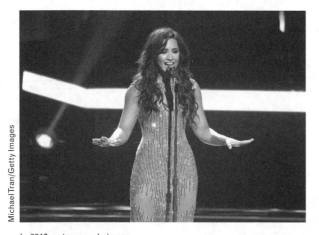

Michael Tran/Getty Images

In 2016, actress and singer Demi Lovato checked into a treatment center to get treatment for bulimia. Both her mother and grandmother had also struggled with this eating disorder.

The Role of Genetics

Biological factors may influence the likelihood of developing an eating disorder (Allison & Faith, 1997; Hewitt, 1997). First, women who have a close relative who suffers from an eating disorder are two to three times more likely to experience anorexia or bulimia than are women without this link. Second, twin studies have shown that these disorders are much more likely to appear in both twins of an identical pair than in fraternal twins. For example, one study examined rates of bulimia in over 2,000 female twins and found that genetic factors may predict bulimia in nearly 55% of cases (Kendler et al., 1991). Similarly, some evidence suggests a genetic link to binge eating disorder; people with a particular variation of a gene linked to both binge eating disorder and obesity are 20% to 30% more likely to binge-eat than people without this gene (Davis, 2015; Micali, Field, Treasure, & Evans, 2015).

People with eating disorders may have impairments in brain neurochemistry that lead to dysfunctional eating patterns. For example, bulimics are less sensitive to serotonin, which cues feelings of fullness, than people with normal eating patterns (Sunday & Halmi, 1996). So, bulimics may eat huge amounts of food because they are unable to recognize feelings of fullness as quickly as others. On the other hand, anorexics show abnormally high levels of serotonin as well as leptin (which regulates eating) (Walsh & Devlin, 1998). However, because these findings are correlational, it is not clear whether abnormal levels of serotonin produce disordered eating or perhaps are caused by disordered eating. One possibility is that these physiological changes are initially caused by irregular eating patterns, but then maintain these irregularities. For example, anorexics have low levels of leptin, which is secreted by fat cells, because they have such low levels of body fat. However, when anorexics increase how much they are eating, their leptin levels climb more quickly than their weight gain, making them feel full too early (hence less able to gain appropriate amounts of weight).

Finally, exposure to particular sex hormones during the fetal period may increase the risk of developing anorexia (Procopio & Marriott, 2007). Moreover, although the risk of developing anorexia in female twins is higher than in male twins, males with a female twin have a higher risk of developing anorexia than other males. In fact, their risk is at a level that is not statistically significantly different from that of females from such a pair. One explanation for males with a female twin's increased risk of anorexia is that some type of hormonal substance is produced during pregnancy with a female fetus that increases the risk of developing anorexia. In turn, this would explain not only the generally greater risk for females than males of developing anorexia but also the greater risk for males with a female twin.

PSYCHOSOCIAL FACTORS CONTRIBUTING TO DISORDERED EATING

LO 8.5

Explain how psychosocial factors contribute to disordered eating

Most research indicates that psychological factors are heavily involved in the acquisition of eating disorders. This section therefore examines how media images, sociocultural norms, personality, and family interactions can contribute to disordered eating.

Media Images

Think quickly—who is the most attractive female movie star? I don't know who you named, but I bet she's very thin. Virtually all media images of women in the United States, including women in movies, on television shows, in music videos, and on the covers of magazines, show very thin women—some would say even dangerously thin: Miss America contestants have body weights 13% to 19% below the expected weight for women of their height (Wiseman, Gray, Mosimann, & Ahrens, 1992), which is one criterion for diagnosing anorexia.

The thinness norm portrayed in media is actually relatively new. Marilyn Monroe, the most revered sex symbol of the 1940s and 1950s, would be considered obese by our current standards. Movie and magazine depictions of women have become consistently thinner in the past 20 years (Silverstein, Perdue, Peterson, & Kelly, 1986). For example, between 1959 and 1978, the weight of Miss America contestants and Playboy centerfolds decreased significantly (Garner, Garfinkel, Schwartz, & Thompson, 1980). Similarly, over the last 20 years, women's magazines have increased the number of articles on weight-loss techniques, presumably in an attempt to "help" women reach this increasingly thin ideal (Andersen & DiDomenico, 1992; Garner et al., 1980). However, and as described in **Research in Action**, exposure to Western media influences preference for such a thin ideal.

Not surprisingly, the presence of such thin women in the media often leads women of normal weight to feel too heavy. Nearly half of women of average weight are trying to lose weight (Biener & Heaton, 1995), as are 35% of normal-weight girls and 12% of

RESEARCH IN ACTION

The Hazards of Thin Media Images of Women

Researchers in one study compared preference for the thin ideal in people living in Nicaragua, but with different levels of access to Western media (Boothroyd et al., 2016). One group of people lived in an urban area, with full access to television; the other two groups lived in small villages, but one of these villages had regular television access and the other did not. The people living in the villages thus shared similar environmental and cultural norms but differed in their exposure to Western media. Men and women in all three groups were asked to rate the attractiveness of various images of women's bodies, which varied in terms of their body size and shape. As predicted, people living in the village with little media access rated the bodies with higher BMIs as more attractive than did those living in the village with media access and those living in the urban area. Women living in the village without media access also reported the lowest levels of dieting behavior. These findings provide strong evidence that exposure to media images of women's bodies leads to a preference for a thinner body ideal in both men and women.

underweight girls (Schreiber et al., 1996). One study of teenage girls found that the "ideal girl" was perceived to be 5 feet, 7 inches tall and 100 pounds (translating into a BMI of less than 16, which is anorexic) (Nichter & Nichter, 1991). Repeated exposure to the extremely thin ideals presented by the media may also lead some women to develop more negative attitudes about their own bodies and can trigger disordered eating behaviors, such as binge eating and vomiting, in women with anorexia (Heinberg & Thompson, 1995; White et al., 2015).

Sociocultural Norms

Given the prevalence of the thinness norm, and its clear association with femininity and attractiveness, women often believe that they must be thin in order to appeal to potential dating partners. In fact, both men and women rate thin women as more feminine and attractive than normal-weight or overweight women (Silverstein et al., 1986), and being thinner is often associated with greater success in dating (Paxton et al., 1991). For example, although the average high school girl is 5 feet, 3 inches tall and 126 pounds, girls of this height who weigh 110 pounds are twice as likely to be dating, and girls who weigh 140 pounds are only half as likely to be dating (Halpern, Udry, Campbell, & Suchindran, 1999). In turn, women often eat less in front of desirable dating partners than in front of undesirable partners in an attempt to appear attractive (Mori, Chaiken, & Pliner, 1987).

Thinness in women is associated not only with greater success in dating but also with general popularity with both men and women. Thinner girls and "average" boys (not too thin, not too heavy) are seen as more popular by their high school peers (Wang, Houshyar, & Prinstein, 2006). Similarly, high school girls who attend school with a higher percentage of female students have higher rates of eating disorders, suggesting that other girls may also influence the development of unhealthy patterns of eating and body ideals (Bould et al., 2016). Relatedly, a study of women who lived in a sorority revealed that those who engaged in more frequent bulimic behavior were more popular than those who engaged in such behavior less frequently, presumably because engaging in this behavior indicates a desire to conform to the thinness norm (Crandall, 1988).

Sociocultural norms for thinness are often communicated via social media, which can have negative consequences on how women feel about their own bodies. For example, researchers in one study examined whether the use of social media was associated with greater feelings of body dissatisfaction (Mabe, Forney, & Keel, 2014). College women were asked to rate how much time they spent on Facebook, how important receiving "likes" for their posts was, and whether they frequently compared their photos to those of their friends. As predicted, simply spending about 20 minutes on Facebook was associated with greater increases in anxiety as well as weight and shape concerns than spending time on the Internet in other ways. Women who spent more time on Facebook reported more symptoms of disordered eating.

Sadly, even girls as young as three to five show signs of adopting the thin ideal (Harriger, Calgero, Witherington, & Smith, 2010). When preschool girls were asked to select which of three body figures (one thin, one average, one fat) they would most like for their best friend, 71% chose the thin figure and only 7.3% chose the fat figure. Researchers then asked the girls to play a game of Candy Land or Chutes and Ladders and to choose which of the body figures they would like to be for the game. Once again, 69% chose the thin piece and only 11% chose the fat piece. This research suggests that this preference for the thinness norm emerges very early in life. However, and as described in **Focus on Diversity**, this preference varies as a function of culture, social class, and race/ethnicity.

FOCUS ON DIVERSITY

The Thin Ideal Is Not Universal

Although in the United States the thin ideal has taken hold, this preference is by no means universal. One large cross-cultural study revealed that less socioeconomically developed countries generally show a stronger preference for heavier figures compared to more developed countries (Swami et al., 2010). This finding is in line with that from prior research showing that in societies in which food is scarce, the ideal female body type is heavy, perhaps because women who are heavier are perceived as healthy and more fertile, and heaviness can be a sign of wealth (Anderson, Crawford, Nadeau, & Lindberg, 1992). For example, in cultures with a very reliable food supply, such as the United States, 40% of people prefer a very thin female body, whereas only 17% show such a preference in cultures with fairly low reliability of food and no cultures show such a preference in cultures with very low reliability of food. Finally, this research revealed that women in more socioeconomically developed countries have higher body dissatisfaction than those in less developed countries. Greater exposure to Western media was also associated with a stronger preference for a thinner figure, suggesting that the very thin images of women in typical Western media portrayals may in fact lead to greater adoption of the thinness norm

as well as higher levels of body dissatisfaction. In line with this view, rates of eating disorders have increased substantially in many Asian countries as Western influences, including media, industries, and technology, have spread into the Asian continent (Pike & Dunne, 2015).

Even within the United States, ethnic groups vary on how much emphasis they place on the thin ideal (Halpern et al., 1999). Adolescent girls from higher socioeconomic status backgrounds have more awareness of the thin ideal and more family/friends who are trying to lose weight (Wardle et al., 2004). They also see a lower BMI as "fat" and are more likely to use weight-control methods, such as not eating particular foods. In fact, compared to White girls and women, Blacks have a heavier ideal weight, are less preoccupied with weight and dieting, and are more satisfied with their weight (Desmond, Price, Hallinan, & Smith, 1989). Similarly, Mexican American women who are higher in acculturation, meaning orientation toward American culture, show higher rates of disordered eating than those who are oriented toward Mexican culture, as do Latino women who have lived a greater percentage of their lives in the United States (Alegria et al., 2007; Cachelin, Phinney, Schug, & Striegel-Moore, 2006).

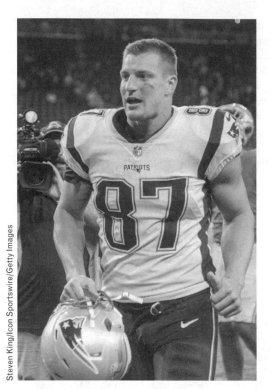

Steven King/Icon Sportswire/Getty Images

Boys and men may feel pressure to conform to the muscular male body type seen in professional athletes.

Although most research on social pressures leading to body image dissatisfaction has focused on the prevailing thin ideal for women, men may also feel pressure to conform to a similarly unrealistic body image norm (Pope, Olivardia, Gruber, & Borowiecki, 1999). However, the male ideal focuses on achieving a muscular ideal. To test the evolution of the "muscular male ideal" over time, researchers examined the measurements of the GI Joe action toy (the action toy with the longest continuous history) produced in 1973, 1975, and 1994. This review revealed a disturbing trend: the GI Joe action figure became much more muscular over time. For example, although there was no change in the height of the action figure, the biceps increased from 2.1 inches (1973) to 2.5 inches (1975) to 2.7 inches (1994). These may seem like small differences, but when translated into measurements for adult male bodies, bicep size would have increased from 12.2 inches to 16.4 inches. The latest GI Joe (the GI Joe Extreme, introduced in 1998) has biceps that translate to 26.8 inches—larger than any bodybuilder in history.

Finally, although the cultural norms in most Western societies seem to support a very thin ideal for women, these norms are not as extreme as people think. In fact, college women's ideal figure is significantly smaller than their current figure (Fallon & Rozin, 1985). In contrast, the gap between men's current and ideal figure is quite small! Women also typically believe men prefer a female figure that is thinner than men actually do. Similarly, my own research has shown that women believe other women are more supportive of the thinness norm than these women actually are (Sanderson, Darley, & Messinger, 2002). For example, women have an average BMI of 22 but believe other women have a BMI of about 20.5, and women exercise about 4 hours a week but believe other women exercise about 5.5 hours a week. Sadly, however, women who feel discrepant from the campus thinness norm—even if such a perception is inaccurate—have a greater frequency of symptoms of eating disorders, such as an extreme focus on thinness, binge eating, and purging.

Family Dynamics

Parents can influence their children's eating behaviors. First, families of women with eating disorders may also be particularly focused on weight and shape. In fact, girls who believe it is important to their parents that they are thin are more likely to be concerned about their weight and to diet than those who do not believe their parents have such preferences (Field et al., 2001). Women whose mothers are preoccupied with weight and dieting behaviors and who criticize their daughters' appearance also report more weight-loss behaviors themselves (Baker, Whisman, & Brownell, 2000; Sanftner, Crowther, Crawford, & Watts, 1996). For example, one study with 89 pairs of mothers and their teenage daughters found that girls who use extreme weight-loss methods (e.g., fasting, crash dieting, skipping meals) are very likely to have mothers who also use such methods (Benedikt, Wertheim, & Love, 1998). Although they may not be directly encouraging their daughters to engage in such behaviors, these mothers are still modeling these attitudes and behaviors. Moreover, while only 14% of the girls in this sample were overweight, 51% of the mothers reported that they encouraged their daughters to lose weight and 39% of the mothers wanted their daughters to be thinner. Mothers who are preoccupied with their own weight are more likely to restrict what their daughters eat and encourage them to lose weight, which in turn leads, over time, to daughters' restrained eating (Francis & Birch, 2005).

On the other hand, families who regularly have meals together tend to have children with lower rates of disordered eating behavior. Specifically, adolescents who report more frequent family meals (as well as making eating as a family a priority, having a positive atmosphere at family meals, and having a more structured family meal environment) are less likely to engage in extreme unhealthy weight control behaviors (Neumark-Sztainer, Wall, Story, & Fulkerson, 2004). For example, 18.1% of girls who reported eating only one or two meals as a family engaged in extreme weight control behaviors, such as vomiting, taking diet pills, and using laxatives/diuretics, compared to 8.8% of girls who reported eating three or four meals a week as a family. In fact, making family meals a priority, even given difficulties in scheduling, was the strongest predictor of rates of disordered eating behavior. The association between more frequent family meals and rates of disordered eating behaviors was stronger for girls than for boys.

The families of anorexics often have some distinct, potentially dysfunctional, dynamics (Kog & Vandereycken, 1985). They may appear normal, and even high achieving, from the outside, but family members have problems with engaging in open communication and managing conflict. Parents also tend to be overinvolved in their daughters' lives and may be demanding and controlling—they often do not encourage autonomy or assertiveness in their children. One study of anorexic patients found that they typically describe their parents as setting extremely high achievement standards and as being often disapproving (Waller & Hartley, 1994).

The families of bulimics also often show particular characteristics, including more conflict and hostility coupled with less nurturance and support within the family group (Wonderlich, Klein, & Council, 1996). Women with bulimia may binge and purge to cope with feelings of isolation and stress, in part because they are unlikely to have supportive interpersonal relationships in their families. Women with bulimia also feel less socially competent in a variety of ways, including in their ability to form close relationships and function well socially (Grisset & Norvell, 1992). They are also rated by observers as less socially effective, including being worse at problem solving, less likely to be a good friend, and less skilled in social interaction.

People with bulimia are more likely to report that their family emphasized keeping in shape and maintaining a low weight. For example, people with bulimia report higher rates of obesity in childhood and adolescence, coupled with parental disapproval of their weight, which may trigger dysfunctional eating patterns (Gonçalves, Machado, Martins, Hoek, & Machado, 2016; Machado et al., 2015).

Personality

Anorexics often have a distinct personality style—they are rigid, anxious, perfectionistic, and obsessed with order and cleanliness (Kaye, 1997). In fact, anorexics have high rates of diagnosis with obsessive-compulsive disorder. Anorexics hold themselves to particularly high standards; hence, they may seem like "the perfect child" to outside observers (Tiller, Schmidt, Ali, & Treasure, 1995). Often they have assimilated a very thin ideal. For example, when asked to judge the weight at which their own bodies and other women's bodies would change from "thin" to "normal" to "fat," anorexics give lighter weights for each of the transition points than do normal weight women, indicating that they set particularly strict standards for attractiveness (Smeets, 1999). These personality characteristics may not be simply a result of their current eating disorder, and hence a reflection of malnutrition, because recovered anorexics who are of normal weight show similar traits.

Women who have bulimia have quite a different set of personality characteristics than those who develop anorexia. Bulimics are often depressed and anxious, leading some researchers to believe that they use food as a way of comforting themselves. Bulimics have often struggled with weight issues for some time and may have a history of binge eating, weight fluctuation, and frequent exercise or dieting (Kendler et al., 1991). Bulimics may lack a clear sense of self-identity or have very negative self-views (Humphrey, 1986, 1988). While anorexia involves extreme levels of control, bulimics typically report feeling out of control while they are binge eating, resulting in guilt and self-contempt following such episodes. Two studies suggest that 20% to 33% of bulimics who are in treatment have made at least one serious suicide attempt (Garfinkel & Garner, 1984). Women with bulimia report higher levels of other types of destructive behaviors, including alcohol use, substance abuse, and kleptomania (compulsive stealing), than women without an eating disorder (Holderness, Brooks-Gunn, & Warren, 1994). Bulimics are also more likely to have experienced sexual abuse during childhood (Wonderlich, Wilsnack, Wilsnack, & Harris, 1996).

What You'll Learn 8.5

Although binge eating disorder (BED) has only recently been identified as a distinct disorder, and thus relatively little research has examined how personality factors are associated with its development, some research suggests that people with BED have more general difficulties in controlling impulses, even those not related to food (Manasse et al., 2015). In turn, people with BED may be particularly likely to engage in unhealthy eating behaviors in response to stress. To test this hypothesis, researchers examined predictors of binge eating in a sample of female twins (Racine et al., 2015). Fourteen percent of these women reported engaging in unhealthy patterns of eating, including binge eating, overeating, or feeling a loss of control over eating. Women with these eating patterns generally were higher in impulsivity, meaning a tendency to act rashly or on a whim. They may therefore be responding to negative emotions, such as stress, by binge eating because they feel unable to manage these unpleasant feelings in a healthier way.

REDUCING DISORDERED EATING

LO 8.6

Compare different strategies for reducing disordered eating

Given the very serious, even fatal, consequences of eating disorders, reducing the rates of such disorders is essential. This section will describe efforts to prevent the development of disordered eating behaviors as well as the treatment of such disorders.

Preventing Disordered Eating

Because eating disorders are so prevalent and so problematic, some high schools and most colleges and universities have programs designed to prevent such problems by giving students knowledge about the hazards of disordered eating in the hopes that having such information will help prevent serious disorders. Unfortunately, research on the effectiveness of such programs has yielded somewhat mixed findings. For example, in one study, sixth- and seventh-grade girls were randomly assigned to receive either 18 hour-long lessons on eating disorders or their regular health class (Killen et al., 1993). The lessons included information on normal growth and development, the dangers of unhealthy dieting strategies, the influence of media images, and strategies for healthy eating and exercise. Although girls who received this intense information did have higher scores on knowledge of eating behavior than those without this program, they did not show changes in their concern about weight.

Other research even points to the potential of disordered eating prevention efforts leading to unintended negative consequences. A study by Mann and colleagues (1997) evaluated the effectiveness of an eating disorder prevention program that was presented to 788 first-year women attending Stanford University. Contrary to expectations, women who attended this program actually had more symptoms of disordered eating one month after than those who did not attend the program, perhaps because the programs inadvertently taught participants strategies for engaging in unhealthy methods of weight loss. This research suggests that eating-disorder prevention programs must be very careful to avoid causing unintended harm to participants.

Fortunately, programs that emphasize the importance of engaging in healthy eating and exercise behaviors and teach strategies for critiquing media images of women can help prevent disordered eating behaviors.

Emphasize Healthy Eating, Exercise, and Body Image

Programs focusing on healthy eating, exercise, and body image can help reduce the likelihood of developing eating disorders. Prevention programs using this approach teach participants about various factors that influence weight and help them make healthy improvements to their current eating and exercise habits (Stice, Marti, Spoor, Presnell, & Shaw, 2008). Such programs lead to decreases in body dissatisfaction and symptoms of eating disorders in high school girls and reduce participants' likelihood of developing an eating disorder as long as two to three years later. Moreover, learning skills and strategies for engaging in healthy eating and exercise may protect high school girls from becoming obese. For example, adolescent girls who participated in a healthy-weight group (which focused on eating a balanced dieting and engaging in regular exercise) showed greater decreases in bulimic symptoms at the one-year follow-up than those in the control group (Stice, Presnell, Groesz, & Shaw, 2005). In addition, girls in the control condition were more likely than girls in the healthy-weight condition to become obese over time; at the one-year follow-up, only 1.2% of girls in the healthy-weight condition had become obese compared to 11.4% of girls in the control condition. These findings suggest that participation in a healthy-weight group protects girls from the increases in weight seen in those in the control condition.

Encouragingly, the benefits of such an intervention can be realized using entirely Internet-based approaches. College women who receive Internet-based programs that provide information related to body image and healthy eating—including information on the thin ideal in the media, emotional eating, and the "freshman 15"—show lower levels of overeating and excessive exercise, increases in body satisfaction, and fewer symptoms of disordered eating (Franko et al., 2005; Winzelberg et al., 2000). These programs also lead to decreases in symptoms of disordered eating. Encouragingly, this type of Internet-based intervention is particularly effective in terms of reducing the risk of developing an eating disorders for women at high risk for developing such a disorder (Jacobi et al., 2007).

Critique Media Images

As described previously, thin images of women in the media can contribute to disordered eating. In turn, programs that help people learn to critique the thin ideal can help prevent disordered eating (Becker, Bull, Schaumberg, Cauble, & Franco, 2008; Stice, Chase, Stormer, & Appel, 2001; Stice, Mazotti, Weibel, & Agras, 2000; Stice, Shaw, Burton, & Wade, 2006). Many such programs are based in **cognitive dissonance theory**, which proposes that when people's thoughts are inconsistent with their behavior or two thoughts are in conflict, they experience unpleasant physiological arousal and in turn will change their behavior or thoughts to restore consistency. Women who publicly critique the dangerously thin images of women in the media may therefore change their own idealization of the thinness norm as well as unhealthy efforts to achieve this norm. Dissonance-based interventions lead to reductions in eating disorder symptoms in both college women (Stice, Rohde, Butryn, Shaw, & Marti, 2015) and high school girls (Stice, Rohde, Shaw, & Gau, 2011). In fact, findings from one study revealed that participation in such a program led to a 60% reduction in the likelihood of developing an eating disorder several years later (Stice et al., 2008).

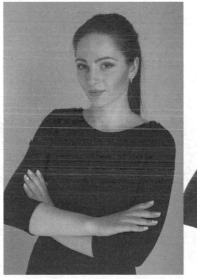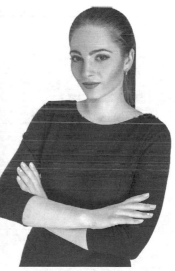

Intervention programs that help participants understand, and critique, the false images of thin women in the media, such as the airbrushed version on the left above, can help reduce body dissatisfaction as well as symptoms of disordered eating.

For example, researchers in one study assigned high school girls to one of two groups (Stice, Rohde, Gau, & Shaw, 2009). Girls in the cognitive dissonance intervention group discussed the nature, origins, and continuation of the thin ideal; wrote a letter to a younger girl discussing the costs of this ideal; and developed strategies for coping with and countering this ideal. Girls in the control condition simply received an educational brochure about negative and positive body image. Researchers then examined the impact of each condition over the next year. As predicted, findings indicated that girls in the dissonance intervention reported greater decreases in idealization of the thinness norm, body dissatisfaction, dieting, and eating disorders symptoms. Moreover, 42% of those in the dissonance intervention reported clinically significant reductions in symptoms of disordered eating a year later, compared to only 24% of those in the brochure condition. This research provides strong evidence that programs that help girls critique the thin ideal may reduce rates of disordered eating. Moreover, and as described in **Focus on Neuroscience**, participating in such an intervention changes how the brain responds to thin images of women in the media.

Dissonance-based interventions can also be effective if delivered via the Internet, which increases their ability to reach more people. However, group-based interventions are more effective than those delivered entirely on the computer (Stice, Durant, Rohde, & Shaw, 2014). For example, one recent study compared the effects of two distinct types of group-led dissonance interventions (one led by clinicians, one led by peers) to those of an Internet-delivered intervention (Stice, Rohde, Shaw, & Gau, 2017). Although women in the Internet-delivered intervention showed greater reductions in eating disorder symptoms than those in the control condition, who simply watched an educational video, they showed smaller reductions than those in either of the two group-based interventions.

Treating Disordered Eating

Although eating disorders are obviously associated with serious health consequences, people with such disorders are often very reluctant to seek treatment (Pike & Striegel-Moore, 1997). They may feel ashamed and embarrassed to admit their behavior and may believe that the

FOCUS ON NEUROSCIENCE

How Exposure to Healthy Body Images Changes the Brain

To examine the effects of dissonance-based eating disorders prevention education, researchers compared patterns of brain activation in women at risk of developing an eating disorder both before and after receiving such education (Stice, Yokum, & Waters, 2015). First, women viewed photos of both thin- and average-sized women while in an fMRI machine. Next, they were randomly assigned to receive either a standard dissonance-based eating disorders prevention program, in which they discussed the costs of pursuing the thin ideal in a group, or an educational brochure. Participants then again viewed both thin- and average-sized images of women while in an fMRI. Initial findings revealed that a part of the brain that processes rewarding experiences was activated when seeing the thin images of women, suggesting that seeing these images causes a positive neurological reaction. However, after exposure to a dissonance-based intervention, women's brains instead showed greater activation in the reward center in response to images of average-sized, healthy women than in response to those of the very thin women. These findings provide objective evidence that dissonance-based messages lead to changes in how the brain responds to thin images of women, which helps explain why such education helps reduce disordered eating.

disorder will simply go away on its own at some point. While bulimics often feel out of control, depressed, and guilty about their eating habits, and hence are motivated to get better, anorexics typically feel in control and even proud of their highly restricted eating habits and hence often resist treatment. People with anorexia may also be afraid that seeking treatment will lead them to gain weight. And in some cases, this is true—because people with anorexia often seek help (or, more often, are forced to seek help) only when they are on the verge of collapsing from starvation, tube or intravenous feeding may be used (in a hospital setting) to try to get their body weight and nutrition under control (Goldner & Birmingham, 1994).

A few approaches can help in treating eating disorders, including cognitive-behavioral therapy, family-based therapy, and drug therapy.

Cognitive-Behavioral Therapy

Cognitive-behavioral therapy may be effective in treating both anorexia and bulimia (Accurso et al., 2016; Knott, Woodward, Hoefkens, & Limbert, 2015; Walsh & Devlin, 1998). This type of therapy focuses on normalizing patients' eating patterns (by encouraging slow eating, regular meals), expanding their food choices (by eliminating "forbidden" foods), and changing their thoughts and attitudes about eating, food, and their bodies (by trying to avoid linking self-esteem with weight). Techniques can include monitoring the thoughts, feelings, and circumstances that lead to binge eating and purging and clarifying distorted views of eating, weight, and body shape. For example, therapists may use cognitive-behavioral therapy to attempt to change faulty beliefs, such as "If I gain one pound, I'll gain a hundred," and "Any sweet is instantly converted into fat." They teach patients that media images of women are often illusions (e.g., models often have their body flaws airbrushed away) as a way of helping them develop more realistic body ideals. Cognitive-behavioral therapy for bulimia is especially effective when coupled with antidepressant drugs, such as Prozac.

Cognitive-behavioral therapy is typically more effective than therapeutic approaches that simply provide listening and support. For example, researchers in one study compared the effectiveness on bulimia of two types of therapy (Garner, Rockert, & Davis, 1993). Sixty bulimic women, ages 18 to 35 years, were randomly assigned to receive either cognitive-behavior or supportive-expressive therapy over 18 weeks, with one 45- to 60-minute session each week. The cognitive-behavior therapy consisted of self-monitoring of food intake, vomiting, and binge eating, as well as monitoring feelings and thoughts surrounding eating. Supportive-expressive therapy, which views eating disorders as a symptom of larger problems, had therapists listen to and help clients identify feelings. Both treatments were equally effective in decreasing the frequency of binge eating, but cognitive-behavior therapy was somewhat better in decreasing the frequency of vomiting (82% reduction versus 64% reduction). Although women in both groups gained some weight, those in the cognitive-behavior therapy group gained more weight (6.6 pounds versus 3.0 pounds respectively). Finally, clients who received the cognitive-behavior therapy also had lower rates of depression, higher rates of self-esteem, and greater satisfaction with their therapy than those in the supportive-expressive therapy.

Family-Based Therapy

Because family interaction patterns are thought to influence the development of disordered eating, many therapists recommend some combination of individual and family therapy in treating eating disorders (Becker et al., 1999; Chen et al., 2016; Goldstein et al., 2016; Murray et al., 2015). People with eating disorders need help changing their social environment in order to fully recover from their unhealthy patterns, and having support and empathy from family members is particularly useful (Garner, Garfinkel, & Bemis, 1982).

Family therapy is therefore generally more effective than other forms of therapy in treating adolescents with eating disorders. For example, researchers in one study compared family-based treatment for adolescents with bulimia to supportive psychotherapy (le Grange, Crosby, Rathouz, & Leventhal, 2007). Family-based therapy focuses on giving parents power to stop unhealthy binging and purging behavior, to see the disorder as separate from their child, and to address how bulimia affects their child's development. Supportive psychotherapy, in contrast, focuses on helping adolescents resolve underlying problems that may contribute to the eating disorder and to think about how these problems affect them and what they can do about them in the future. Participants in each condition received 20 therapy sessions over six months of treatment. At the end of treatment, 39% of those in family therapy had stopped engaging in disordered eating behaviors, compared to only 18% of those receiving supportive therapy. These effects were generally maintained as long as six months after treatment, with 29% of those receiving family-based therapy showing a reduction in symptoms of bulimia compared to only 10% of those receiving supportive therapy. These findings suggest that family-based therapy may be particularly beneficial for adolescents with bulimia. Similarly, and as shown in Figure 8.4, family-based therapy is more effective at reducing symptoms of disordered eating than cognitive-behavioral therapy for adolescents with bulimia.

Other Therapeutic Approaches

Interpersonal therapy, which focuses on the interpersonal sources of stress that lead to disordered eating, can also be effective (Agras, 1993). This type of therapy can help disordered eaters identify interpersonal problems that cause stress, such as an obsession with perfectionism (in the case of anorexics) and negative self-image (in the case of bulimics).

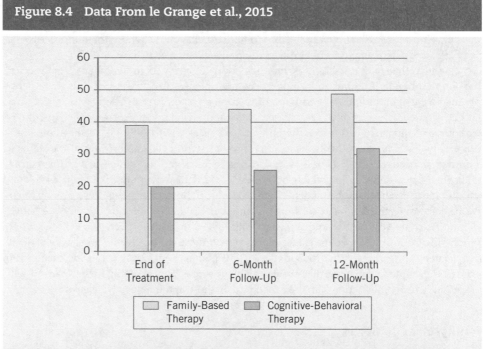

Figure 8.4 Data From le Grange et al., 2015

Researchers in this study compared the effectiveness of family-based and cognitive-behavioral therapy at eliminating binge eating and purging behavior in adolescents with bulimia. As shown, family-based therapy was more effective in reducing symptoms than cognitive-behavioral therapy immediately after treatment ended as well as six months later (the difference between the two groups at the 12-month follow-up was not statistically significant).

Source: Data from le Grange, Lock, Agras, Bryson, & Jo (2015).

People with eating disorders may also benefit from therapy that focuses on acceptance and managing emotions (Rowsell, MacDonald, & Carter, 2016). Emotion-acceptance behavior therapy (EABT) combines standard behavioral interventions for treating disordered eating with specific strategies to increase emotion awareness, decrease emotion avoidance, and encourage resumption of valued activities and relationships outside the eating disorder (Wildes, Marcus, Cheng, McCabe, & Gaskill, 2014). This approach is associated with significant improvements in weight, disordered eating symptoms, and emotion avoidance that were maintained over the six-month follow-up. Group therapy that focuses on managing the problematic emotions associated with disordered eating behaviors is also effective in reducing the frequency of binge episodes, improvements in mood, and improvements in emotion regulation and self-efficacy, as well as lower weight in obese patients (Compare & Tasca, 2014; Wnuk, Greenberg, & Dolhanty, 2014). Emotion-focused therapy is also associated with greater weight decline in obese patients with binge eating disorder.

Drug Therapy

Recent evidence suggests drug treatment may help in treating disordered eating, including binge eating disorder (Guerdjikova, Mori, Casuto, & McElroy, 2016; McElroy et al., 2016). Medication can also be useful in treating binge eating disorder, but only if used in combination with psychotherapy (Grilo, Reas, & Mitchell, 2016).

Conclusions

As described in this section, a number of different therapeutic approaches, including group therapy, can be effective for treating disorders eating, and such treatment is especially effective when the patient feels connected to the therapist (Accurso et al., 2015; Polnay, James, Hodges, Murray, Munro, & Lawrie, 2014). Outpatient therapy can help reduce symptoms, and may be particularly likely to be successful when such disorders are diagnosed at an earlier stage (Freudenberg et al., 2015; Toulany et al., 2015). In fact, one analysis comparing the effectiveness of different types of treatment (inpatient, outpatient, etc.) for anorexia revealed no difference (Madden, Hay, & Touyz, 2015).

Unfortunately, recovering from eating disorders is often a long process and may involve repeated treatment; patients and their families should not expect instant results. Many anorexics continue to be underweight and may require repeat hospitalizations, and about one third of bulimics who have fully recovered experience a relapse within two years (Olmsted, Kaplan, & Rockert, 1994). However, and encouragingly, about two thirds of women with anorexia or bulimia will eventually recover from their disorder (Eddy et al., 2016).

Table 8.4 Information YOU Can Use

- If you want to lose weight, develop short-term goals for changing what you eat and increasing physical activity—and make sure to monitor your progress and reward yourself for small successes.

- Simple strategies can help people lose weight and maintain that weight loss. If you are trying to lose weight, try cooking meals at home instead of eating out, keeping healthy foods around for snacking, and engaging in regular exercise.

(Continued)

Table 8.4 (Continued)

- Make sure to model healthy eating and exercise behavior for your children. Children form their initial attitudes toward eating and exercise from watching their parents, and these early attitudes and habits have a lasting influence.

- Don't be fooled by the very thin images of women in the media—most women are much heavier than the models and actresses portrayed in magazines, television, and movies. Moreover, many of the images of women seen in the media are altered in some way so that even these photos aren't portraying accurate information about women's body shape and size.

- Eating disorders can have very serious short- and long-term consequences, yet many people who suffer from such disorders don't get help. If you, or someone you know, has an eating disorder, talk to someone you know—a parent, a professor, a counselor—to get advice on how to seek help.

SUMMARY

Understanding Obesity

- Although historically researchers relied on the use of tables that plot normal weight ranges for people of various heights or calculated the percentage of body fat, the most common measure of obesity today is body mass index (BMI). A BMI between 19 and 24 is considered ideal; 25 to 29 is moderately overweight; and people with indexes greater than 30 are considered obese.

- Obesity is associated with substantial consequences, including physical, psychological, and social. People who are obese are at an increased risk of developing many different types of health problems, including cancer and diabetes. In women, obesity is also linked with fertility problems and poor pregnancy outcomes. Most important, people who are overweight have higher rates of mortality and are particularly at risk of dying from cardiovascular disease. Obese people also suffer negative social and psychological consequences.

- Genetic factors clearly play a role in obesity; they are estimated to predict about 40% to 70% of the variation in BMI. Genes may influence how much—and even what—people want to eat. Genes may also influence metabolism, the rate the body uses energy to carry out basic physiological processes, such as respiration, digestion, and blood pressure.

Psychosocial Factors Contributing to Obesity

- One of the earliest hypotheses about why and when people eat is the internal-external hypothesis, which proposes that people often fail to listen to their internal cues for eating (namely, hunger), and instead pay attention to external cues, such as food taste, smell, and variety. According to restraint theory, people are generally motivated to eat as a function of internal physiological signals that cue hunger. However, when people are trying to lose weight—either because they are obese or because they are dieting—they deliberately ignore these internal signals and instead use cognitive rules to limit their caloric intake. This approach can be successful in helping people restrict their eating, but it can also backfire and lead to overeating. Considerable research indicates that people may eat to influence how they feel, that is, for mood regulation. People eat more when they experience negative affect (e.g., bored, angry, sad, stressed), presumably in an attempt to make themselves feel better.

- Situational factors influence not only how much we eat but also what we eat. People eat more when they are with other people than when they are alone, and are particularly likely to eat more when eating with family and friends. Even subtle environmental factors, such as the size of the dish food is served on and the brightness of the room, influence how much we eat. Cultural factors such as the availability and amount of food may also contribute to obesity

Reducing Obesity

- Preventing obesity must begin in childhood because obese children are very likely to become obese adults. A number of different strategies can help prevent obesity in children, including avoiding using food as a reward, limiting television, encouraging physical activity, and helping children get adequate sleep.

- Various strategies can help overweight and obese people lose weight. These include setting short-term goals, creating rewards, monitoring behavior, making small changes, and getting social support. Larger-scale societal changes can also play a role in treating obesity. In extreme cases, drugs and surgical techniques may be used.

Understanding Disordered Eating

- The three most common types of eating disorders are anorexia nervosa, bulimia nervosa, and binge eating disorder. Anorexia nervosa involves a drastic reduction in a person's food intake and an intentional loss of weight (which eventually leads to amenorrhea), an intense focus on achieving and maintaining a very thin body size, and an excessive fear of gaining weight. Bulimia nervosa is characterized by recurrent episodes of binge eating followed by purging. These episodes are typically triggered by some type of negative emotion, such as anxiety, tension, or even tiredness. Binge eating disorder is characterized by repeatedly eating large quantities of food, often very quickly and to the point of discomfort, and feeling out of control during these episodes. All three types of disordered eating are associated with serious medical consequences.

- Biological factors may influence the likelihood of developing an eating disorder. These factors include particular genes, impairments in brain neurochemistry that lead to dysfunctional eating patterns, and/or exposure to particular sex hormones during the fetal period.

Psychosocial Factors Contributing to Disordered Eating

- Virtually all media images of women in the United States show very thin women. Not surprisingly, the presence of such thin women in the media often leads women of normal weight to feel too heavy, and can thus trigger disordered eating behavior.

- Given the prevalence of the thinness norm and its clear association with femininity and attractiveness, women often believe that they must be thin in order to appeal to potential dating partners. Thinness in women is associated not only with greater success in dating but also with general popularity with both men and women.

- Parents influence their children's eating behaviors in a number of ways, such as by placing a strong emphasis on physical appearance. The families of anorexics often set high standards but have problems with engaging in open communication and managing conflict. The families of bulimics tend to show more conflict and hostility as well as less nurturance and support.

- Anorexics often have a distinct personality style—they are rigid, anxious, perfectionistic, and obsessed with order and cleanliness, and may seem like "the perfect child" to others. People with bulimia are often depressed and anxious, struggle with weight issues, and engage in other types of destructive behaviors. Some research suggests that people with binge eating disorder have more general difficulties in controlling impulses.

Reducing Disordered Eating

- Research on the effectiveness of programs to prevent disordered eating has yielded somewhat mixed findings, in part because some evidence suggests such programs may even lead to unintended negative consequences. However, programs focusing on healthy eating, exercise, and body image can help reduce the likelihood of developing eating disorders. Furthermore, programs that help people learn to critique the thin ideal can help prevent disordered eating.

- A number of different approaches may be used for treating eating disorders. Cognitive-behavioral therapy focuses on normalizing patients' eating patterns, expanding their food choices, and changing their thoughts and attitudes about eating, food, and their bodies. Because family interaction patterns are thought to influence the development of disordered eating, many therapists recommend some combination of individual and family therapy in treating eating disorders, and such approaches tend to be more effective. Other therapeutic approaches, such as interpersonal therapy, emotion-acceptance behavior therapy, and drug therapy, may also be effective.

UNDERSTANDING AND MANAGING PAIN

Learning Objectives

9.1 Describe the definition, consequences, and measurement of pain and theories explaining pain

9.2 Explain the impact of psychosocial factors on pain

9.3 Summarize physical methods of managing pain

9.4 Summarize psychological methods of managing pain

9.5 Explain the impact of placebos on pain

What You'll Learn

9.1 How chronic pain can lead to substance abuse

9.2 Why marathon runners forget their pain later on

9.3 How looking at a picture of your dating partner changes your response to pain

9.4 Why simply walking can ease chronic lower back pain

9.5 Why expensive drugs are more effective than cheap drugs

Preview

Pain is, perhaps unfortunately, a relatively common part of life. We've all experienced minor pains, such as pain caused by a paper cut, headache, or back pain. Many of us have experienced—or will experience—more substantial types of pain, such as the pain caused by breaking a bone, undergoing surgery, or giving birth. In this chapter, you'll learn how psychological factors contribute to the intensity of the pain we experience, how psychological factors can help us manage pain, and how, in the case of the placebo effect, people's mere beliefs about the effectiveness of a drug or treatment can in fact reduce pain.

UNDERSTANDING PAIN

LO 9.1

Describe the definition, consequences, and measurement of pain and theories explaining pain

Pain affects more Americans than diabetes, heart disease, and cancer combined, with an estimated 126 million people (nearly 56% of all American adults) experiencing some type of pain in the last three months (Nahin, 2015). Although in some cases this pain is relatively minor, an estimated 25.3 million adults experience chronic, daily pain, and 23.4 million report experiencing a lot of pain. In fact, headache pain is one of the leading causes of visits to the emergency department (National Center for Health Statistics, 2006).

The most common types of pain are low back pain, severe headache or migraine pain, and neck pain (National Center for Health Statistics, 2006). More than 25% of American adults—meaning one in every seven Americans—report experiencing back pain in the last three months, and over 14% report experiencing a migraine or severe headache (Burch, Loder, Loder, & Smitherman, 2015).

However, demographic factors influence the experience—or at least the reporting—of pain. Pain is more common in women than men. For example, 19% of American women, but only 9% of American men, report having experienced a migraine or severe headache in the last three months (Burch et al., 2015). Women also report higher levels of jaw pain, neck pain, and low back pain than men (Plesh, Adams, & Gansky, 2011). Although there are no differences by race/ethnicity in the prevalence of headache pain, a higher percentage of Whites report experiencing low back pain, neck pain, and jaw pain compared to Blacks and Hispanics (Plesh et al., 2011).

Defining Pain

Although we all know what pain is, it can actually refer to many different sensations—a sharp pain when we step on a sliver of glass, the dull ache of a tension headache, the blistering of a sunburn, even the small but very irritating pain of a paper cut. The International Association for the Study of Pain (IASP) defines pain as "an unpleasant sensory and emotional experience associated with actual or potential tissue damage, or described in terms of such damage" (International Association for the Study of Pain, 1979).

Acute pain is intense but time-limited pain that is generally the result of tissue damage or disease, such as a broken bone, a cut or bruise, or the labor of childbirth (Turk, Meichenbaum, & Genest, 1983). This type of pain typically disappears over time (as the injury heals) and lasts less than six months. Because acute pain is intense, people suffering from it are highly motivated to seek out its causes and to treat it. Many of the pain control techniques that we discuss later in this chapter are very effective at treating acute pain.

In contrast, **chronic pain** often begins as acute pain (in response to a specific injury or disease), but does not go away after a minimum of six months (Turk et al., 1983). Lower-back pain, headaches, and the pain associated with arthritis and cancer are all examples of chronic pain. Chronic pain can be divided into several different subcategories. *Recurrent acute pain* is caused by a benign, or harmless, condition and refers to pain that is sometimes intense but that also sometimes disappears. Migraine headaches are one example of this type of pain. *Intractable-benign pain* is, as its name suggests, benign but persistent. Although it may vary in intensity, it never really disappears. Lower-back pain is a particularly common type of intractable-benign pain. Finally, *progressive pain* is pain that originates from a malignant condition; hence, it is continuous and worsens over time. The pain caused by arthritis or cancer, for example, is a type of progressive pain.

Medical care professionals distinguish between acute and chronic pain because these different types of pain often have different causes and hence need to be treated in different ways. Acute pain generally is caused by physical damage to the body, which then improves over time as body tissues, bones, and muscles heal. In contrast, most types of chronic pain are caused at least in part by behavioral factors (although this is not necessarily true, especially for progressive pain), and this type of pain lasts long after specific tissue damage has healed. This does not mean that chronic pain is "all in your head," but rather that psychological factors may contribute in some way to physical pain. Because chronic pain is extremely resistant to treatment, it lingers for some time, leading to a number of negative consequences (Melzack & Wall, 1982). People in constant pain may feel depressed and helpless, have difficulty sleeping, and experience weight loss or weight gain. Many people with chronic pain lose their jobs, lose friends, and have dysfunctional relationships with family (because they require or request constant assistance and attention and/or push people away completely).

Consequences of Pain

Chronic pain imposes serious costs on individuals' ability to function in daily life. Approximately 8.1% of people experience severe pain—most often caused by headaches—that disrupts their ability to function (Fröhlich, Jacobi, & Wittchen, 2006). An estimated 20% of Americans report that pain or physical discomfort disrupts their sleep a few nights a week or more (National Center for Health Statistics, 2006).

Chronic pain also has implications for health care utilization and employers. Chronic low back pain is the leading cause of disability in Americans under 45 years old, is the second most frequent cause of visits to doctors' offices (after the common cold), causes 12% of all sick leave, and costs $16 billion a year in direct medical costs (for surgery, disability, physician/hospital visits) (Arena & Blanchard, 1996; National Center for Health Statistics, 2006). Similarly, migraine headaches cost $6.5 billion to $17.2 billion annually in lost labor costs, with 8.3% of those who suffer from such headaches missing work and 43.6% reporting reduced effectiveness at work (Holroyd & Lipchik, 1999; Schwartz, Stewart, Simon, & Lipton, 1998). In fact, the annual cost of pain, including health care expenses, lost income, and lost productivity, is an estimated $560 billion to $635 billion a year (Gaskin & Richard, 2012). In sum, pain has major consequences for people and for society.

As described in **Chapter 6: Injury and Injury Prevention**, opioid addiction is a substantial problem in the United States. Almost 2 million Americans abuse prescription opioids each year, and 91 die every day from an opioid overdose (National Center for Health Statistics, 2016). For many of these people, substance abuse initially begins as a way to manage chronic pain, which then escalates to drug addiction. Researchers in one recent study examined the link between chronic pain and substance use, including use of any type of illegal drug (heroin, marijuana, cocaine, etc.), excessive alcohol use, or the misuse of prescription drugs (Alford et al., 2016). Of those testing positive for such substance use, 87% suffered from chronic pain, and half of these rated their pain as severe. Although only half of those using illegal drugs reported their use was to help with alleviating chronic physical pain, 79% of those drinking alcohol to excess and 81% of those misusing prescription drugs reported their intention was to help reduce physical pain. These findings illustrate the clear link between experiencing pain and engaging in substance abuse.

Although no one likes to experience pain, feeling pain is actually beneficial to long-term health and survival (Vertosick, 2000). Pain is a warning signal that your body is experiencing a problem, and it thereby motivates you to change your behavior. For example, if you touch a hot stove and burn your finger, you learn to not touch the stove again. Similarly, if you hurt your ankle, you will try to avoid putting weight on that foot, and thereby prevent further damage. People who are born with an insensitivity to pain, and who therefore experience little or no sensation of pain, often suffer numerous health problems and die at a relatively young age (Manfredi et al., 1981). Because they don't experience pain,

What You'll Learn
9.1

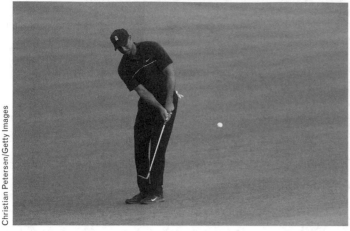

Christian Petersen/Getty Images

In June 2017, golfer Tiger Woods entered treatment to help manage his use of prescription medications for pain. Woods has undergone four knee operations as well as four back operations, and he used prescription medication during his recovery from these surgeries. For many people, addiction to such medication begins simply as a way to manage chronic pain.

they do not have the opportunity to learn from small mistakes (e.g., they never learn that falling on pavement leads to abrasions and cuts and the potential development of infection), and hence they may suffer from constant bumps, bruises, and cuts. Their inability to feel pain also means they don't seek medical care when they should, so relatively small problems can become much larger ones (e.g., they don't see a doctor when they experience severe stomach pains, and therefore could develop a ruptured appendix). Although at times you may wish you'd never experience pain, as you can see, *not* feeling pain can have many negative consequences.

Theories Explaining Pain

Although the consequences of pain are clearly substantial, for both the individual and for society, the precise mechanisms regarding how we experience pain are still not fully known. This section reviews early theories explaining pain as well as more contemporary explanations.

Early Theories

One of the earliest theories of pain was **specificity theory** (Melzack & Wall, 1982), which posits that there are specific sensory receptors for different types of sensations, such as pain, warmth, touch, and pressure. The classic description of this theory was presented by René Descartes in 1664 and compared the experience of pain to a bell-ringing mechanism in a church—a person on the ground floor of the church pulls a rope, and this tug of the rope travels up to the bell in the belfry at the top of the tower, causing the bell to ring. Similarly, according to specificity theory, once a person experiences an injury, a direct chain carries these messages of pain to the brain, which then sets off an "alarm"; hence, the person experiences pain.

Another early theory was the **pattern theory** (Melzack & Wall, 1982), which describes pain as resulting from the type of stimulation received by the nerve endings and theorizes that the key determination of pain is the intensity of the stimulation. A small stimulation of the nerve endings could be interpreted as touch, whereas a more substantial stimulation could be interpreted as pain. This theory explains why touching a warm heating pad feels pleasant but touching a very hot pan in the oven feels painful.

Although both specificity and pattern theory may have some components that are correct, current evidence suggests that both of these theories have limitations. First, people can experience pain without having tissue damage (Melzack & Wall, 1988). Phantom-limb pain, which is often experienced as a severe burning or cramping, is the experience of feeling pain in a limb that has been amputated. Because the limb is nonexistent, obviously this type of pain cannot have a purely physical basis. One study found that 72% of amputees experience pain in their phantom limb eight days after surgery, 65% have pain six months later, and 60% continue to have pain two years later. Second, people can have tissue damage and feel no pain (Fordyce, 1988). Athletes who are in the middle of a competition, for example, may experience a severe injury and yet report feeling no pain until later. In sum, lots of evidence suggests that the link between physiological stimulation and the experience of physical symptoms is indirect. Both the specificity and pattern theories fail to account for the role of psychology in the experience of pain.

Figure 9.1 Model Showing How Pain Signals Reach the Brain

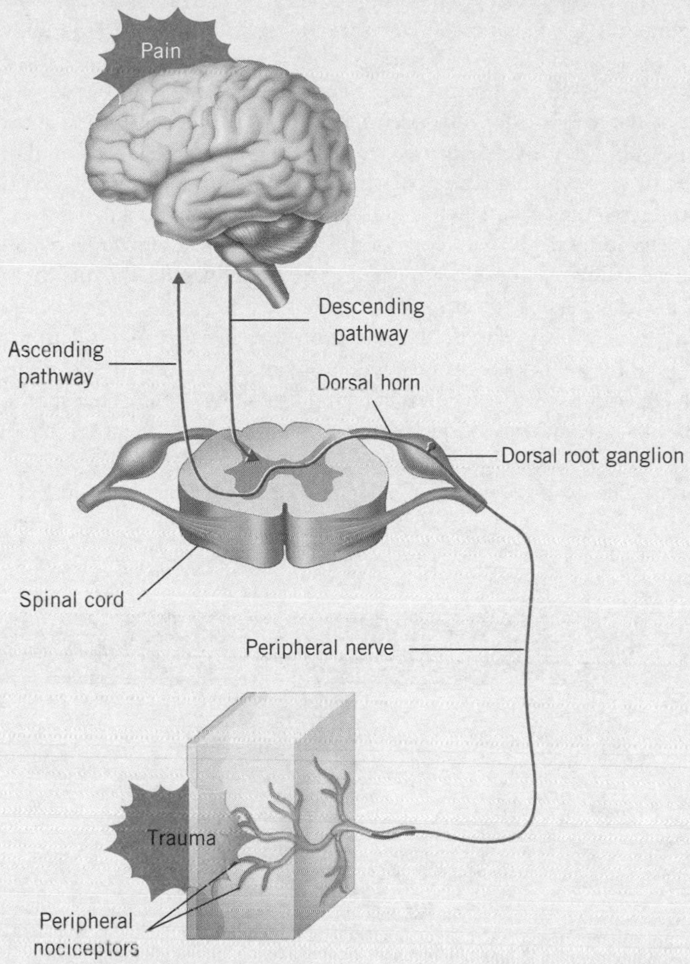

Pain

Descending pathway

Ascending pathway

Dorsal horn

Dorsal root ganglion

Spinal cord

Peripheral nerve

Trauma

Peripheral nociceptors

This figure shows how pain signals are normally transmitted by nerve fibers from the point of injury to the dorsal section of the spinal cord, and then ultimately to the brain.

Illustration: © SAGE Publishing. All Rights Reserved. Created by Body Scientific International.

Gate Control Theory of Pain

The **gate control theory** of pain, developed by Ronald Melzack and Patrick Wall (1965, 1982, 1988), attempts to correct for the limitations of prior theories by including the role of psychological factors in the experience of pain. According to this theory, when body tissues are injured, such as when you get cut or scraped, nerve endings, or *nociceptors*, in the damaged area transmit impulses to a particular part of the dorsal horn section of the spinal cord called the *substantia gelatinosa* (see Figure 9.1). Some nerve fibers, A-delta fibers, are small and myelinated (covered with a fatty substance that acts as insulation); therefore, they carry information very rapidly. These fibers transmit sharp, localized, distinct pain sensations. Other nerve fibers, C-fibers, are unmyelinated (uncoated) and transmit the sensation of diffuse, dull, or aching pain much more slowly.

Once these nerve impulses reach the substantia gelatinosa, one of two things may happen. If the sensations are sufficiently intense, the nerve impulses are sent all the way up to the brain, where they are experienced as pain—the more signals that reach the brain, the more pain the person experiences. These signals also travel to the *somatosensory cortex* of the brain, which generally allows a person to figure out exactly where on the body he or she is experiencing pain. The pain from stubbing your toe is interpreted in one part of the somatosensory cortex, whereas the pain from a paper cut on your finger is interpreted by a different area. The size of the area in the somatosensory cortex devoted to a particular region of the body determines how sensitive we are to pain experienced in that region. The area corresponding to the fingers, which are particularly sensitive, is quite large. On the other hand, the area corresponding to the back, which is not very sensitive, is quite small.

However, according to the gate control theory, not all of the pain signals carried by the nerve fibers successfully reach the brain (see Figure 9.2). Specifically, this theory posits that there is a gate in the substantia gelatinosa that either lets pain impulses travel on to the brain or blocks their progress. Any competing sensation that increases stimulation to the site of potential pain could serve to block transmission of pain sensations, or close the gate. This is why rubbing a leg cramp, scratching an itch, and putting an ice pack on a sprained ankle may all reduce pain: this type of stimulation activates the large A-beta fibers, which are responsible for modulating pain sensations by closing the gate.

The brain can also control whether the gate is open or shut by sending signals down to the spinal cord. Specifically, the *central control mechanism* influences how much information is transmitted from the brain to the spinal cord. When a person feels anxious or scared, for

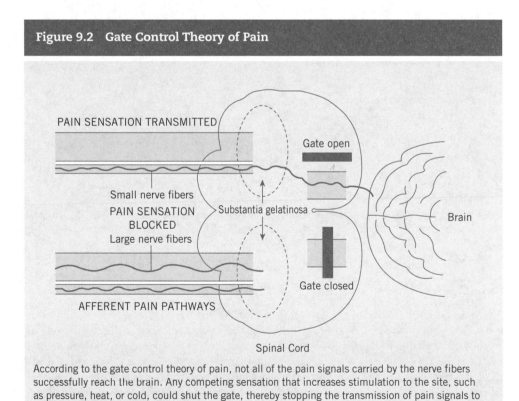

Figure 9.2   Gate Control Theory of Pain

PAIN SENSATION TRANSMITTED

Gate open

Small nerve fibers

PAIN SENSATION BLOCKED

Large nerve fibers

Substantia gelatinosa

Brain

Gate closed

AFFERENT PAIN PATHWAYS

Spinal Cord

According to the gate control theory of pain, not all of the pain signals carried by the nerve fibers successfully reach the brain. Any competing sensation that increases stimulation to the site, such as pressure, heat, or cold, could shut the gate, thereby stopping the transmission of pain signals to the brain. Psychological factors, such as distraction and relaxation, can also send messages from the brain down to the spinal cord to shut the gate.

Source: http://medical-dictionary.thefreedictionary.com/Gate+control+theory+of+pain, taken from Linton (2001).

example, the brain opens the gate and thereby increases the potential to experience pain. On the other hand, when a person is distracted or relaxed, the brain shuts the gate, thereby decreasing the potential to experience pain. This is why a person may experience something that should be very painful (e.g., an athlete who dislocates a shoulder during a game) but not consciously feel the pain immediately because the brain stopped the transmission of pain signals long enough for the person to "escape" (or at least finish the game). As we discuss later in the chapter, this is one of the explanations for the influence of hypnosis on pain relief—it may encourage the brain to close the gate.

Although the precise gating mechanism is not entirely understood, a portion of the midbrain, called the *periaqueductal gray*, seems to be involved in the experience of pain. Several studies, with both animals and humans, have shown that activating the periaqueductal gray area, such as through the use of mild electrical stimulation, can entirely block the experience of pain. For example, following electrical stimulation of this area of the brain, rats could withstand the pain of abdominal surgery without any other type of anesthetic (Reynolds, 1969).

The gate control theory clearly differs from other theories in a number of ways. First, it describes pain as caused by a physiological stimulation as well as psychological factors. Specifically, it views pain as resulting partially from a person's perception or interpretation, not simply as a physiological sensation. This theory explains why the same event can be interpreted by different people as more or less painful, and why sometimes pain is not experienced immediately. This theory also describes the person as having some control over the experience of pain. Specifically, people can take concrete steps to reduce their experience of pain, such as by distracting themselves, relaxing their muscles, or using an ice pack or heating pad. (You'll learn more about strategies for reducing pain later in this chapter.)

The Role of Neurotransmitters

Neurochemical processes are also involved in the experience of pain (Rabin, 1999). Specifically, the neurons release chemicals called *neurotransmitters* that can increase or decrease the amount of pain experienced. Some neurotransmitters, such as *substance P* and *glutamate*, excite the neurons that send messages about pain, therefore increasing the experience of pain. Other chemicals in the body, such as *bradykinin* and *prostaglandins*, are released by the body's cells when damage occurs; they, too, excite the neurons that carry information about pain as well as mobilize the body to repair the damage in a variety of ways, including causing inflammation at the site of the injury and increasing the immune system's functioning. These chemicals increase the experience of pain. Other neurotransmitters, such as *serotonin* and *endorphins*, work by slowing or blocking the transmission of any nerve impulses, which reduces the experience of pain. Endorphins, for example, bind to receptors in the periaqueductal gray area of the midbrain, dramatically reducing pain. (Although endorphins are naturally produced in our bodies, opiate drugs, such as morphine, can serve a similar function in the brain, and therefore reduce pain.)

Neuromatrix Theory

Ronald Melzack (1993) has also proposed an extension to gate control theory that places an even stronger emphasis on the influence of the brain in the perception of pain. According to his **neuromatrix theory**, a network of neurons is distributed throughout the brain, which processes the information that flows through it. Although the neuromatrix typically acts to process sensory information transmitted from the body, the neuromatrix can process experiences even in the absence of sensations. Using brain-imaging technology, researchers have learned that people who have had a limb amputated show a reorganization of how the brain processes stimulation of various body parts (Flor et al., 1995). For example, the parts of the brain that previously responded to the arm and hand may, in the case of a person who has lost that limb, now respond to facial stimulation. Moreover, the greater the reorganization, the more intense phantom limb pain is felt. This theory helps explain the phenomenon of phantom limb pain, in which the brain tells the body it is experiencing pain even in the absence of direct sensations.

Measuring Pain

In order to assess (and hopefully ease) pain, it is important to know where it is and what it feels like. Researchers use a number of different strategies to assess pain, including self-report measures, behavioral measures, and physiological measures.

Self-Report Measures

Self-report measures of pain basically ask people to describe their pain (Turk et al., 1983). The advantage of this approach is that pain has many outward behavioral manifestations, but only the person experiencing it can tell how intense the feeling really is. In some cases, professionals interview patients (and sometimes their family members) about issues related to the pain, such as when it began, the treatments they have tried, the impact it has had on the patient's professional and personal life, and how the patient typically handles it. In other cases, patients report their experience of pain by responding to a written questionnaire. For example, the West Haven–Yale Multidimensional Pain Inventory assesses the impact of pain on patients' lives, the response of others to patients' expression of pain, and the extent to which pain disrupts patients' daily lives (Kerns, Turk, & Rudy, 1985). Another type of self-report pain inventory, the McGill-Melzack Pain Questionnaire, asks people to choose various words to describe their pain, the area of the body in which they feel pain, the timing of the pain, and the intensity or strength of the pain (Melzack & Torgerson, 1971). This measure also assesses three different aspects of pain, including sensations (e.g., cramping, stabbing, aching), feelings (e.g., exhaustion, terror), and intensity (e.g., unbearable, intense, annoying).

Although self-rating scales are easy to use and at least in some cases can capture diverse types of pain, such measures clearly have limitations. First, self-report measures of pain often require fairly high levels of verbal skills (Chapman et al., 1985). Patients must have the ability to understand and make small distinctions between types of pain, such as the difference between lacerating versus cutting, pulsing versus throbbing, and scalding versus searing. Self-report measures are therefore less useful for children and people who are not fluent speakers of English (although see Figure 9.3 for a self-report measure of pain that requires few, if any, verbal skills). Moreover, people's memory for pain isn't perfect, and therefore asking people to recall pain experienced may not be so accurate—different people will recall pain at different levels (Stone, Schwartz, Broderick, & Shiffman, 2005).

Most important, people sometimes misrepresent how much pain they are feeling. In some cases, people exaggerate to get sympathy or attention (as you'll learn later in this chapter). For example, children learn quickly that expressing pain can lead to positive consequences (e.g., special adhesive strips, hugs and kisses, grape-flavored medicine). Similarly, professional athletes may express pain loudly immediately following a push or hit by another player in an effort to draw a foul or penalty. In other cases, people may attempt to downplay their experience of pain. One study found that male patients report experiencing less pain to females than they report to males (Levine & DeSimone, 1991)!

Finally, people's memory of pain may change over time, meaning that the intensity of pain they report experiencing at the time of an event may be quite different from what they report later on. For example, to test how people's memory of pain changes over time, researchers asked marathon runners to rate their pain immediately after they finished the race (Bąbel, 2016). Participants were then recontacted three or six months later and asked to again rate the pain of the marathon. Can you predict what the researchers found? People consistently forget the

**What You'll Learn
9.2**

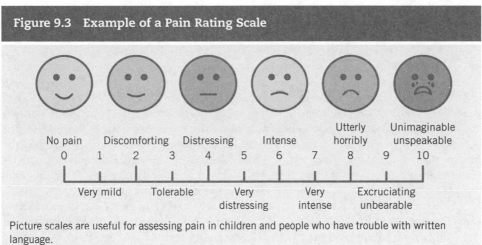

Figure 9.3 Example of a Pain Rating Scale

No pain | Discomforting | Distressing | Intense | Utterly horribly | Unimaginable unspeakable
0   1   2   3   4   5   6   7   8   9   10

Very mild | Tolerable | Very distressing | Very intense | Excruciating unbearable

Picture scales are useful for assessing pain in children and people who have trouble with written language.

Source: © iStockPhoto.com/sparkusdesign.

severity of the pain: although just after finishing the race, participants reported feeling about a 5.4 (on a scale of 1 to 11) level of pain, three months later they "remembered" feeling about a 4.2 and six months later they "remembered" feeling only about a 3.2. Similarly, and as described in **Research in Action**, women's memory of the pain of childbirth is more strongly influenced by their peak experience of pain than by the average pain they experience during labor.

Behavioral Measures

Behavioral pain measures assess the outward manifestations of pain, including physical symptoms (such as limping and rubbing), verbal expressions (such as sighing and groaning), and even facial expressions (such as grimacing and frowning; Craig, Prkachin, & Grunau, 1992;

RESEARCH IN ACTION

Why Labor Pain Is Misremembered

Researchers in one study examined how women remember the pain of childbirth, which is, for many women, one of the most painful experiences they will endure (Chajut, Caspi, Chen, Hod, & Ariely, 2014). To test this question, researchers asked women who were in labor to rate their pain every 20 minutes on a scale of 1 (meaning no pain) to 100 (meaning the worst pain imaginable). They were therefore able to calculate the peak pain women experienced, their pain at the end of labor, and the average pain they experienced throughout labor, as well as the overall duration of labor. Then, the researchers called the same women two days after the birth, and again two months after the birth, and asked them to rate their

overall labor pain. This method allowed researchers to determine how women's experience of pain during childbirth was remembered over time. Can you predict what they found? The best predictors of the pain they experienced, as reported both days and months later, were the peak pain they experienced—meaning their highest pain rating—and the end rating—meaning their final pain rating. The duration of labor, meaning how long it lasted, had no impact on their memory of the pain. These findings indicate that particularly salient moments of pain play a substantial impact on our memory of pain, whereas the length of pain—although salient to us at the moment—has little impact on how we think about that pain later on.

Keefe & Block, 1982). In some cases, these observations are made by health care workers, and in other cases they are made by people familiar with the patient. For example, nurses may ask patients recovering from surgery to perform a variety of tasks, such as touching their toes, standing up, and sitting down. As an indirect measure of pain, the nurses may then rate how easily the patient performs each of these tasks.

Generally, behavioral pain measures are accurate in assessing pain. Different people seem to be able to rate pain behaviors in fairly similar ways (Keefe & Block, 1982), such as in five general clusters: guarding (abnormally stiff or rigid movement), bracing (a stationary position in which one part of the body maintains an abnormal distribution of weight), rubbing (touching, rubbing, or holding part of the body), grimacing (facial expressions such as clenching the teeth or furrowing the brow), and sighing (deep exhalations of breath). Behavioral approaches are an especially good way of measuring pain in children, who often are unable to accurately report on their experience of pain using self-report methods.

Although behavioral measures of pain can be very useful, judging people's pain can be hard. Researchers in one study examined the reports of pain in children undergoing painful procedures, their parents, and their nurses (Rajasagaram, Taylor, Braitberg, Pearsell, & Capp, 2009). Although there were no differences between the pain reported by children and their parents, the nurses' scores were significantly lower than both the parents' and the children's scores, which may mean that children aren't receiving adequate pain medication.

Judging the amount of pain a person is experiencing is particularly difficult since people sometimes misrepresent their pain, either by pretending to feel more or less pain than they really are or by pretending to feel less pain than they really do (Block, Kremer, & Gaylor, 1980; Romano et al., 1992). People sometimes are motivated to show they are experiencing pain as a way of getting something (or getting out of something)—you might grab your knee and walk stiffly in an attempt to avoid playing a tennis match you fear you will lose. One study found that patients often report being unable to do various activities (e.g., walking, lifting, standing), but observations by unobtrusive staff revealed patients could do more than they admitted (Kremer, Block, & Gaylor, 1981). On the other hand, sometimes people go to some lengths to (falsely) show they are not feeling pain, perhaps to avoid undergoing an unpleasant medical procedure or to avoid appearing weak to others. Athletes who are eager to get back into a game, for example, may demonstrate to their coach that they are able to perform, even though this action causes them substantial pain.

Physiological Measures

Psychophysiological measures of pain are based on the assumption that the experience of pain should be associated in distinct ways with physiological responses, such as muscle tension, heart rate, and skin temperature (Nigl, 1984). Researchers have used a number of different physiological measures to determine whether pain is associated with such responses. For example, electromyography (EMG) can be used to measure muscle tension in patients with headaches and lower back pain (Chapman et al., 1985). Other researchers, under the assumption that more substantial pain is associated with higher spikes in brain waves, have used electroencephalograms (EEGs) to measure electrical activity in the brain. Still other researchers have relied on autonomic nervous system responses, including increases in heart rate, blood pressure, and respiration, as a way of quantifying the amount of pain experienced.

However, most research using these measures has failed to demonstrate a consistent relationship between physiological responses and the experience of pain (Chapman et al., 1985). For example, EMG levels are sometimes higher in patients with low back pain, but other times they are lower. People also adapt to painful stimuli over time—a person may initially show a very rapid heart rate in response to pain, but then over time, the heart rate decreases in response to the same stimulus. There is no consistent link between the experience of pain and physiological reactions; therefore, physiological measures of pain have limited use.

THE IMPACT OF PSYCHOSOCIAL FACTORS ON PAIN

LO 9.2

Explain the impact of psychosocial factors on pain

Although everyone has experienced pain, the amount of discomfort that people feel from a given injury or disease varies from person to person—one person may find that having a stomachache makes it impossible to get out of bed, whereas another person may find such pain a relatively small annoyance and continue with regular activities. In fact, people vary considerably in how much pain they can stand—some estimates are that some people can stand eight times as much pain as others (Rollman & Harris, 1987). Moreover, many pain complaints have no clear physical basis: it is estimated that up to 85% of people seeing a doctor with a complaint of back pain have no apparent physical basis for the pain (White & Gordon, 1982). This lack of physical cause suggests that psychological factors have some role in producing such pain. This section examines several theories about how psychological factors influence the expression and/or experience of pain, including stress, learning, cognition, and mood states.

Stress

As described in *Chapter 4: Understanding Stress*, stress, including the stress caused by family or marital conflict, financial pressures, and major life events, influences psychological and physical well-being in numerous ways. Pain can also be influenced by stress (Holm, Holroyd, Hursey, & Penzien, 1986; Klapow, Slater, Patterson, & Atkinson, 1995). For example, only 7% of those who experience low stress report experiencing frequent headache pain, as compared to 17% of those with moderate stress and 25% of those with high stress (Sternbach, 1986). People who experience more stress on a given day not only report increases in pain on that day but also report increases in health care use (including hospitalizations, ER visits, calls to doctors, and medication) and work absence (Gil et al., 2004). Similarly, children with recurrent abdominal pain (meaning pain that has no clear physical cause) report more daily stressors, both in and out of school, than those without such pain (Walker, Garber, Smith, Van Slyke, & Claar, 2001); they also tend to describe their daily stress as more severe and report other symptoms (e.g., headache, fatigue) more often than other children. Finally, stress can lead to the experience of pain over time. In line with this view, patients undergoing knee surgery who were under high levels of stress experienced greater pain one year later (Rosenberger, Kerns, Jokl, & Ickovics, 2009).

Work stress is also associated with the experience of pain. People who have low job satisfaction, poor relationships with coworkers, and stress at work are more likely to have chronic pain, as are those who perceive their work goals as conflicting with their nonwork goals (Karoly & Ruehlman, 1996). In fact, the level of work burnout, a response to chronic exposure to work-related stress, is the most important predictor of overall pain, as well as neck/shoulder and back pain, even when researchers take into account other measures likely to be associated with pain (Grossi, Thomtén, Fandiño-Losada, Soares, & Sundin, 2009). Although these studies are correlational, meaning burnout may not necessarily cause stress, longitudinal research provides stronger evidence that the experience of work stress leads to the development of pain over time. For example, people who experience burnout are more likely to develop musculoskeletal pain (neck, shoulder, and/or low back pain) three to five years later (Melamed, 2009). Thus, burnout seems to contribute to the development of pain in apparently otherwise healthy individuals.

How exactly does stress lead to pain? One possibility is that experiencing stress leads people to engage in behaviors, such as tensing their muscles, that in turn cause pain. For example, while my husband, Bart, was studying for the bar exam, he developed a severe pain in his jaw. After he underwent a number of medical tests (e.g., for Lyme disease and others), a physician suggested that he might be grinding his teeth at night while he slept, which would lead to jaw pain. So, Bart was experiencing real pain, but the pain was caused by a behavior, which in turn was caused by stress. Moreover, and as described in **Chapter 4: Understanding Stress**, people who experience high levels of stress may stop taking care of themselves (they may overeat or exercise less) and distance themselves from their family and friends, all of which reduces their social support and thereby increases their experience of stress and pain. Finally, stress can lead directly to physiological problems, such as dilation of arteries surrounding the brain and tension in muscles in the head, neck, and shoulders, both of which may lead to headaches (Turner & Chapman, 1982).

Learning

As described in detail in **Chapter 3: Theories of Health Behavior**, people learn health-related behaviors in part by watching those around them and also by receiving rewards and punishments for particular behaviors. These two processes also influence the experience of pain, as you'll learn about in this section.

Modeling

According to social learning theory, children learn how to respond to pain by observing how their parents and other role models act when undergoing medical procedures and responding to pain (Bandura, 1986). For example, the best predictor of children's distress while receiving their regular immunizations is how their parents respond, meaning that they are picking up cues about how painful the shots will be from watching their parents' reactions (Racine et al., 2016). Similarly, children model how their parents respond to pain, including the coping strategies they use and the behaviors they engage in and/or avoid (Stone & Wilson, 2016). In line with this view, teachers rate the children of chronic pain patients as displaying more illness-related behaviors, such as complaining and whining about pain, visiting the school nurse, and avoiding certain behaviors, than other children (Rickard, 1988).

Cross-cultural research demonstrates that we also learn appropriate norms for responding to potentially painful experiences as well as how much pain it is appropriate to express. A study of chronic pain patients revealed that Hispanics and Italians reported experiencing more pain, worry, anger, and tension about their pain and also perceived their pain as interfering more with their work (Bates, Edwards, & Anderson, 1993). In contrast, "old Americans" (meaning those whose families had lived in the United States for some time) and Polish people felt they should suppress experiences of pain and were less expressive and emotional about their pain. Cross-cultural research also shows that people in different countries vary in how much impairment low back pain causes them. Specifically, Americans report experiencing greater work and social impairment than Italians and New Zealanders, who in turn report experiencing more problems than Japanese, Mexican, and Colombian individuals (Sanders et al., 1992). These findings indicate that one's culture plays an important role in the interpretation and experience of pain.

Reward

People may also learn to experience, or at least express, pain as a way of receiving some type of secondary gain or reinforcement (Turk, 1996). In some cases, people experiencing pain are allowed to avoid doing things they really don't want to do—a type of negative reinforcement; perhaps you remember complaining of a stomachache on a morning you were supposed to take a test in school, hoping that your parents would let you stay home. In other cases, experiencing pain leads to very desirable consequences, such as attention and expressions of concern from others—a type of positive reinforcement. One study examined the amount of pain a person complained about as a function of whether the person was told his or her spouse or a hospital clerk was listening behind a one-way mirror (Block et al., 1980). Those with spouses who were generally caring and helpful complained more when they were told that their spouse was behind the mirror, whereas those with less helpful spouses complained more when they were told a clerk was behind the mirror. Similarly, children tend to show more anxiety during medical procedures when their parents are present than when their parents are not, presumably because children are more motivated to engage in behaviors, such as making noise and complaining, that will elicit their parents' attention when in their company (Gross, Stern, Levin, Dale, & Wojnilower, 1983; Shaw & Routh, 1982). In line with this view, infants whose parents reassure them during a painful medical procedure, such as by saying "It will soon be over," show more distress (Wolff et al., 2009).

Perhaps the most obvious benefit someone might receive from experiencing pain is financial, such as a disability payment. Considerable research shows that people who receive financial benefits for experiencing pain report having more pain and find pain treatments less effective (Fordyce, 1988; Rohling, Binder, & Langhin-Rich-sen-Rohling, 1995). One study reported a case in which a disabled factory worker had received $251 per week for his full-time work in a woolen mill but began receiving $257 per week while on disability (Block et al., 1980). Can you imagine his incentive to stop feeling pain? This doesn't mean that all people who are experiencing pain—or receiving some type of benefit from the experience of such pain—are simply faking it, but it does mean that at times psychological factors can influence how much pain people feel (or how much they report feeling).

People also learn to avoid certain activities based on their fear that engaging in a particular behavior will lead to pain (Turk & Flor, 1999). For example, getting a cavity filled is typically somewhat painful, whereas simply getting your teeth cleaned is not. Someone who has had a cavity filled could then develop a general fear of going to the dentist, even if he or she is not scheduled to have painful dental work done. Unfortunately, once a link between two behaviors is established (even in error), people's anxiety about experiencing pain again often leads them to avoid that activity completely—and they never learn that engaging in the activity would not cause the pain they anticipate. A study of low-back-pain patients found that 83% of them were unable to complete a series of exercises (e.g., leg lifts, bending at the waist) because of fear of pain, whereas only 5% of them were actually physically unable to complete the exercises (Council, Ahern, Follick, & Kline, 1988).

Cognition

One of the first people to demonstrate the power of cognition in the experience of pain was Dr. Henry Beecher, who treated injured soldiers during World War II. Although all of the soldiers had received surgery for severe wounds, only 49% reported experiencing "moderate" or "severe" pain, and only 32% accepted medication when it was offered (Beecher, 1959). In contrast, when Dr. Beecher later interviewed other patients in his office who had experienced similar types of surgery, 75% reported experiencing at least "moderate" pain, and 83% requested medication. According to Beecher, the cause of these differences is

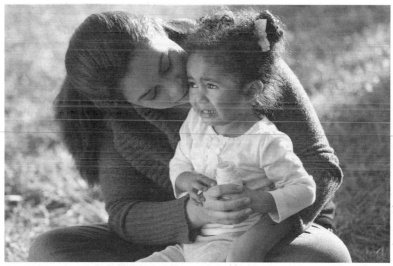

Children often show more pain when their parent is present than when they are alone or with other children, probably because parents reinforce crying with hugs, kisses, and special bandages.

© iStockphoto.com/kali9

that the soldiers most likely compared their injuries to those of others around them who were dying; hence, they felt relatively good about their state of health, whereas those in civilian life probably compared their injuries to their own and others' normal states of health and hence felt much worse than normal. Moreover, the soldiers may have also felt in some way rewarded by becoming injured, namely, getting to leave the war. The civilians, in contrast, were less likely to perceive such an obvious benefit from their surgery. This section will describe how various cognitive factors influence the experience of pain.

Cause of Pain

How people think about, or attribute the causes of, their pain has a substantial impact on the experience of pain (Keefe, Brown, Wallston, & Caldwell, 1989; Turk & Flor, 1999). Specifically, those who believe that their pain is caused by a very serious debilitating condition perceive pain as worse than those who believe the pain is caused by a more minor (and fixable) problem. For example, although chronic pain patients with cancer and chronic pain patients without cancer do not differ in self-reported pain severity, those whose pain is caused by cancer report feeling greater disability and engaging in fewer activities (Turk et al., 1998). People who blame themselves for their injury also experience more pain (Kiecolt-Glaser & Williams, 1987).

On the other hand, people who perceive a clear benefit resulting from the experience of pain perceive such pain as less intense than those without such an "upside," which may explain why people voluntarily undergo painful activities and procedures (e.g., having a navel pierced, getting a tattoo, climbing Mount Everest). They may also remember such pain later on as less intense than it actually was at the time.

Beliefs About Pain

Moreover, people's beliefs about pain, and in particular their anxiety about pain, influences how much pain they report experiencing (Marván & Cortés-Iniestra, 2001; Palermo & Drotar, 1996; Turk & Flor, 1999). Specifically, people who focus their attention on the unpleasant aspects of a procedure, who anticipate negative outcomes, and who think negative thoughts may experience or report more pain (Gil, Williams, Keefe, & Beckham, 1990; Keefe, Hauck, Egert, Rimer, & Kornguth, 1994). For example, people who are very anxious about scheduled dental procedures report experiencing more pain three months after the procedure than they actually felt (as reported by them immediately following the procedure; Kent, 1985). When we experience a physical problem (e.g., migraine, broken leg), our anticipation about its consequences may make the pain seem that much greater. In fact, the *anticipation* of pain can in some cases be worse than the pain itself.

In line with this view, people who catastrophize, meaning they ruminate about and magnify their pain yet feel helpless to manage it, tend to experience higher levels of pain. Specifically, catastrophizing is associated with greater pain intensity, use of more pain medication, and greater work disability and absenteeism (Esteve, Ramírez-Maestre, & López-Martínez, 2007; Litt, Shafer, & Napolitano, 2004; Nijs, Van de Putte, Louckx, Truijen, & De Meirleir, 2008; Severeijns, Vlaeyen, van den Hout, & Picavet, 2004). People who catastrophize also report experiencing greater pain intensity following back surgery and require more pain medication (Papaioannou et al., 2009). You can test your own tendency to catastrophize using **Table 9.1: Test Yourself**.

The use of other passive strategies, such as self-criticism—blaming oneself for the pain—and overgeneralizing—believing the pain will never end and will ruin other aspects of one's life—is also associated with experiencing higher levels of pain (Klapow et al., 1995; Mercado, Carroll, Cassidy, & Cote, 2000). For example, people who suffer from chronic headaches appraise the stressful events they experience more negatively than do controls, use less

Table 9.1 Test Yourself: How Much Do You Worry About Pain?
Please respond to the following statements using a scale of 0 (meaning not at all) to 4 (meaning all the time).
1. I keep thinking about how much it hurts.
2. I can't seem to keep it out of my mind.
3. I anxiously want the pain to go away.
4. I become afraid that the pain may get worse.
5. I wonder whether something serious may happen.
6. I think of other painful experiences.
7. I worry all the time about whether the pain will end.
8. I feel I can't stand it anymore.
9. It's awful and I feel that it overwhelms me.
These items assess people's tendency to ruminate about pain (items 1 to 3), tendency to magnify the experience of pain (items 4 to 6), and feelings of helplessness to control pain (items 7 to 9). Add up your scores on each of these three subscales to see how you typically react to pain.

Source: Sullivan, Bishop, & Pivik (1995).

effective coping strategies (avoidance and self-blame) to cope with these events, and feel less control over the event (Holm et al., 1986). In fact, studies of patients with low back pain and arthritis indicate that the use of passive strategies is a stronger predictor of pain than disease-related variables, such as severity of the disease and obesity (Flor & Turk, 1988; Keefe et al., 1987).

Ability to Cope

People's expectations about their ability to cope with pain also influence how much pain they experience (DeGood, 2000; Jensen, Karoly, & Harris, 1991; Turk & Flor, 1999). In fact, people's expected ability to cope with pain is a strong predictor of both the intensity and duration of pain (Bachiocco, Scesi, Morselli, & Carli, 1993) as well as the amount of disability caused by pain (Bunketorp, Lindh, Carlsson, & Stener-Victorin, 2006). Similarly, women's beliefs about their ability to go through childbirth without medication are a strong predictor of their success at doing so (Manning & Wright, 1983). Expectations about the ability to cope with pain may influence pain in part through their impact on the strategies people use to cope with pain. For example, children who believed they would be unable to manage their gastrointestinal pain showed passive coping—including believing that the pain was going to get worse and there was nothing they would be able to do about it—experienced more pain as well as more disability, depression, and symptoms three months later (Walker, Smith, Garber, & Claar, 2005). Similarly, people who are uncertain about the nature and cause of their illness also experience greater pain, in part because illness uncertainty leads to less effective coping with pain symptoms (Johnson, Zautra, & Davis, 2006).

Although much of the research described thus far is correlational, meaning it is impossible to determine whether cognition actually *causes* the experience of pain, experimental research provides additional evidence that people's thoughts about pain do influence the amount of pain they feel. Researchers in one study examined the impact of threatening information on coping and pain tolerance (Jackson et al., 2005). Prior to engaging in a cold pressor test, college students were randomly assigned to one of three conditions: a threat condition in which they read an orienting passage warning them about symptoms and consequences of frostbite, a reassurance condition in which they read a passage about the safety of the cold pressor test, or a control condition in which no orienting passage was read before the experimental task. Only 15.6% of participants in the threat group completed the test to its four-minute duration, compared with 55.6% in the reassurance group and 45.2% of those in the control group. Even though groups did not differ on the amount of pain they reported experiencing, threatened participants catastrophized more about the pain and reported less use of cognitive coping strategies (reinterpreting pain sensations, ignoring pain, diverting attention away from pain to other experiences, and using coping self-statements) than other respondents. In turn, the threatening information about the pain led people to use poorer coping strategies, which then influenced pain tolerance. Thus, thinking about pain as threatening in fact leads to less effective coping, which in turn reduces individuals' capacity to bear pain.

Mood State

Considerable research reveals that negative emotions, and in particular depression and anxiety, are associated with the experience of pain (Beesdo et al., 2010; Cui, Matsushima, Aso, Masuda, & Makita, 2009; Kato, Sullivan, Evengård, & Pedersen, 2006; Lee & Tsang, 2009; Sherbourne et al., 2009). First, people who are experiencing pain are more likely to report feeling anxious and/or depressed. For example, 33.7% of those in chronic pain report feeling anxious or depressed, as compared to only 10.1% of those who are not in chronic pain (Gureje, Von Korff, Simon, & Gater, 1998). Similarly, people who have chronic back pain are more likely to have an anxiety or depressive disorder (Sullivan, Reesor, Mikail, & Fisher, 1992), and people with irritable bowel syndrome (IBS), a chronically painful disease, have higher rates of major depression, panic disorder, and agoraphobia (Kato, Sullivan, Evengård, & Pedersen, 2006; Walker, Katon, Jemelka, & Roy-Byrne, 1992). People with higher levels of anxiety and depression also experience a greater intensity of pain (Mok & Lee, 2008; Rosemann, Laux, Szecsenyi, Wensing, & Grol, 2008).

Although much of this research is correlational, meaning it is impossible to tell the precise relationship between anxiety, depression, and pain, the bulk of evidence suggests that experiencing chronic pain tends to lead to depression, and not the reverse—in other words, people who live in chronic pain develop depression, anxiety, and anger (Magni, Moreschi, Rigatti-Luchini, & Merskey, 1994). For example, one study followed patients with chronic low back pain for six months following treatment at an intensive rehabilitation clinic (Barnes, Gatchel, Mayer, & Barnett, 1990). Although patients with chronic pain had higher than normal scores on several measures of psychological well-being (hypochondria, neuroticism, depression) at the start of the program, these scores decreased to normal levels following treatment, which again suggests that pain is the cause of these psychological problems, not the result. Similarly, research with chronic pain patients reveals that experiencing pain leads to increases over time in depression, anxiety, and anger (Feldman, Downey, & Schaffer-Neitz, 1999).

However, depression may lead to pain over time, which suggests that pain may lead to depression as well as the reverse. For example, a study of people undergoing dialysis revealed that those experiencing symptoms of depression at the start of treatment were more likely to report severe pain at the two-and-a-half year follow-up (Yamamoto et al., 2009). These findings suggest that the association between depression and the experience of pain probably works in both directions.

Social Support

As you may remember from *Chapter 5: Managing Stress*, people who have higher levels of social support experience a number of beneficial health outcomes, including fewer major and minor illnesses, faster recovery from illness and surgery, and longer life expectancy. It therefore isn't surprising that people with higher levels of social support experience lower levels of pain (Holm et al., 1986; Klapow et al., 1995).

How exactly do higher levels of social support lead to reduced pain? One explanation is that support partners help people use better strategies for coping with their pain. In line with this view, people with rheumatoid arthritis who are satisfied with the social support they receive use more adaptive coping mechanisms, which in turn leads to lower levels of daily pain (Holtzman, Newth, & Delongis, 2004). Similarly, chronic-pain patients who are satisfied with the social support they receive are less likely to use maladaptive coping strategies, such as complaining to others about how much pain they feel, which in turn leads to lower levels of pain (López-Martínez, Esteve-Zarazaga, & Ramírez-Maestre, 2008).

Yet another explanation is that the presence of supportive friends and family members allows people to express emotions, which helps them cope with pain. Based on prior research demonstrating the benefits of emotional disclosure for chronically ill individuals, chronic pain patients were randomly assigned to either express their anger constructively or write about their goals nonemotionally in a letter-writing format on two occasions (Graham, Lobel, Glass, & Lokshina, 2008). Participants in the anger expression group experienced greater improvement in terms of their control over pain, pain severity, and level of depression. These findings suggest that expressing anger may be helpful for chronic pain sufferers. On the other hand, people who try to suppress emotions may experience heightened pain intensity, perhaps in part because suppressing pain leads to increases in muscle tension as well as in blood pressure (Burns, Quartana, & Bruehl, 2007; Quartana, Burns, & Lofland, 2007). Over time, such attempts to repeatedly suppress the experience of pain can even lead to long-term sensitivity to chronic pain (Elfant, Burns, & Zeichner, 2008).

What You'll Learn
9.3

Interestingly, even reminders of social support can lead to reductions in pain. For example, women who hold hands with their romantic partner or simply look at a photograph of their partner report experiencing lower levels of pain during a laboratory procedure involving heat than do women who hold a stranger's hand (Master et al., 2009). In line with this view, viewing pictures of a romantic partner activates parts of the brain that are associated with the experience of reward, suggesting that this type of positive activation may have a direct influence on reducing the experience of pain in the brain (Younger, Aron, Parke, Chatterjee, & Mackey, 2010). These findings suggest that beneficial effects of social support on pain reduction may come at least in part due to the mere presence of a loved one, perhaps as a reminder of the availability of such support.

Although this section has focused on the benefits of social support from loved ones in terms of reducing pain, there are times in which people actually benefit more from receiving support from strangers. Researchers in one study randomly assigned people having minor surgery to text-message with a close friend or family member, text-message with a stranger, play a mobile phone game (for distraction), or receive a standard care control condition (Guillory, Hancock, Woodruff, & Keilman, 2015). Interestingly, while text-messaging with either a family member, friend, or stranger all led to lower levels of required pain medication than standard care, only people who text-messaged with a stranger required lower levels of pain medication than those who used distraction. In this case, texting with a friend or family member may have led to both sides sharing anxiety about the procedure, which likely is less helpful than messages from strangers that are entirely focused on supporting the patient. In line with this view, messages from strangers were more emotionally positive, and thus were likely more effective in reducing anxiety, than those from the patient's family member or friend, which were more likely to focus on the surgery itself.

PHYSICAL METHODS OF MANAGING PAIN

LO 9.3

Summarize physical methods of managing pain

Because the earliest theories of pain focused entirely on its physical causes, researchers concentrated on developing purely physical pain control techniques. Physical approaches to controlling pain include more traditional methods, such as medication and surgery, as well as more recent methods that include complementary and alternative approaches, such as acupuncture, biofeedback, and relaxation. This section reviews a number of different physical methods of controlling pain, including physical stimulation, physical therapy/exercise, medication, and surgery.

Physical Stimulation

Physical stimulation, or **counterirritation**, refers to irritating body tissue to ease pain. At first this seems counterintuitive—why, *increase* pain as a way to *reduce* it? However, as described earlier in this chapter, the gate control theory of pain suggests that increasing pain by increasing stimulation of nerves in one region is a way to get the gate to close, thereby reducing the perception of pain (Melzack & Wall, 1982). This is why you put your finger in your mouth after you burn it on a hot stove and why you grab your foot after stubbing your toe. All of the physical stimulation methods of pain control are based on this general principle.

Transcutaneous Electrical Nerve Stimulation (TENS)

The **transcutaneous electrical nerve stimulation (TENS)** technique of pain reduction involves placing electrodes on the skin and administering continuous electrical stimulation (Melzack & Wall, 1982). Patients wear a small portable unit that attaches the electrodes to the skin; the degree of stimulation can be increased or decreased depending on need. This stimulation does not hurt and typically leads to a feeling of numbness in the area, which can be effective in reducing pain for some chronic conditions, such as musculoskeletal pain and diabetic nerve pain, as well as pain during dental procedures and following surgery (Bril et al., 2011; DeSantana, Walsh, Vance, Rakel, & Sluka, 2008; Kasat et al., 2014).

However, controlled research studies now raise questions about the effectiveness of this approach. There is no clear evidence that TENS is effective at treating knee problems or back pain (Rutjes et al., 2009). These findings have led the American Academy of Neurology to recommend people not use TENS to manage chronic low back pain.

Acupuncture

Acupuncture, in which needles are inserted at specific points on the skin, is another type of physical stimulation technique that may help control pain. This technique is ancient and widely used in Asian medicine. It is based on the idea that the body's energy flows in 14 distinct channels (Richardson & Vincent, 1986; Vincent & Richardson, 1986) and a person's health is supposedly dependent on the balance of energy flowing through them. Imbalances can be corrected by inserting tiny needles into the skin and twirling them. Acupuncture is used to treat a variety of different types of pain, including pain following dental surgery, painful menstruation, tennis elbow, low back and headache pain, and carpal tunnel syndrome (Brattberg, 1983; Helms, 1987; Richardson & Vincent, 1986). Acupuncture is also an effective way of reducing children's chronic pain (Johnson et al., 2015). In some cases, acupuncture can even be effective in reducing pain during surgery (Melzack & Wall, 1982).

Massage Therapy

Massage therapy, a technique in which people receive deep-tissue manipulation by a trained therapist, has recently received considerable attention. Multiple studies point to the benefits of massage therapy in reducing the experience of pain, including the pain of childbirth, post-surgery pain, and arthritis pain (Field, 1998). In fact, chronic migraine patients who receive massage therapy report experiencing less pain and more headache-free days than those who receive medication for migraines. Massage therapy is also more effective than progressive muscle relaxation at reducing pain and increasing range of motion in people with chronic lower back pain. Massage therapy can even reduce physical discomfort and improve mood disturbances in women with breast cancer (Listing et al., 2009).

Chiropractic Therapy

Like massage therapy, **chiropractic therapy** focuses on manipulating the bones, muscles, and joints to improve body alignment. Approximately 8% of Americans visit chiropractors each year, usually with complaints of back pain (Clark, Black, Stussman, Barnes, & Nahin, 2015). Although the medical community is skeptical about the benefits of this approach, some research finds that spinal manipulation is as effective as more traditional medical treatments for back pain (Shekelle, Adams, & Chassin, 1992).

Conclusions

One important question about the use of physical stimulation methods is whether their use leads to long-term pain relief. Massage therapy, for example, is effective in reducing ongoing pain, but this approach has no long-term effectiveness once it is discontinued (Field, 1998).

The specific mechanisms that account for the effects of physical stimulation are also unclear. One possibility is that these techniques simply distract patients from their real pain. For example, people who are undergoing acupuncture may focus intensely on the feeling of the needles going into their skin and may stop concentrating on other pain. Another possibility is that their effects are largely due to patients' *beliefs* that they will work (a placebo effect) (Dowson, Lewith, & Machin, 1985). In line with this explanation, although 47% of back pain patients who received TENS did report significant improvements in functioning as well as reduced pain, these benefits were reported by 42% of those who received sham TENS (in which no actual stimulation was given; Deyo, Walsh, & Martin, 1990). Similarly, a study examining the effects of acupuncture for treating migraines revealed no differences between the acupuncture and the sham acupuncture groups (Linde et al., 2005). However, both of these interventions were more effective than the waiting list control, suggesting that some of the beneficial effects seen with acupuncture may be a reflection of people's beliefs about the effectiveness of acupuncture and not due to any specific physical properties of this treatment.

But this is not to say that the power of physical stimulation methods is simply all in the mind. For example, 53% of patients reported experiencing less pain following acupuncture as compared to only 33% of those in a placebo group (who received fake electrical nerve stimulation), which suggests that acupuncture may lead to some type of actual physical effect on the body that reduces pain (Dowson et al., 1985). As discussed later in this chapter, if people simply believe they have control over their pain, and that the pain will decrease, this can lead to physiological changes in the body, including the release of endorphins in the brain that do in fact inhibit the experience of pain (He, 1987). Relatedly, physical stimulation

© iStockphoto.com/leezsnow

An estimated 8.3% of all Americans see a practitioner for chiropractic therapy, and nearly 7% see a practitioner for massage therapy (Nahin et al., 2016). Have you ever tried one of these complementary health approaches for managing pain?

methods of pain control lead to improvements in immune functioning and stress hormones, which could in turn reduce pain (Hernandez-Reif, Field, Krasnegor, & Theakston, 2001; Rapaport, Schettler, & Bresee, 2010). Moreover, these methods also can reduce pain in animals, including monkeys and rats, indicating that their effects are not entirely due to expectations (Melzack & Wall, 1982).

Physical Therapy/Exercise

Because certain types of pain are exacerbated by weak muscles, a lack of flexibility, and muscle tension, physical therapy and exercise can help reduce and even prevent pain (Davies, Gibson, & Tester, 1979; Steffens et al., 2016). People with chronic low back pain, for example, may experience this pain because their abdominal muscles are weak and they are overusing their back muscles to compensate. Similarly, patients with arthritis who engage in regular exercise may maintain the flexibility of their joints, and surgical patients who participate in physical therapy may restore muscle strength. This increased flexibility and muscle strength can in turn decrease the experience of pain. In turn, physicians who previously prescribed bed rest for people with back pain now urge patients with back pain to become active as soon as possible. Women with fibromyalgia who receiving training in aerobic and flexibility exercise or strength training show significantly greater improvements in terms of function and reduced pain than those who receive only general information on self-help, suggesting that exercise is an important strategy for improving functioning and decreasing pain (Rooks et al., 2007).

In some cases, exercise can be as—or even more—effective than traditional methods of therapy. For example, one study of patients with lower back pain assigned some to aerobic exercise treatment, others to behavior therapy, and a third group to aerobic exercise plus behavior therapy (Turner, Clancy, McQuade, & Cardenas, 1990). Patients in the behavior therapy condition received information about the power of social reinforcement in maintaining or reducing pain, and both they and their spouses were asked to keep track of pain behaviors and to try not to reward pain complaints but instead reward pain-free behaviors. The combined group showed the greatest benefits initially, but all three treatments were effective in reducing pain at the one-year follow-up. Similarly, patients with low back pain who engage in general physical activities to improve health show reductions in back pain and improvements in mood, whereas those who focus on completing exercises specifically designed to decrease back pain experience more pain (Hurwitz, Morgenstern, & Chiao, 2005).

**What You'll Learn
9.4**

Researchers in one study compared the effectiveness of two distinct types of treatment for patients with chronic low back pain (Shnayderman & Katz-Leurer, 2013). People with chronic low back pain were randomly assigned to either a walking group, which involved walking on a treadmill at a moderate level of intensity, or a back-exercise group, which involved completing specific low back exercises. People in both conditions engaged in their designated activity twice a week for six weeks. People in both groups showed equivalent improvements on walking speed, pain, and disability, suggesting that any type of exercise may help reduce pain and improve functioning.

Medication

The most common way to control pain is with *analgesic drugs*, such as aspirin, acetaminophen, and ibuprofen, which reduce fever and inflammation at the site of wounds and work to decrease pain by interfering with the transmission of pain signals (Whipple, 1987; Winters, 1985). Analgesics are very effective in reducing mild to moderate levels of pain, such as headache and arthritis pain. *Narcotics*, such as codeine and morphine, work by binding to the opiate receptors, thereby inhibiting the transmission of pain signals (Aronoff, Wagner, &

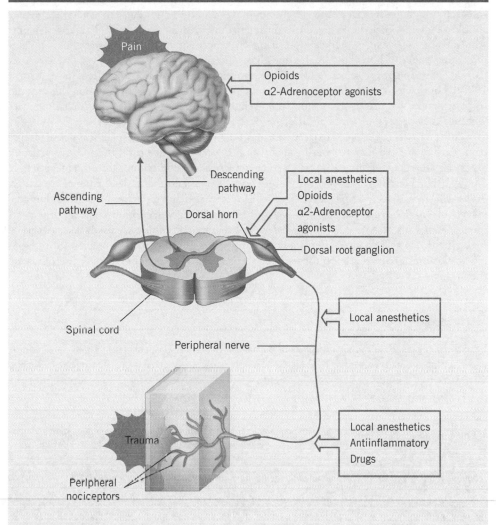

This model shows how different medications interfere with the transmission of pain signals in different ways.

Illustration: Figure reillustrated by Body Scientific International.

Spangler, 1986). These drugs are very effective in reducing severe pain. *Local anesthetics*, such as novocaine and lidocaine, can be applied directly to the site at which pain occurs; they work by blocking nerve cells in that region from generating impulses, which is why your mouth feels numb after a shot of novocaine. Other pharmacologic methods of pain control rely on blocking the transmission of pain impulses up the spinal cord. For example, during childbirth many women choose to have a spinal epidural, an injection of narcotics or local anesthetics in the spinal cord, which blocks the experience of pain from the point of injection down. As shown in Figure 9.4, different medications to control pain interfere with the transmission of pain signals in different ways.

Doctors' beliefs about the benefits of pain medication for particular patients and in particular circumstances play a substantial role in whether they prescribe such drugs. For example, for many years infant boys were circumcised without any anesthesia due to the belief that infants don't experience pain in the same way as adults (Anand & Craig, 1996). However, research now suggests that even very young infants do experience pain; hence, ethically they should be given some type of anesthesia during painful medical procedures. Moreover, infants who do not receive pain medication during circumcision show more distress during later injections than do those who receive anesthesia, presumably because early experiences with pain make people more sensitive to pain later in their lives (Taddio, Katz, Ilersich, & Koren, 1997). Physicians also tend to hold different—and erroneous—beliefs about the amount of pain people from different ethnic and racial backgrounds experience, which influences whether they prescribe pain medication, as described in **Focus on Diversity**.

Although the use of drugs to treat pain may be essential in treating specific types of intense pain, such as for patients recovering from surgery or in hospice care, the use of particular types of pain-relieving drugs can produce dependence and addiction (Dowell, Haegerich, & Chou, 2016). Health professionals therefore now recommend that unless patients are undergoing cancer treatment or palliative (end-of-life) care, patients reporting pain should first be given non-opioid drugs (such as anti-inflammatories) along with nonpharmacological treatments, such as exercise and cognitive-behavioral therapy. If opioids are used, doctors should prescribe the lowest possible effective dosage, provide only the quantity needed for the specific duration of pain, and monitor patients to make sure the benefits of such use outweigh the harms.

Surgery

In extreme cases, when other methods of pain control have failed, surgical pain control can be used to manage pain (Melzack & Wall, 1982). Surgical pain control typically involves severing or destroying the nerves that transmit pain signals, thereby reducing the perception of pain. This technique is especially common in the treatment of chronic back pain. In the United

FOCUS ON DIVERSITY

How Ethnicity Influences Physicians' Beliefs About Pain

To examine why people of color tend to receive less medication for treating pain, researchers in one study tested whether medical professionals hold different beliefs about patients' need for pain medication as a function of their race (Hoffman, Trawalter, Axt, & Oliver, 2016). Specifically, White medical students and residents read two hypothetical medical cases—a kidney stone and a leg fracture—for both a White and a Black patient, and then rated the amount of pain they thought the patients would experience and recommended pain treatments. They also measured whether people held inaccurate beliefs about biological differences between Blacks and Whites, such as that Black people's skin is thicker than White people and that Black people's nerve endings are less sensitive than White people's. Sadly, their findings revealed that half of the medical professionals believed at least one false statement about racial differences, and that people who held such false beliefs were more likely to report lower pain ratings for the Black patient than the White patient. People who held such false beliefs were also less accurate in their treatment recommendations, which helps explain why people of color may receive inadequate pain relief (Cleeland et al., 1994; Ng, Dimsdale, Shragg, & Deutsch, 1996).

States, over 100,000 laminectomies (in which pieces of a herniated disk are removed) and over 400,000 spinal fusions (in which pieces of vertebrae are fused together) are performed each year (Rajaee, Bae, Kanim, & Delamarter, 2012). Surgery is much more common in the United States than in other industrialized countries, despite cross-cultural similarities in back pain.

Surgical methods of pain control have very limited benefits, however. First, procedures can lead to other problems, including numbness, memory loss, and even paralysis in the region involved in the surgery. Even more problematic is that surgery sometimes provides only short-term pain relief: it may sever a particular pathway in the body that is transmitting pain signals, thereby initially eliminating or reducing pain, but because the nervous system can regenerate and pain messages can travel to the brain in different ways, patients may begin to experience pain again weeks or months following surgery (Melzack & Wall, 1982). Surgery should be considered a last resort when all other techniques have failed.

PSYCHOLOGICAL METHODS OF MANAGING PAIN

LO 9.4

Summarize psychological methods of managing pain

Given the considerable evidence suggesting that the experience of pain is influenced by psychological factors, as well as the limitations of some of the physical methods of pain management, researchers have also examined psychological methods of controlling pain. This section reviews several different psychological methods of managing pain, including behavioral, cognitive, and combined cognitive-behavioral.

Behavioral

Many strategies to reduce pain involve people changing their behavior in some way. Let's examine various behavioral approaches to reducing pain, including relaxation, biofeedback, and behavior therapy.

Relaxation

As its name implies, the relaxation approach to pain management works by helping people learn to relax and thereby reduce their stress, anxiety, and pain (Blanchard, Appelbaum, Guarnieri, Morrill, & Dentinger, 1987; Johnson, Crespin, Griffin, Finch, & Dusek, 2014). One relaxation method is called *progressive muscle relaxation*, in which patients focus on tensing and then releasing each part of their body (hands, shoulders, legs, etc.) one at a time (Carlson & Hoyle, 1993; Jacobson, 1938). This process helps patients distinguish states of tension from states of relaxation and therefore trains patients in ways to calm themselves in virtually any stressful situation. People who are guided through progressive muscle relaxation are able to withstand much more pain than those without such assistance (Cogan, Cogan, Waltz, & McCue, 1987). Moreover, the effects of relaxation training can be quite long-lasting (Blanchard et al., 1987).

Similarly, in the technique of **systematic desensitization**, a person is asked to describe the specific source of his or her anxiety and then to create a hierarchy of different stimuli (which cause increasing levels of arousal) associated with that anxiety (Wolpe, 1958). The therapist then asks the patient to focus on the least-anxiety-provoking image; the therapist changes the focus to a less-stressful stimulus whenever the patient experiences any anxiety during the technique. Gradually, when the patient is able to think about a low-level stimulus without feeling anxiety, the therapist continues to progressively higher-level, more-anxiety-provoking stimuli; over time, this enables people to build up their tolerance to specific stressful situations.

Another relaxation-based strategy for reducing pain is **guided imagery**, which pairs deep muscle relaxation with a specific pleasant image (Johnson et al., 2014; Menzies & Jallo, 2011; Menzies & Taylor, 2004). This approach is designed to help people relax but also to focus their mind on something other than the pain, which in turn should lead to decreases in pain (see Table 9.2). To test the effectiveness of guided imagery training, researchers randomly assigned adolescents and young adults who were undergoing spinal surgery to treat scoliosis to receive either standard care or standard care along with a DVD that provided training in relaxation and guided imagery (Charette et al., 2015). Patients who received the guided imagery training reported lower levels of pain both when discharged from the hospital and a month later. Guided imagery training also increases people's perceptions of their ability to cope with migraine pain (Ilacqua, 1994).

Biofeedback

In **biofeedback**, people are trained, using electric monitors, to monitor and change selected physiological functions, such as their heart rate, finger temperature, muscle activity, and brain wave patterns (Arena & Blanchard, 1996). How does this process work? First, a particular biological response, such as heart rate or muscle tension, is measured and the results are shown immediately to the patient. The patient is then asked to engage in different thoughts or behaviors in an attempt to influence that particular physiological response. He or she might be instructed, for example, to think relaxing thoughts or to tense his or her muscles, and then to see how these thoughts and behaviors influence his or her physiological responses. By providing constant feedback on how such thoughts and behaviors influence physiological

Table 9.2 Tension-Reducing Imagery Practice (TRIP)

1. Decide to take a mini-TRIP by stopping all other activities and thoughts. Decide where your trip will take you (e.g., the beach, the mountains, your backyard, an abstract location or experience).

2. Take a deep breath.

3. Purse your lips and slowly exhale your first deep breath through the small opening between your lips. As you slowly exhale, say the word *relax* to yourself.

4. After this first deep breath, let your jaw relax and go slack. Future deep breaths will be taken normally.

5. Relax your jaw and then allow the feeling of relaxation to travel downward from your jaw to the rest of your body. Allow the feeling of relaxation to wash like a wave over your entire body. As the wave travels down your body, make each breath you take a deep one.

6. Begin your imagery. Make the image as rich as possible by using all of your senses. For example, if you are imagining a beach, allow yourself to see the clouds, the water, the sand, and the sky. Hear the waves, the seagulls, and the wind. Feel the sand on your feet, the sea breeze on your face, and the waves wetting your ankles. Smell the ocean mist and the sweet coconut smell of suntan oil, and taste the salt on your lips. Bring this image into your mind quickly and intensely, so that your mind is highly distracted for a brief period of time.

The mini-TRIP can be a useful way of coping with pain during relatively short medical procedures, such as injections, spinal taps, and dental procedures.

Source: Williams (1996).

reactions, over time patients can learn to change their physiological responses by changing their thoughts or behavior.

Biofeedback is an effective way to control many different types of chronic pain, including headache and back pain (Compas, Haaga, Keefe, Leitenberg, & Williams, 1998; Turner & Chapman, 1982). For example, one study compared biofeedback to cognitive-behavioral therapy and medical treatment for chronic back pain and found that biofeedback was superior to the other two approaches (Flor & Birbaumer, 1993). Moreover, the effects of biofeedback can be quite long-lasting (Blanchard et al., 1987).

Although biofeedback is an effective way of decreasing various types of pain, it has a number of drawbacks limiting its usefulness. Specifically, biofeedback is time-consuming and expensive, given the necessary equipment and time to learn the technique (Roberts, 1987). Patients must have considerable practice in order to learn how to influence their physiological responses, and this requires time on the part of a technician as well as access to very expensive equipment. Moreover, while biofeedback can work to reduce pain, comparison studies suggest that it is often no better than simpler techniques, such as relaxation (Bush, Ditto, & Feuerstein, 1985); therefore, it is not widely used for managing pain.

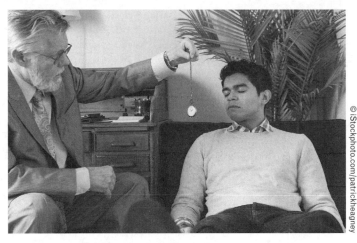

Although biofeedback teaches people how to influence their physiological responses and, thus, how to control certain types of pain, it is time-consuming and expensive, so other methods of behavioral and cognitive pain control may be more practical.

Behavior Therapy

As described previously, people who are in pain often receive certain relative benefits, such as attention from others, assistance with tasks, and avoidance of undesirable activities (Turk, 1996). Operant-conditioning approaches to the reduction of pain therefore focus on eliminating the "perks" of pain (Fordyce, Brockway, Bergman, & Spengler, 1986). This approach, developed by Wilbert Fordyce, focuses on reinforcing positive behaviors (e.g., increased activity) and ignoring negative behaviors (e.g., complaints of pain). One behavior therapy technique trains family members in how to respond to a patient's complaints of pain, namely, by ignoring reports of pain and disability. Research by Joan Romano and her colleagues (1992) demonstrated that spouses of chronic pain patients were much more likely to discourage their partners from engaging in physical tasks than those whose spouses were not chronic pain patients. For example, they were much more likely to say, "I'll do that—you rest now," and "Don't overdo it." Over time, family members are causing the patient to be dependent and may decrease patients' self-efficacy and self-esteem. Behavioral therapy programs often try to help family members understand the role they play in perpetuating pain behaviors. Behavior therapy programs also try to reduce patients' dependence on pain medication by providing drugs only at fixed intervals, as opposed to on demand, which also rewards complaints of pain. Moreover, the dose of pain medication given is gradually decreased over time without the patient knowing, so eventually he or she simply may be taking an inert substance. This approach helps reduce the patient's physical dependence on medication.

Behavioral approaches can work very well to decrease various types of chronic pain (Compas et al., 1998; Turner & Clancy, 1988). For example, one study examined chronic-pain patients who spent six to eight weeks in a hospital undergoing various types of behavior therapy (having their pain behaviors ignored, engaging in physical therapy, reducing pain-related medicines, participating in work opportunities; family members were also taught to not reinforce pain behaviors; Roberts & Reinhardt, 1980). At the end of treatment, patients were using fewer drugs, reported feeling less pain, and spent less time inactive. Another study of 148 patients with chronic back pain examined the effectiveness of an operant-conditioning program alone (they were given behavioral goals and spouses were trained to reinforce only healthy behaviors) as compared to an operant-conditioning plus cognitive coping skills program (patients received education about the role psychological factors play in the experience and management of pain) (Kole-Snijders et al., 1999). Compared to the waiting-list control condition, both operant conditioning alone and operant conditioning plus cognitive coping skills led to less negative affect, less pain behavior, and higher pain coping and pain control. Although operant-conditioning techniques can be very effective in decreasing pain, they are most effective when they are supported by cooperative family members.

Behavioral intervention may be particularly effective when combined with drug treatment. Researchers in one study examined whether a combined pharmacological and behavioral intervention improves both depression and pain in primary care patients with musculoskeletal pain as well as depression (Kroenke et al., 2009). Two hundred and fifty patients who had low back, hip, or knee pain for three months or longer and at least moderate depression severity were randomly assigned to the intervention, which included 12 weeks of antidepressants followed by 12 weeks of a pain self-management program and then six months of a continuation phase of therapy, or to usual care. At the 12-month follow-up, 37.4% of the intervention patients had substantially reduced signs of depression, compared to only 16.5% of the usual-care patients. In addition, 41.5% of the intervention patients experienced a reduction in pain compared to only 17.3% of the usual-care patients. These findings suggest that antidepressant therapy followed by a pain self-management program may be a particularly effective way to reduce both depression and pain.

Conclusions

There are several possible explanations for how behavioral techniques work to decrease pain. First, various forms of relaxation may reduce muscle tension, which can then decrease the experience of pain (for headaches, back pain, ulcers, etc.; Turner & Chapman, 1982). Second, these techniques may give people power to cope with stress, which reduces pain. As discussed earlier, people who believe they can cope with pain actually feel less pain, perhaps because this expectation leads to the use of more effective pain management strategies (DeGood, 2000; Jensen, Turner, Romano, & Karoly, 1991; Turk & Flor, 1999). In line with this view, research reveals that optimists generally cope with pain better than pessimists, at least in part because optimists generally cope with a painful stimulus by mentally disengaging from the pain (Geers, Wellman, Helfer, Fowler, & France, 2008). In sum, behavioral techniques may work to reduce pain at least in part by giving patients the expectation that their pain will decrease, which in turn can lead to physiological changes in the body that can decrease the experience of pain.

Cognitive

Cognitive methods focus on helping people understand how their thoughts and feelings influence the experience of pain as well as helping people change their reactions to and perceptions of pain and their ability to manage that pain (Fernandez, 1986). First, helping people see the consequences of maladaptive thoughts can be effective in reducing pain. For example, people may learn that feeling stress and anxiety could enhance pain; therefore, they might focus on reducing these feelings as a way of decreasing the experience of pain. Giving people specific strategies for controlling pain is another way of helping to change their thoughts about pain. Patients could, for example, focus on believing pain is manageable and having confidence in their ability to cope with it (e.g., they might think, "This really isn't so bad. I can get through this"). Finally, cognitive approaches to pain control can work by helping people think about pain in new ways, a technique called *cognitive redefinition*. For example, a woman might be trained to think about the pain of labor as her baby pushing its way into the world, which puts it in a more positive light.

Hypnosis

Hypnosis refers to an altered state of consciousness or trance state that individuals can experience under the guidance of a trained therapist (Chaves, 1994). People under hypnosis may be particularly responsive to statements made by the hypnotist. Hypnosis is thought to help decrease pain by helping people dissociate, or separate, the physical sensations their body is experiencing from their conscious awareness of these feelings (Hilgard, 1975; Hilgard & Hilgard, 1983). Alternatively, or perhaps additionally, hypnosis may change people's expectations about their ability to control pain.

Hypnosis can be effective in controlling pain, including the pain associated with dental work, childbirth pain, back pain, burn pain, headaches, and arthritis pain (Barber, 1998; Hilgard & Hilgard, 1983; Jensen & Patterson, 2014). For example, breast cancer patients who received a 15-minute hypnosis session prior to surgery reported less pain intensity, pain unpleasantness, nausea, fatigue, discomfort, and emotional upset than those who receive a session on empathic listening (Montgomery et al., 2007). Moreover, patients in the hypnosis group required less use of pain medication. Hypnosis can also effectively reduce pain during medical procedures for children and adolescents (Liossi, White, & Hatira, 2006).

Although some researchers believe very strongly in the power of hypnosis in helping people cope with pain, others believe that hypnosis does not really represent a unique approach to pain relief. Hypnosis may work to relieve pain simply because people believe it will work (e.g., the placebo effect) or because they want to please the experimenter (which is really a type of experimenter expectancy effect). In line with this view, people who are most susceptible to hypnosis may experience substantial pain relief, whereas those who are low in hypnotizability often show no benefits of hypnosis over a placebo (Miller, Barabasz, & Barabasz, 1991; Smith, Barabasz, & Barabasz, 1996; ter Kuile et al., 1994). Hypnosis may also work to decrease pain by distracting patients and helping them relax, which in turn reduces their awareness of pain. For example, one study found that there was no difference in pain reduction between people who were hypnotized and those who were not when all participants were told that they were selected because they would be highly responsive to the pain reduction treatment they would receive (Spanos & Katsanis, 1989). The power of suggestion may therefore be a more important predictor of pain relief than the power of hypnosis. Finally, still other research suggests that while hypnotic treatment can be effective in reducing pain, it is no more effective than cognitive-behavioral therapy (Edelson & Fitzpatrick, 1989; Stam, McGrath, & Brooke, 1984). Although there are reports of people undergoing cardiac surgery, cesarean sections, and appendectomies with no anesthesia other than hypnosis, these cases are considered anecdotal because they were not conducted using controlled, scientific methods. In sum, hypnosis probably works for some people better than or as well as other psychological methods of pain control, but there is little evidence that hypnosis itself has unique pain-relieving qualities and can thus be used in place of other methods of pain control.

Meditation

Meditation is a cognitive strategy that involves people relaxing their bodies and focusing their attention on a single thought, sometimes while verbalizing a single word or thought (Wallace & Benson, 1972). For example, a person experiencing chronic back pain might concentrate on and repeat a single word, such as "relax" or "breathe or "calm." Each time he or she exhales, the word is repeated. Practicing meditation is easiest in a quiet place so that unwanted stimulation is reduced. Meditation also requires a passive attitude, meaning allowing thoughts and feelings to enter the mind and then leave without making an effort to focus on such distractions in any way.

Meditation can help reduce chronic pain, such as low back pain, as well as pain during medical procedures (Carson et al., 2005; Jacob, 2016; Jensen, Day, & Miró, 2014). As shown in Figure 9.5, patients with lower back pain show more improved physical functioning and pain reduction following treatment with meditation, compared to the usual treatment condition (Cherkin et al., 2016). Similarly, patients trained to meditate showed lower levels of pain and used less pain medication than those who used traditional medical treatment (Kabat-Zinn, Lipworth, & Burney, 1985).

A relatively new type of cognitive strategy for managing pain is *mindfulness*, in which people are taught to pay conscious attention to their thoughts, emotions, and bodily sensations (Bishop et al., 2004; Kabat-Zinn, 2003). To examine how mindfulness meditation leads to reductions in pain, researchers in one study injected healthy, pain-free volunteers with either a drug called naloxone (which blocks the pain-relieving effects of opioids) or a saline placebo (Zeidan et al., 2015). Half of the people in each of these two conditions then received training in meditation for four days (20 minute a day). Researchers then exposed all participants to a painful heat (placed on a small area of the arm) in order to measure pain tolerance. People who were trained in meditation—regardless of whether they had received the naloxone—rated the heat as less painful compared to their initial ratings of that pain (at the start of the study). Specifically, participants who received naloxone rated the pain as 24% lower

Figure 9.5   Data From Cherkin et al., 2016

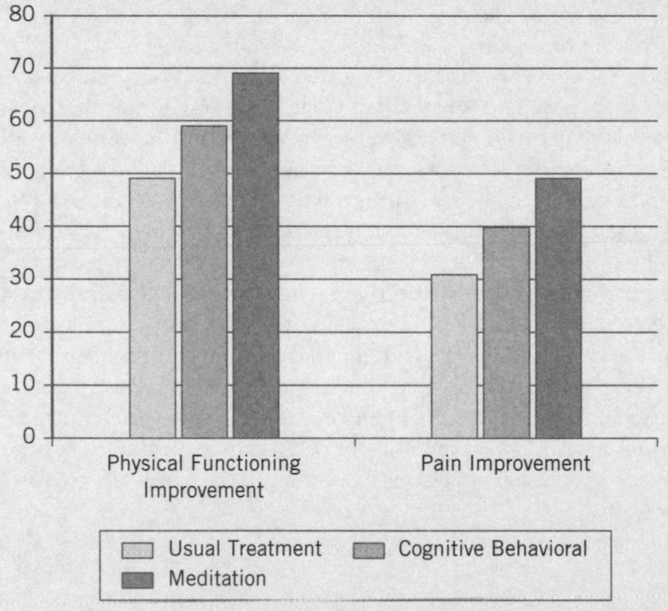

Of patients with lower back pain, a higher percentage of those treated with meditation showed improvement in both physical functioning and pain improvement at the one-year follow-up compared to the percentage of those showing improvement who received the usual care; meditation training was as effective as cognitive-behavioral therapy.

Source: Data from Cherkin, Sherman, Balderson, Cook, Anderson, Hawkes, . . . Turner (2016).

than their baseline measurement of that same pain, and those who received the placebo rated the pain as 21% lower. These findings indicate that even when the body's opioid receptors are blocked, meditation still helps people cope with painful stimuli. In contrast, people in both of the nonmeditation groups rated the pain as more intense compared to their initial ratings.

Distraction

Some techniques simply focus on trying to distract the patient to get his or her mind off the pain based on the idea that patients will not be able to concentrate on the pain because they are focusing on something else (McCaul & Marlatt, 1984). For chronic pain patients, even a simple activity such as reading a book, watching television, or listening to music can help distract them from their pain. In line with this theory, patients with persistent pain who cope by distracting themselves experience less-intense pain (Cui et al., 2009). Similarly, people who look at paintings they see as beautiful show lower ratings of pain in an experimental setting compared to those who look at paintings they find less appealing (De Tommaso, Sardaro, & Livrea, 2008). More important, real-world studies find similar results about the benefits of distraction. For example, patients who listen to music while recovering from spine surgery report lower levels of pain, and require less pain medication, than those who receive the standard care (Holc, Hirsch, Ball, & Meads, 2015; Mondanaro et al., 2017). As described in **Focus on Development**, distraction may be especially useful in helping children manage pain.

Explaining the Mechanisms

How exactly do cognitive approaches work to reduce the experience of pain? First, these approaches give people practical strategies for reducing pain. Giving women information on helpful positions they can use during labor (e.g., standing as opposed to lying down), for example, can actually help reduce the pain of labor when employed (Melzack, 1993). Second, cognitive approaches give people information about what to expect, such as the types of sensations they may experience, which can decrease anxiety and thereby help the body relax in ways that reduce pain. This may be why women who attend childbirth-training classes experience greater reductions in pain during labor than those who don't attend classes (Melzack, Taenzer, Feldman, & Kinch, 1981).

FOCUS ON DEVELOPMENT

How Music and Audiobooks Reduce Postsurgical Pain

Distraction can be an especially important technique for reducing pain in very young infants and children, who may have trouble using other methods of pain control (Cohen, 2002; Cohen, Blount, Cohen, Schaen, & Zaff, 1999). For example, researchers in one study examined whether different forms of audio distraction would help children manage pain following major surgery (Sunitha Suresh, De Oliveira, & Suresh, 2015). Children were randomly assigned to a music, audiobook, or silence (control) condition. As predicted, children in both audio groups had lower levels of pain than those in the control condition. Similarly, children who play an interactive video game are better able to withstand pain than those who simply watch a movie (a less engaging form of distraction) or receive no form of distraction (Dahlquist et al., 2007). Other forms of distraction, such as humor and small talk, can even help children with leukemia cope better during painful procedures (Blount et al., 1989).

Cognitive approaches to pain control may also work by increasing people's perceived control over the pain, which helps lessen its perceived severity (Zucker et al., 1998). Similarly, one study of patients with chronic pain who were enrolled in a pain program found that increases in perceived control over pain were associated with decreases in depression, perceived disability, and pain intensity at the 6- and 12-month follow-ups (Jensen, Turner, & Romano, 2001). Moreover, patients who received cognitive therapy to cope with irritable bowel syndrome showed no decreases in the frequency of daily hassles following the therapy but showed decreases in the distress such hassles caused them, suggesting that patients learned effective strategies for coping with these events (Payne & Blanchard, 1995). These findings suggest that changing patients' cognitions about pain can be an effective approach to changing perceived pain.

Finally, learning skills for managing pain may even lead to the release of pain-relieving endorphins. In one compelling study showing the physiological benefits of learning cognitive skills for managing pain, all participants first underwent a very painful procedure called the cold pressor test, which involves submerging one's hand in a bucket of very cold ice water for as long as a person can stand it (Bandura, O'Leary, Taylor, Gauthier, & Gossard, 1987). After completing this first test, the students were randomly assigned to one of three treatment conditions: a cognitive-coping group, a placebo pill group, and a control group. Students in the cognitive-coping group were taught different ways to think about their pain, such as thinking about something other than the pain, thinking about the pain as completely separate from their bodies, and thinking encouraging thoughts about how well they were coping with the pain. The students in the placebo group were given an inert pill that they were told would prevent and/or alleviate their pain. All students then repeated the cold pressor test to see whether their pain tolerance had increased. Findings showed, as predicted, that those who were taught cognitive coping had a much higher pain tolerance than those in the other two conditions. Specifically, students in the cognitive-coping condition showed an increase in pain tolerance of nearly 60%, whereas those in the placebo and control conditions showed only very small increases (less than 10%).

The researchers were then interested in testing exactly how training someone in cognitive-coping skills for managing pain leads to such a remarkable increase in pain tolerance. Specifically, they were interested in examining whether this type of training increases the activation of endorphins in the body, which in turn leads to the reduction of pain. To test this part of their hypothesis, the researchers gave half of the subjects in each condition an injection of a drug called naloxone, which blocks the pain-reducing effects of endorphins, and the other half of the subjects received a saline injection, which should have had no influence on the activation of endorphins. These findings showed that there was no difference in pain tolerance as a function of whether students received the naloxone or saline for those who were in the control or placebo conditions. Apparently, people in these conditions did not experience the benefits of endorphins for reducing pain, and therefore it didn't matter whether the potential effects of endorphins were blocked (in the case of those receiving the naloxone injection) or not (in the case of those receiving the saline injection). However, students in the cognitive-control condition who received saline had a much higher pain tolerance than those in this condition who received the naloxone, suggesting that participants in this condition did have higher levels of endorphins—and hence were able to withstand much more pain when these endorphins were not blocked (in the case of the saline) than when they were blocked (in the case of the naloxone). Giving someone training in cognitive techniques for controlling pain actually increases the level of endorphins in the body, which in turn reduces the feeling of pain.

Cognitive-Behavioral

The prior two sections separately described the role of behavioral and cognitive strategies for managing pain. However, many pain management programs use several techniques in combination, and, not surprisingly, including multiple approaches tends to be particularly effective (Compas et al., 1998; Flor, Fydrich, & Turk, 1992). For example, 66% of children with recurring abdominal pain who receive training in both behavioral and cognitive strategies for managing pain report no pain at the six-month follow-up compared to only 27% of those who receive standard treatment (Sanders, Shepherd, Cleghorn, & Woolford, 1994). Perhaps most important, cognitive-behavioral therapy is as effective as antidepressant medication in reducing headache activity, medication use, and headache-related disability in people who suffer from chronic tension headaches (Holroyd et al., 2001).

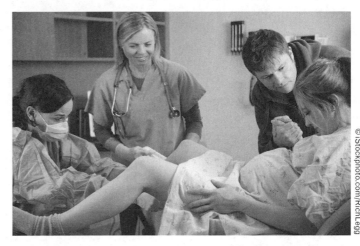

Cognitive and behavioral strategies for managing pain are routinely taught in childbirth education classes to help women withstand pain during labor.

Combined cognitive and behavioral strategies can also be effective in helping people manage relatively short-term pain. For example, childbirth education involves training in both behavioral and cognitive strategies for managing the pain of labor and childbirth (Lamaze, 1970; Melzack & Wall, 1982). This education includes information on behavioral strategies for relieving pain, including positions to try during labor, massage techniques that a partner can do to help reduce pain, and special breathing exercises. This education also includes training in distraction. For example, couples are encouraged to choose a "focal object," such as a stuffed animal, special photo, or other personally meaningful object, to concentrate on during labor, and thus help distract women from the pain. Finally, women are taught to think about pain in a new way—to think about each (incredibly painful) contraction as working to bring the baby's arrival that much closer.

THE IMPACT OF PLACEBOS ON PAIN

A **placebo** is a medicine or treatment that affects someone even though it contains no specific medical or physical properties relevant to the condition it is supposedly treating (Liberman, 1962). In this section, you'll learn about the power of the placebo effect, explanations for its influence, and factors that impact its effectiveness.

The Power of Placebos

Placebo medicines and treatments can produce very real and even lasting effects on virtually every organ system in the body and many diseases, including chest pain, arthritis, hay fever, headaches, ulcers, hypertension, postoperative pain, seasickness, and pain from the common cold (Benedetti & Amanzio, 1997). In one review involving more than 1,000 patients treated for a variety of conditions, Henry Beecher (1955) reported that an average of 35% of patients benefited from placebo treatments, with the effectiveness of placebos ranging from 15% to 58%. For example, 67% of surgical patients who receive morphine report feeling some reduction in pain; so do 42% of those given a placebo instead of the actual morphine they were told they were receiving (Beecher, 1959).

In a particularly remarkable demonstration of the power of placebos, in some cases patients have had "placebo surgery," in which they are cut open but nothing medical is done to them (Beecher, 1959; Diamond, Kittle, & Crockett, 1960). Amazingly enough,

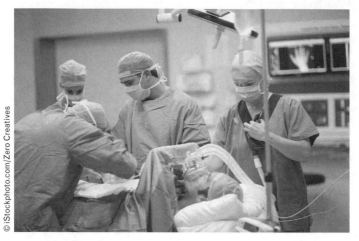

Surgery can clearly have a major impact on physical health—but is part of this effect merely caused by patients' belief in the power of surgery?

many patients show some benefits simply from having some type of surgery. For example, Leonard Cobb, a cardiologist working in Seattle in the 1950s, performed fake surgery in which surgeons made incisions in people's chests but did not tie off patients' arteries, as was typically done in surgery for angina at the time (Cobb, Thomas, Dillard, Merendino, & Bruce, 1959). However, this fake procedure was just as effective at decreasing chest pain as the actual procedure—which was quickly abandoned. Similarly, one study compared Parkinson's disease patients who simply had holes drilled in their skulls (the placebo surgery) to those who experienced a real procedure in which holes were drilled in their skulls and then fetal cells were implanted in their brain. Fetal-tissue transplantation is thought to reactivate some brain functions and thereby reverse motor problems associated with this disease. Patients who received the placebo surgery showed significant improvement in their motor functioning (although not as substantial as that shown by patients who actually received the cell implant) (Talbot, 2000).

More recent research provides additional support for the power of "placebo surgery" in both reducing pain and improving physical functioning. For example, patients with painful vertebral fractures who underwent vertebroplasty, a common treatment for such fractures, or a sham procedure both reported significant—and equivalent—reductions in pain as well as increases in physical functioning, quality of life, and perceived improvement at each follow-up assessment (Buchbinder et al., 2009). Similarly, patients with vertebral fractures who underwent either vertebroplasty or a simulated procedure reported similar improvement in disability and pain scores one month later (Kallmes et al., 2009). The improvements in pain and pain-related disability associated with vertebrate fractures in patients treated with vertebroplasty were similar to those seen for patients in a control group. In sum, this research provides powerful evidence that the placebo effect can even influence people's response to surgical procedures.

Explaining the Placebo Effect

Although the placebo effect can clearly have lasting effects on people's response to both drugs and procedures, the research described thus far hasn't revealed the specific mechanisms that explain these effects. The leading explanation is that placebos change people's behavior as well as their physiological response.

The Role of Behavior

People's beliefs about the power of a pain treatment may in turn impact their behavior (Benedetti & Amanzio, 1997). Specifically, when people are given a pain treatment they fully expect to work, they may change their behavior in ways that in turn lead to the desired reduction of pain. For example, if you have a bad headache and take an aspirin that you fully believe will alleviate the headache, you may relax because you know the pain will soon disappear; therefore, this conscious attempt to relax may lead to a decrease in your headache pain. In sum, just the belief that the treatment will work may lead to a decrease in anxiety, which may lead directly to a reduction in pain.

Similarly, patients who believe the treatment they have been given may change their behavior in ways that reduce pain. In a particularly remarkable demonstration of the power of placebos on improved functioning, patients with osteoarthritis of the knee were randomly assigned to one of three groups: standard arthroscopic surgery, a rinsing of the knee joint (but not scraped as occurs during standard surgery), or a control condition (they would simply be cut with the scalpel to create incisions and scars (Moseley et al., 2002). The patients were then assessed regularly over two years to determine whether "actual surgery" was indeed better than "placebo surgery" for reducing pain and increasing function (walking, climbing stairs, etc.). Results show that there were no differences in degree of pain or function among patients in the three groups at any point during the follow-up. Although the researchers weren't able to determine precisely what led to the equivalent improvement for men in all three conditions, one possibility is that all of the participants believed they had received surgery to improve their functioning and thereby regularly followed recovery instructions. Their behaviors, which may have included getting regular exercise to increase movement and working with a physical therapist to improve function, may in turn have led to reduced pain and improved functioning.

The Role of Physiology

Placebos may also lead to physiological changes in the body, which in turn inhibit the experience of pain (Bandura et al., 1987; Benedetti & Amanzio, 1997; Levine, Gordon, & Fields, 1978) (see Figure 9.6). Some research suggests that the endorphin system is activated when people simply believe they are receiving a painkiller, even when they are receiving a placebo (Benedetti & Amanzio, 1997). For example, researchers in one study randomly assigned dental patients to receive an injection of naloxone (which is known to reduce the effect of endorphins in providing pain relief) followed by a placebo, a placebo followed by an injection of naloxone, or simply two placebos (Levine et al., 1978). As predicted, those who got a placebo first and then naloxone reported greater pain than those who got a placebo both times, presumably because naloxone reduced the effectiveness of the endorphins (created by the placebo). Similarly, in a study with patients having their wisdom teeth removed, half were given real ultrasound therapy (known to reduce pain) during their procedure, while the others thought

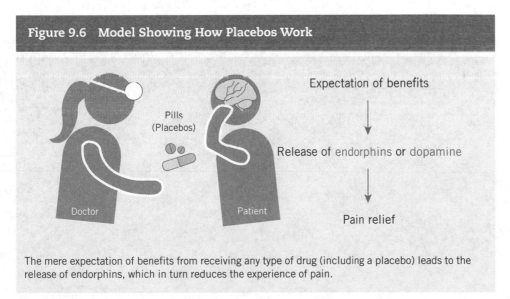

Figure 9.6 Model Showing How Placebos Work

Pills (Placebos)

Doctor   Patient

Expectation of benefits

↓

Release of endorphins or dopamine

↓

Pain relief

The mere expectation of benefits from receiving any type of drug (including a placebo) leads to the release of endorphins, which in turn reduces the experience of pain.

Source: Adapted from Pinch, B., & Choi, K. (2016, September 16). More than just a sugar pill: Why the placebo effect is real. http://sitn.hms.harvard.edu/flash/2016/just-sugar-pill-placebo-effect-real/.

they were receiving this therapy when in reality the machine was unplugged (Hashish, Hai, Harvey, Feinmann, & Harris, 1988). Patients in both cases showed a decrease in pain, jaw tightness, and swelling, indicating that all of these physical effects were caused simply by the expectation that they were receiving a pain-reducing therapy. Moreover, and as described in **Focus on Neuroscience**, placebos may influence how the brain responds to pain.

Factors Influencing the Placebo Effect

As you learned earlier in this section, the strength of the placebo effect varies in different studies. Three factors that influence the effectiveness of a placebo are the practitioner's beliefs, the patient's expectations, and environmental cues.

Practitioner's Beliefs

The behavior of the practitioner can clearly influence the effectiveness of a placebo (Fuentes et al., 2014; Gracely, Dubner, Deeter, & Wolskee, 1985; Roberts, Kewman, Mercier, & Hovell, 1993). When a placebo is administered by an enthusiastic and friendly practitioner who seems interested in and sympathetic to the patient, the placebo is more effective than when it is delivered by an angry or rejecting practitioner. For example, in one study with surgery patients, half were visited the night before their surgery by the anesthesiologist, who told them in a brusque manner that everything would be fine (Talbot, 2000). The other patients were also visited by the same anesthesiologist, who this time sat on their beds, held their hands as he talked, and was very warm and friendly. As predicted, those who saw the kind and friendly practitioner required much less pain medication and were even discharged earlier from the hospital than those who had interacted with the brusque and cold practitioner.

A practitioner's expectations about the effectiveness of the placebo can also influence responsiveness. In fact, estimates are that between 25% and 70% of the effectiveness of a placebo is due to the doctor's attitudes about the placebo. For example, patients whose doctors thought they were getting a pain-relieving drug reported feeling significantly less pain than those whose doctors thought they would receive a pain-enhancing drug—even though in reality all patients were given a placebo (Gracely et al., 1985). The placebo effect as well as

FOCUS ON NEUROSCIENCE

The Impact of Placebos on Brain Activity

Considerable evidence now suggests that taking a placebo leads to changes in brain activity, which helps explain how such expectations actually cause reductions in pain. In one study, researchers gave participants painful electric shocks to their wrists after applying either what they were told was an analgesic cream (which would reduce, but not eliminate, the pain) or an ineffective cream (which would serve as the control; Wager et al., 2004). In reality, the cream was the same in both conditions and had no properties that would reduce the experience of pain. The researchers then measured the participants' brain activity using functional magnetic resonance imaging (fMRI). As predicted, participants who believed they were receiving an analgesic showed decreased brain activity in areas of the brain that respond to pain, including the thalamus, insula, and anterior cingulate cortex. This study provides powerful evidence that the placebo effect reduces pain at least in part by changing how the brain responds to pain.

the practitioner expectancies effect are major reasons why clinical drug trials now use double-blind procedures in which neither the patient nor the practitioner knows who is getting an active or a placebo drug.

Patients' Expectations

One factor that influences the effectiveness of placebos is patients' expectations about the effects of the treatment (Skelton & Pennebaker, 1982; Stewart-Williams, 2004). In other words, patients who expect a given reaction to a placebo may look for signs that show the treatment or drug is working. For example, participants who were told that they would be hearing some noise that might cause their skin temperature to change—some were told it would rise, others were told it would fall—reported feeling such a change in precisely the direction they were told to expect it (Pennebaker & Skelton, 1981). Expectations also influence other types of physiological reactions, including heart rate and amount of nasal congestion and stuffiness. In fact, one study on the role of the placebo effect in influencing people's reactions to antidepressant medication found that 75% of the effectiveness of such drugs is caused by patients' expectations that they will work as opposed to any psychological changes in brain chemistry (Kirsch & Sapirstein, 1999).

Environmental Cues

Placebos may also work as a result of broad principles in learning, such as classical conditioning (Benedetti & Amanzio, 1997). Many of the factors that increase the effectiveness of placebos are linked with environmental cues that suggest pain relief, such as sitting in a doctor's office, receiving a pill, or feeling an injection. Over time, people may learn to associate these types of stimuli with feeling better; therefore, placebos may work simply by triggering these associations. For example, if you always take an aspirin, which reduces the pain, when you have a headache, you may experience the same reduction in pain if you take a pill that you think is aspirin but is actually just an inert sugar pill. This connection between taking a pill and feeling better helps explain a recent study showing that taking a placebo reduces pain even when people are fully aware they are taking a placebo (Carvalho et al., 2016). As shown in Figure 9.7, people who are told about the placebo effect and then take two capsules twice daily from a bottle marked "placebo pills" report greater reductions in pain, pain-related disability, and bothersomeness three weeks later than people who are in the control condition (and don't receive any pills).

In line with this view, all placebo treatments are not equal in their effectiveness—some are more effective than others (Benedetti & Amanzio, 1997). Those administered through injection have greater effects than those taken orally; capsules are more effective than pills. Even the brand name of the pill can influence its effectiveness: one study showed an increase of 10% in effectiveness through the use of a known name versus an unknown name (which helps explain why people often select the higher-priced name-brand drugs over cheaper alternatives even though the chemical properties of the drugs are virtually identical). The placebo effect is also stronger when a drug is administered by a doctor in a hospital setting than when given by a family member at home. In sum, having a placebo that looks, tastes, and feels like "real medicine" is likely to increase patient confidence, and thereby its effectiveness.

Similarly, because we associate higher-priced drugs with greater effectiveness, people respond better in terms of pain relief to drugs that cost more. In one simple demonstration of the effect of drug cost on its ability to reduce pain, researchers first gave all participants a light electric shock on their wrists (Waber, Shiv, Carmon, & Ariely, 2008). Next, participants were told they would be receiving a newly approved painkiller to measure whether it would reduce their experience of pain. Half of the participants were told the pill cost $2.50 per dose, whereas the others were told the drug had been marked down and cost only 10 cents. After the participants took the drug (which was, in all cases, a pill containing no actual medicine), the researchers

**What You'll Learn
9.5**

then repeated the electric shock test and asked people whether they felt less pain. Can you predict their findings? Eighty-five percent of the people who took a pill costing $2.50 reported feeling less pain, compared to only 61% of people who took a pill costing just 10 cents.

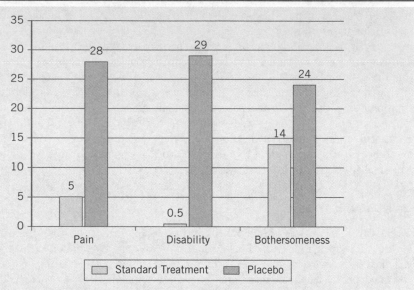

Figure 9.7   Data From Carvalho et al., 2016

Chronic back pain patients who receive a 15-minute explanation of the placebo effect and then receive "placebo pills" show more improvement than those in the control condition, who receive no pills. These findings suggest that there are actual benefits of taking pills—even if you understand that they are placebo pills!

Source: Data from Carvalho, Caetano, Cunha, Rebouta, Kaptchuk, & Kirsch (2016).

Table 9.3   Information YOU Can Use

- Stress matters a lot for pain—which is why you may develop migraines or nausea during particularly stressful times. Taking steps to reduce stress in your environment—or even change how you perceive potentially stressful events—can therefore help reduce pain.

- Your own thoughts, feelings, and behaviors influence how much pain you experience—which means that you can take some steps that reduce pain. Simply minimizing stress and focusing on maintaining a good mood helps decrease the experience of pain.

- Engaging in regular exercise can prevent, or at least reduce, the pain caused by headaches, back pain, and stomachaches. So, think about going for a jog or taking a yoga class as a way to minimize the experience of pain.

- When you are undergoing a painful experience, use psychological strategies to reduce the pain you feel. Try to relax your body, distract yourself, and/or think about pain in a new way—all of these approaches can help you feel better in the face of pain.

- Your expectations about pain relief can in fact lead to physiological changes in your body and even your brain that influence the experience of pain, which explains why the placebo effect is so powerful. Thus, when you take a medication or undergo a treatment to reduce pain, believing in its effectiveness can in fact improve its ability to reduce pain.

Understanding Pain

- Acute pain is intense but time-limited pain that is generally the result of tissue damage or disease. Chronic pain often begins as acute pain (in response to a specific injury or disease) but does not go away after a minimum of six months.

- Chronic pain imposes serious costs on individuals' ability to function in daily life. It also has implications for health care utilization and employers. Opioid addiction, which often begins with prescription pain-relieving drugs, is a substantial problem in the United States.

- Specificity theory posits that there are specific sensory receptors for different types of sensations, such as pain, warmth, touch, and pressure. In contrast, pattern theory describes pain as resulting from the type and intensity of stimulation received by the nerve endings. The leading theory explaining pain is now gate control theory of pain. According to this theory of pain, not all of the pain signals carried by the nerve fibers successfully reach the brain. Any competing sensation that increases stimulation to the site could shut the gate, thereby stopping the transmission of pain signals to the brain. Psychological factors, such as distraction and relaxation, can also send messages from the brain down to the spinal cord to shut the gate. Neurochemical processes, and neurotransmitters, are also involved in the experience of pain. According to neuromatrix theory, a network of neurons is distributed throughout the brain, which processes the information that flows through it.

- Self-report measures of pain basically ask people to describe their pain. Behavioral pain measures assess the outward manifestations of pain, including physical symptoms, verbal expressions, and facial expressions. Psychophysiological measures of pain assess specific biological responses, such as muscle tension, heart rate, and skin temperature, and brain activity.

The Impact of Psychosocial Factors on Pain

- People who report greater stress in their daily lives experience more pain. Experiencing stress may lead people to engage in behaviors that cause pain. People who experience high levels of stress may also stop taking care of themselves, which increases their experience of stress and pain. Stress can also lead directly to physiological problems that cause pain.

- People learn health-related behaviors in part by observing how others around them act when undergoing medical procedures and responding to pain. People may also learn to experience, or at least express, pain as a way of receiving some type of secondary gain or reinforcement.

- How people think about pain, or to what they attribute their pain and its outcome, impacts their experience of pain. Beliefs about pain, and in particular anxiety about pain, also influence how much pain people report experiencing. People who catastrophize, self-criticize, and overgeneralize experience more pain. People's expectations about their ability to cope with pain also influence how much pain they experience.

- Negative emotions, such as depression and anxiety, are associated with the experience of pain. Although most evidence suggests that experiencing chronic pain tends to lead to depression, depression may also lead to pain over time.

- People with more social support experience lower levels of pain. Support partners may help people use better strategies for coping with their pain. Alternatively, the presence of supportive friends and family members allows people to express emotions, which helps them cope with pain.

Physical Methods of Managing Pain

- Physical stimulation, or counterirritation, involves irritating body tissue to ease pain. These techniques include transcutaneous electrical nerve stimulation (TENS; placing electrodes on the skin and administering continuous electrical stimulation), acupuncture (needles are inserted at specific points on the skin), massage therapy (deep-tissue manipulation), and chiropractic therapy (manipulation of the bones, muscles, and joints to improve body alignment).

- Because certain types of pain are exacerbated by weak muscles, a lack of flexibility, and muscle tension, physical therapy and exercise can help reduce and even prevent pain. In some cases, exercise can be as effective as or even more effective than traditional methods of therapy.

- The most common way to control pain is with *analgesic drugs*, which reduce fever and inflammation at the site of wounds and interfere with the transmission of pain signals. *Narcotic drugs* work by binding to the opiate receptors and thereby inhibiting the transmission of pain signals, whereas local *anesthetics* block nerve cells in a particular region from generating impulses. Other pharmacologic methods of pain control rely on blocking the transmission of pain impulses up the spinal cord.

- In extreme cases, surgical pain control can be used to manage pain. Surgical pain control typically involves severing or destroying the nerves that transmit pain signals, thereby reducing the perception of pain.

Psychological Methods of Managing Pain

- Many strategies to reduce pain involve people changing their behavior in some way. Relaxation approaches include progressive muscle relaxation (patients focus on tensing and then releasing each part of their body), systematic desensitization (patients gradually become more comfortable with different types of stimuli), guided imagery (deep muscle relaxation is paired with a specific pleasant image), and biofeedback (people learn to monitor and change selected physiological functions). Behavior therapy, which focuses on reinforcing positive behaviors and ignoring negative behaviors, may also be used to decrease various types of chronic pain.

- Cognitive methods focus on helping people understand how their thoughts and feelings influence the experience of pain as well as helping people change their reactions to and perceptions of pain and their ability to manage that pain. These methods include hypnosis (people dissociate, or separate, the physical sensations their body is experiencing from their conscious awareness of these feelings), meditation (people relax and focus their attention on a single thought), mindfulness (people pay conscious attention to their thoughts, emotions, and bodily sensations), and distraction (people try to get their mind off the pain).

- Many pain management programs use both cognitive and behavioral strategies to reduce pain, which tends to be particularly effective.

The Impact of Placebos on Pain

- Placebos, meaning a medicine or treatment that affects someone even though it contains no specific medical or physical properties relevant to the condition it is supposedly treating, can produce very real and even lasting effects. Placebos can reduce pain and improve physical functioning.

- Placebo effects may occur because people's beliefs about the power of a pain treatment impact their behavior. Specifically, when people are given a pain treatment they fully expect to work, they may change their behavior in ways that in turn lead to the desired reduction of pain. Placebos may also lead to physiological changes in the body, which in turn inhibit the experience of pain.

- The behavior of the practitioner, and his or her expectations about a particular drug or treatment, influence its effectiveness, as do patients' expectations about the effects of the treatment. Many of the factors that increase the effectiveness of placebos are linked with environmental cues that suggest pain relief, such as sitting in a doctor's office, receiving a pill, or feeling an injection. Over time, people may learn to associate these types of stimuli with feeling better; therefore, placebos may work simply by triggering these associations.

UNDERSTANDING AND MANAGING CHRONIC ILLNESS

Learning Objectives

10.1 Describe the prevalence and costs of chronic disease

10.2 Compare the common types of chronic disease

10.3 Summarize the consequences of chronic disease

10.4 Explain factors influencing reactions to chronic disease

10.5 Describe strategies for coping with a chronic disease

What You'll Learn

10.1 How neighborhoods can influence the likelihood of developing diabetes

10.2 Why having a chronic disease is harder on younger than on older people

10.3 Why caring for a pet helps children with diabetes

10.4 Why people who are HIV-positive benefit from practicing positive emotions

10.5 How brisk walking may improve memory in people with Alzheimer's disease

Preview

Chronic diseases—such as arthritis, diabetes, and cancer—are the most common cause of health problems in the United States. About half of all adults have at least one chronic health condition, and 25% of Americans have two or more such conditions (Ward,

(Continued)

(Continued)

Schiller, & Goodman, 2014). In this chapter, you'll learn about the prevalence, costs, and consequences of chronic diseases, as well as factors that influence how people react to having a chronic health condition. Most important, you'll learn how interventions can help people manage having a chronic disease.

UNDERSTANDING CHRONIC DISEASES

LO 10.1

Describe the prevalence and costs of chronic disease

As described in *Chapter 1: Introduction*, historically most people died from **acute diseases**, which generally develop quickly and last only a relatively short time. Pneumonia, tuberculosis, and typhoid fever are all examples of acute diseases that were responsible for many deaths in the early 1900s (Grob, 1983). Other acute diseases include the common cold, strep throat, and the flu. This type of disease is often caused by exposure to a virus or an infection but can also be caused by an injury, such as a broken bone or burn.

Chronic diseases differ from acute diseases in several ways. First, chronic diseases often have a slow onset, and the disease intensity increases over time. Many people with HIV infection do not even know when they were exposed to the disease, and often they are infected for months or years before they notice any symptoms. Second, chronic conditions often have multiple causes, including people's behavioral choices or lifestyles. As discussed in *Chapter 7: Substance Use and Abuse* and *Chapter 8: Obesity and Disordered Eating*, behavioral choices regarding eating, exercise, smoking, and alcohol use are responsible for much of the illness, disability, and premature death related to chronic diseases. Third, whereas acute conditions often can be cured with medication or some other intervention, chronic conditions can only be managed—people with chronic diseases sometimes get worse and sometimes stay the same, but they can't be cured.

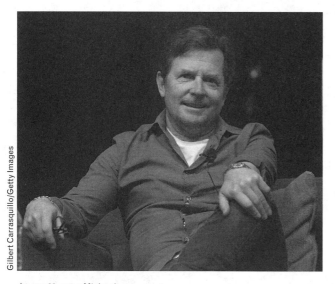

At age 29, actor Michael J. Fox was diagnosed with Parkinson's disease, a chronic disorder that impacts the central nervous system. Common symptoms of Parkinson's disease include shaking, rigidity, and difficulty with walking, as well as problems with thinking and behavior.

Gilbert Carrasquillo/Getty Images

Prevalence of Chronic Disease

Although children and adolescents are more likely to experience acute diseases, they are at risk of developing certain chronic diseases (Torpy, Campbell, & Glass, 2010). The most common chronic diseases experienced during childhood and adolescence are asthma, cystic fibrosis, and diabetes. These diseases may be caused by genetic factors, environmental factors, or a combination of both genetic and environmental factors. For example, cystic fibrosis, a serious lung disease for which there is no cure, is caused entirely be genetic factors, as described in **Focus on Neuroscience**. Genetics also influence the likelihood of developing asthma, Alzheimer's disease, and diabetes, although environmental factors also play a role (Mathias, 2014; Ober & Yao, 2011; Onengut-Gumuscu et al., 2015).

Health in general declines with age, and thus the likelihood of having a chronic disease increases with age. Because the immune system's responsiveness decreases in older age, older individuals are more susceptible to mild illnesses that younger people may effectively fight off (Rabin, 2000). Chronic diseases are therefore far more prevalent in older adults. In fact, 88% of adults over age 65 with serious health conditions have a chronic condition (Hoffman, Rice, & Sung, 1996).

Chronic diseases tend to be more common in people of color than in Whites. For example, diabetes rates are 77% higher among Blacks, 66% higher among Latinos, and 18% higher among Asians than among Whites (Centers for Disease Control and Prevention, 2017t). Rates of HIV and asthma are also higher in Blacks and Latinos than in Whites and Asian Americans (Centers for Disease Control and Prevention, 2017l, 2017o). These racial and ethnic differences in the prevalence of chronic diseases are often a function of socioeconomic status (SES); people in lower SES classes are more likely to live in environments that contribute to the development of such diseases and less likely to receive regular preventive care. (You'll learn more about race/ethnic differences in specific chronic diseases, and some explanations for such differences, in the next section.)

Costs of Chronic Disease

Chronic diseases exert a substantial cost on individuals and on society. As shown in Table 10.1, seven of the top 10 causes of death are chronic diseases (National Center for Health Statistics, 2017). (Two of these diseases—heart disease and cancer—will be discussed in detail in *Chapter 11: Leading Causes of Mortality*.) One recent study suggests that if diabetes were eliminated as a disease, the number of deaths in the United States each year would decline by 12% (Stokes & Preston, 2017).

Even non-life-threatening chronic diseases cause serious health problems. Diabetes is the leading cause of kidney failure and new cases of blindness and may also cause amputations (Centers for Disease Control and Prevention, 2017a). People with diabetes are also less likely to survive a heart attack than people without this condition, even when taking into account other factors, such as age, sex, other illnesses, and emergency treatment they receive (Alabas et al., 2016). Arthritis is the most common cause of disability; many adults with arthritis have

Table 10.1 Leading Causes of Death	
Disease	**Number of Deaths**
Heart disease	614,348
Cancer	591,700
Chronic lower respiratory disease	147,101
Unintentional injuries	135,928
Stroke	133,103
Alzheimer's disease	93,541
Diabetes	76,488
Flu and pneumonia	55,227
Kidney disease (nephitis)	48,146
Suicide	42,826
Chronic conditions now cause a majority of deaths in the United States each year.	

Source: Data from the Centers for Disease Control and Prevention (2017), https://www.cdc.gov/nchs/fastats/leading-causes-of-death.htm.

difficulty engaging in routine activities in daily life (Barbour et al., 2017; Brault, Hootman, Helmick, Theis, & Armour, 2009).

Chronic diseases, and the health-related behaviors that contribute to such diseases, account for the majority of health care costs in the United States. In fact, 86% of all health care spending is on people with one or more chronic health conditions (Gerteis et al., 2014). Chronic diseases lead to high medical costs, but also have substantial costs in terms of decreased work productivity when people are unable to work, or are less productive at work, due to their health. Diabetes and asthma together cost an estimated $116 billion a year in decreased productivity (Centers for Disease Control and Prevention, 2017e).

COMMON TYPES OF CHRONIC DISEASE

LO 10.2

Compare the common types of chronic disease

Although chronic diseases all share certain commonalities, as described previously, different types of chronic diseases have distinct symptoms, onset timing, and long-term side effects. For example, *epilepsy* is a common neurological condition characterized by recurrent seizures, which can limit a person's ability to participate in daily activities and thus reduce overall well-being. *Parkinson's disease (PD)* is a movement disorder in which people experience tremors, problems with balance, and muscle symptoms, and hence may have trouble completing routine daily tasks. This section will examine four common types of chronic diseases—diabetes, arthritis, HIV/AIDS, Alzheimer's—which differ substantially in their causes, symptoms, and management.

Diabetes

Diabetes is extremely common. Over 30 million Americans—meaning 1 in every 11 people—has diabetes (Centers for Disease Control and Prevention, 2017f). Moreover, an additional

84 million people have prediabetes, a serious health condition that increases a person's risk of developing diabetes as well as heart disease and stroke. Most of these people are not aware of their risk.

Understanding Diabetes

Diabetes is a disorder in which the body is unable to properly convert glucose (sugar) into usable energy. *Type 1 diabetes*, which accounts for only about 5% of diabetes cases, occurs when the body can't produce enough insulin. Insulin, a hormone produced by the pancreas, allows blood sugar (glucose) to enter cells, where it provides energy. *Type 2 diabetes*, the most common type of diabetes, occurs when the body can't properly use insulin. When glucose can't enter the cells, it builds up in the blood and causes hyperglycemia. This can cause serious health problems, including heart disease, stroke, kidney failure, and blindness. Diabetes can also reduce blood flow to the legs and feet, which increases the risk of infections. In some cases, damage caused by infections can require amputations of the toes, feet, or legs.

Gestational diabetes is a temporary form of diabetes, which occurs in a small percentage of pregnant women. This type of diabetes is caused by the woman's inability to produce an adequate amount of insulin while pregnant. Although gestational diabetes typically goes away after giving birth, women who develop this condition during pregnancy are at increased risk of developing Type 2 diabetes later on.

Risk Factors for Diabetes

As described in the prior section, both age and genetic factors impact a person's likelihood of developing diabetes. Only 4% of people younger than 45 have diabetes, whereas 17% of those ages 45 to 64 and 25% of those ages 65 and older have diabetes (Centers for Disease Control and Prevention, 2017q). People with a genetic predisposition and/or family history of diabetes are at increased risk of developing diabetes.

Although there are no gender differences in the prevalence of diabetes, there are also substantial differences in likelihood of developing diabetes as a function of race/ethnicity. Specifically, only 7.4% of Whites have been diagnosed with diabetes, compared to 8% of Asian Americans, 12.1% of Hispanic/Latino Americans, and 12.7% of Blacks. Diabetes is especially prevalent in Native Americans; an estimated 15.1% of Native Americans have diabetes (Centers for Disease Control and Prevention, 2017q). Specifically, only 7.1% of Whites have been diagnosed with diabetes, compared to 8.4% of Asian Americans, 11.8% of Hispanic/Latino Americans, and 12.6% of Blacks. Diabetes is especially prevalent in Native Americans; an estimated 33% of Native Americans have diabetes. Gestational diabetes also occurs more frequently in Blacks, Hispanic/Latino Americans, and Native Americans than in Whites and Asian Americans. Perhaps most concerning is the rapid increase in the prevalence of diabetes among children of color, including Black, Asian or Pacific Islander, Latino, and Native American children, compared to White children (Mayer-Davis et al., 2017). Rates of Type 2 diabetes are increasingly at particular high rates among Latino children.

What causes these racial/ethnic differences in prevalence of diabetes? As you'll soon learn, this increased likelihood of developing diabetes as a function of ethnicity is due largely to the increased prevalence of other fixable risk factors that are more prevalent in people of color. For example, Blacks are 40% more likely than Whites to have high blood pressure, and Native Americans are 60% more likely to be obese than Whites, and both high blood pressure and obesity increase the likelihood of developing diabetes. Such differences in rates of diabetes and diabetes risk factors are largely a function of social and environmental conditions; people of color are more likely to live in neighborhoods with less access to healthy foods and safe places to exercise (Spanakis & Golden, 2013).

Although age, race/ethnicity, and genetic factors are fixed, meaning they can't be changed, other factors that increase the risk of diabetes can be changed. People who are obese, as well as those who engage in low levels of physical activity, are substantially more likely to develop diabetes (Centers for Disease Control and Prevention, 2017b). For example, children and adolescents who are obese are four times as likely to develop diabetes as those who have a BMI within the normal range (Abbasi, Juszczyk, van Jaarsveld, & Gulliford, 2017). Engaging in regular physical activity, such as walking briskly or bicycling for the recommended 150 minutes a week, can reduce the risk of developing Type 2 diabetes by as much as 26% (Smith, Crippa, Woodcock, & Brage, 2016).

Researchers in several studies have examined whether neighborhood factors that encourage physical activity and healthy eating reduce the risk of obesity, and in turn, diabetes. For example, one study rated neighborhoods in terms of their "walkability," which included measures of how many stores, schools, and services (banks, libraries, etc.) were located within a 10-minute walk as well as how easily the streets connected on one another for pedestrians (Creatore et al., 2016). They then evaluated rates of overweight, obesity, and diabetes over an 11-year period. As predicted, neighborhood walkability was associated with lower rates of obesity and diabetes. Similarly, people who live in neighborhoods with ready access to healthy foods (meaning a high prevalence of grocery stores and fruit and vegetable markets) and recreation facilities—such as bowling, golf, tennis, and water activities—also have a reduced risk of diabetes (Christine et al., 2015). These findings suggest that environmental factors also contribute to the risk of developing diabetes.

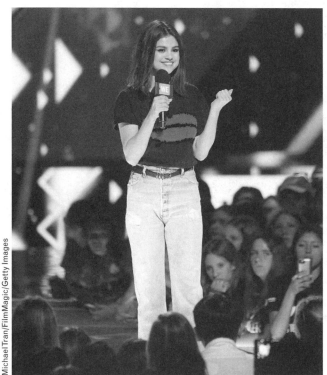

Michael Tran/FilmMagic/Getty Images

In 2016, singer Selena Gomez canceled her world tour due to side effects of lupus, a chronic disease in which the immune system attacks healthy tissues. Symptoms of lupus include fatigue, weight loss, fever, rash, painful joints, anemia, and hearing loss. People with lupus are also at increased risk of experiencing a stroke or heart attack.

What You'll Learn
10.1

Arthritis

As estimated 54 million American adults—meaning 23% of all adults—have some form of **arthritis** (Centers for Disease Control and Prevention, 2017p). The most common form of arthritis is *osteoarthritis*, a degenerative disease causing swelling and pain in any joints but most commonly in the knees, hips, lower back, and neck. Other diseases within this category include *rheumatoid arthritis* (an autoimmune disorder causing swollen and painful joints), *gout* (a painful type of arthritis caused by the buildup of uric acid in the blood), *lupus* (an autoimmune disease in which the immune system attacks healthy cells and tissues), and *fibromyalgia* (a musculoskeletal condition causing muscle and joint pain and fatigue).

Understanding Arthritis

The term arthritis refers to more than 100 different types of diseases and conditions that affect the joints, and/or tissues surrounding the joints, in some way. Common symptoms of diseases within this category include pain, swelling, and stiffness in the joints, although the specific location, patterning, and severity of these symptoms varies depending on the specific form of the disease. Certain diseases within this category, such as rheumatoid arthritis and lupus, can impact the immune system and/or various organs and thus lead to a broader range of symptoms.

Risk Factors for Arthritis

As described previously, the risk of developing arthritis increases with age. Only 7.1% of people ages 18 to 44 have been diagnosed with arthritis, compared to 29.3% of those ages 45 to 64 and 49.6% of those ages 65 and older (Barbour, Helmick, Boring, & Brady, 2017).

Other demographic factors also influence the likelihood of developing arthritis. Women are somewhat more likely to be diagnosed with arthritis than men; 26% of women and 19.1% of men have arthritis (Barbour et al., 2017). Whites and Native Americans are more likely to be diagnosed with arthritis than people in other racial ethnic groups; an estimated 26.3% of Whites and 24.6% of Native Americans have been diagnosed with arthritis, compared to 21.8% of Blacks and only 12.1% of Latinos and 11.1% of Asian Americans.

Other risk factors for arthritis are caused by lifestyle factors. For example, people who are overweight or obese are more likely to develop arthritis, presumably because excess weight places additional pressure on the joints. Only about 16% of underweight or normal-weight adults have arthritis, compared to nearly 23% of people who are overweight and 31% of people who are obese (Barbour et al., 2017). In line with this finding, arthritis commonly occurs with other chronic diseases; about half of American adults with heart disease or diabetes have arthritis, which are both linked with obesity.

Certain types of arthritis may be caused by other factors. For example, people who experience an injury to a particular joint are at greater risk of developing arthritis in that joint later on. Infections can also lead to some types of arthritis. People with jobs that involve particular types of repetitive movements, such as squatting or knee bending, are also at increased risk of arthritis.

HIV/AIDS

Acquired immunodeficiency syndrome (AIDS), which is caused by the human immuno-deficiency virus (HIV), was first identified as a syndrome in 1981 (Foege, 1983). An estimated 1.1 million people in the United States are HIV-positive, with about 15% of these people being unaware of their infection (Centers for Disease Control and Prevention, 2017l). Over 39,000 new cases of HIV are diagnosed in the United States each year, and an estimated 12,000 people die of AIDS in the United States each year.

AIDS is a very serious, and life-threatening, disease throughout the world. Nearly 37 million people around the world are living with HIV, and over a million people die from AIDS-related illnesses each year.

Understanding HIV/AIDS

HIV, which causes AIDS, is a retrovirus. Retroviruses replicate by injecting themselves into host cells and literally taking over the genetic workings of these cells. They can then produce virus particles that infect new cells. After HIV enters the bloodstream, it invades the T cells, incorporates its genetic material into the cells, and then starts destroying cells' ability to function. As discussed in *Chapter 4: Understanding Stress*, T cells are responsible for recognizing harmful substances in the body and for attacking such cells, in part by releasing NK cells. Although HIV is able to stay in the body in a latent and dormant state, it gradually starts replicating itself and in the process begins destroying the T cells.

The progression from HIV to AIDS varies in time but follows a distinct pattern of four stages (McCutchan, 1990). During the first stage, which may last for a period of one to eight weeks, people experience relatively mild symptoms, such as fever, headache, and sore throat. This initial stage is then followed by a latent period, in which people experience few, if any, symptoms; this stage can last as long as 10 years. During the third stage, people develop a specific group of symptoms, including night sweats, painful skin rash, swollen lymph nodes, and white spots in the mouth. Finally, as the patient's immune system begins to have trouble fighting off various infections, people may experience problems with the lungs, gastrointestinal tract, nervous system, bones, and the brain (see Figure 10.1). This stage is marked by a dramatic reduction in T cell counts—which may be 200 or less per cubic millimeter of blood compared to a rate of 1,000 in a healthy person. People infected with HIV may also experience more severe symptoms, such as shortness of breath, substantial weight loss, personality shifts, and dementia (mental confusion and memory loss). Because HIV basically destroys the immune system, people with AIDS often die of opportunistic infections, such as pneumonia, tuberculosis, and a type of cancer called Kaposi's sarcoma.

Risk Factors for HIV/AIDS

In the United States and other Western cultures, HIV transmission occurs through behavioral choices, such as engaging in unprotected sex and sharing needles when injecting drugs. Therefore, individuals who decide to protect themselves from HIV, and follow through on these intentions, are quite safe. Even in cases in which one member of a couple is HIV-positive, HIV transmission is extremely rare as long as the couple consistently uses condoms (De Vincenzi, 1994; Rodger et al., 2016).

In the 1980s, in the early stages of the HIV epidemic, the vast majority of people with AIDS were men who had sex with men (as discussed in *Chapter 2: Research Methods*).

Figure 10.1 Model of HIV Infection in the Body Over Time

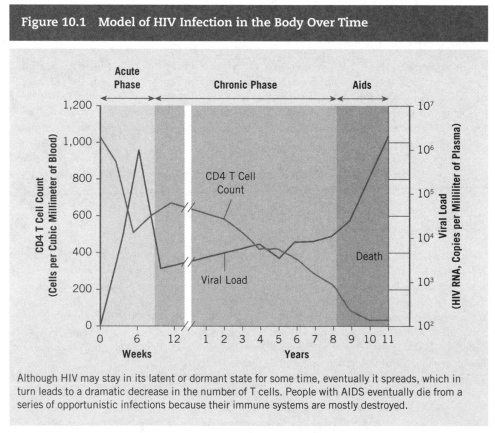

Although HIV may stay in its latent or dormant state for some time, eventually it spreads, which in turn leads to a dramatic decrease in the number of T cells. People with AIDS eventually die from a series of opportunistic infections because their immune systems are mostly destroyed.

Source: Reproduced by permission of Scientific American. Copyright Scientific American © 1998.

Men having sex with men is still the largest route of transmission of HIV in the United States, accounting for 67% of new HIV diagnoses each year (Centers for Disease Control and Prevention, 2017k). Heterosexual transmission accounts for 24% of new infections, and injection drug use accounts for 9% of diagnoses each year.

There are also substantial race/ethnicity differences in likelihood of acquiring HIV. Only about 5% of Whites and Asians have been diagnosed with HIV, compared to 8.8% of Native Americans, 16.4% of Latinos, and 44.3% of Blacks (Centers for Disease Control and Prevention, 2016d). Although Blacks make up only 12% of the United States population, they make up 45% of HIV diagnoses and 53% of deaths caused by AIDS each year (Seth, Walker, Hollis, Figueroa, & Belcher, 2015). Some explanations for this very high rate of HIV among Blacks are described in **Focus on Diversity**.

Alzheimer's Disease

Alzheimer's disease is the most common cause of dementia and the sixth leading cause of death in the United States (Heron, 2016; Taylor, Greenlund, McGuire, Lu, & Croft, 2017). Alzheimer's currently affects an estimated 5.5 million Americans, but rates are increasing rapidly as life expectancy continues to increases. In fact, by 2050, the number of Americans with Alzheimer's is expected to reach 14 million (see Figure 10.2).

Understanding Alzheimer's Disease

Alzheimer's disease is a brain disorder that damages and, over time, destroys brain cells, causing serious problems with memory, thinking, language, and behavior. It is a progressive

FOCUS ON DIVERSITY

Explaining Race Differences in HIV/AIDS

Each year over 17,000 Blacks in the United States are diagnosed with HIV, and the majority of these cases are in gay or bisexual men (Centers for Disease Control and Prevention, 2017j). Gay and bisexual men are in general more at risk of acquiring HIV than women or heterosexual men for several reasons, including their tendency to have a greater number of sexual partners, the frequency of their engagement in receptive anal sex, and the relatively high rate of HIV within sexual networks. However, Black gay and bisexual men account for more HIV cases than any other group of Americans. For example, one study of young men who have sex with men found that Black men were seven times more likely to become HIV-positive over a three-year period than White men (Halkitis, Kapadia, & Ompad, 2015). This increased risk is explained by multiple factors. First, Black men have higher rates of incarceration, which increases the likelihood of engaging in risky sexual behavior. They also tend to

have relatively small and exclusive sexual networks (made up largely of other gay and bisexual Black men), in which a single person with HIV may infect multiple other people. Third, Black gay and bisexual men are less likely to be aware of their HIV status—in part because they are less likely to have access to regular health care—which decreases their likelihood of receiving treatment and increases their likelihood of spreading the disease to others. HIV-related stigma also contributes to the higher rate of HIV within this population. Admitting to homosexuality can be very hard for Black men, who may encounter homophobia within their family and broader community, which may lead Black men to identify as heterosexual but to secretly engage in sex with men (Brooks, Etzel, Hinojos, Henry, & Perez, 2005). Unfortunately, this fear of stigma and discrimination reduces Black men's likelihood of engaging in HIV-preventive behaviors, such as using condoms and seeking HIV testing.

Figure 10.2   Data From Hebert et al., 2013

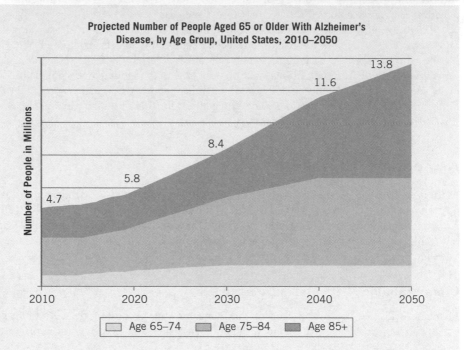

Projected Number of People Aged 65 or Older With Alzheimer's Disease, by Age Group, United States, 2010–2050

Rates of Alzheimer's disease are increasing rapidly, in part because an increasing number of people are living into their 80s and beyond.

Source: Data from Hebert, Weuve, Scherr, & Evans (2013).

disease, meaning symptoms develop slowly but get significantly worse over time. Although memory problems are typically one of the first signs of Alzheimer's, other signs of this disease include getting lost, having difficulty handling money and paying bills, losing and misplacing items, and repeating questions. Over time, people with Alzheimer's may show personality and mood changes and have difficulty carrying out normal daily life activities.

In the final stages of Alzheimer's, in which cognitive and physical impairments are substantial, people need virtually constant care, which places a tremendous burden on caregivers. Nearly 16 million Americans take care of family and friends with Alzheimer's and other forms of dementia each year, providing over 18 billion hours of unpaid care (Centers for Disease Control and Prevention, 2017c). People who provide care to a spouse with Alzheimer's disease experience substantial stress, and report lower levels of happiness and enjoyment in life, as well as higher levels of sadness and loneliness (Adams, 2008). In addition, total costs for health care, including long-term care and hospice, for people with Alzheimer's and other forms of dementia are estimated to be $236 billion a year.

Risk Factors for Alzheimer's Disease

The single biggest risk factor for Alzheimer's disease is age. Ten percent of people ages 65 and older have Alzheimer's disease, and the percentage of people with this disease doubles every five years after age 65 (Hebert, Weuve, Scherr, & Evans, 2013). Although people younger than 65 may develop Alzheimer's disease (which is called early-onset Alzheimer's), it is much less common in younger people.

Alzheimer's disease is also more common in women than in men; an estimated two thirds of people with this disease are women (Hebert et al., 2013). One explanation for women's increased risk of developing Alzheimer's, given the increased likelihood of developing Alzheimer's with age, is women's longer life expectancy. However, even among people of the same age, women have a greater likelihood of having Alzheimer's, indicating that age alone does not explain this difference. Similarly, although early research suggested life experiences, and in particular women's historically lower level of education compared to men, could explain women's risk of developing Alzheimer's, more recent research examining whether a lower level of education increases the risk of dementia provides mixed evidence for this theory (Sharp & Gatz, 2011). Most researchers believe that biological differences likely explain this gender difference. In line with that view, recent evidence suggests that women's brains may be more prone than men's to experience damage that can trigger cognitive impairments (Gallart-Palau et al., 2016).

People of color are also at greater risk of developing Alzheimer's disease than Whites. Compared to Whites, Black people are twice as likely to develop Alzheimer's and Latinos are one and a half times more likely to develop this disease (Alzheimer's Association, 2016). These racial and ethnic differences in the prevalence of Alzheimer's disease are likely a reflection of differences in health conditions, such as diabetes and cardiovascular disease, which increase the likelihood of developing Alzheimer's and are more prevalent among people of color. Specifically, risk factors for heart disease and stroke, such as high blood pressure and high cholesterol, also increase the risk of Alzheimer's disease, and these risk factors are more prevalent in people of color. Socioeconomic factors—such as poverty, level of education, and discrimination—that impact general cognitive functioning may also help explain racial/ethnic differences in the prevalence of Alzheimer's disease (Glymour & Manly, 2008).

Considerable evidence demonstrates that genetic factors also influence the likelihood of developing Alzheimer's disease (Huang et al., 2017; Sims et al., 2017). Although specific genes that directly cause Alzheimer's have yet to be identified, several genes that are associated with an increased likelihood of developing Alzheimer's disease are known. In addition, particular genes may influence the progression of Alzheimer's symptoms, including rate of loss of memory and thinking skills (Boots et al., 2017).

Finally, some evidence points to the role of behavioral choices, including diet and exercise, in influencing the risk of Alzheimer's. For example, one longitudinal study of older adults revealed that both engaging in regular exercise and following a Mediterranean-style diet (meaning a diet based largely in fruits, vegetables, legumes, cereals, and fish, with low levels of meat and dairy) were associated with a lower risk of developing Alzheimer's disease (Scarmeas et al., 2009). Similarly, older adults who engage in regular physical activity are less likely to develop Alzheimer's, and among those with the disease, engaging in regular physical activity improves not only mobility but potentially general cognition (Ginis et al., 2017). These findings indicate that regardless of fixed factors, such as age, gender, ethnicity/race, and genetics, behavioral choices may also contribute to an individual's risk of developing Alzheimer's disease.

CONSEQUENCES OF CHRONIC DISEASE

LO 10.3

Summarize the consequences of chronic disease

Because chronic diseases can be managed but never cured, people with such a diagnosis face a lifetime of managing the symptoms and treatment of the disease. People diagnosed with a chronic illness therefore experience a number of consequences, including physical, sexual, social, and psychological problems.

Physical Problems

Many people with chronic diseases experience some type of physical debilitation, such as paralysis, disfigurement, incontinence, and pain (Devins & Binik, 1996). People with diabetes, for example, are at increased risk of developing heart disease, blindness, sexual dysfunction, kidney failure, and problems with circulation that can lead to amputation (Bishop, Roesler, Zimmerman, & Ballard, 1993). Symptoms of multiple sclerosis (MS), a neurological disorder, include impaired vision, weakness, tremors, incoordination, and bowel and bladder difficulties (Franklin & Nelson, 1993). Even non-life-threatening chronic diseases can lead to physical problems. For example, people with arthritis (a chronic, systemic, inflammatory condition causing pain and swelling of the joints) often experience constant pain from inflammation of the joints and have difficulty managing daily tasks, such as getting dressed, walking, or standing (Scott & Hochberg, 1993). One man with diabetes described how the physical problems caused by this disease impaired his ability to attend significant family functions, saying, "I have a problem in walking around and because of this I cannot attend programs like weddings in the family and I feel very sad about this" (Stuckey et al., 2014, p. 2468).

In other cases, the disease itself is not debilitating, but the treatment for it is quite destructive to health. An individual with kidney failure, for example, may need to undergo hemodialysis, in which his or her blood is circulated through an artificial kidney for several hours each week. Medications that are used to treat hypertension lead to a number of unpleasant side effects, such as impotence, weight gain, and drowsiness (Taylor & Aspinwall, 1993). Similarly, anticonvulsant drugs, which provide the main treatment for epilepsy, have several unpleasant side effects, such as drowsiness, nausea, mood change, and skin rash (Oles & Penry, 1987). Although one of the most commonly used drugs to treat HIV is *zidovudine (AZT)*, its use is associated with numerous unpleasant side effects, including anemia, headaches, itching, and even mental confusion.

The physical problems caused by the symptoms or treatment for a chronic disease may affect people's employment, which in turn can have major financial implications (Taylor & Aspinwall, 1993). In some cases, the symptoms of chronic illness cause people to be unable to work, or at least to do certain tasks. People with epilepsy, for example, often have trouble holding a job because they are not allowed to drive. People who are chronically ill may find themselves offered less demanding positions or passed over for promotion because employers think investing time and resources in them is a waste. These economic problems can be particularly difficult because insurance companies often do not cover all the costs associated with health problems.

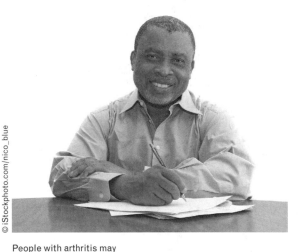

© iStockphoto.com/nico_blue

People with arthritis may have difficulty gripping objects, including pens, utensils, doorknobs, and faucets. This type of impairment may severely impact a person's ability to manage many daily life tasks.

Sexual Problems

Many people with chronic diseases experience some type of sexual problems. Such problems may be caused by the chronic disease itself, or by people's response to the disease; not surprisingly, people who feel depressed about their condition or develop poor body image are less interested in engaging in sexual behavior (Reininghaus, Reininghaus, Fitz, Hecht, & Bonelli, 2012). More than two thirds of men and women with diabetes report having sexual dysfunction (Rutte et al., 2015). Sexual dysfunction, including problems with feeling desire and reaching orgasm, is also highly prevalent in people with arthritis (Coskun, Coskun, Atis, Ergenekon, & Dilek, 2014; Tristano, 2014). One study of women with lupus found that over half of the women reported avoiding engaging in sexual contact (intercourse as well as foreplay) with their husbands during episodes of lupus (Druley, Stephens, & Coyne, 1997). Unfortunately, women who avoid such contact experience more negative affect, and overall poorer well-being, suggesting that avoidance of sexual behavior can have broader consequences.

Social Problems

One of the most difficult aspects of coping with a chronic illness is the effect it can have on interpersonal relationships (Taylor & Aspinwall, 1993). Social problems can include the loss of relationships, a lack of helpful support, and negative psychological reactions from others.

Loss of Relationships

Friends may withdraw from the patient, either because of their own fears about acquiring the illness or because they cannot bear to face the physical changes in the patient. People often hold negative beliefs and biases about those with chronic illnesses, including perceiving them as helpless, depressed, and even deserving of their fate (Devins & Binik, 1996). For example, people with diabetes may be lectured for eating sugar, or perceived as drunk if they experience an episode of hyperglycemia (low blood sugar; Stuckey et al., 2014). Some people with chronic illnesses therefore report feeling shunned by others and experiencing a loss of social support—ironically, just at the time when they are most in need of such support.

People with a chronic disease may also feel isolated from others if they lack a network of people who are experiencing a similar health challenge. Researchers in one study examined how people who were newly diagnosed with HIV coped with this news (Webel et al., 2014). Those who were under age 50 at the time of their diagnosis reported feeling more stress and disconnection from family and friends than those who were older. One explanation for this finding is that younger people are less likely to know others in their social network who are living with a chronic disease, and thus it is harder for them to find good social support. Compared to older people, younger adults also feel more stigma about having a disease and thus may be less likely to reveal their diagnosis to others, which also reduces their ability to receive support.

People with chronic diseases therefore sometimes choose to hide their conditions from others, in part because of concerns about being pitied and/or abandoned, and may thereby withdraw from many social relationships. This approach is particularly likely in cases when people have illnesses with high levels of stigma, such as epilepsy and AIDS. People with AIDS are often worried about rejection and abandonment (Marks, Richardson, Ruiz, & Maldonado, 1992; Simoni, Mason, Marks, Ruiz, & Al, 1995). And these fears are not unreasonable—one study found that one in five women who told their partners about their HIV-positive status were abandoned. In some cases, this disclosure even leads to physical violence and abuse (Rothenberg & Paskey, 1995). One study of sexually active HIV-positive people found that 41% had not disclosed their HIV status even to their sexual partners (Kalichman & Nachimson, 1999). Interestingly, people who report that religion is an important part of their lives are more likely to hide their HIV-positive status from their partners (Préau, Bouhnik, Roussiau, Lert, & Spire, 2008), as are those who are older (Emlet, 2006).

Lack of Helpful Support

Even when family members and friends want to help, they simply may not have realistic conceptions of what the patient is going through. People with chronic diseases may be reluctant to share how they are feeling and what type of help they need because they do not want to be perceived as a burden for family members (Stuckey et al., 2014). Unfortunately, this creates a vicious cycle because family members do not always know how to help, so the person with diabetes can feel more isolated and disconnected.

In some cases, people with a chronic illness have family and friends with unrealistically high expectations about how patients should cope with and manage their illnesses (Hatchett, Friend, Symister, & Wadhwa, 1997). For example, family and friends may believe that the patient could do more tasks to help around the house or that the patient's feelings of depression and anxiety are too pessimistic. Patients with arthritis whose spouses are impatient and critical of how they are coping with their illness use less-effective coping strategies and, in turn, experience more anxiety and depression (Manne & Zautra, 1989). Moreover, 85% of people with chronic disease report experiencing unwanted attempts by family members to influence their health-related behavior, which is associated with less behavior change as well as decreases in psychological adjustment (Thorpe, Lewis, & Sterba, 2008).

In other cases, family members and friends have unrealistically low expectations about how people cope with having a chronic illness (Burish & Bradley, 1983; Mohr et al., 1999). They may be overly protective or indulgent, which in turn can cause patients to feel or become dependent. For example, one study of physically disabled people found that nearly 40% had experienced emotional distress as a result of receiving unwanted help from their spouses (Newsom & Schultz, 1998). In this case, overprotection, even though well-intentioned, was associated with depression even as long as a year later. This pattern also interrupts the normal reciprocity in relationships, which can be a stressful disturbance. For example, family members might encourage the patient to simply "take it easy" and may try to discourage patients from talking about or thinking about the disease. Finally, family members can offer unhelpful advice or encouragement, such as, "It will turn out all right"—these sentiments are typically well meant but can raise false hopes and hence are inappropriate. You can rate what types of support you would find unhelpful if experiencing a chronic disease using **Table 10.2: Test Yourself**.

Negative Psychological Reactions

Family members of people with chronic illnesses also may experience negative psychological reactions. One of the major problems that families experience is dealing with the increased dependency of the ill person (Burish & Bradley, 1983). The patient may need assistance with a variety of tasks, including personal hygiene, medical care, financial responsibilities, and household chores, which can be time-consuming and emotionally upsetting for family members to accomplish. These changes in family roles can lead to great imbalances in family relationships, which increases guilt on the part of the patient and adds resentment on the part of family members. Caregivers of patients with cancer and multiple sclerosis who feel the relationship is inequitable experience more emotional exhaustion and have more feelings of anger at and detachment from the patient (Ybema, Kuijer, Buunk, DeJong, & Sanderman, 2001). Caregivers even may suffer health problems of their own, especially if they must take care of the ill person for a long time and that person is in very poor health (Wight, LeBlanc, & Aneshensel, 1998).

Family members also suffer their own losses when a loved one is diagnosed with a chronic illness; hence, they may experience negative psychological consequences, including depression and anxiety. These feelings are particularly likely when the patient has or will have a high level of functional impairment. For example, spouses of patients with chronic disease may experience a decrease in social activities, such as spending time with family and friends, seeing movies, and engaging in athletic activities. Chronic diseases can therefore lead to lower levels of marital satisfaction. In line with this view, both people with diabetes and their spouses report lower levels of relationship enjoyment and higher levels of marital tension (Iida, Stephens, Franks, & Rook, 2013).

Table 10.2 Test Yourself: How Helpful Is the Social Support You Receive?

Sometimes even when people may have good intentions, they say or do something that upsets you. I am going to list some of these things. Think about the period of time since you were diagnosed up until today. How often did the following situations arise with your family or friends (1 = never and 5 = very often)?

1. Changes the subject when I try to discuss my illness

2. Tells negative stories about other people who have cancer

3. Doesn't understand my situation

4. Avoids me

5. Appears afraid to be around me

6. Minimizes my problems

7. Seems to be hiding feelings

8. Acts uncomfortable when I talk about my illness

9. Trivializes my problems

10. Tells me I look well when I don't

This scale assesses the types of negative social interactions people with chronic diseases may encounter.

Source: Helgeson, Cohen, Schulz, & Yasko (2000).

Although most research on the social consequences of having a chronic disease has focused on the impact on the patient and the spouse, other family members, including parents, children, and siblings, are also affected. Parents who have a child with a chronic disease are, not surprisingly, deeply influenced. An estimated 20% to 30% of parents of children or adolescents with diabetes show symptoms of anxiety or depression (Whittemore, Jaser, Chao, Jang, & Grey, 2012). Distress is particularly high in cases in which a child's disease is life-threatening. For example, parents of a child with cystic fibrosis (a common genetic disease that affects the lungs and pancreas and virtually always leads to death in childhood or early adulthood) had more conflict with their spouse on child-rearing practices and fewer positive daily interactions with their spouse than did parents with a healthy child (Quittner et al., 1998). This was particularly true for women, who seemed to feel the burden of having a chronically ill child more than their husbands did. Couples with a chronically ill child also spent less time engaging in recreational activities, such as watching TV and going to the movies; couples with a sick child spent about 23% of their time engaging in recreational activities as compared to 33% of the time for those with a healthy child.

Psychological Problems

Virtually all people who are diagnosed with any chronic disease experience, at least initially, some psychological problems. Let's examine the most common such reactions.

Shock and Disbelief

People who are diagnosed with a chronic illness often experience an initial sense of shock and disbelief (Janoff-Bulman, 1992; Moos, 1977). Receiving a diagnosis of a chronic disease is stressful for virtually all people, in part because such a diagnosis shatters people's core beliefs about a "just world," namely, that life is fair and just, and can be particularly difficult to deal with because there is "no end in sight." Similarly, over 50% of college students with a chronic illness experience symptoms of posttraumatic stress, although relatively few meet the criteria for PTSD (Barakat & Wodka, 2006). People who learn they have a highly disabling chronic disease, such as Parkinson's disease or Huntington's disease, may have to put aside some plans and dreams, such as deciding not to have children or pursue a new career. Disbelief, denial, and anger are therefore common immediate reactions to receiving a diagnosis of chronic illness, and are particularly common in younger people, for whom receiving such a diagnosis is especially disturbing and surprising.

Depression and Anxiety

Many people with chronic illnesses experience depression, which is caused at least in part by the major loss of control that comes with having a chronic disease (Stuckey et al., 2014; Zashikhina & Hagglof, 2007). In fact, estimates are that about 35% of individuals with disabilities suffer from depression, as compared with 12% in the nondisabled population. In line with this view, many patients with multiple sclerosis—a disease of the central nervous system that leads to loss of function in limbs, bowel, and bladder, pain, and a loss of cognitive functioning—feel depressed and useless (Mohr et al., 1999). Similarly, women with diabetes are nearly twice as likely to experience postpartum depression as those without diabetes (Kozhimannil, Pereira, & Harlow, 2009). In some cases, such responses to chronic diseases can have very serious, even life-threatening consequences. For example, adults with asthma have an increased likelihood of suicidal ideation and suicide attempts (Goodwin & Eaton, 2005).

Depression is, not surprisingly, particularly common in cases of severe and life-threatening illnesses (Taylor & Aspinwall, 1993). Over half of those who are HIV-positive report symptoms of depression, and one in four report having contemplated suicide (Cooperman & Simoni, 2005; Kalichman, Heckman, Kochman, Sikkema, & Bergholte, 2000; Yi et al., 2006). Depression can even influence life expectancy. Patients with chronic diseases who are high in depression show more symptoms of their illness and a shorter life expectancy (Kellerman, Christensen, Baldwin, & Lawton, 2010; Kemeny et al., 1994; Patterson et al., 1996).

Anxiety, which is caused in part by the great uncertainty caused by a diagnosis of chronic disease, is another common psychological problem (Devins & Binik, 1996; Stuckey et al., 2014). As you might expect, upon learning of their status, HIV-positive individuals show considerable increases in anxiety, depression, and mood disturbances, which may persist for several weeks. In some cases, experiencing the symptoms of a disease can cause great anxiety—patients with asthma, for example, often worry that they will die during an attack, which naturally heightens anxiety.

However, many of the negative psychological consequences of having a chronic disease are most apparent immediately after diagnosis. Over time, most people adjust to their disease and its management and show signs of adaptation. In fact, one study found that there were no differences in rates of depression between healthy people and those with various chronic illnesses, such as arthritis, diabetes, and kidney disease, after the first three months following diagnosis (Cassileth et al., 1984).

Positive Effects

Although the psychological consequences of developing a chronic disease are primarily negative, people often experience some positive effects, such as feeling closer and more in touch with family and friends, having a greater appreciation of life, and changing life goals and priorities (Collins et al., 2001; Mohr et al., 1999; Schwartzberg, 1993; Stuckey et al., 2014; Updegraff, Taylor, Kemeny, & Wyatt, 2002). Receiving a diagnosis of chronic illness can encourage people to live life to the fullest and focus on achieving their dreams instead of delaying them. As writer Michael Kinsley, who has Parkinson's disease, notes, "It's like having a get-out of jail free card from the prison of delayed gratification. Skip the Democratic convention to go kayaking in Alaska? Absolutely. Do it now, in case you can't do it later." (2001). Moreover, and as described in **Focus on Development**, people with a chronic disease may be better able to cope with the relatively minor stresses of daily life.

Receiving a chronic illness diagnosis can even lead people to engage in health-promoting behavior. One study with nearly 3,000 HIV-positive people found that following their diagnosis, 43% increased their exercise, 59% improved their diet, and 49% of smokers decreased their smoking (Collins et al., 2001). Many people with diabetes report engaging in similar types of broad lifestyle changes (Stuckey et al., 2014). Not surprisingly, these improvements in health-related behavior can lead to better physical outcomes, including fewer side effects and slower disease progression, as you'll learn about later in this chapter.

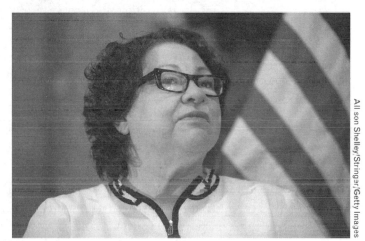

Allson Shelley/Stringer/Getty Images

Supreme Court Justice Sonia Sotomayor was diagnosed with Type 1 diabetes at age seven. She credits having this disorder with giving her discipline, developed from years of managing her disease, which helped her succeed in her academic studies.

FACTORS INFLUENCING REACTIONS TO CHRONIC DISEASE

LO 10.4

Explain factors influencing reactions to chronic disease

The extent of difficulty people have in coping with a chronic illness varies as a function of illness factors, personal factors, and social factors. This section examines three distinct factors that impact how people cope with a chronic illness: illness intrusiveness, coping strategies, and social support.

Illness Intrusiveness

Chronic diseases vary in the extent to which they interrupt or interfere with a person's daily life. Illnesses that require major lifestyle changes, either due to preventing their symptoms or following treatment, are more intrusive in a person's life, and thereby are more difficult to cope with. For example, people with asthma who see their illness as more intrusive show higher levels of anxiety and depression (Carpentier, Mullins, & Van Pelt, 2007).

In many cases, people must make major changes in lifestyle in order to avoid exacerbating their conditions. These changes might include avoiding unhealthy foods, stopping smoking, and starting an exercise program. For example, patients with diabetes must limit the sugar in their diets, and patients with coronary heart disease (CHD) must eat healthier foods and give up cigarettes. In some cases, people are even told to avoid certain locations and activities. People with asthma, for example, often must avoid spending time outside when pollen counts are high, and those who have experienced a heart attack may be asked to avoid stressful situations, strenuous activities, and heavy lifting. In turn, these changes can lead to anxiety, depression, and social withdrawal, particularly in cases in which managing the disease interferes with a person's daily life, including work, social, and recreational activities (Devins et al., 1990; Talbot, Nowven, Gingras, Belanger, & Audet, 1999).

People with chronic diseases must also engage in relatively complex behaviors to monitor their conditions and manage their treatment regimens (Devins & Binik, 1996). For example, a person with diabetes must monitor blood glucose levels to avoid both sugar shortage and insulin shock and must administer (by injection) appropriate amounts of insulin regularly. However, many people with diabetes find this constant maintenance tedious and fail to follow their treatment regimen. Similarly, people who are HIV-positive should start antiretroviral therapy, a combination of different medicines designed to decrease the spread of HIV. But these drugs need to be taken every day, and thus require strict adherence to avoid developing a resistance to these drugs.

What You'll Learn 10.3

Researchers in one study examined factors associated with children's ability to self-manage their diabetes (Maranda & Gupta, 2016). Children between the ages of 9 and 19 were asked whether they had a pet at home, and, if so, whether they were actively involved in its care. Researchers also gathered information from their doctor on whether they were successfully keeping their glucose levels in an acceptable range. Children who reported caring for one or more pets at home were 2.5 times more likely to have control over their glucose levels than those who did not care for a pet, even after researchers took into account children's age, socioeconomic status, and duration of the disease. Although this study did not directly test how caring for a pet helps children manage their diabetes, researchers believe it may increase children's general feelings of responsibility, provide a daily routine, and/or improve their overall mood.

Another factor that influences the experience of having a chronic disease is the patients' continued dependence on health care professionals and biomedical technology (Devins & Binik, 1996). Patients with severe kidney disease, for example, must undergo dialysis, a procedure in which the blood is cleaned to remove excess salts, water, and waste products, three times a week for an average of four to six hours per session. Although they may experience frustration with their disease and treatment, which can influence their feelings toward health care workers, maintaining communication is an important part of managing their illness. Patients must also deal with medical professionals with great regularity and can experience difficulties in these relationships (e.g., understanding a physician's communications, expressing feelings, maintaining a sense of control over treatment options). You'll learn more about some of these issues in patient–practitioner relationships in *Chapter 13: Managing Health Care*.

Coping Strategies

As discussed in *Chapter 5: Managing Stress*, people cope with stressful situations in very different ways, which in turn lead to very different outcomes. This section examines various strategies people may use, including problem-focused coping, emotion-focused coping, and perceiving control over the disease.

Problem-Focused Coping

Problem-focused coping strategies focus on dealing directly with the source of the stress and trying to reduce its impact (Aspinwall & Taylor, 1997; Carver, Scheier, & Weintraub, 1989). For people with a chronic disease, this type of coping could include coming up with a strategy to solve a particular side effect, gathering advice on how to treat the disease, or taking action to reduce the effects of the disease. For example, a person with diabetes could avoid experiencing a drop in blood sugar by regularly eating small meals to keep blood sugar at a consistent level, and a person with asthma could make sure to check pollen counts before deciding whether to exercise outside that day.

Because problem-focused coping helps eliminate or reduce an aspect of the disease or its treatment, these approaches are often helpful in reducing the negative effects of chronic diseases. Specifically, people with a chronic disease who seek information about the illness and its treatment show lower levels of depression and better overall adjustment (Felton & Revenson, 1984; Fleishman & Fogel, 1994; Macrodimitris & Endler, 2001). For example, people with multiple sclerosis who rely more on problem-focused coping are less depressed and felt better about their health (Pakenham, 1999). Similarly, adults with diabetes who use more direct and problem-focused coping strategies experience lower levels of anxiety and depression than those who engage in wishful thinking (e.g., wishing the situation would go away or be over) and withdrawal (e.g., sleeping more than usual, avoiding being with people) (Macrodimitris & Endler, 2001). The use of problem-focused coping may even lead to better physical outcomes. In line with this view, HIV-positive men who use problem-focused coping show greater immune system activity (Goodkin et al., 1992).

Emotion-Focused Coping

Emotion-focused coping strategies focus on managing the reaction to stress, although not the cause of the stress itself (Carver et al., 1989). This approach is most useful in cases in which people believe they have little or no ability to directly reduce or avoid the stressor. However, emotion-focused coping can include many distinct approaches, including denying and avoiding the diagnosis completely, accepting the diagnosis but reappraising it in a positive way, and adopting religious and/or spiritual beliefs. (Seeking social support is another type of emotion-focused coping, and will be addressed in the following section.)

DENIAL AND AVOIDANCE. Emotion-focused coping can include both escape–avoidance (trying to avoid the situation) and distancing (trying to stop thinking about the problem). Both of these types of emotion-focused coping rely on avoiding the stressor. These forms of emotion-focused coping are generally associated with negative outcomes, including higher levels of depression and anxiety (Fleishman & Fogel, 1994; Leserman, Perkins, & Evans, 1992; Macrodimitris & Endler, 2001). Patients with spinal cord injuries, for example, show greater distress when they focus on wishful thinking (e.g., imagining the accident didn't happen) as opposed to a realistic acceptance of their condition (Buckelew, Baumstark, Frank, & Hewett, 1990). This type of unrealistic optimism, such as trying to mentally "undo" an event, inhibits the person from adapting to the condition and in turn adopting new, more realistic goals and expectations about the future.

Denial may also decrease people's willingness to follow medical advice or seek prompt treatment and can therefore lead to negative health outcomes. For example, adolescents with diabetes who use avoidant coping—such as downplaying the seriousness of their disease and trying not to think about it—feel more overwhelmed by their disease later on (Iturralde, Weissberg-Benchell, & Hood, 2017). They also show less adherence to medical recommendations for managing diabetes, such as not testing their blood glucose levels and carrying quick-acting sugar products to treat low blood sugar, which can result in serious health problems. Similarly, early treatment following HIV infection can substantially improve longer-term health outcomes.

Although avoidance coping is generally a destructive coping technique, this approach can be especially adaptive in the short term, at least in the case of some diseases. Specifically, immediately after receiving a diagnosis of chronic illness, denying this reality may help people cope with the very threatening and upsetting news (Taylor & Aspinwall, 1993). Pretending to not have the disease and attempting to let it affect daily life as little as possible reduces the threat of the illness and thereby decreases anxiety, which can help people cope with the devastating news diagnosis. This strategy may be especially helpful in the case of diseases without a cure, such as Parkinson's and Huntington's.

POSITIVE REAPPRAISAL. Emotion-focused coping can also include positive reappraisal, meaning trying to think about a negative situation in a new way. Not surprisingly, people who are able to find benefits in having a chronic disease experience more positive mood and quality of life (Leserman et al., 1992; Pakenham, 2005). For example, people with diabetes who see benefits to their disease have fewer symptoms of depression and feel better able to cope with the challenges of this disease (Stuckey et al., 2014; Tran, Wiebe, Fortenberry, Butler, & Berg, 2011). Positive reappraisal may also have important benefits for improving symptoms and disease progression. For instance, among men who are HIV-positive, those who find some meaning in their condition, such as shifting their values and priorities, show slower declines in their T cell levels and survive for longer periods of time (Bower, Kemeny, Taylor, & Fahey, 1998).

What You'll Learn
10.4

Interestingly, simply adopting a stronger focus on the positive in one's life can lead to improvements in psychological and physical well-being. To examine whether focusing on the positive would benefit physical health, researchers in one recent study assigned people who were recently diagnosed with HIV to one of two conditions (Moskowitz et al., 2017). Half of the participants were taught a set of skills over five weekly sessions to help them experience more positive emotions. These skills included the following:

- Recognizing a positive event each day, and either logging it in a journal or telling someone else about it

- Keeping a daily gratitude journal

- Listing a personal strength each day and how they had used this strength recently

- Setting an attainable goal each day and noting their progress toward reaching it

- Doing a small act of kindness each day

- Practicing mindfulness through a daily 10-minute breathing exercise

Participants in the control group completed interviews—which focused on social support, use of complementary and alternative medicine, physical activity, and finding meaning—with a trained facilitator for five weeks. Fifteen months after the intervention, 91% of those in the positive emotion group had a reduced level of HIV in the body, compared to only 76% of those in the control condition. Moreover, whereas initially about 17% of people in both the positive-emotions and control groups were using antidepressants, at the 15-month follow-up there was no increase in antidepressant use among those who received training in positive emotions but 35% of those in the control condition now reported using antidepressants. These findings point to the benefits of helping people with chronic diseases focus on ways of feeling happier in their daily lives, and how such a focus can lead to benefits in both psychological and physical health.

ADOPTING RELIGIOUS/SPIRITUAL BELIEFS. Another form of emotion-focused coping used by some people with a chronic disease is adopting religious and/or spiritual beliefs. For example, 25% of adults who are diagnosed with HIV/AIDS report being more religious, 41% report being "more spiritual," and 75% report that this illness has strengthened their faith (Cotton, Puchalski, et al., 2006; Cotton, Tsevat, et al., 2006). The use of religious coping is particularly likely to occur shortly after diagnosis, when people are gathering their coping resources (Gall, Guirguis-Younger, Charbonneau, & Florack, 2009).

For many people, the adoption of religious and spiritual beliefs is associated with improved health-related quality of life as well as psychosocial functioning (Gall, Kristjansson, Charbonneau, & Florack, 2009; Wildes, Miller, de Majors, & Ramirez, 2009; Zavala, Maliski, Kwan, Fink, & Litwin, 2009). Moreover, even in cases in which religious beliefs do not directly affect adjustment to having a chronic disease, people may experience an enhanced sense of social support from a community with whom they share those beliefs, which in turn leads to better well-being (Howsepian & Merluzzi, 2009).

Perceiving Control

Several studies have examined the influence of people's perceived controllability of the disease on psychological distress and well-being. For example, asthma patients who are confident in their ability to control symptoms experience better asthma control and quality of life (Lavoie et al., 2008). Similarly, HIV-positive men who feel they have control over their disease outcome and believe they can accept their disease show better adjustment and lower levels of depression (Thompson, Nanni, & Levine, 1994).

In contrast, people who believe that the disease will progress and that they have low control over its development experience negative psychological and physical outcomes. For example, one study with HIV-positive men found that those who attributed negative events to themselves had a faster rate of immune decline over the next 18 months than those without this type of attribution pattern (see Table 10.3; Segerstrom, Taylor, Kemeny, Reed, & Visscher, 1996). Similarly, women with a pessimistic outlook show lower NK cell activity and T cell levels and hence are less able to fight off their HIV progression (Byrnes et al., 1998). People who are HIV-positive and hold negative expectations about their ability to control the disease also show a faster progression to AIDS and develop symptoms of HIV earlier than those without such beliefs (e.g., diarrhea, weight loss, high fever, night sweats), even when researchers take into account other variables, such as health behaviors, depression, age, and treatment (Reed, Kemeny, Taylor, & Visscher, 1999; Reed, Kemeny, Taylor, Wang, & Visscher, 1994). They also die, on average, nine months earlier.

Understanding the Mechanisms

Although this section has described the association between various forms of coping and both psychological and physical outcomes for people with chronic diseases, much of this research demonstrates an association between particular coping styles and outcomes but not the mechanisms explaining this relationship. One potential explanation is that people who adopt positive coping styles, and perceive high levels of control over their illness, are then more motivated to engage in health-promoting behaviors, such as following medical regimens and adapting a healthy lifestyle. These behaviors, in turn, lead to a stronger immune system, fewer symptoms, and slower disease progression. Alternatively, other factors account

Table 10.3	Examples of Negative and Positive Attributions in HIV-Positive Men

Negative

I lost a couple of friends because I am HIV-positive.

Sometimes at work I just feel isolated because I'm the only person that's gay there.

I would imagine that my T cell count would get lower because over time that's the way it goes.

Positive

To actually die of AIDS or AIDS-related complications is less likely because I think effective therapies will continue to be developed.

I've never felt much isolation because I've always benefited from having other people there . . . who share their feelings, support, and love with me.

I am less likely than other HIV-positive gay men to experience health problems related to AIDS. I think most gay men were promiscuous. . . . I just was not very promiscuous.

HIV-positive men who tend to make negative attributions show a faster decline in immune system functioning than those who tend to make positive attributions.

Source: Segerstrom et al. (1996).

for the association between the use of particular coping styles and positive outcomes. For example, among women living with HIV/AIDS, those with more emotional support show higher levels of personal growth (Siegel, Schrimshaw, & Pretter, 2005). Similarly, people with chronic diseases who have adequate financial resources or comprehensive health insurance may find coping with a diagnosis less stressful, which in turn leads to better psychological and physical well-being. In sum, many of these studies reveal a *correlation* between particular coping styles and particular outcomes but do not necessarily demonstrate that the use of a specific coping style *causes* a particular outcome.

Social Support

As described in ***Chapter 5: Managing Stress***, social support is a very important predictor of psychological well-being in patients with chronic illness (Taylor & Aspinwall, 1993). Studies with patients with AIDS indicate that those who receive higher levels of social support from their family and friends experience lower levels of anxiety, depression, and anger (Hays, Turner, & Coates, 1992; Namir, Alumbaugh, Fawzy, & Wolcott, 1989; Pakenham, Dadds, & Terry, 1994). Similarly, people with diabetes who receive support from people around them are better able to cope with the psychosocial challenges of this disease (Stuckey et al., 2014).

Social support is also associated with better physical well-being in patients with chronic illness (Taylor & Aspinwall, 1993). Chronic disease patients who receive more social support report experiencing better physical health, including experiencing fewer symptoms, recovering more rapidly from surgery, and requiring less pain medication (Ashton et al., 2005; Namir et al., 1989). For example, patients with knee osteoarthritis whose spouses are more empathically responsive to their pain expression show better physical function over the next 18 months compared with those whose spouses are less empathically responsive (Wilson, Martire, & Sliwinski, 2017). Moreover, among people who are HIV-positive, those who have higher levels of social support show slower progression to AIDS, even when researchers take into account age, health-related behaviors, and medication use (Leserman et al., 1999;

Pakenham et al., 1994; Theorell et al., 1995). These findings provide powerful evidence that the presence of social support can slow the progression of a chronic disease.

Social support improves psychological and physical well-being for people with chronic diseases in a number of distinct ways. First, and as discussed previously, receiving a diagnosis of a chronic illness is associated with various types of stress, and people who have high levels of social support are clearly better able to buffer the effects of such stress (Brown, Wallston, & Nicassio, 1989; Rini, Jandorf, Valdimarsdottir, Brown, & Itzkowitz, 2008). Second, social support may lead to the use of healthier coping strategies, such as positive reappraisal and perceived control. In line with this view, HIV-positive men who are satisfied with the level of support from their social networks report using more adaptive coping strategies (Leserman et al., 1992). People who receive more social support are also more likely to engage in health-promoting behaviors (Heckman, Kelly, & Somlai, 1998). For example, gay men with high levels of social support engage in less sexual risk taking (Darbes & Lewis, 2005). In some cases, family members and friends may even adopt healthier behaviors themselves as a sign of support, such as in the case of a person with diabetes who needs to maintain a healthier diet and engage in regular physical activity (Stuckey et al., 2014). Social support also improves adherence to medical recommendations, which in turn leads to better health outcomes. For example, a study of patients with kidney disease revealed that those with higher levels of support were more likely to follow their doctors' orders (such as controlling weight) and continue with dialysis (Untas et al., 2010). As described previously, HIV-positive men with large social networks live longer (Patterson et al., 1996). Interestingly, social support in some cases can cause emotional distress yet also be beneficial for physical health, as described in **Research in Action**.

RESEARCH IN ACTION

Why a Nagging Spouse May Be Good for Men's Health

Researchers in one study examined data from over 12,000 married people over the course of five years to assess whether marital quality predicted the development of diabetes over time (Liu, Waite, & Shen, 2016). Both members of the couple completed measures of marital quality, depression, and health-related behaviors (BMI, smoking, alcohol use, and physical activity). In addition, the researchers collected blood samples to test for levels of blood sugar to measure diabetes risk. Five years later, researchers again collected the same measures from all participants. Their findings revealed striking—and unexpected—gender differences in the link between marriage quality and risk of diabetes. Specifically, for women, having a good marriage at the start of the study was associated with a lower likelihood of developing diabetes five years later. These findings are in line with those from other research showing that good relationships are often associated with better health, and that women—who may be more sensitive to the quality of a relationship than men—may particularly benefit from such positive bonds. For men, on the other hand, an increase in negative marital quality was associated with a lower likelihood of developing diabetes and, for those who acquired diabetes, better management of the disease. Although these findings were unexpected, they may indicate that wives who nag their husbands to watch their health, such as pushing them to engage in regular exercise and avoid unhealthy foods, may be perceived as irritating, but this nagging is actually beneficial for men's health over time. Similarly, men whose wives push them to follow treatment recommendations may find such reminders annoying, but as a result show greater adherence, which in turn leads to better health. These findings therefore suggest that for men, an unhappy marriage may both reduce the risk of developing diabetes and, for those with diabetes, slow disease progression.

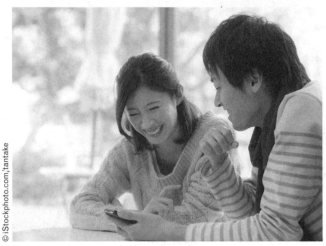

Simply having someone to share thoughts and feelings with helps people with chronic diseases relieve stress, which in turn can lead to improved physical health.

Perhaps most important, social support allows people with chronic diseases to express and process their emotions (Stanton, Parsa, & Austenfeld, 2002). Being able to share their thoughts and feelings about the disease and its treatment helps reduce the stress associated with having this disease. Such disclosure can, at least in some cases, have valuable health benefits. For example, HIV-positive men who show higher levels of emotional disclosure and processing of trauma experience greater immunological benefits in terms of number of NK cells, which in turn leads to survival advantages (O'Cleirigh, Ironson, Fletcher, & Schneiderman, 2008). HIV-positive men who hide their sexual orientation, on the other hand, and are thereby less able to receive support from others, experience negative health outcomes, including a faster progression to AIDS (Cole, Kemeny, Taylor, Visscher, & Fahey, 1996).

Interestingly, even expressing thoughts and feelings about the disease in writing—and not to another person—can lead to beneficial health outcomes. As shown in Figure 10.3, people with asthma or arthritis who write about stressful life experiences show improvements in their symptoms four months later. They also show improvements in lung function (for people with asthma) and disease severity (for people with arthritis), whereas those in the control group show no such changes.

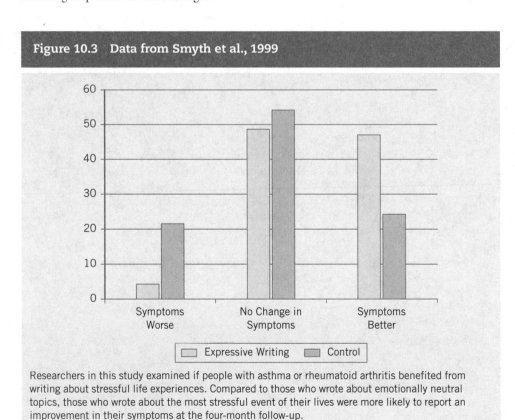

Figure 10.3   Data from Smyth et al., 1999

Researchers in this study examined if people with asthma or rheumatoid arthritis benefited from writing about stressful life experiences. Compared to those who wrote about emotionally neutral topics, those who wrote about the most stressful event of their lives were more likely to report an improvement in their symptoms at the four-month follow-up.

Source: Data from Smyth, Stone, Hurewitz, & Kaell (1999).

STRATEGIES FOR MANAGING A CHRONIC ILLNESS

Given all the problems associated with having a chronic disease, how can people adjust effectively to such a diagnosis? Research suggests several different approaches that may have positive effects on patients' psychological adjustment as well as physical symptoms. These approaches include providing information and education, encouraging physical activity, training in cognitive-behavioral techniques, and utilizing social support groups.

LO 10.5

Describe strategies for coping with a chronic disease

Provide Information and Education

One of the most common approaches to helping people adapt to a chronic disease is providing information about the psychological and physical symptoms of their disease and its treatment (Taylor & Aspinwall, 1993). Patients and their families who receive this knowledge feel more "in control" of the disease and its course; they also show greater adherence to medical regimens that help them manage their conditions. Education programs to help people cope with asthma, for example, teach patients about the physiology and mechanisms of breathing, what happens during as asthma attack, and how medicine works to counteract such an attack (Lehrer, Feldman, Giardino, Song, & Schmaling, 2002). They also learn behavioral techniques for preventing and controlling asthma attacks, including common triggers for such an attack. Providing this type of education decreases patients' anxiety about asthma and reduces the use of medical services; not surprisingly, patients with asthma who participate in an education program show fewer symptoms. Similarly, patients with diabetes who receive information from a health care provider about various aspects of managing the disease (such as having eye and foot exams, blood pressure checks, and urine tests to measure kidney function) report greater satisfaction with their health care and overall health (Corathers et al., 2017).

Education interventions can also lead to improvements in physical health. For example, people recently diagnosed with diabetes who participated in a brief self-management intervention, which emphasized the importance of planning ahead to carry out self-care behaviors, achieved sustained health improvements (Thoolen, Ridder, Bensing, Gorter, & Rutten, 2009). The intervention led to improvements in diet and physical activity behavior, and significant weight loss at the one-year follow-up.

Educational interventions can be especially useful when they involve collaboration with health care professionals. For example, researchers in one study examined whether coordinated care management of multiple conditions improved disease control in patients with diabetes and/or coronary heart disease (Katon et al., 2010). Patients were randomly assigned to the usual-care group or to the intervention group, in which a nurse, working with each patient's primary care physician, provided clear guidelines for managing the risk factors associated with multiple diseases. Compared to those in the control, patients in the intervention group showed greater improvement one year later in terms of cholesterol, blood pressure, and depression. Patients in the intervention group also reported experiencing a better overall quality of life as well as greater satisfaction with the care they received. Similarly, patient support programs (PSPs), meaning interventions for patients requiring ongoing medication to manage symptoms and/or disease progression, provide counseling, training, support, and reminders to approve adherence to medical recommendations (Ganguli, Clewell, & Shillington, 2016). PSPs improve treatment adherence and quality of life and reduce functional impairments caused by the disease.

Encourage Physical Activity

Engaging in regular physical activity helps reduce symptoms of chronic diseases, including functional impairment and pain (Hoffmann et al., 2016). For example, older adults with knee osteoarthritis who engage in even as little as 45 minutes of moderate activity, such as brisk walking, show improved functioning compared to those who do less (Dunlop et al., 2017). Similarly, although people with asthma are often reluctant to exercise due to concern about triggering an asthma attack, people with asthma who are randomly assigned to engage in moderate levels of aerobic exercise—walking on a treadmill for 30 minutes twice a week—report reduced severity of asthma symptoms and improved quality of life (França-Pinto et al., 2015). Engaging in other types of physical activity, such as yoga, is also associated with increases in physical functioning and decreases in pain (Moonaz, Bingham, Wissow, & Bartlett, 2015).

Because regular exercise helps promote weight loss, such activity may be especially beneficial for people with particular chronic diseases. People with knee osteoarthritis who maintain a healthy weight, for example, are better able to protect their joints. Similarly, for people with diabetes, engaging in regular exercise helps decrease not only weight but also blood pressure, blood glucose, and cholesterol, which in turn reduces the risk of heart disease and nerve damage.

Exercise may also reduce negative psychological consequences of chronic diseases, such as stress, anxiety, and depression (Moonaz et al., 2015). In line with this view, one study of men who were HIV-positive found that engaging in either an aerobic exercise or resistance weight-training intervention was associated with increases in positive well-being and decreases in psychological distress (Lox, McAuley, & Tucker, 1996). Similarly, people with Parkinson's disease who participate in an exercise program—involving cardiovascular as well as resistance training—show lower levels of depression than those in the control group (Park et al., 2013).

What You'll Learn

10.5

Recent evidence suggests that engaging in regular exercise may also help improve cognitive functioning in older adults with dementia. Researchers in one study examined the effects of a 12-week walking program with older adults, ages 60 to 88 (Chirles et al., 2017). Half of the people in this study were healthy older adults; the others had been diagnosed with mild cognitive impairments. All participants completed an exercise intervention, which included walking four times a week for 30 minutes over three months. Both before and after this exercise intervention, participants completed standard memory tests and underwent fMRI brain scans so that researchers could examine any changes that might be caused by the intervention. Both groups of people showed improved scores on memory tests, suggesting that engaging in regular exercise may boost cognitive performance generally in older adults. But most important, participants with mild cognitive impairment showed increased functional connection between brain regions after completing the exercise program. (There were no such changes for participants without this impairment.) These findings provide strong evidence that engaging in physical activity may help reestablish connections within the brain that may disappear as symptoms of Alzheimer's disease progress.

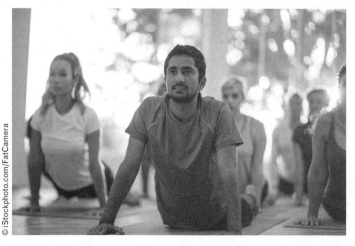

Patients with chronic disease benefit from interventions that reduce stress, such as meditation, yoga, and mindfulness training.

© iStockphoto.com/FatCamera

Perhaps most important, engaging in regular physical activity may potentially slow disease progression. For example, engaging in regular aerobic exercise can help improve immune functioning and thereby delay the progression of HIV infection (LaPerriere et al., 1990; Solomon, 1991). Similarly, patients with Parkinson's disease who exercise for 150 minutes a week show slower declines in quality of life and mobility over two years compared to people who do not exercise or exercise less frequently (Rafferty et al., 2017).

Interventions that emphasize increasing physical activity as well as making other types of lifestyle changes, such as eating a healthier diet, are particularly beneficial for people with chronic diseases that are heavily influenced by lifestyle factors. For example, people with diabetes who receive an intensive lifestyle intervention (weekly group and individual counseling for the first six months, plus twice-monthly contact for the next three and a half years) show substantially more improvements in weight loss and increased physical fitness than those who receive only three group sessions focused on support and education per year (Gregg et al., 2012). Most important, and as shown in Figure 10.4, a higher percentage of patients who receive a lifestyle intervention show either partial or complete remission, meaning they no longer are seen as having diabetes. Although intensive lifestyle interventions are expensive, they can lead to substantial reductions in the prevalence of chronic diseases, which in turn reduces overall treatment costs.

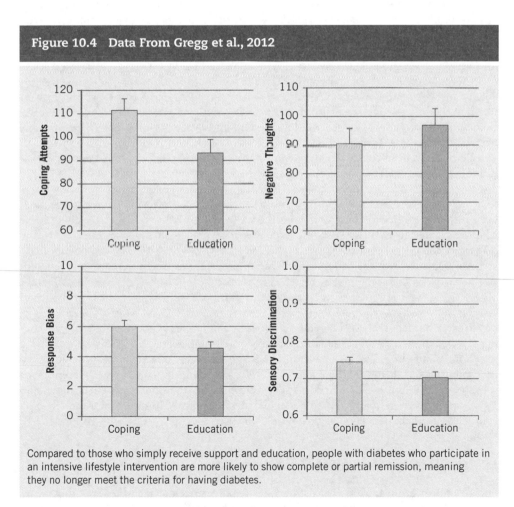

Figure 10.4   Data From Gregg et al., 2012

Compared to those who simply receive support and education, people with diabetes who participate in an intensive lifestyle intervention are more likely to show complete or partial remission, meaning they no longer meet the criteria for having diabetes.

Source: Data from Gregg, Chen, Wagenknecht, Clark, Delahanty, Bantle, . . . Pi-Sunyer (2012).

Train in Cognitive-Behavioral Techniques

Cognitive-behavioral approaches focus on challenging individuals' irrational beliefs about their condition and providing training in coping skills to handle their illness (Devins & Binik, 1996; Parker, 1995). For example, a therapist or doctor could challenge the belief held by a person with epilepsy that he or she will never get married.

Such approaches are especially effective when they provide specific strategies for managing stress. As described previously, people who are diagnosed with a chronic disease often experience considerable stress, and stress can increase both symptoms and disease progression (thereby setting up a vicious negative cycle) (Kemeny, 1994). For example, asthma attacks and epileptic seizures may be brought on by stress, and hence training in various techniques to help manage stress can decrease the likelihood of experiencing such symptoms (Lehrer et al., 2002; Parker, 1995). (Specific techniques for reducing stress and pain are described in detail in **Chapter 5: Managing Stress** and **Chapter 9: Understanding and Managing Pain**.) Stress may also increase the speed at which HIV is replicated, causing a quicker progression to AIDS (Leserman et al., 1999; Remor, Penedo, Shen, & Schneiderman, 2007).

Cognitive-behavioral training is an effective strategy for improving mental health in people with a chronic disease (Agras, Taylor, Kraemer, Southam, & Schneider, 1987; Crepaz et al., 2008). Studies with people with HIV indicate that people who receive training in stress management (including help with thinking through daily stressors in a new way, relying more on social support, and increasing assertiveness while decreasing anger) and relaxation (including progressive muscle relaxation, meditation, and guided imagery) show lower levels of anxiety, anger, and stress and improved quality of life (Antoni et al., 2000; Cruess et al., 2000; Scott-Sheldon, Kalichman, Carey, & Fielder, 2008). Similarly, people with inflammatory bowel disease, an intestinal disorder that causes persistent pain and diarrhea, who receive training in mindfulness-based stress reduction show improvements in depression, anxiety, and overall quality of life (Neilson et al., 2016).

Perhaps even more important, cognitive-behavioral interventions can improve physical well-being in people with chronic diseases. Patients with sickle cell anemia, a rare blood disease that causes severe pain, who receiving training in relaxing and distraction show lower levels of negative thinking and pain than those who simply receive education about their disease (Gil et al., 1996). Such training can have long-term effects, suggesting that people who are trained in using such skills are then able to implement them in their daily lives (Gil et al., 2000).

Although some of the cognitive-behavioral interventions described thus far are intensive in terms of time and money, briefer interventions can also be effective. For example, people living with HIV/AIDS who receive a 12-session coping improvement group intervention delivered via teleconference report fewer psychological symptoms, lower levels of life-stressor burden, increased coping self-efficacy, and less frequent use of avoidance coping (Heckman et al., 2006). Similarly, people with chronic heart problems who receive six telephone counseling sessions to identify and address illness-related fears show improved psychological well-being (McLaughlin et al., 2005). Specifically, patients who receive such calls show a 27% improvement in depression symptoms, a 27% improvement in anxiety, and a 38% improvement in home limitations compared with controls. In sum, even relatively brief counseling can help patients adjust to chronic illness.

Utilize Social Support Groups

Social support groups, which consist of other people suffering from the same illness, are another effective way of helping people cope with chronic diseases (Devins & Binik, 1996).

This approach gives people an opportunity to compare coping strategies and solutions to daily problems and provide social support to each other. They can share emotions and discuss topics such as physical problems, communication with physicians, relationships with family members, finding meaning in life, and facing death. One meta-analysis examining the effects of social support groups on people living with HIV found such participation was associated with a number of positive outcomes, including lower levels of depression, anxiety, and HIV-related symptoms (Bateganya, Amanyeiwe, Roxo, & Dong, 2015).

These groups may be particularly effective when participants have the opportunity to share their own successful coping strategies with others. Researchers in one study randomly assigned patients with kidney disease to either a problem-disclosure group (people described their difficulties in coping with the illness), a self-presentation group (people described the strategies they used to cope effectively with their disease), or a control group (people saw a videotape on effective coping with dialysis) (Leake, Friend, & Wadhwa, 1999). At the one-month follow-up, people in the self-presentation group had lower rates of depression and fewer physical symptoms than people in the control group or the problem disclosure group. Apparently talking about how well you are coping, as opposed to focusing on how many problems you are having, may be an effective way of helping patients with chronic disease manage their illnesses, presumably because this approach helps patients generate their own coping strategies.

Table 10.4 Information YOU Can Use

- People with chronic diseases really benefit from receiving social support, both in informal ways (from family and friends) and through organized social support. Given the benefits of social support for coping with a chronic disease, seek out such support if you are diagnosed with a chronic disease, and find ways to provide such support to your loved ones with a chronic condition.

- People who can see the benefits of having a chronic disease, and find meaning in this diagnosis, experience better physical and psychological well-being. So, if you or a loved one is diagnosed with such a disease, try to focus on the positives and not just the negatives.

- Stress impacts the likelihood of developing a chronic disease and the ability to cope with such a diagnosis. Therefore, make sure to reduce the amount of stress in your life whenever possible, and take deliberate—and healthy—steps to manage the stress you experience.

- College students are at high risk for becoming infected with HIV or another sexually transmitted disease, so make sure to protect yourself. Use condoms whenever you have sex, even if the person doesn't seem risky, you are highly physically aroused, or you don't know how he or she will react to this request. Protecting yourself from such infection is just too important.

- Virtually all chronic conditions are influenced by behavioral choices, so make sure to make wise health-related decisions to protect yourself from developing such a disease: eat a healthy diet, engage in regular physical activity, use alcohol in moderation, and, most important, don't smoke.

Understanding Chronic Diseases

- Acute diseases generally develop quickly and last only a relatively short time. In contrast, chronic diseases often have a slow onset, may have multiple causes, and can't be cured.

- Although children and adolescents are more likely to experience acute diseases, they are at risk of developing certain chronic diseases, such as asthma, cystic fibrosis, and diabetes. Chronic diseases are far more prevalent in older adults.

- Chronic diseases exert a substantial cost on individuals and on society; in fact, seven of the top 10 causes of death are chronic diseases. Non-life-threatening chronic diseases cause serious health problems, including blindness, amputations, and disability. Chronic diseases, and the health-related behaviors that contribute to such diseases, account for the majority of health care costs in the United States

Common Types of Chronic Disease

- Diabetes is a disorder in which the body is unable to properly convert glucose (sugar) into usable energy. *Type 1 diabetes* occurs when the body can't produce enough insulin, whereas *Type 2 diabetes*, the most common type of diabetes, occurs when the body can't properly use insulin. *Gestational diabetes* is a temporary form of diabetes caused by a woman's inability to produce an adequate amount of insulin while pregnant. Genetic factors contribute to the risk of diabetes, as does age and ethnicity, with older people and people of color having a greater likelihood of developing diabetes. People who are obese and engage in low levels of physical activity are also at greater risk.

- The term arthritis refers to more than 100 different types of diseases and conditions that affect the joints and/or tissues surrounding the joints. Symptoms of diseases within this category include pain, swelling, and stiffness in the joints. The risk of developing arthritis increases with age. Women are somewhat more likely to be diagnosed with arthritis than men, and Whites and Native Americans are more likely to be diagnosed with arthritis than people in other racial ethnic groups. Additional risk factors for arthritis include obesity, other chronic diseases, injuries, infections, and repetitive movements.

- AIDS is a set of symptoms and illnesses that are caused by the human immunodeficiency virus (HIV), a virus that attacks the body's immune system. HIV transmission occurs through engaging in unprotected sex and sharing needles when injecting drugs. Men having sex with men is the largest route of transmission of HIV in the United States. Whites and Asians are at substantially lower risk of acquiring HIV than Native Americans, Latinos, and, especially, Blacks.

- Alzheimer's disease is a progressive brain disorder that damages and destroys brain cells, causing serious problems with memory, thinking, language, and behavior. The single biggest risk factor for Alzheimer's disease is age. Alzheimer's disease is also more common in women than in men, and in people of color than in Whites. Both genetic factors and environmental factors, such as diet and exercise, influence the risk of developing Alzheimer's.

Consequences of Chronic Disease

- Many people with chronic diseases experience some type of physical debilitation, such as paralysis, disfigurement, incontinence, and pain. In other cases, the disease itself is not debilitating, but the treatment for it is quite destructive to health. The physical problems caused by the symptoms or treatment for a chronic disease may affect people's employment, which in turn can have major financial implications.

- Many people with chronic diseases experience some type of sexual problem.

- One of the most difficult aspects of coping with a chronic illness is the effect it can have on interpersonal relationships. Friends may withdraw from the patient, and people with chronic diseases may withdraw from many social relationships. Even when family members and friends want to help, they simply may not have realistic conceptions of what the patient is going through. Spouses as well as other family members of people with chronic illnesses may also experience negative psychological reactions when a loved one is diagnosed with a chronic illness.

- People who are diagnosed with a chronic illness often experience an initial sense of shock and disbelief. Depression, especially in cases of severe and life-threatening illnesses, and anxiety are also common psychological problems. However, many of the negative psychological consequences of having a chronic disease are most apparent immediately after diagnosis and fade over time.

- People often experience some positive effects from having a chronic disease. Receiving a chronic illness diagnosis can even lead people to engage in health-promoting behavior.

Factors Influencing Reactions to Chronic Disease

- Illnesses that require major lifestyle changes are more intrusive in a person's life, and thereby are more difficult to cope with. People with chronic diseases must also engage in relatively complex behaviors to monitor their conditions and manage their treatment regimens, and they depend on health care professionals and biomedical technology.

- People cope with stressful situations in very different ways, which in turn lead to very different outcomes. Problem-focused coping strategies focus on dealing directly with the source of the stress and trying to reduce its impact. These approaches are often helpful in reducing the negative effects of chronic diseases. Emotion-focused coping strategies focus on managing the reaction to stress, although not the cause of the stress itself. Emotion-focused coping strategies that rely on avoiding the stressor are generally associated with negative outcomes. However, positive reappraisal and adopting religious and spiritual beliefs generally lead to improvements in psychological and physical well-being. People who believe that they have control over their disease experience better psychological and physical outcomes.

- Social support improves psychological and physical well-being for people with chronic diseases. First, people with high levels of social support are better able to buffer the effects of the stress caused by a chronic disease. Social support may lead to the use of healthier coping strategies as well as engaging in health-promoting behaviors. Perhaps most important, social support allows people with chronic diseases to express and process their emotions.

Strategies for Managing a Chronic Illness

- Providing information about the psychological and physical symptoms of a disease and its treatment can help people cope with this diagnosis. Patients and their families who receive this knowledge feel more "in control" of the disease and show greater adherence to medical regimens that help them manage their conditions. Education interventions that involve collaboration with health care professionals are especially useful.

- Engaging in physical activity helps reduces symptoms of chronic diseases, including functional impairment and pain. Exercise also leads to weight loss, which may be especially beneficial for those with particular chronic diseases. Exercise may reduce negative psychological consequences of chronic diseases, lead to improved cognitive functioning, and even slow disease progression.

- Cognitive-behavioral approaches focus on challenging individuals' irrational beliefs about their condition and providing training in coping skills to handle their illness. Such approaches are especially effective when they provide specific strategies for managing stress. Cognitive-behavioral training is an effective strategy for improving both mental and physical health in people with a chronic disease.

- Social support groups help people cope with chronic diseases. This approach gives people an opportunity to compare coping strategies and solutions to daily problems, share emotions, and discuss topics specific to their disease. These groups may be particularly effective when participants can share their own coping strategies with others.

11

LEADING CAUSES OF MORTALITY

Coronary Heart Disease and Cancer

Learning Objectives

11.1 Describe the biology of coronary heart disease and its risk factors

11.2 Explain how psychosocial factors contribute to coronary heart disease

11.3 Summarize strategies for reducing the risk of recurring heart attacks

11.4 Describe the biology of cancer and its risk factors

11.5 Explain how psychosocial factors contribute to cancer

11.6 Summarize strategies for coping with cancer

What You'll Learn

11.1 Why living in—or even visiting—New York City could be a bad idea

11.2 How even a single angry outburst can cause a heart attack

11.3 Why feeling lonely increases the risk of experiencing a stroke

11.4 How stress at work may hurt your health

11.5 Why married people with cancer live longer

Preview

Virtually everyone reading this book has been—or will be—touched by coronary heart disease (CHD) and/or cancer. These two diseases are the leading causes of death and are responsible for approximately half of all deaths in the United States each year (Kochanek, Murphy, Xu, & Tejada-Vera, 2016). In this chapter, you'll learn about risk factors for both diseases, how psychosocial factors contribute to their development, and strategies that help people cope with treatment.

CORONARY HEART DISEASE

LO 11.1

Describe the biology of coronary heart disease and its risk factors

Until the 20th century, **cardiovascular diseases**, meaning diseases that involve the heart and blood vessels, were not a major health problem. However, **coronary heart disease** (CHD), the most common type of heart disease, is now the leading cause of death for both men and women (National Center for Health Statistics, 2017). Over 600,000 people die of heart disease in the United States each year, which means about 25% of all deaths each year are due to heart disease. This section will describe the biology of CHD and various factors that increase the risk of developing this disease.

Figure 11.1 Model of the Cardiovascular System

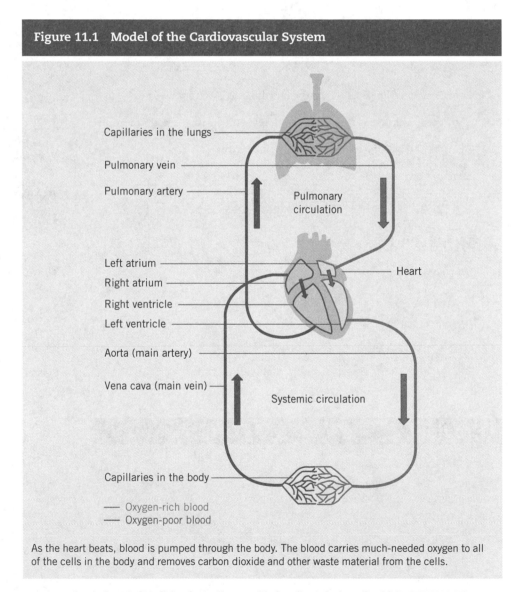

Capillaries in the lungs

Pulmonary vein

Pulmonary artery

Pulmonary circulation

Left atrium

Right atrium

Right ventricle

Left ventricle

Heart

Aorta (main artery)

Vena cava (main vein)

Systemic circulation

Capillaries in the body

— Oxygen-rich blood
— Oxygen-poor blood

As the heart beats, blood is pumped through the body. The blood carries much-needed oxygen to all of the cells in the body and removes carbon dioxide and other waste material from the cells.

Source: National Library of Medicine, https://www.ncbi.nlm.nih.gov/pubmedhealth/PMHT0023062/.

Understanding Coronary Heart Disease

Under normal conditions, the heart contracts and releases, which pumps blood throughout the body (Smith & Pratt, 1993) (see Figure 11.1). The blood carries necessary oxygen to all the cells in the body and removes carbon dioxide and other waste material from the cells. However, over time the artery walls can become clogged with a buildup of fatty substances, such as *low-density lipoprotein (LDL) cholesterol* and other substances. (In contrast, *high-density lipoproteins*, or *HDLs*, remove LDL cholesterol from the bloodstream, and thereby reduce the risk of arterial clogging.) When this buildup occurs, the area through which blood can flow decreases and the likelihood of a blood clot increases (see Figure 11.2). This process is known as **atherosclerosis**.

Moreover, over time arteries can lose their elasticity and become thick and stiff (commonly called hardening of the arteries). This process, known as **arteriosclerosis**, makes it difficult for them to expand and contract with the blood pressure, and thus leads to a decrease in blood flow to organs and tissues.

Although both atherosclerosis and arteriosclerosis can be present in the body without a person experiencing any symptoms for some time, they can eventually lead to very

Figure 11.2   Model Showing Artery Blocked With Plaque

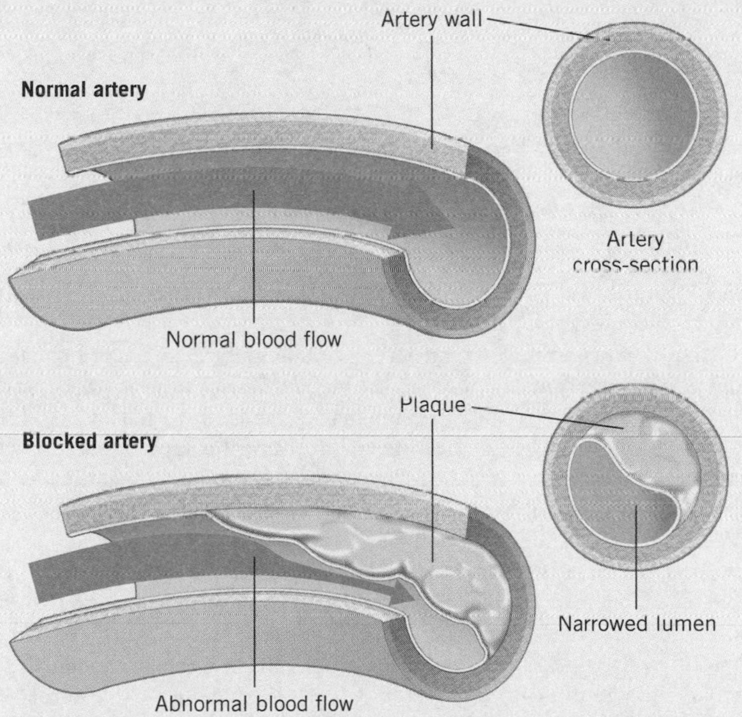

As cholesterol and fats build up in the arteries, the walls of the arteries become thicker and thicker, leaving little room for blood to flow. Over time, arteries can become completely blocked, which causes a heart attack.

Source: Figure reillustrated by Body Scientific International, from National Heart, Lung, and Blood Institute, https://www.nhlbi.nih.gov/health/health-topics/topics/atherosclerosis.

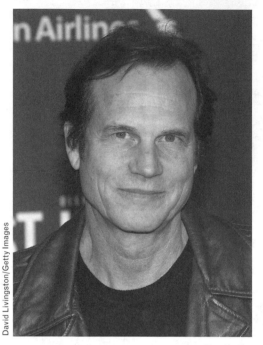

serious problems. First, a person may develop **angina**, a feeling of pain and tightness in the chest as the heart is deprived of oxygen. This type of attack may pass quickly but is often a sign that future cardiovascular problems will develop. In more serious cases, in which there is a complete blockage of the coronary arteries, a person may experience a **myocardial infarction**, or heart attack. Heart attacks often occur because a blood clot formed around the built-up cholesterol blocks the passage of blood to the heart. This deprivation of oxygen causes permanent damage to the heart muscles.

Atherosclerosis and arteriosclerosis can lead to **strokes**. Strokes can occur when the plaque that forms on the artery wall becomes detached and then travels in the bloodstream. If one of these blood clots lodges in the circulatory system so that it deprives the brain of oxygen, the person experiences a stroke, which damages neurons in the brain that can never be replaced. People who have suffered a stroke may therefore experience some type of long-term damage, such as speech impairment or difficulty in moving parts of their bodies. Strokes can also lead to death; in fact, strokes are the fifth leading cause of death in the United States (National Center for Health Statistics, 2017).

Actor Bill Paxton, who appeared in such films as *Aliens*, *Titanic*, *Twister*, and *Apollo 13*, died of a stroke in February 2017. He was 61 years old.

Risk Factors

Although anyone could potentially develop CHD, some people are at greater risk than others. Medical conditions, genetics, and demographic factors all influence the likelihood of developing CHD.

Medical Conditions

Three medical conditions are consistently linked with an increased risk of developing CHD: hypertension, high cholesterol, and diabetes.

Hypertension is a condition in which a person's blood pressure is at a consistently high level. Blood pressure represents the force of the blood against the artery walls, and when this pressure is too high, the artery walls can get damaged, which in turn leads to CHD. Because high blood pressure makes the heart beat more forcefully, this type of continuous wear and tear on the heart can weaken it, which also can contribute to CHD. In fact, an estimated 54% of strokes and 47% of cases of heart disease worldwide are caused by high blood pressure (Lawes, Vander Hoorn, & Rodgers, 2008).

As described earlier, a buildup of fatty substances, including cholesterol, can lead to clogged or blocked arteries. People with high levels of cholesterol—either due to genetics or through diet—are therefore at greater risk of experiencing CHD. In fact, a person's total cholesterol level at age 22 is a good predictor of his or her likelihood of experiencing CHD or stroke and age of death (Klag et al., 1993). People with cholesterol levels in the top 25% are twice as likely to die of a heart attack than those with cholesterol levels in the bottom 25%.

As described in *Chapter 10: Understanding and Managing Chronic Illness*, people with diabetes lack adequate levels of insulin, a hormone which helps the body create adequate energy from food. A lack of insulin causes sugars to build up in the blood, which increases the risk of CHD. People with diabetes are twice as likely to die from heart disease as people without this condition (Centers for Disease Control and Prevention, 2014).

Genetics

Genetic factors clearly contribute to the likelihood of developing CHD, at least in part because such factors influence medical conditions associated with CHD (such as cholesterol levels, blood pressure, and diabetes) (Neufeld & Goldbourt, 1983). For example, compared to people without CHD, people with CHD are more than twice as likely to report having a parent or sibling with some type of heart disease, such as angina, CHD, or a myocardial infarction (Shea, Ottman, Gabrieli, Stein, & Nichols, 1984). People with a family history of CHD, such as those who have a parent or sibling who has experienced a heart attack, are also at greater risk of developing this disease (Lloyd-Jones et al., 2004; Murabito et al., 2005).

Although in many cases it is difficult to disentangle whether family history predicts CHD due to questions of nature versus nurture, adoption studies provide further evidence that genetics do play a role. For example, having a biological parent with CHD increases the risk of developing this disease by 40% to 60%, whereas there is no increased risk even if both adoptive parents have CHD (Sundquist et al., 2011). However, family habits—including eating, exercise, and smoking—do contribute to the likelihood of developing CHD, as you'll learn in the next section.

Demographic Factors

A variety of demographic factors influence the risk of developing CHD (Smith & Pratt, 1993). For example, the likelihood of developing CHD increases with age, for example, presumably because over time the arteries are more likely to become clogged or hardened.

Gender also influences a person's likelihood of developing CHD; men are at greater risk of experiencing CHD than women, which is one of the reasons why men have a shorter life expectancy than women (Smith & Pratt, 1993). One explanation for this gender difference is that testosterone, which circulates in higher levels in men than in women, is associated with aggression and competitiveness, and these behaviors may increase a person's risk of developing cardiovascular disease. However, men and women were relatively equally likely to die of heart disease until the 1920s, suggesting that hormone levels alone are unlikely to explain this gender gap (Nikiforov & Mamaev, 1998). Another possibility is that men engage in more behaviors that lead to CHD than women, including smoking, drinking alcohol, and eating high-fat foods. However, even when men and women have the same level of risky behaviors, men are still more likely than women to die of CHD (Fried et al., 1998). Although research is clearly needed to show exactly why, it is important to recognize that cardiovascular problems are not just a "male problem." In fact, CHD is the leading cause of death in women as well as men—women simply develop such problems about 15 years later than men.

There are also clear differences in the frequency of CHD as a function of race and ethnicity, with Blacks showing more risk than Whites, who in turn show more risk than Hispanic Americans (Mozaffarian et al., 2016). Moreover, heart disease death rates are higher among Blacks than Whites (Kung, Hoyert, Xu, & Murphy, 2008). As described in **Focus on Diversity**, a number of factors contribute to these differences in risk of CHD by race/ethnicity.

Although cardiovascular disease is a leading cause of death in many countries, people living in South Asian countries, such as India, Pakistan, Nepal, Bangladesh, and Sri Lanka, are at particular risk of experiencing a heart attack (Joshi et al., 2007). Moreover, people living in these countries tend to have a first heart attack at younger ages than those living in Western countries; the mean of first age in South Asian countries is 53 years, compared to 58.8 years in other countries. The increased risk is largely explained by the increased prevalence of risk factors, such as smoking and diabetes, as well as lower levels of protective factors, such as regular physical activity and consumption of fruits and vegetables, in these countries. These findings provide powerful evidence that changing behaviors, especially early in life, could lead to substantial reductions in heart attack risk among South Asians.

PSYCHOSOCIAL FACTORS CONTRIBUTING TO CORONARY HEART DISEASE

LO 11.2

Explain how psychosocial factors contribute to coronary heart disease

In the last section, you learned about various fixed factors that increase the risk of developing CHD. However, psychosocial factors are the most significant factors contributing to CHD. These includes behavioral choices, stress, environment, personality, and loneliness.

Behavioral Choices

Behavioral choices play a substantial role in the development of CHD. For example, a longitudinal study of over 23,000 men found that those who didn't smoke, engaged in regular exercise, and maintained recommended weight were 59% less likely to experience heart problems and 69% less likely to die compared to men with all of these risk factors (Lee, Sui, & Blair, 2009). This section describes the role of four distinct behaviors in increasing the risk of developing CHD: smoking, alcohol use, diet, and exercise.

Smoking

As discussed in *Chapter 7: Substance Use and Abuse*, cigarette smoking influences CHD in a number of ways, including by increasing the heart rate, increasing blood pressure, and constricting the blood vessels, which causes problems over time and particularly during times of stress (Smith & Pratt, 1993). Smoking also decreases the production of HDL cholesterol, which protects against heart attacks. Smoking basically increases wear and tear on the heart and accelerates atherosclerosis. In fact, a person who smokes is twice as likely to die from CHD than someone who doesn't smoke (Fried et al., 1998; Twisk, Kemper, Van Mechelen, & Post, 1997). Moreover, nonsmokers who live with smokers are about 20% more likely to develop CHD than nonsmokers who live with other nonsmokers (Werner & Pearson, 1998).

Alcohol Use

Although smoking is associated with a substantially increased risk of developing CHD, moderate levels of alcohol use—meaning one to two drinks a day—are associated with a *decreased* risk of CHD (Maclure, 1993; Rimm et al., 1991). Specifically, compared to men who rarely drink alcohol, those who drink two to six drinks a week are 34% to 53% less likely to die from CHD (Camargo et al., 1997). Moderate levels of alcohol consumption lead to decreases in *high-density lipoproteins*, or *HDLs*, which, as you learned earlier in this section, remove LDL cholesterol from the bloodstream, and thereby reduce the risk of arterial clogging (Gaziano et al., 1993).

Although some people may experience benefits in terms of CHD from drinking one or two drinks a day, heavier consumption of alcohol is associated with a number of serious health consequences (Pearson, 1996). Excessive alcohol use raises blood pressure, and increases the level of triglycerides, which leads to hardening of the arteries. Moreover, people with particular medical conditions, such as hypertension or liver disease, or those with a genetic predisposition to alcohol addiction, should avoid consuming even moderate amounts of alcohol.

Diet

As described previously, people with hypertension and high cholesterol are at increased risk of developing CHD. Both of these medical conditions are influenced, at least in part, by diet

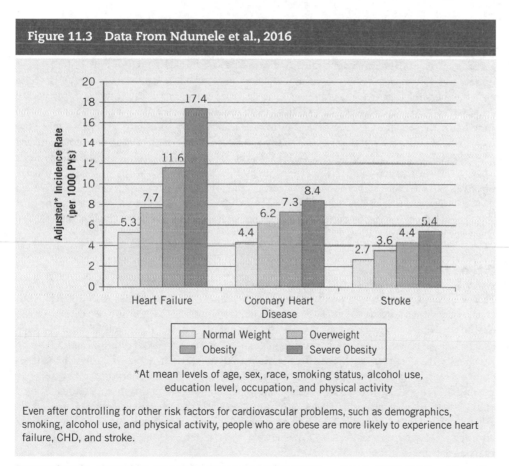

Figure 11.3 Data From Ndumele et al., 2016

*At mean levels of age, sex, race, smoking status, alcohol use, education level, occupation, and physical activity

Even after controlling for other risk factors for cardiovascular problems, such as demographics, smoking, alcohol use, and physical activity, people who are obese are more likely to experience heart failure, CHD, and stroke.

Source: Ndumele , Matsushita, Lazo, Bello, Blumenthal, Gerstenblith, . . . Coresh (2016). Retrieved from the *Journal of the American Heart Association.*

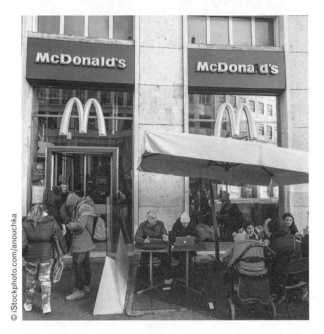
© iStockphoto.com/anouchka

(Smith & Pratt, 1993). People who eat foods that are high in cholesterol and fats (especially saturated fat and trans fat) are at greater risk of developing CHD (Stamler, Wenthworth, & Neaton, 1986). Diets that are high in sodium (salt) can raise blood pressure levels, and thereby increase the risk of CHD. Eating foods high in fats, cholesterol, and salt also increases the risk of obesity, which in turn is linked with high blood pressure and diabetes as well as CHD. As shown in Figure 11.3, people who are obese are more likely to experience various cardiovascular problems.

On the other hand, some types of food seem to protect people from developing CHD (Stampfer, Rimm, & Walsh, 1993). For example, women who consume high levels of vitamin E are at reduced risk of CHD (Stampfer et al., 1993), as are people who have a diet high in fiber (Katan, Grundy, & Willett, 1997). Some research even suggests that people who eat deep-sea fish regularly have a lower likelihood of experiencing a heart attack (Albert et al., 1998).

Do you know what you're consuming when you eat at McDonald's (or another fast food restaurant)? A Big Mac has 34 grams of fat and 590 calories, an order of medium-size fries has 22 grams of fat and 450 calories, and a medium Coca-Cola Classic has 0 grams of fat and 220 calories. Remember, for someone eating 2,000 calories per day (a rough average), today's nutritional guidelines recommend including 65 grams of fat per day.

Exercise

People who engage in regular exercise are less likely to develop CHD, or to experience a heart attack or stroke (Myers, 2003; Smith & Pratt, 1993). Physical activity helps reduce blood pressure and promotes healthy weight, which are both linked to lower risk of CHD. Exercise also has beneficial effects on cholesterol; it decreases levels of LDL (the harmful type of cholesterol) and increases levels of HDL (the helpful type). One study of over 45,000 people found that those who biked regularly—either for leisure or to commute to work—were 11% to 18% likely to have developed CHD 20 years later (Blond et al., 2016). Moreover, biking was associated with a reduced risk of CHD even when the researchers took into account other risk factors, such as BMI, hypertension, high cholesterol, and diabetes. People who are physically fit also show faster recovery in terms of heart rate from stressful experiences, which reduces wear and tear on the heart (Forcier et al., 2006), as you'll learn more about in the next section. These findings illustrate the importance of engaging in regular physical activity as a strategy for reducing the risk of CHD.

Stress

Stress, including pressure caused by work, interpersonal conflict, traumas, and financial concerns, may contribute to CHD (Kop, Gottdiener, & Krantz, 2001; Sumner et al., 2015). For example, people who work in jobs that have constant demands but low levels of control—such as working on an assembly line or waiting tables—are at greater risk of developing CHD than those who have less stressful jobs (Bosma, Stansfeld, & Marmot, 1998). People who experience chronic job strain are more likely to experience recurrent coronary heart disease, even when researchers take into account other variables associated with this disease (Aboa-Éboulé et al., 2007). Even relationship stress can lead to both CHD and cardiac events (Coyne et al., 2001; Matthews & Gump, 2002). Women with CHD who experience high levels of marital conflict are three times as likely to experience a heart attack as those who are in low-conflict marriages (Orth-Gomér et al., 2000).

Some researchers have examined another type of stress that may lead to CHD—the stress of constant racial discrimination (Krieger & Sidney, 1996; Krieger et al., 1998). As described previously, Blacks have higher rates of CHD and hypertension than do Whites, and one explanation is that these differences are caused at least in part by constant exposure to discrimination and racism. In line with this view, Blacks who reported experiencing racial discrimination and accepting unfair treatment had significantly higher blood pressure than those who reported experiencing such discrimination but challenging unfair treatment (Krieger & Sidney, 1996). However, this association between accepting racial discrimination and high blood pressure was found in working-class Blacks but not among Black business professionals (Krieger & Sidney, 1996; Krieger et al., 1998). This finding suggests that stress may be greatest among those who are trying to overcome adversity but who have limited socioeconomic resources to do so. Moreover, although racial discrimination may indeed influence rates of hypertension and CHD in Blacks, this association is also influenced by gender and SES.

Although racial discrimination is a consistent source of stress for people of color, even relatively short-lived stressful experiences are associated with an increased risk of cardiovascular problems. Researchers in one study examined whether a temporary stressor is linked to bad health outcomes (Christenfeld, Glynn, Phillips, & Shrira, 1999). Specifically, they calculated the rates of death caused by CHD for three distinct groups of people: New York City residents who died in the city, New York City residents who died while traveling outside the city, and non–New York City residents who died while visiting the city. As predicted, people who lived in New York City had a very high death rate as a result of CHD while living in the city—in fact, their death rate from CHD was 55% higher than the national average. In contrast, New York City residents who were traveling outside of the city were 20% less likely to die from CHD than if they were in the city. Visitors to New York City experienced the same types of problems, with a death rate from CHD 34% higher than the national average. Is this pattern true in all cities? No. Researchers found no differences in CHD for people who lived in or visited other major cities, including Los Angeles, Chicago, Houston, Philadelphia, Dallas, San Diego, Phoenix, Detroit, San Antonio, and San Jose, as compared to the national average. Although the researchers were unable to determine what leads to the greater death rate from CHD, one possibility is that the stress of spending time in New York City—which has a greater population density than any other region of the country—accounts for this association.

What You'll Learn
11.1

How exactly does stress increase the risk of CHD? As discussed in **Chapter 4: Understanding Stress**, people who are under stress show an acceleration of the heartbeat, a strengthening of the heart's contractions, and higher blood pressure. Moreover, epinephrine is released during times of stress, which decreases the time needed for blood to coagulate and causes blood vessels to constrict. Chronic stress can therefore lead to excessive wear and tear on the cardiovascular system, which over time can lead to considerable damage to the heart and arteries (Sapolsky, 1994). Alternatively, or perhaps additionally, people who experience stress engage in unhealthy behaviors—smoking, alcohol use, poor eating habits—as a way of coping, which in turn increases the risk of cardiovascular problems.

Environment

A number of environmental factors are associated with an increased likelihood of developing cardiovascular diseases. For example, the number of heart attacks in a given community drops substantially after a smoking ban is implemented, which presumably reduces people's exposure to smoke (likely for smokers as well as nonsmokers) (Cesaroni et al., 2008). Specifically, after the city of Rome instituted a public smoking ban (which included all indoor public places, such as offices, restaurants, and retail shops), coronary events dropped 11.2% for people ages 35 to 64 and 7.9% for people ages 65 to 74.

Another environmental factor linked with an increased risk of developing—and dying from—cardiovascular disease is living in an inner city (Nayyar & Hwang, 2015). One explanation for this association is that city living may reduce people's ability to exercise outside—due to a lack of safe parks and concern with violence—and ability to buy healthy foods—due to a lack of options for buying healthy foods. However, determining the precise mechanisms explaining this relationship are difficult, in part because people with lower levels of education and income are more likely to live in an inner city and are also more likely to lack access to regular preventative medical care.

Another explanation for the greater prevalence of CHD in inner cities is that air pollution, which is more common in urban areas, leads to these negative health outcomes. In line with this view, air pollution—even at levels considered safe by federal guidelines—increases the risk of experiencing a stroke by 34% (Wellenius et al., 2012). Exposure to air pollution also increases the risk of death in people with cardiovascular disease. Heart attack survivors living less than 328 feet from a roadway have a 27% higher risk of dying within 10 years than survivors living at least 3,277 feet from the roadway (Rosenbloom, Wilker, Mukamal, Schwartz, & Mittleman, 2012). Moreover, on days in which air pollution is higher in a given urban area, rates of hospital admissions for cardiovascular events, such as heart attacks, are higher (Powell, Krall, Wang, Bell, & Peng, 2015).

Personality

Although anyone can develop cardiovascular problems, some people seem to be at greater risk than others from experiencing such problems. Let's examine the personality traits most strongly linked with CHD: Type A behavior pattern, hostility, anger expression, and Type D personality.

Type A Behavior Pattern

As discussed in *Chapter 5: Managing Stress*, for many years the Type A behavior pattern was thought to predict occurrence of CHD (Friedman & Rosenman, 1959; Rosenman & Friedman, 1961; Suinn, 1975). People who are Type As—meaning those who are competitive, time-urgent, and hostile—are more likely to experience a heart attack and to show signs of hypertension. One explanation is that Type A people show heightened levels of physiological arousal, including elevated heart rate, higher blood pressure, and increased catecholamines and corticosteroids, in stressful situations (Jorgensen, Johnson, Kolodziej, & Schreer, 1996; Smith, 1992). While a Type B person might calmly sit in the car and listen to music during a traffic jam, a Type A person might experience this situation as very upsetting and arousing. Over time this constant physiological arousal can damage the heart and blood vessels and increase the formation of blood clots, which in turn can lead to cardiovascular disease as well as heart attacks.

Hostility

Although Type A is the personality variable most often associated with CHD, recent research suggests that a specific component of the Type A personality, hostility, is a particularly strong predictor (Barefoot, Dodge, Peterson, Dahlstrom, & Williams, 1989; Miller, Smith, Turner, Guijarro, & Hallet, 1996; Smith, 1992). In fact, level of hostility, but not Type A behavior, predicts the likelihood of developing CHD and suffering a heart attack (Chida & Steptoe, 2009; Shekelle, Gale, Ostfield, & Paul, 1983). One prospective study assessed hostility in 200 healthy women and then followed these women over 10 years (Matthews, Owens, Kuller, Sutton-Tyrrell, & Jansen-McWilliams, 1998). Even after controlling for variables such as smoking, women who had higher hostility scores in the earlier test were more likely to show symptoms of cardiovascular disease 10 years later. Similarly, in studies of patients with CHD, those who are higher in hostility have more severe heart disease and are twice as likely to die as those low in hostility (Williams et al., 1980; Wong, Sin, & Whooley, 2014). You can test your own level of hostility in **Table 11.1: Test Yourself**.

Physiological reactions explain why people who are high in hostility tend to have worse health. Specifically, hostile people have consistently higher heart rates and blood pressure than those who are low in hostility, they show extreme cardiovascular reactions to stressful situations, and they take longer to have their bodies return to normal functioning following a stressful interaction (Raikkonen, Matthews, Flory, & Owens, 1999; Smith, 1992; Suarez, Kuhn, Schanberg, Williams, & Zimmermann, 1998).

Anger Expression

Still other research suggests that feeling hostile doesn't lead to negative health outcomes, but that engaging in hostile behaviors creates such outcomes. In other words, expressions of anger, including raising a voice while arguing and yelling back when someone yells at you, increase the risk of developing CHD (Siegman, 1993). In line with that view, people who frequently experience anger are three times as likely to suffer a heart attack as those who rarely experience anger (Chida & Steptoe, 2009; Williams et al., 2000).

Researchers in one study examined the link between single outbursts of anger and the likelihood of triggering serious cardiovascular problems, such as heart attacks and strokes (Mostofsky, Penner, & Mittleman, 2014). Their findings revealed that in the two hours immediately following an angry outburst, a person's risk of experiencing a heart attack increased nearly 5%, and the risk of experiencing a stroke increased by 3%, compared to when the person wasn't angry. People who had some type of preexisting condition, such as preexisting cardiovascular risk factors or frequent angry outbursts, were at even higher risk.

How does the expression of anger lead to CHD? When a person yells, his or her heart rate increases, and, although the person may not be aware of it, blood pressure also increases. In turn, people who regularly experience this higher level of physiological arousal may be at greater risk of developing cardiovascular problems because they have so much wear and tear

What You'll Learn
11.2

Table 11.1   Test Yourself: How Hostile Are You?

Answer the following questions yes or no.

1. No one cares much what happens to me.
2. I have often met people who were supposed to be experts who were not better than I.
3. Some of my family have habits that bother and annoy me very much.
4. I often have had to take orders from someone who did not know as much as I did.
5. It makes me feel like a failure when I hear of the success of someone I know well.
6. People often disappoint me.
7. It is safer to trust nobody.
8. I have often felt that strangers were looking at me critically.
9. I tend to be on my guard with people who are somewhat more friendly than I expected.
10. My way of doing things is apt to be misunderstood by others.

Now add up all your "yes" items. Higher scores indicate higher levels of hostility.

Source: Cook & Medley (1954).

on their blood vessels and heart (Siegman, Anderson, Herbst, Boyle, & Wilkinson, 1992). Changes in blood flow could also cause blood clots, which increases the risk of heart attacks and strokes.

Type D Personality

Although for many years researchers focused on the role of Type A behavior pattern in leading to CHD, growing evidence now points to another personality factor that is linked with cardiovascular problems. Specifically, people with Type D—meaning distressed—personality are three times more likely to experience future cardiovascular problems, such as heart failure, heart surgery, or a heart attack (Denollet, Schiffer, & Spek, 2010). People with Type D personality have persistent negative emotions (e.g., anxiety, depression, irritation), pessimism, and social inhibition (meaning they don't share these negative feelings with others).

Other types of negative emotions, such as anxiety and depression, are also linked with an increased risk of developing, and dying from, CHD (Kubzansky, Cole, Kawachi, Vokonas, & Sparrow, 2006; Markowitz, Matthews, Kannel, Cobb, & D'Agostino, 1993). For example, men who are high in hopelessness are four times more likely to die from cardiovascular diseases than those who are low in hopelessness (Everson, Goldberg, Kaplan, & Cohen, 1996). People who consistently experience such negative emotions over time are at particular risk of developing cardiovascular problems. Researchers in one longitudinal study of nearly 7,000 people found that people who showed signs of anxiety and depression in childhood are at greater risk for developing heart disease at age 45 (Winning, Glymour, McCormick, Gilsanz, & Kubzansky, 2015). Moreover, people who experienced consistent distress throughout their entire lives had the highest level of risk for developing CHD. This association held true even when researchers took into account various other factors that could explain this link, including socioeconomic status and health behaviors.

The specific mechanism that leads people with Type D personality to have more negative health outcomes is not known (Denollet, Schiffer, & Spek, 2010; Steptoe & Molloy, 2007). One possibility is that people with this personality trait show heightened physiological responses to stress, such as increased heart rate, blood pressure, and cortisol, which leads to greater wear and tear on the cardiovascular system. Other evidence suggests that people with Type D personality are less likely to have regular medical checkups, adhere to medical regimens, and share symptoms with medical professionals, all of which in turn increases their risk of experiencing more serious problems (Schiffer, Denollet, Widdershoven, Hendriks, & Smith, 2007).

Positive Emotions

Finally, although most research has focused on the negative effects of some types of emotions on CHD, some researchers have examined the benefits of positive emotions (Kubzansky & Thurston, 2007). For example, people who are higher in emotional vitality—characterized by a sense of energy, positive well-being, and effective emotion regulation—have a reduced risk of coronary heart disease. Emotional vitality may therefore help protect people against developing CHD.

Loneliness

**What You'll Learn
11.3**

Another factor that increases the risk of developing cardiovascular problems is feeling socially isolated or lonely (Holt-Lunstad & Smith, 2016). In fact, one recent meta-analysis found that a lack of social connections is associated with an increased risk of having a stroke and developing coronary artery disease (Valtorta, Kanaan, Gilbody, Ronzi, &

Hanratty, 2016). Specifically, feeling lonely and/or socially isolated was associated with a 29% increased risk of experiencing a heart or angina attack and a 32% increased risk of having a stroke. Similarly, and as described in *Chapter 5: Managing Stress*, people who feel more connected to their neighbors are less likely to experience a heart attack (Kim, Hawes, & Smith, 2014). For people who are recovering from a heart attack, higher social support is associated with lower levels of depression and improved health one year later (Bucholz et al., 2014).

Although the specific mechanisms that explain this relationship are unknown, researchers posit three distinct possibilities (Valtorta, Kanaan, Gilbody, Ronzi, & Hanratty, 2016). First, people who are lonely may engage in poorer health-related behaviors, such as smoking and poor diet. They may also experience more sleep problems, which deprives their body of beneficial opportunities for physiological restoration (Hawkley & Cacioppo, 2010). Finally, loneliness may be associated with negative physiological reactions to stress, such as higher blood pressure and weaker immune responses (Steptoe, Owen, Kunz-Ebrecht, & Brydon, 2004). All of these factors could lead people who are lonely and social isolated to be at increased risk of developing cardiovascular problems.

STRATEGIES FOR REDUCING THE RISK OF RECURRING HEART ATTACKS

Every year, over half a million Americans have a first heart attack and over 200,000 people who have already had at least one heart attack experience another attack (Centers for Disease Control and Prevention, 2017i). Because of the significant rate of CHD in the United States, many intervention programs have specifically targeted heart attack survivors in an effort to help reduce their risk of experiencing another heart attack and dying of cardiovascular disease.

LO 11.3

Summarize strategies for reducing the risk of recurring heart attacks

Health Education Programs

One type of treatment for CHD focuses on helping people change their health-related behavior (Dusseldorp, van Elderen, Maes, Meulman, & Kraaij, 1999; Smith & Pratt, 1993). Health education programs focus on changing people's behavior, including by showing them how to reduce their sodium and fat intake, lower their weight, and stop smoking. Because smoking and high-fat diets can cause the heart to operate less efficiently, making changes in these behaviors reduces the risk of CHD. Health education programs also encourage people to start exercising, which decreases the risk of cardiovascular disease in several ways, including reducing weight and improving the efficiency of the heart (Rovario, Holmes, & Holmsten, 1984). Health education programs also provide patients with information about the medications they could take and encourage patients to follow prescribed medical regimens. Such programs may be particularly beneficial for single people, who are at greater risk of experiencing another heart attack than married people, at least in part because they are less likely to engage in health-promoting behavior (e.g., engaging in exercise, eating a healthy diet, seeking medical advice) (Nielsen, Faergeman, Larsen, & Foldspang, 2006).

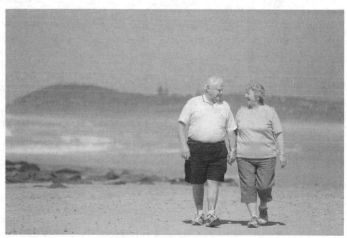

©iStockphoto.com/davidf

People who make even simple behavioral changes, such as starting to engage in regular physical activity, can reduce their risk of developing cardiovascular problems.

These programs can be quite effective in reducing CHD. People who make dietary changes show substantial reductions in cardiovascular risk factors (Brunner et al., 1997), and those who engage in regular exercise following a heart attack show lower blood pressure and lower heart rates (Rovario, Holmes, & Holmsten, 1984). Health-promotion programs are particularly effective at decreasing CHD risk when they also include cholesterol-lowering medication (Maher, Brown, Marcovina, Hillger, & Zhao, 1995). Lifestyle interventions can also lead to reductions in the rate of diabetes, which is often linked to CHD (Knowler et al., 2002).

Health education programs also provide people with clear information about the early signs and symptoms of a heart attack, which increases their ability to seek prompt medical care. Patients learn, for example, to call 911 as soon as they experience any signs of a heart attack, and to call an ambulance instead of driving themselves to the hospital. As described in **Research in Action**, even minutes can make the difference between life and death in the case of a heart attack.

Stress Management Strategies

Another common approach to reducing the risk of CHD is through stress management programs (Dusseldorp, van Elderen, Maes, Meulman, & Kraaij, 1999). These programs focus on training patients in techniques for managing stress, such as relaxation

RESEARCH IN ACTION

How Marathon Races Impact Heart Attack Survival

One of the most crucial factors predicting survival from a heart attack is prompt medical attention; heart muscle dies very quickly during a heart attack—when the heart is deprived of blood and oxygen—so receiving prompt medical attention is extremely important. Thus, another factor that could impact survival from a heart attack is speed of reaching a hospital. To examine this question, researchers examined death rates in 11 cities in the United States that host a marathon (Jena, Mann, Wedlund, & Olenski, 2017). Specifically, the researchers compared data collected over a 10-year period on the death rates of older Americans, those ages 65 and older, who were hospitalized on the day of the race versus those hospitalized five weeks earlier or five weeks later. They also compared death rates of people living near the marathon (using zip codes) to those of people living well outside the race route, who presumably would be less impacted by street closings. As predicted, people who lived near the race route and suffered a heart attack on the day of a marathon were more likely to die within a month than those who lived in a different city. They were also more likely to die within a month than those who lived in the same city but farther away. The researchers believe this increased risk of death is due to delays in reaching the hospital caused by the street closures. Although the delay caused by such closures on average only amounts to about an additional 4.4 minutes in an ambulance on marathon days, even very small delays can make the difference between life and death. Moreover, although the researchers examined other factors that could have led to increased death rates due to marathon traffic—such as whether people were sent to more distant hospitals, whether people waited to see if their condition was more severe before seeking help, or whether staffing levels at the hospital were lower during marathon days—none of these factors explained their findings.

training, and can reduce cardiac events and increase survival. For example, men who participated in a weekly stress management group for four months experienced fewer negative health events—including heart attacks, bypass surgery, and death—than those who simply received medicine for their condition and those who exercised (Blumenthal et al., 2002).

Other studies point to the availability of trained professionals as a resource in helping heart attack survivors manage stress. Researchers in one study assigned some patients to receive regular calls from a nurse for one year following their heart attack (Frasure-Smith & Prince, 1989). The nurse asked them whether they were experiencing stress and then either talked through the problems with the patient or referred them to another health care professional (therapist, physician, social worker). Patients who received such follow-up contact had lower rates of mortality over the seven-year follow-up as compared to those who received standard care.

Several studies have attempted to decrease individuals' risk of CHD by teaching them techniques and methods for changing negative cognitions, behaviors, and emotions, such as by teaching people more adaptive ways to cope with stress (Friedman et al., 1986). For example, patients might examine the triggers for their angry outbursts and then learn cognitive and behavioral techniques to help them reduce their competitiveness, hostility, and cynicism. This type of program is very effective in reducing the risk of a second heart attack—in fact, rates of death caused by CHD were twice as high in the control group as in the treatment group. Similarly, highly hostile men with CHD who receive a hostility-reduction intervention—including training in listening, problem-focused coping, and enhancing self-awareness—have lower blood pressure at a two-month follow-up (Gidron, Davidson, & Bata, 1999). Patients with CHD who undergo a hostility management group therapy program also have a much shorter hospital stay following the session, suggesting that such training may result in reduced health care costs (Davidson, Gidron, Mostofsky, & Trudeau, 2007).

Combined Strategies

Finally, programs that combine health education and stress management techniques by focusing on lifestyle changes (including smoking, diet, exercise, and stress) may be quite effective at reducing rates of cardiovascular problems (e.g., heart attacks, bypasses, and death) (Lisspers et al., 2005). For example, CHD patients who participate in a very intensive program—including severe dietary restrictions, assistance in quitting smoking and increasing exercise, and training in relaxation and other stress management techniques—have significantly less blockage of their coronary arteries one year later compared to those in a control group (Ornish et al., 1990, 1998). Moreover, findings from a five-year follow-up indicated that patients who completed this program had fewer coronary problems. Similarly, researchers in another study randomly assigned people with CHD to one of two conditions: a combined-intervention group (including diet, exercise, stress management, and group support) or a standard care group (Pischke, Scherwitz, Weidner, & Ornish, 2008). Compared to people in the control group, those in the combined-intervention group showed reductions in psychological distress and hostility, which were maintained as long as five years later. Moreover, people who received the combined-intervention group also reported improvements in diet, weight reduction, and stress management, which in turn led to improvements in cardiovascular outcomes. Although this types of approach is clearly successful in decreasing CHD, it is very costly in terms of time, energy, and expense and is therefore not likely to be a particularly useful approach in the general population.

CANCER

LO 11.4

Describe the biology of cancer and its risk factors

After heart disease, **cancer** is the leading cause of death in the United States, with close to 600,000 Americans dying from this disease each year (www.cancer.gov; Centers for Disease Control and Prevention, 2017v). Each year an estimated 1,685,210 new cases of cancer will be diagnosed in the United States; close to 40% of all Americans will be diagnosed with cancer at some point in their lives. Although there are more than 200 types of cancer, the most common cancers are breast cancer, lung and bronchus cancer, prostate cancer, colon and rectum cancer, bladder cancer, melanoma of the skin, non-Hodgkin lymphoma, thyroid cancer, kidney and renal pelvis cancer, leukemia, endometrial cancer, and pancreatic cancer. As shown in Figures 11.4 and 11.5, lung cancer is the leading cause of cancer death in both men and women (Howlader et al., 2017).

Figure 11.4 Leading Causes of Cancer Deaths in Men

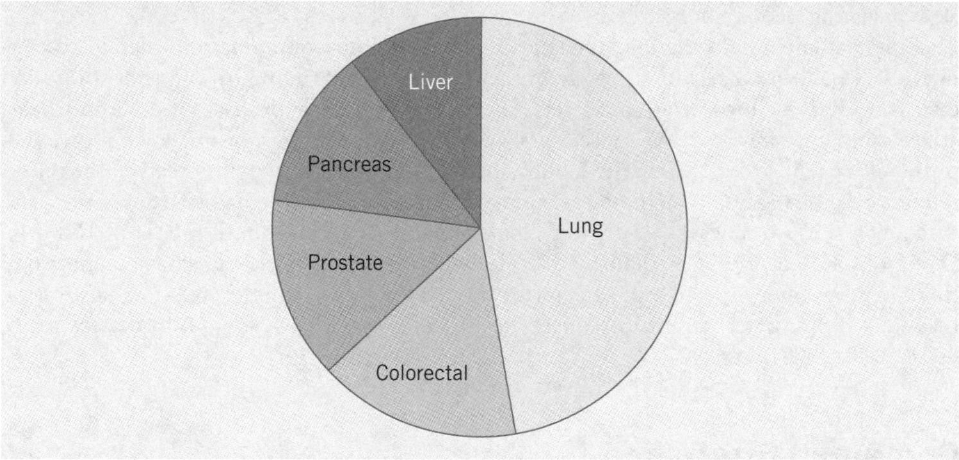

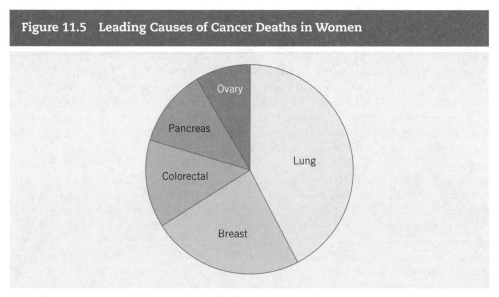

Source: Data from Cancer Facts & Figures (2017), American Cancer Society.

Figure 11.5 Leading Causes of Cancer Deaths in Women

Source: Data from Cancer Facts & Figures (2017), American Cancer Society.

Understanding Cancer

Cancer is the uncontrollable growth and spread of abnormal cells, which form tumors (Brownson, Reif, Alavanja, & Bal, 1993). Benign tumors consist of cells that are similar to the nearby cells, and they grow relatively slowly and are mostly harmless. On the other hand, malignant tumors (commonly called cancers) consist of cells that are different from their surrounding cells and grow very rapidly. Malignant tumors often grow beyond their original location and invade other body organs (metastasize), spreading cancer throughout the body (see Figure 11.6). Tumors can cause intense pain when they put pressure on normal tissues and nerves and block the flow of fluids in the body (Melzack & Wall, 1982). If these tumors are not stopped (either by removing them with surgery or stopping their growth with radiation or chemotherapy or other therapies), they can obstruct vital organs (as in intestinal cancer), cause organs to fail (as in liver or kidney cancer), or lead to hemorrhaging or strokes.

Most cancers are caused by genetic mutations, which may gradually occur over time. Some of these mutations are simply a function of age—as cells continue to multiply, the chance of mutations occurring increases over time. This is why cancer is more common in older people than in younger people. Cancer can also be caused by a **carcinogen**, meaning any substance capable of converting normal cells into cancerous ones. Carcinogens change the cell's DNA, which in turn leads to cancer. For example, exposure to ultraviolet light while sun-tanning can cause a chemical reaction in cells that alters both the components and the shape of the DNA molecule in cells. Although sometimes these changes are found and repaired by the cell, or the cell is killed before it can reproduce, other times these alterations

Figure 11.6   Model Showing Cancer

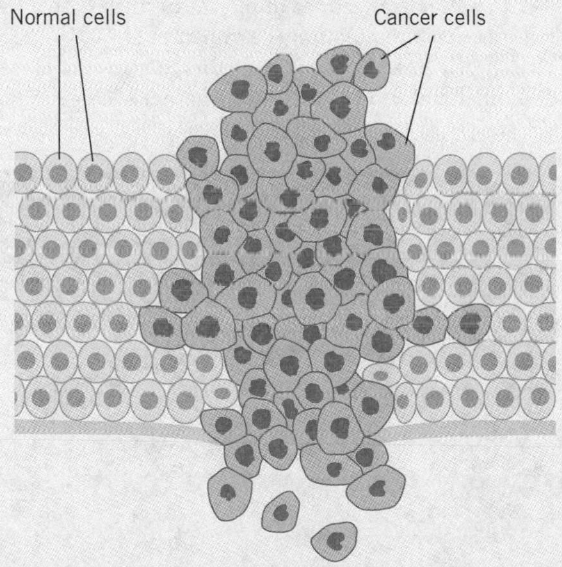

Cancer can be caused by random and naturally occurring mutations or by carcinogens, both of which lead to changes in cells' DNA. These changes disrupt the normal functioning of both the oncogenes, which work to control cell growth and reproduction, and the suppressor genes, which work to inhibit uncontrolled growth. In turn, cancer can spread out of control.

Source: Illustration from © Shutterstock/Alila Medical Media.

go unnoticed and lead to cancer. In normal cells, two different types of genes act to regulate cell growth: *oncogenes* work to control cell growth and reproduction, and *suppressor genes* work to inhibit uncontrolled growth. However, when either of these types of genes is damaged by a mutation—either caused by random chance or exposure to a carcinogen—uncontrolled cell growth and reproduction can occur. For example, benzopyrene, a chemical in cigarette smoke, damages cancer suppressor genes and may therefore lead to lung cancer (Denissenko, Pao, Tang, & Pfeifer, 1996). Similarly, mutations in two genes that are responsible for repairing damage to cell DNA, BRCA1 and BRCA2, are associated with an increased risk of developing breast cancer.

Risk Factors

Some of the factors associated with acquiring cancer are largely fixed and unchangeable. These include genetics, age, and race/ethnicity.

Genetics

An estimated 5% to 10% of all cancers, and 8.5% of pediatric cancers, are influenced by inherited genetic factors (www.cancer.gov; Zhang et al., 2015). In these cases, people have a genetic predisposition to developing a particular type of cancer. For example, a woman whose mother or sister has breast cancer is at nearly twice the risk of developing breast cancer as someone without such a genetic link (Claus, Risch, & Thompson, 1993; Colditz et al., 1993). Finally, genes may influence how cancer patients respond to particular types of treatment, which has important implications for survival, as described in **Focus on Neuroscience**.

Current research provides the strongest evidence for a genetic link for breast, ovarian, colorectal, and prostate cancer (Lichtenstein et al., 2000; Phelan et al., 2017; Prat, Ribé, & Gallardo, 2005; Rebbeck et al., 2015). For example, an estimated 16% of early-onset colon cancer cases are linked to a genetic mutation (Pearlman et al., 2017). However, only 2% to 5% of breast cancers are clearly linked to genetic factors, such as the presence of BRCA1 and BRCA2, indicating that other factors also influence whether such genes are expressed.

FOCUS ON NEUROSCIENCE

How Genes Influence the Value of Chemotherapy

Although the link between particular genes and the likelihood of developing cancer has been known for years, recent research provides evidence that particular genes influence the effectiveness of different types of cancer treatments (Sparano et al., 2015). Specifically, researchers have now developed a test that examines 21 genes from a cancer tumor; this test measures how active the genes are, meaning how likely the cancer is to spread. For patients at low risk, based on this test, undergoing chemotherapy does not increase survival, and patients can therefore avoid the unpleasant side effects of this treatment. In one study, of breast cancer patients who had a low score on this gene test and received standard hormone therapy (treatment with the drug tamoxifen) but did not undergo chemotherapy, 98% were alive at the five-year follow-up. This type of research provides valuable information to cancer patients about the best treatment options, and future research will provide more information health professionals can use to offer this type of personalized medical care and thereby improve treatment outcomes.

Age

People who are older are also at greater risk of developing cancer, perhaps in part because the genetic mutations that cause cancer are more likely to occur over time. However, cancer is the second leading cause of death in children ages 1 to 14 years (after accidents), so this is not simply a disease of the old.

Race/Ethnicity

Ethnicity is also associated with the development of cancer, with Blacks being at a greater risk of developing cancer than Whites (Meyerowitz, Richardson, Hudson, & Leedham, 1998). In fact, Blacks have the highest overall rate of cancer, a rate caused largely by the very high incidence of lung and prostate cancer among Black men. In addition, Blacks who are diagnosed with cancer have an overall survival rate that is lower than that seen in White and Latino patients (Woodward et al., 2006). On the other hand, Latinos and Asian Americans in the United States have relatively low rates of cancer.

Most evidence suggests that these race differences in frequency of cancer are caused by nongenetic factors, such as knowledge, behavior, and access to health care. For example, as compared to Blacks, Whites know more about the risks and signs of cancer, have lower blood pressure, and eat less dietary fat (Meyerowitz, Richardson, Hudson, & Leedham, 1998; Winkleby, Robinson, Sundquist, & Kraemer, 1999). Such differences may also be caused by differences in socioeconomic factors. As you'll learn in *Chapter 13: Managing Health Care*, socioeconomic status (SES) influences people's access to health care. People with a lower SES are less likely to have jobs that provide health insurance and thus are less likely to have access to regular medical care. In turn, they are more likely to get diagnosed with cancer (and other diseases) at later stages, which reduces treatment options and survival rates. As described in the next section, people with a lower SES are also more likely to engage in behaviors that increase their risk of developing cancer, such as smoking, eating unhealthy foods, and not getting enough exercise. Finally, race differences in cancer survival may also reflect the types of tumors seen in patients of different ethnicities. In line with this view, the specific types of tumors seen in patients with colon cancer differ as a function of race, which may help explain why Blacks, compared to Whites, tend to develop this type of cancer at an earlier age and are at a higher risk of dying from this cancer (Yoon et al., 2015).

PSYCHOSOCIAL FACTORS INFLUENCING THE DEVELOPMENT OF CANCER

Although demographic variables such as age and race as well as genetic factors are associated with the likelihood of developing cancer, substantial evidence points to the link between psychosocial factors and the acquisition of cancer too. In fact, an estimated 90% to 95% of all cancers are caused by environmental and lifestyle factors, including smoking, diet, alcohol, sun exposure, and pollutants (Anand et al., 2008). This section examines three such factors.

LO 11.5

Explain how psychosocial factors contribute to cancer

Behavioral Choices

Lifestyle factors are a strong predictor of the development of cancer, with some evidence suggesting that 85% of all cancers could be prevented by changing people's behavior (Brownson et al., 1993; Spring, King, Pagoto, Van Horn, & Fisher, 2015). What types of things do people do that lead to cancer?

Smoking

An estimated 25% to 30% of all cancer deaths are a result of smoking (Anand et al., 2008). In fact, 87% of lung cancer cases—the type of cancer responsible for the most deaths in the United States each year—are attributed to cigarette smoking. Smokers are also at increased risk of developing other types of cancer, including cancer of the mouth, throat, larynx, kidney, cervix, bladder, and pancreas, as well as leukemia and lymphoma. One study even found that women who smoked were 25% more likely to die of breast cancer than those who never smoked (Calle, Miracle-McMahill, Thun, & Heath, 1994). Moreover, women who started smoking before age 16 are at a much greater risk of dying from breast cancer than those who start smoking after age 20, and women who smoke more cigarettes per day have a greater likelihood of acquiring breast cancer than lighter smokers. Simply being regularly exposed to secondhand cigarette smoke increases a person's risk of developing cancer (Fielding & Phenow, 1988).

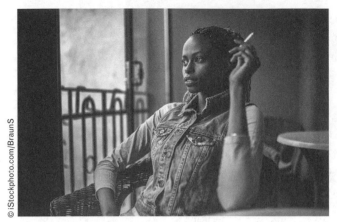

Smoking is the single biggest behavioral choice predicting cancer. If you currently smoke, do everything in your power to stop. The sooner you quit, the lower your risk of developing cancer.

Diet

After smoking, being overweight or obese is the single biggest preventable cause of cancer; an estimated 30% to 35% of cancer-related deaths are linked to diet (Anand et al., 2008). Obesity is linked to 13 types of cancer, including bowel, breast, colorectal, endometrial, kidney, and pancreatic. One explanation for this link is that carrying excess body fat changes levels of sex hormones (estrogen and testosterone), increases levels of insulin, and leads to inflammation, all of which are associated with increased cancer risk. However, how a person carries excess fat may be a better predictor of cancer risk than simply BMI (Freisling et al., 2017). Specifically, carrying excess body fat around the waist is linked with an increased risk of obesity-related cancers as well as bowel cancer.

Although we don't know exactly how particular foods influence cancer risk, there is also evidence that what you eat influences your likelihood of getting cancer. Women who eat more high-fat foods, such as milk, cheese, and butter, have an increased likelihood of developing breast cancer (Toniolo, Ribloi, Protta, Charrel, & Coppa, 1989), and men who eat diets that are high in dietary cholesterol have twice the risk of developing lung cancer than those who eat little excess cholesterol (Shekelle, Rossof, & Stamler, 1991). Similarly, people who eat large quantities of foods that are high in animal (saturated) fat, such as red meat, are at increased risk of developing several different types of cancers, including colon, rectum, and prostate cancers (Slattery, Boucher, Caan, Potter, & Ma, 1998). Patients with colon cancer who eat a diet high in meat, fat, refined grains, and dessert also have a higher risk of recurrence and mortality than those who eat a diet characterized by high intake of fruits and vegetables, poultry, and fish (Meyerhardt et al., 2007).

On the other hand, people who eat large quantities of fruits, vegetables, and foods high in fiber are much less likely to develop colon and rectal cancer (Slattery et al., 1998; Zhang et al., 1999), perhaps in part because these foods work to quickly rid the body of cancer-causing fats. For example, one large-scale study found that women who consumed five or more servings of fruits and vegetables each day were 23% less likely to develop breast cancer than those who ate two or fewer servings per day. Similarly, people who have diets high in *antioxidants*, such as foods containing vitamin A and vitamin C, have lower rates of lung and stomach cancer, perhaps because these vitamins help block the work of carcinogens (Hunter et al., 1993; Yong et al., 1997).

Alcohol

Alcohol use, and especially excessive alcohol use, increases the risk of developing many different types of cancer, including head and neck (such as larynx and throat), esophageal, pancreas, liver, breast, and colorectal (Baan et al., 2007; Collaborative Group on Hormonal Factors in Breast Cancer, 2002; Connor, 2017; Fedirko et al., 2011; Grewal & Viswanathen, 2012; Heuch, Kvale, Jacobsen, & Bjelke, 1983; IARC Working Group on the Evaluation of Carcinogenic Risks to Humans, 2012). For example, people who consume 3.5 or more alcoholic drinks a day are two to three times more likely to develop a head or neck cancer than people who don't drink (Baan et al., 2007). Moreover, the more alcohol a person drinks over time, the greater his or her risk of developing an alcohol-related cancer. For every additional 10 ounces of alcohol consumed a day (slightly less than one drink), a woman's risk of developing breast cancer increases 12% (Allen et al., 2009).

The specific processes by which alcohol causes cancer are not known, although researchers have proposed a number of different explanations (Boffetta & Hashibe, 2006; Purohit, Khalsa, & Serrano, 2005). One possibility is that when the body processes the ethanol found in alcohol, it creates a toxic chemical (acetaldehyde), which is a carcinogen. Alcoholic beverage may also themselves contain various carcinogenic elements. Alternatively, or perhaps additionally, alcohol may disrupt the body's ability to absorb various nutrients—such as vitamins A, C, D, and E—that help protect the body from cancer. Alcohol may also lead to increases in estrogen, a hormone that increases the risk of breast cancer.

Other Lifestyle Choices

Other lifestyles choices also influence people's risk of developing cancer. Sun exposure is clearly recognized as a major cause of skin cancer, yet many people who tan regularly do not use sunscreens at all (Brownson et al., 1993; Koh et al., 1997; Spring et al., 2015). And even people who do use sunscreen often use a lower-than-recommended level of protection.

Some patterns of sexual behavior are also associated with cancer (Spring et al., 2015). For example, women who have multiple sexual partners, a history of STDs, and begin having sex at an early age are at increased risk of developing cervical cancer (Brownson et al., 1993).

Exercise

What's the good news? Engaging in regular exercise seems to offer some protection against various types of cancer, including breast cancer (Bernstein, Henderson, Hanisch, Sullivan-Halley, & Ross, 1994; Rockhill et al., 1999; Thune, Brenn, Lund, & Gaard, 1997), prostate cancer (Lee, Paffenbarger, & Hsieh, 1992), and colon cancer (Slattery, Schumacher, Smith, West, & Abd-Elghany, 1990; White, Jacobs, & Daling, 1996). For example, one study found that young women who engaged in regular physical exercise—at least four times a week—were half as likely to develop breast cancer as those who did not engage in regular exercise (Bernstein et al., 1994). Although this study was conducted by matching women who exercised regularly to those who did not based on age, race, and whether they had children, and then comparing the rate of breast cancer in both groups, it does not definitively show that exercise decreases a woman's risk of cancer. Perhaps women who exercise regularly are generally healthier (e.g., less likely to smoke, more likely to eat healthy foods) and therefore less likely to develop cancer.

Engaging in regular exercise is also associated with positive outcomes in people who have been diagnosed with cancer. One recent review of lifestyle predictors associated with reducing the risk of recurring breast cancer found that engaging in regular physical activity—at least 30 minutes of moderate exercise five days a week—and avoiding weight gain during and after treatment were the best predictors of long-term outcomes, such as likelihood of recurrence and death (Hamer & Warner, 2017).

Stress

What You'll Learn
11.4

Stress, including a history of stressful life experiences as well as separation from or loss of a loved one, is associated with acquiring cancer (McKenna, Zevon, Corn, & Rounds, 1999). Studies comparing patients with cancer to those without cancer have found that those with cancer report significantly more negative life events, such as loss of loved ones and marital problems, than those without cancer. For example, children with cancer are quite likely to have experienced a number of life changes, such as personal injury and change in the health of a family member, in the year preceding their diagnosis (Jacobs & Charles, 1980). Although some of these studies are retrospective and therefore it is difficult to tell whether patients' cancer diagnosis at one point leads them to look at the past in a more negative light, one meta-analysis on the predictors of cancer demonstrated that both the experience of stressful life events and the loss of a loved one are associated with an increased likelihood of developing cancer (McKenna et al., 1999).

To examine the link between work stress and the development of cancer, researchers in one recent study interviewed men about their experience of work stress (Blanc-Lapierre, Rousseau, Weiss, El-Zein, Siemiatycki, & Parent, 2017). The most stressful jobs were firefighter, aerospace engineer, and mechanic foreman, although people with the same job varied in how much they perceived stress. The factors causing stress included job insecurity, dangerous work conditions, interpersonal conflict with colleagues, and a difficult commute. Most important, the findings indicated that those who reported exposure to prolonged work-related stress—meaning for at least 15 years—were more likely to have been diagnosed with cancer. Diagnoses of lung, colon, rectal, stomach cancer, and non-Hodgkin lymphoma were all more common in men reporting chronic work stress.

How exactly does stress lead to cancer? As discussed in *Chapter 4: Understanding Stress*, stress clearly weakens the immune system, which thereby decreases the body's ability to detect and kill abnormal cancer cells (Delahanty & Baum, 2001). Research with both humans and rats shows that stressful events, such as exams, divorce, and job loss (in humans) and rotation on a turntable, uncontrollable shocks, and flashing lights (in rats) reduces the number of immune cells in the blood. For example, people who have recently been separated from their spouses have lower levels of natural killer (NK) cells and helper T cells (Kiecolt-Glaser & Glaser, 1989), as do people who are taking care of a terminally ill relative (Kiecolt-Glaser, Dura, Speicher, Trask, & Glaser, 1991). Stress may also reduce the body's ability to fix DNA errors, meaning that random errors that would normally be found and repaired by the body are instead allowed to remain in the body (Glaser, Thorn, Tarr, Kiecolt-Glaser, & D'Ambrosio, 1985). Sadly, and as described in **Focus on Development**, these findings help explain why children who experience abuse are more likely to later develop cancer.

Personality

Many people, including those with cancer, believe that this disease is caused at least in part by personality factors (Roberts, Newcomb, Trentham-Dietz, & Storer, 1996). A number of personality dimensions, including depression, extraversion, and difficulty expressing emotions, are often associated with the development of cancer (Dattore, Shontz, & Coyne, 1980; Perskey, Kempthorne-Rawson, & Shekelle, 1987; Shaffer, Duszynski, & Thomas, 1982; Shaffer, Graves, Swank, & Pearson, 1987). In fact, some researchers describe people with such traits, namely, those who present a pleasant and cheerful face to the world, show passivity in the face of stress, and tend to suppress negative emotions, as having a "Type C," or cancer-prone, personality (McKenna et al., 1999). Many of these studies, however, have used cross-sectional designs, in which they examine people with and without cancer at a single point in time, and therefore they cannot determine whether the presence of such traits caused the cancer or vice versa. After all, it is therefore not surprising that people with cancer would show distinct types of personality traits, including a tendency to try to suppress their difficult emotions about the disease as well as depression. However, other studies using longitudinal designs have often revealed similar results. For example, Shaffer and colleagues (1982) examined attitudes toward family by following a group of healthy medical students and then followed these participants to measure illness over time for 30 years. Those with impaired self-awareness, a lack of emotional expression, and feelings of self-sacrifice and self-blame were 16 times more likely to develop cancer than the others. Similarly, another study revealed that men who were depressed at one point in time were twice as likely to die from cancer 20 years later than those who were not depressed (Shekelle et al., 1981).

A meta-analysis, a combination of various studies on the link between personality and cancer, provided only moderate evidence for the role of personality traits leading to cancer (McKenna et al., 1999). First, people who rely heavily on denial and repression as a way of coping with problems are at a somewhat greater risk of developing cancer. This type of coping pattern is associated with an overall weakened immune system, which could be one explanation for the link between denial, repression, and cancer. Second, there is limited evidence that people with a conflict-avoidant personality style are more likely to develop cancer. This type of coping is similar to that of denial and repression and may also therefore impact the immune system. Finally, current research provides no evidence that other personality dimensions, including depression/anxiety, introversion/extraversion, and expression of anger, are associated with acquiring cancer.

FACTORS INFLUENCING COPING WITH CANCER

LO 11.6

Summarize strategies for coping with cancer

Receiving a cancer diagnosis is very difficult for virtually everyone. Many people experience symptoms of depression and anxiety following such a diagnosis (Gandubert et al., 2009). In fact, 28% of patients newly diagnosed with cancer meet the criteria for acute stress disorder within the first month, and 22% meet the criteria for posttraumatic stress disorder (PTSD) at the six-month follow-up (Kangas, Henry, & Bryant, 2005). Although some of the initial reactions fade over time, even long-term cancer survivors may continue to worry about recurrence (Skaali et al., 2009). However, different factors influence how people react to such a diagnosis, including the treatment they receive, the coping strategies they use, and their level of social support. Various interventions may also help cancer patients cope with their diagnosis and treatment, as you'll learn in the final section.

Treatment

Many of the treatments used to fight cancer, including chemotherapy—which involves administering toxic chemicals to the body in an attempt to kill the cancerous cells—and radiation—in which beams of radiation are used to destroy tissue in a particular area—have unpleasant side effects, including fatigue, diarrhea, vomiting, hair loss, loss of appetite, and nausea. In some cases, these effects can be quite long-lasting. For example, although breast cancer survivors do not differ from women who have never had cancer in many measures of quality of life, survivors report more difficulties with physical functioning and more physical symptoms than do women without cancer even five years later (Helgeson & Tomich, 2005).

Some types of cancer treatment, including treatment for prostate, urinary, and colorectal cancer, can lead to changes in bowel, urinary, and/or sexual function (Moyer & Salovey, 1996; Sanda et al., 2008). Patients with colon cancer may require a colostomy, or surgical opening in the abdomen from which feces are evacuated from the body. Patients may experience feelings of shame as they are forced to handle their bodily wastes on a daily basis and may worry that others easily recognize their condition. Prostate cancer patients are particularly likely to experience sexual dysfunction following surgery, which can lead to marital distress—especially if partners didn't talk about this experience (Badr & Carmack Taylor, 2009).

Surgery, one of the most common treatments for some types of cancer, can lead to various types of disability and disfigurement, including amputation of a limb (in the case of bone cancer), removal of part or all of one or both breasts (in the case of breast cancer), or removal of a testis (in the case of testicular cancer). Women who are diagnosed with breast cancer must cope with their concerns about body image, particularly if their treatment involves removal of one or both breasts (Carver et al., 1998; Spencer et al., 1999). These concerns are particularly salient for younger women. Encouragingly, women who undergo lumpectomies, in which only the cancerous tumor is removed from the breast, generally have fewer problems with marital and sexual adjustment than those who undergo mastectomies, in which one or both breasts are removed totally (Moyer, 1997; Taylor, Bandura, Ewart, Miller, & DeBusk, 1985).

Coping Strategies

Although a cancer diagnosis is difficult for virtually everyone, people respond to this information in very different ways. For example, women who are high on agreeableness and low on negative affect experience lower levels of depression following a cancer diagnosis than do women without such personality traits (Den Oudsten, Van Heck, Van der Steeg, Roukema, & De Vries, 2009). Not surprisingly, the coping strategies people utilize are associated with psychological as well as physical outcomes.

Perceiving Control

Although people who are diagnosed with cancer typically experience considerable fear and uncertainty about the future, those who believe they have some control over the disease experience lower levels of psychological distress and a higher overall quality of life (Bárez, Blasco, Fernández-Castro, & Viladrich, 2009; Beckjord, Glinder, Langrock, & Compas, 2009; Dunkel Schetter, Feinstein, Taylor, & Falke, 1992; Helgeson, Snyder, & Seltman, 2004;

Rozema, Völlink, & Lechner, 2009). One study with patients with breast cancer revealed that women who believed that they and their doctors had control over the cancer experienced better adjustment (e.g., less anxiety, fear, depression, anger) to their disease (Taylor, Lichtman, & Wood, 1984). These beliefs are largely illusions (e.g., cancer is largely uncontrollable and unpredictable) but serve a valuable role in psychological adaptation and are therefore quite functional. For example, women with breast cancer who are more involved in decision making regarding cancer treatment and follow-up (including surgery, radiation, chemotherapy) show improved health-related quality of life as long as 10 years after diagnosis, at least in part because involvement in such decision making increases perceptions of control (Andersen, Bowen, Morea, Stein, & Baker, 2009).

Expecting the Best

People who approach a cancer diagnosis with optimistic expectations about the outcome show better psychological adjustment, including lower levels of anxiety and depression, than those who dwell on potential negative outcomes (Carver et al., 1993; Deimling, Wagner, Bowman, Sterns, & Kahana, 2006; Dunkel Schetter et al., 1992; Helgeson et al., 2004). For example, women with breast cancer who are determined to beat the disease and refuse to give up show lower levels of emotional distress (Classen, Koopman, Angell, & Spiegel, 1996). People who are optimistic experience lower levels of anxiety and depression at least in part because they are less likely to blame themselves and withdraw from others (Epping-Jordan et al., 1999). These findings are in line with those described in *Chapter 5: Managing Stress* that people who cope with stressful life events with an optimistic and active style tend to experience fewer psychological problems.

People's style of coping with cancer can even influence survival (Greer, 1991). Specifically, those who simply "give in" and stop fighting the disease, or deny its existence, often die more rapidly than those who maintain a more aggressive and active approach. For example, one study classified women based on their response to the cancer diagnosis: stoic acceptance, helplessness/hopelessness, optimistic spirit, or denial (Pettingale, Morris, Greer, & Haybittle, 1985). These patients were then followed for 10 years. Among those with stoic acceptance, 31% had died after 5 years and 75% had died after 10 years, and among those with helplessness, 80% had died after 5 years. In contrast, among those with an optimistic spirit, 10% had died after 5 years and 30% after 10 years, and those who responded with denial had a 10% death rate after 5 years and a 50% death rate after 10 years. Although this study was based on a small sample of women, it certainly suggests that psychological factors may influence the length of survival in patients with cancer.

Focusing on the Positive

A substantial percentage of people who have cancer report finding some positive aspects of their diagnosis (Jansen, Hoffmeister, Chang-Claude, Brenner, & Arndt, 2011; Mols, Vingerhoets, Coebergh, & van de Poll-Franse, 2009). Two relative common positive aspects are **benefit finding**, meaning recognizing beneficial aspects of an adverse situation, and **posttraumatic growth**, meaning experiencing significant positive growth after struggling with a major life crisis. These positive aspects could include increased feelings of personal strengths, a richer spiritual life, a change in life priorities, and closer relationships (Collins, Taylor, & Skokan, 1990; Tedeschi & Calhoun, 1996; Tennen & Affleck, 2002).

Not surprisingly, people who cope with cancer by finding some positive aspects experience better outcomes (Dunkel Schetter et al., 1992). Specifically, people with cancer who report more benefit finding have less distress, more positive affect, and an overall increased quality of life (Rinaldis, Pakenham, & Lynch, 2010). In fact, breast cancer patients who report benefit finding have lower distress and depression even four to seven years later (Carver &

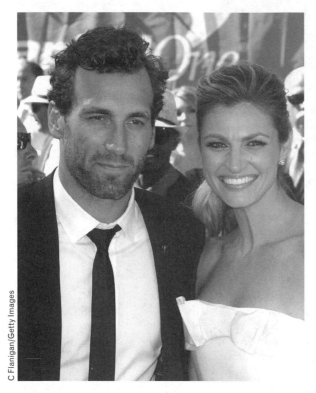

C Flanigan/Getty Images

Sportscaster and *Dancing With the Stars* host Erin Andrews reports that her diagnosis with cervical cancer in September 2016 brought her closer to her then-boyfriend (now husband) Jarret Stoll, saying, "It was a huge step for my relationship with my boyfriend at the time. Because you don't know if a guy is going to want to sit in with an oncologist and see, 'OK, so this is your cervix, and this is your uterus, and we are cutting out this part. . . .'" This type of benefit-finding following a cancer diagnosis is associated with positive psychological outcomes.

Antoni, 2004). Similarly, women with breast cancer who are high in posttraumatic growth show lower levels of distress over time; this is especially true for women who undergo a mastectomy (Wang et al., 2017).

Blaming One's Self

Although this section has focused thus far on coping strategies that lead to lower levels of psychological distress, the use of particular strategies can have negative outcomes. People who blame themselves for getting cancer—which about 40% of people do following diagnosis—experience higher levels of anxiety and depression (Glinder & Compas, 1999; Taylor et al., 1984). Those who feel responsible for their illness often experience considerable guilt for the pain they are causing themselves as well as their loved ones. People whose cancer is more clearly linked with their behavioral choices are especially at risk of engaging in self-blame, and, in turn, showing poor psychological adjustment. For example, people with lung cancer—a type of cancer most often caused by smoking—are more likely to engage in self-blame than people with breast or prostate cancer, which are less commonly caused by behavioral choices (Else-Quest, LoConte, Schiller, & Hyde, 2009).

In some cases, however, negative feelings may result in positive outcomes. For example, cancer patients who experience feelings of anger and guilt may be inspired to set new goals, such as starting to go for brisk walks and engage in regular physical activity (Castonguay, Wrosch, & Sabiston, 2017). In turn, these health-promoting activities help people avoid the typically negative physiological effects of negative feelings on health outcomes.

Conclusions

Finally, although this section has described how coping strategies influence psychological adjustment, it is also possible that psychological adjustment influences coping strategies. Specifically, people who feel better adjusted may find it easier to use effective strategies. In line with this view, the quality of life in women with breast cancer is a stronger predictor of coping strategies than the reverse (Danhauer, Crawford, Farmer, & Avis, 2009). This finding suggests that the link between coping strategies and quality of life may in fact work in both directions.

Social Support

Not surprisingly, people with cancer who receive more social support from friends and family report better psychological adjustment (Alferi, Carver, Antoni, Weiss, & Duran, 2001; Badr & Taylor, 2008; Dunkel Schetter et al., 1992; Helgeson et al., 2004). For example, people who feel they receive an adequate amount of emotional social support, such as having people available to listen and share concerns, show lower distress over time (Helgeson & Cohen, 1996). Similarly, people who feel able to share their feelings with their spouse following a cancer diagnosis report lower levels of cancer-related distress (Badr, Carmack,

Kashy, Cristofanilli, & Revenson, 2010). Instrumental support, such as help with chores, transportation, and assistance with child care, is also helpful, especially for people with a poor prognosis for recovery, presumably because they have more trouble managing these practical tasks. These findings about the benefits of social support help explain research showing that married people and women tend to cope better with cancer than unmarried people and men, who tend to receive lower levels of social support (Goldzweig et al., 2009).

Although all types of social support are associated with better adjustment to cancer, positive social interaction support—meaning the availability of people with whom to have fun, relax, and get one's mind off cancer for a while—is the strongest predictor of overall quality of life (Kroenke et al., 2013). Moreover, this type of support was also related to physical outcomes, including lower levels of nausea, pain, and needed bed rest, as well as higher levels of energy. These findings indicate that support is particularly valuable when it truly allows a person to forget about her or his cancer and just have a good time.

More important, people with cancer who have higher levels of social support may survive for longer periods than those without such support (Goodwin, Hunt, Key, & Samet, 1987; Reynolds & Kaplan, 1990). Researchers in one study examined whether patients who were married when they were diagnosed with cancer would live longer than those who were single (Aizer et al., 2013). To test this question, they examined over 700,000 people who were diagnosed with cancer between 2004 and 2008. Even after taking into account other factors related to survival, such as age, sex, race, and income, single people were 17% more likely to have metastatic cancer, meaning cancer that had spread beyond its original site (which is more difficult to treat). They were also 53% less likely to receive the appropriate treatment. These findings suggest that married cancer patients live longer because the support provided by their spouse increases their likelihood of following recommended treatment regimens. Other research suggests that married people also get diagnosed at earlier stages, which also leads to better outcomes (Goodwin et al., 1987).

What You'll Learn
11.5

However, marriage isn't the only type of social support that benefits survival. Cancer patients with more social ties—including marriage but also friendships, other family members, and community networks—have lower rates of disease recurrence and cancer death than those who are more socially isolated (Kroenke, Michael, Poole, et al., 2017; Kroenke, Michael, Shu, et al., 2017). Specifically, a study of women with breast cancer found that compared to social integrated people, socially isolated women were 43% more likely to experience a cancer recurrence and 64% more likely to die from cancer. One explanation for the benefits of social support on survival is that socially isolated women show more cancer-related risk factors, including obesity, smoking, low physical activity, and high alcohol use. They are also less likely to receive chemotherapy. These factors may increase the likelihood of a recurrence and faster disease progression.

How exactly does social support lead to improved adjustment to chronic disease? One possibility is that social support is associated with better coping strategies. Women with early-stage breast cancer who receive unsupportive behavior from their partner show more use of avoidant coping and, in turn, higher levels of distress (Manne, Ostroff, Winkel, Grana, & Fox, 2005). On the other hand, cancer patients who receive more social support from friends show higher levels of fighting spirit, suggesting that receiving support may lead patients to see cancer as a challenge and to take an active role in therapy and recovery (Cicero, Lo Coco, Gullo, & Lo Verso, 2009). Social support may also help patients find positive meaning in their diagnosis. In line with this view, cancer survivors who receive more emotional support in the months following the diagnosis report experiencing more positive consequences of the illness eight years later (Schroevers, Helgeson, Sanderman, & Ranchor, 2010).

Another possibility is that social support provides an opportunity for patients to process information about their diagnosis. For example, patients with cancer who have high levels of social support are likely to have people with whom they can share their fears and concerns about the disease. People who can express their emotions about having cancer report less stress, anxiety, depression, and distress than those who aren't able to express these emotions (Schmidt & Andrykowski, 2004; Stanton, Kirk, Camerson, & Danoff-Burg, 2000). Similarly, prostate cancer patients who discuss treatment options with social networks prior to beginning treatment show higher levels of social support and emotional expression as well as decreases in negative affect after treatment (Christie, Meyerowitz, Giedzinska-Simons, Gross, & Agus, 2009). In sum, greater time spent talking with family and friends about treatment options may provide opportunities for patients to cope with the emotions related to their cancer diagnosis, which may improve feelings of distress over time.

Interventions

Many people with cancer benefit—both psychologically and physically—from participating in some type of formal intervention group. These groups provide training in specific strategies for managing the pain and symptoms of cancer as well as its treatment. Such interventions may provide education, stress management techniques, cognitive-behavioral strategies, and/or social support.

Education

Education on managing symptoms and treatment can lead to improvements in both psychological and physical functioning. Cancer patients who participated in eight 45-minute education sessions, which provided information on how to manage the disease and its treatment, showed lower levels of pain and higher reports of physical functioning as long as three years later (Helgeson, Cohen, Schulz, & Yasko, 1999, 2001). People particularly benefit from learning strategies for managing the side effects of chemotherapy, which can include nausea, vomiting, and general physical distress. Specifically, training in hypnosis, progressive muscle relaxation training, guided imagery, and systematic desensitization decreases both physical and psychological side effects of chemotherapy, and may lead to increases in caloric intake (Carey & Burish, 1988; Morrow, Asbury, Hamman, & Dobkin, 1992). Perhaps most important, this type of training leads to greater immune system functioning 6 to 12 months later, which may increase survival.

Cancer patients also benefit from simply knowing what to expect during treatment. For example, patients who received detailed information (including a tour of the oncology ward, a videotaped presentation about chemotherapy, and a take-home booklet) had lower levels of nausea and vomiting, were less depressed and hostile, and experienced less disruption in their daily lives while in chemotherapy treatment compared to those who received relaxation training as well as those who received only a brief (25-minute) information session (Burish, Snyder, & Jenkins, 1991). In sum, providing education about the disease, its symptoms, and its treatment may increase patients' sense of self-efficacy and control, and thereby improve psychological and physical functioning.

Stress Management

Given the anxiety many people have following a cancer diagnosis, receiving training in relaxation can help reduce this stress, and thereby improve psychological as well as physical well-being. For example, patients with cancer who engage in regular meditation show lower levels of anger, depression, and anxiety than those without such training (Speca, Carlson, Goodey, & Angen, 2000). Similarly, patients who receive mindfulness-based stress reduction training show lower rates of depression, anxiety, and fear of recurrence as well as higher levels of energy, physical functioning, and physical role functioning (Lengacher et al., 2009). This type of training also helps patients reduce negative symptoms, such as insomnia, associated with the cancer diagnosis and its treatment (Garland et al., 2014). Relaxation training may be particularly beneficial for coping with the stress of chemotherapy. Patients who receive relaxation training report feeling less anxious and depressed during chemotherapy sessions (Lyles, Burish, Krozely, & Oldham, 1982). They also report less nausea during and after chemotherapy, suggesting such training may help cancer patients cope with the adverse effects of treatment.

Other forms of stress management also lead to improvements in psychological and physical well-being for cancer patients. For example, compared to those in a waiting list control condition, women with breast cancer who participate in weekly yoga classes show improvements in mental health, depression, positive affect, and fatigue (Danhauer et al., 2009). Such classes are particularly beneficial for women with higher negative affect and lower emotional well-being. Perhaps most important, relaxation training may also lead to improved physiological functioning. Specifically, compared to women who received standard care, those who participated in yoga sessions, which included training in relaxation and meditation, while undergoing radiation treatment for breast cancer reported lower levels of fatigue as well as better physical functioning and overall health (Chandwani et al., 2014). They also showed lower levels of cortisol, a marker of stress associated with worse outcomes for cancer patients.

Cognitive-Behavioral Strategies

Many effective interventions provide training in both the cognitive and behavioral skills needed to cope with cancer. For example, they may emphasize the value of holding positive expectations and relying on social support as well as relaxing and reducing anxiety. These interventions can lead to reduced depression and improvements in psychological well-being, including general optimism and ability to find benefits in having cancer (Antoni et al., 2001; Gudenkauf et al., 2015). Cognitive-behavioral training also reduces the impact of side effects of cancer treatment, such as fatigue (Montgomery et al., 2009). The effects of such interventions may be quite long-lasting. As shown in Figure 11.7, women who receive cognitive-behavioral stress management show improved well-being and lower rates of depression even 8 to 15 years later (Stagl et al., 2015).

Some research even suggests that cancer patients who receive training in how to manage cancer-related stress show a longer time until recurrence and greater survival rates (Stagl et al., 2015). For example, breast cancer patients who received an intervention focused on managing stress and improving health-related behaviors were twice as likely to be alive at the 11-year follow-up as those who simply received standard treatment (Andersen et al., 2008; Andersen, Bowen, Morea, Stein, & Baker, 2009). Moreover, of those who experienced a recurrence, those who received the intervention were cancer-free about six months longer. These findings provide substantial evidence that broad-based interventions, which include training in stress management as well as other health-promoting behavior, increase survival.

Social Support Groups

Many patients with cancer choose to participate in social support groups with other patients and find considerable value in spending time with others who truly understand and empathize with the experience of having a life-threatening disease. Some research even indicates that participation in such a group may impact survival (Spiegel, Bloom, Kraemer, & Gottheil, 1989). For example, researchers in one study randomly assigned women with advanced breast cancer to receive a weekly 90-minute group therapy session for one year or no therapy. The patients were then followed for 10 years. Those who received the group therapy lived nearly twice as long as those in the control condition (36.6 versus 18.9 months, respectively). These

Figure 11.7 Data From Stagl et al., 2015

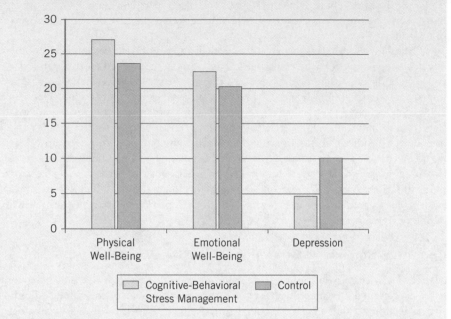

Breast cancer patients who receive group-based training in cognitive-behavioral skills for managing stress show higher levels of physical and emotional well-being, and lower levels of depression, at the 8- to 15-year follow-up than women who receive standard care.

Source: Data from Stagl Bouchard, Lechner, Blomberg, Gudenkauf, Jutagir, . . . Antoni (2015).

results suggest that psychotherapy can help slow the progression of cancer, although it does not cure it. Some evidence suggests that participating in a social support group can improve patients' immunological response, which could help explain the longer life expectancy of those in the group therapy support group, previously mentioned (Fawzy et al., 1990).

However, a subsequent study refuted these findings (Goodwin et al., 2001). In this study 245 women with breast cancer were randomly assigned either to a weekly supportive-expressive group therapy group or to a control group that received no group support. Although women in the therapy group reported less pain and fewer psychological symptoms, especially those who were depressed at the start of the study, there was no difference in length of survival. Women in both conditions lived an average of 17.5 months.

One explanation for the differences in outcomes is that the studies were carried out approximately 20 years apart (Spiegel, 2001). Medical treatment for cancer as well as techniques for detecting cancer improved dramatically between the 1970s and 1990s, which in turn led to decreases in the rate of breast cancer deaths over time. Cancer has also become more understood and accepted during this period—patients with cancer experience lower levels of stigma and alienation, which may mean that social support groups are less beneficial. Finally, whereas now social support groups often are seen as a valued strategy for coping with chronic diseases, this acceptance was not abundant in the 1970s. Dr. David Spiegel, the author of the original study, recalls that in the 1970s it was difficult to convince patients to attend the (presumably worthless) group therapy sessions, whereas in the 1990s, patients not assigned to receive this type of treatment were disappointed. Future research is clearly needed to examine whether, when, and for whom group therapy can work to improve physical and psychological well-being.

Although evidence for the overall value of social support groups for improving both the quality and length of life for people with cancer is mixed, such groups may be beneficial at least for some people. For example, one study with patients with cancer found that those who received low levels of emotional support from their partners benefited in terms of physical functioning from participation in a peer discussion group, but those who already had high levels of support at home showed no such change or decreases in physical functioning following participation (Helgeson, Cohen, Schulz, & Yasko, 2000). Although this finding was unexpected, it may be that those who participated in the group talked about their problems more at home, which in turn led to more negative interactions. It could also be that they changed their expectations about the type of support they should receive at home, and that made them sad. Similarly, women with unsupportive partners who want to express their emotional reactions to a cancer diagnosis may particularly benefit from social support interventions (Manne, Ostroff, & Winkel, 2007).

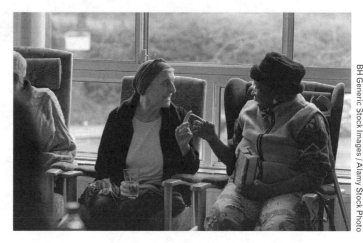

BH Generic Stock Images / Alamy Stock Photo

Although research findings are mixed on whether participating in a cancer support group increases life expectancy, many people with cancer find such groups helpful.

Finally, although social support groups may be effective at least in part because they allow participants to express emotions with others who understand, this opportunity may be more beneficial for some people than for others. For example, several studies have demonstrated that people with cancer benefit in terms of reducing cancer-related symptoms and improving psychological and physical well-being from engaging in expressive writing (Merz, Fox, & Malcarne, 2014; Milbury et al., 2014). However, a recent study with Chinese American women with breast cancer found that writing about cancer facts led to higher overall quality of life than writing about thoughts and feelings regarding cancer (Lu, Wong, Gallagher, Tou, Young, & Loh, 2017). This finding is in line with other research indicating that Anglo-American women with breast cancer feel a greater need for social support during treatment than do Chinese American or Japanese American women (Wellisch et al., 1999). In sum, future research should also examine whether cancer patients from different ethnic and/or cultural backgrounds may benefit from different types of interventions.

Table 11.2 Information YOU Can Use
• Many of the factors that increase the risk of developing CHD are within your control, such as eating a healthy diet, maintaining a healthy weight, and getting enough physical activity. Use some of the strategies described in **Chapter 8: Obesity and Disordered Eating** to make sure you are making healthy food choices and staying within a healthy weight.
• The very best way you can reduce your risk of developing CHD and cancer—the two leading causes of death in the United States—is by not smoking. If you don't smoke now, good for you (and keep it up). If you do smoke, make every effort to stop; quitting reduces your risk of developing these, and other, very serious health conditions. Use the strategies described in **Chapter 7: Substance Use and Abuse** to help you quit.

(Continued)

Table 11.2 (Continued)

- Most evidence suggests that stress increases the risk of developing CHD and cancer as well as the likelihood of experiencing a repeat heart attack or cancer recurrence. Learn strategies for reducing stress in your own life, such as relaxation, meditation, and cognitive reappraisal. *Chapter 5: Managing Stress* provides detailed information on these, and other, methods of reducing stress.

- If you have a friend or family member who is living with CHD or cancer, provide social support to help them during this difficult time. Offer to accompany them to an appointment, help with errands or household tasks they may not be able to do themselves, or sit with them and watch television. People with life-threatening illnesses who receive such support show improved psychological and physical adjustment (and may even live longer).

- Since minutes truly matter for people experiencing a heart attack, learn the signs: chest discomfort (pressure, squeezing, fullness), discomfort in other parts of the upper body (arms, back, neck, jaw, stomach), shortness of breath, breaking out in a cold sweat, nausea, or lightheadedness. Don't wait to get help if you or someone with you experiences any of these heart attack warning signs. Call 911.

SUMMARY

Coronary Heart Disease

- Under normal conditions, the heart contracts and releases, which pumps blood throughout the body, and carries oxygen and removes carbon dioxide and other waste material from the cells. Over time the artery walls can become clogged with fatty substances, which decreases the area through which blood can flow and increases the likelihood of a blood clot. This process is known as atherosclerosis. Moreover, over time arteries can lose their elasticity and become thick and stiff, which is known as arteriosclerosis. Both atherosclerosis and arteriosclerosis can lead to very serious problems, including angina, a myocardial infarction (heart attack), or stroke.

- Three medical conditions are consistently linked with an increased risk of developing CHD: hypertension, high cholesterol, and diabetes. Genetic factors also contribute to the likelihood of developing CHD. In addition, various demographic factors influence the risk of developing CHD, including age, gender, and race/ethnicity.

Psychosocial Factors Contributing to Coronary Heart Disease

- Behavioral choices play a substantial role in the development of CHD. Smoking contributes to CHD by increasing the heart rate and blood pressure, constricting the blood vessels, and decreasing the production of HDL cholesterol. Although moderate levels of alcohol use are associated with a decreased risk of CHD, heavier consumption of alcohol increases the risk of CHD. People who eat foods that are high in cholesterol, fats, and/or sodium are at greater risk of developing CHD, as are people who are obese. People who engage in regular exercise are less likely to develop CHD or to experience a heart attack or stroke.

- Stress, including pressure caused by work, interpersonal conflict, traumas, and financial concerns, may contribute to CHD. Persistent racial discrimination may also lead to CHD, as may relatively short-lived stressful experiences, such as living in or visiting New York City.

- A number of environmental factors are associated with an increased likelihood of developing cardiovascular diseases. These include being exposed to cigarette smoke and living in an inner city.

- Although for many year people with Type A behavior pattern were thought to be at increased risk of developing CHD, more recent evidence now points to the role of hostility, anger expression, and Type D personality in increasing the risk of developing cardiovascular problems. On the other hand, people who experience high levels of positive emotions are at reduced risk of developing such problems.

- Another factor that increases the risk of developing cardiovascular problems, including a heart attack or stroke, is feeling social isolated or lonely.

Strategies for Reducing the Risk of Recurring Heart Attacks

- One type of treatment for CHD focuses on helping people change their health-related behavior, including showing them how to reduce their sodium and fat intake, lower their weight, and stop smoking. Health education programs also encourage people to start exercising, encourage patients to follow prescribed medical regimens, and provide information on the early signs and symptoms of a heart attack.

- Another common approach to reducing the risk of CHD is through training patients in techniques for managing stress. These methods include training in relaxation as well as strategies for changing negative cognitions, behaviors, and emotions.

- Other programs combine health education and stress management techniques by focusing on lifestyle changes (including in regard to smoking, diet, and exercise) as well as stress.

Cancer

- Cancer is the uncontrollable growth and spread of abnormal cells, which form tumors. Benign tumors consist of cells that are similar to the nearby cells, and they grow relatively slowly and are mostly harmless. Malignant tumors (commonly called cancers) consist of cells that are different from their surrounding cells and grow very rapidly, including beyond their original location. Most cancers are caused by genetic mutations, which may gradually occur over time.

- Some of the factors associated with acquiring cancer are largely fixed and unchangeable. These include genetic factors and age. Ethnicity is also associated with the development of cancer, with Blacks being at a greater risk of developing cancer than Whites. Most evidence suggests that these race differences in frequency of cancer are caused by nongenetic factors, such as knowledge, behavior, and access to health care.

Psychosocial Factors Influencing the Development of Cancer

- Lifestyle factors, such as smoking, being overweight or obese, and alcohol use, contribute to the development of cancer. Other lifestyles choices, such as sun exposure and sexual behavior, also influence people's risk of developing cancer. Engaging in regular exercise seems to offer some protection against various types of cancer.

- Stress, including a history of stressful life experiences as well as separation from or loss of a loved one, is associated with acquiring cancer. Stress weakens the immune system, which thereby decreases the body's ability to detect and kill abnormal cancer cells. Stress may also reduce the body's ability to fix DNA errors, meaning that random errors that would normally be found and repaired by the body are allowed to remain instead in the body.

- A number of personality dimensions, including depression, extraversion, and difficulty expressing emotions, are often associated with the development of cancer. People with such traits, namely, those who present a pleasant and cheerful face to the world, show passivity in the face of stress, and tend to suppress negative emotions, are described as having a "Type C," or cancer-prone, personality. However, there is limited evidence for the role of personality traits leading to cancer.

Factors Influencing Coping With Cancer

- Many of the treatments used to fight cancer have unpleasant side effects, which influence how people cope with cancer. These include changes in bowel, urinary, and/or sexual function as well as various types of disability and disfigurement.

- Although a cancer diagnosis is difficult for virtually everyone, people respond to this information in very different ways. People who believe they have some control over the disease experience lower levels of psychological distress and a higher overall quality of life, as do those who approach a cancer diagnosis with optimistic expectations about the outcome and can find some positive aspects of their diagnosis. On the other hand, people who blame themselves for getting cancer experience higher levels of anxiety and depression. Some evidence even suggests that the coping strategies used may impact survival.

- People with cancer who receive more social support from friends and family report better psychological adjustment. Positive social interaction support—meaning the availability of people with whom to have fun, relax, and get one's mind off cancer for a while—is an especially strong predictor of overall quality of life. People with cancer who have higher levels of social support may even survive for longer periods than those without such support.

- Many people with cancer benefit—both psychologically and physically—from participating in some type of formal intervention group. These groups provide training in specific strategies for managing the pain and symptoms of cancer as well as its treatment. Such interventions may provide general education, stress management techniques, cognitive-behavioral strategies, and/or social support.

12

TERMINAL ILLNESS AND BEREAVEMENT

Learning Objectives

12.1 Describe early models of death and dying

12.2 Compare different approaches to managing a terminal diagnosis

12.3 Explain the death with dignity movement

12.4 Summarize the bereavement process

12.5 Describe strategies for coping with bereavement

What You'll Learn

12.1 How hospice care reduces family members' depression and anxiety

12.2 Why people with strong religious beliefs prefer more aggressive end-of-life medical care

12.3 Why having "unfinished business" can make coping with loss of a loved one even harder

12.4 Why men are more likely to remarry following the death of their spouse than are women

12.5 How death of a spouse increases one's own risk of dying in the next year

Preview

What did you learn about death from your parents? If you are like most college students, the answer is probably very little. Although death eventually happens to us all, most people are very uncomfortable with this topic. The topic of death is often considered taboo in our society. For example, we use euphemisms for death (e.g., she passed away, he

(Continued)

kicked the bucket, she bought the farm), delay making wills, and put off discussions of how we'd like to be buried. And because it causes anxiety, thoughts of death are usually pushed out of our minds whenever possible. Yet we will all experience at some point the death of a loved one, and understanding how terminally ill people face this diagnosis, and how survivors cope with such an immense loss, has major implications for both psychological and physical health, as you'll learn in this chapter.

EARLY MODELS OF DEATH AND DYING

LO 12.1

Describe early models of death and dying

As described in *Chapter 1: Introduction*, the leading causes of death in 1900 were acute diseases, such as pneumonia, tuberculosis, and influenza, and these diseases often killed people at very early ages. But given the technological advancements of the last 100 years, these diseases largely have been brought under control and people nowadays typically die from chronic conditions. At least in the United States, the vast majority of people die from heart disease and cancer (Xu, Murphy, Kochanek, & Arias, 2016). Because chronic diseases are the leading causes of death today, death comes after a period of gradually declining health, and terminally ill people are often aware that they are dying. This section describes both early models explaining how people cope with a terminal illness as well as some critiques of such approaches.

Stages of Death and Dying

The best-known model for explaining how people cope with dying was developed in the late 1960s by Dr. Elisabeth Kübler-Ross (1969). Based on interviews with 200 terminally ill patients, Dr. Kübler-Ross concluded that the process of dying involves a series of five stages that differ in content and emotional intensity. These **stages of death and dying** are normal and predictable ways of coping with death, although people differ in how they experience them.

According to Kübler-Ross's model, terminally ill people go through a series of five distinct stages. First, they experience a stage of *denial*. A very common initial reaction to receiving a diagnosis of a terminal illness is, "It can't be me—this must be a mistake." When people receive news that they have a terminal illness, it is stunning, and they may experience an initial state of numbness. They simply can't face the situation and believe the prognosis is a mistake or impossible. Although this period typically doesn't last very long, this initial denial may allow the person to come to terms with the situation psychologically.

After the initial stage of numbness and denial has worn off, a common reaction is *anger*. People feel that their prognosis is unfair and may search for reasons (e.g., "Why me? What have I done?"). The person may express anger toward God, the medical staff, family members, or friends. Other feelings, such as rage, envy, and resentment, are also common. This stage can be hard for the family because the person's anger may be displaced, but it represents an attempt by the ill person to regain control of life.

Over time, anger transitions into *bargaining*, namely, an attempt to trade good behavior for good health. In this stage, ill persons are trying to delay the inevitable. They may start attending church regularly, take their medicine without complaint, or give generously to charity in an attempt to make a pact for more time or bargain with God. For example, a person may try to bargain for time to reach a valued milestone, such as a child's wedding or graduation or their own birthday or anniversary.

When bargaining fails to change the prognosis, people often experience a state of *depression*, a feeling of anticipatory grief in which the person grieves about the upcoming losses he or she will experience in death. This stage is about self-grieving, and it is important for family members and medical staff to accept the person's depression and share in the sadness. The dying person feels many losses, including that of body image, time, money, independence, social status, and relationships, and experiencing depression is a common and understandable response. This stage is often coupled with a growing realization, based on the individual's physical state, that he or she is really dying. In turn, the person may feel weak, fatigued, ashamed, guilty, fearful, or many other anxieties. This is "the worst of the worst."

The final stage of dying is *acceptance*: people finally acknowledge that death is inevitable and believe they can face it calmly. During this stage, people often cut off contact with all but a few close friends and family members in an attempt to disengage. Dr. Kübler-Ross believes that given enough time and help during the prior stages, patients can reach a stage in which they are no longer angry or depressed but rather accepting of their fate. This stage, which Kübler-Ross describes as "quiet expectation," should not, however, be perceived as a happy stage—in contrast, this stage is more appropriately described as a time of quiet resignation, as if the patient has given up his or her struggle and is resting prior to death.

Task Work Models

According to Charles Corr's **task work model** for coping with dying, people who are terminally ill focus on four distinct types of tasks (Corr, 1992). First, they must cope with physical tasks, such as managing their pain and physical symptoms, satisfying the body's needs, and reducing distress. Second, they must focus on psychological tasks, including maintaining independence, feeling secure in the support they receive from others, and even in managing day-to-day tasks that are rewarding (e.g., taking a bath, eating a favorite food); they often need to feel in control. Third, people who are dying are concerned with social tasks, such as enhancing their interpersonal relationships, which often become limited to just a few very close persons, or interacting with hospital workers, social workers, and physicians. Finally, dying people focus on spiritual tasks, including thinking through issues of meaningfulness, hope, connectedness, and transcendence. For example, they may wonder what happens to their spirit following death and the contributions they have made in their life.

Kenneth Doka (1993) describes phase-specific tasks that people with life-threatening illnesses encounter. People in the prediagnostic phase experience symptoms of their illness or disease. They may, for example, notice a lump or feel an unusual pain. Once the condition is diagnosed, they are in the acute phase of the illness. In this stage they try to understand the disease and to cope with it. After this initial focus of coming to terms with the illness, people enter the chronic phase, in which they must manage the illness and its various effects. As discussed in *Chapter 13: Managing Health Care*, these effects could include carrying out medical regimens, coping with feelings regarding the illness, and managing the symptoms and side effects of the illness and its treatment. In cases in which the disease can be managed, people enter the recovery phase. During this stage, they deal with their anxiety about recurrence of the illness as well as any lingering physical effects. However, if the illness is incurable, the person eventually enters the terminal phase, in which he or she copes with managing the often increasingly difficult symptoms, preparing for death, and finding meaning in life and death.

Both of these task-based approaches offer several valuable guidelines (Kastenbaum, 2000). They view dying as a normative event within the total lifespan as opposed to an event of a very different and distinct domain. They view dying people as continuing to strive to accomplish valued goals. These task-based approaches also focus attention on a broad range of problems that dying people may encounter, not simply on the physical process of dying. This should help people pay attention to the diverse sets of needs of terminally ill patients, not just on managing their pain and/or prolonging their lives.

Critiques of Early Models

Although the most famous of these models is the one developed by Dr. Kübler-Ross, this model has been criticized for several reasons (Feifel, 1990; Rainey, 1988). First, this research didn't demonstrate "actual" stages or an orderly progression. In other words, it is not clear that people go from one stage to the next in a particular order—maybe people jump around from one phase to another, or cycle, or maybe experience stages simultaneously. In fact, all people do not go through all the stages. Some patients struggle against death (or even deny it) until the very end, whereas others seem to face death with resignation (Tang et al., 2016). Second, other researchers suggest that this model excludes some stages, such as anxiety, and fails to adequately describe others. The stage of denial, for example, could include a range of different reactions (e.g., "I am not ill; I am not dying; I will get better").

Another critique of all of these early models is that they ignore the role of various factors that could influence how people respond to a diagnosis of a terminal illness. As you might predict, factors such as gender, age, and race/ethnicity may play a substantial role in how people respond to such a diagnosis. For example, people who have strong religious views may experience less depression, in part due to their belief in an afterlife (Edmondson, Park, Chaudoir, & Wortmann, 2008). Similarly, and as described in **Table 12.1: Test Yourself**, people in general vary in their overall acceptance of death and dying, which likely influences how they react to learning they have a terminal illness.

Table 12.1   Test Yourself: Acceptance of Death and Dying Inventory
Answer each of the following items on a 1 to 4 scale (1 means agree not at all, 2 means agree somewhat, 3 means agree for the most part, 4 means agree almost totally).

1. Ultimately, I am at peace with the fact that even people who are close to me have to die.

2. Basically, I am ready to accept that even people who are close to me will be dead one day.

3. I have a positive attitude to the process of dying as part of my life.

4. As painful as it is, I have a positive attitude toward the fact that people who are important to me will be dead one day.

5. Somehow, the knowledge of my death is a part of my life that I view positively.

6. My death is a part of a wider scheme of things that I treat positively.

7. I have a positive attitude to the process of dying as a necessary stage in my life.

8. Basically, I am ready to accept that I have to die one day.

9. The fact that I will die someday is something absolutely natural for me.

10. I accept the death of people who are close to me.

11. The dying process contributes toward rounding off my life.

12. To me, the dying process means the completion of my life.

Sum your scores on each of these 12 items to determine your overall acceptance of death and dying.

Source: Macdougall & Farreras (2016).

Finally, although these early models focused primarily on the psychological and physical challenges people face as they cope with death and dying, some research now indicates that such a diagnosis can also lead to distinct benefits. For example, some evidence suggests that people who are close to death may also experience some unexpected positives (Goranson, Ritter, Waytz, Norton, & Gray, 2017). Researchers in this study assessed the blogs of patients with terminal cancer or ALS and examined the use of positive language—including words and tone—in their writing. Their findings revealed that people's writings become more positive—and less negative—as they approach death. Similarly, some terminally ill cancer patients report experiencing posttraumatic growth, such as a shift in priorities, closer relationships with others, and spiritual development (Tang et al., 2015).

MANAGING A TERMINAL DIAGNOSIS

LO 12.2

Compare different approaches to managing a terminal diagnosis

Historically, most people have died in their own homes, but this trend has clearly changed during the last century—there is a growing shift from people dying at home to people dying in hospitals and nursing homes (Levy, 1983). In fact, although a majority of Americans would prefer to die at home, most instead die in hospitals (63%), with another 17% dying in some type of institutionalized setting, such as a nursing home or long-term care facility (Foley, 1995; Isaacs & Knickman, 1997). This trend toward death occurring in an institution is driven in part by a focus, even among people with a terminal illness, on prolonging life through medical techniques and interventions. However, as you'll learn in this section, growing evidence points to the value of a holistic approach for coping with a terminal illness. The final section will describe the particular challenges faced by terminally ill children.

Medical Approach

The medical approach focuses on curing people, delivering technical skills and interventions, and thereby preventing death (MacLeod, 2001). In turn, medical professionals often emphasize the value of lifesaving equipment, such as tube feeding and mechanical ventilation, in prolonging people's lives. However, hospitals often place relatively little emphasis on the care of terminally ill patients, who represent a failure of medical techniques in curing their disease or injury (Benoliel, 1988; Rainey, 1988). Doctors and nurses therefore aren't particularly interested in or comfortable with taking care of terminally ill patients, nor do they typically receive training on how do so effectively. In fact, one large-scale study of 9,105 adults hospitalized with a life-threatening diagnosis found that even within the last two days of life, many patients received aggressive lifesaving treatment, such as mechanical ventilation, and doctors were often unaware of patients' preferences regarding such procedures (SUPPORT Principal Investigators, 1995). In sum, hospitals are designed to diagnose and treat disease, which is good for people with curable conditions but not as good for those who are dying of chronic, incurable diseases.

Given the emphasis placed by the medical approach on curing illness and disease, medical professionals are often uncomfortable giving realistic news about a poor prognosis, which means patients and their families may have an inaccurate sense of their likelihood of survival and life expectancy. Instead, nurses and doctors who interact with dying patients may use false reassurance and distancing techniques (Maguire, 1985). For example, doctors and nurses may tell the person he or she will get better soon, even when they know that this is unlikely, as a way of avoiding giving negative news. One study of physicians caring for patients with cancer found that 22.7% would not provide any estimates of survival time, and

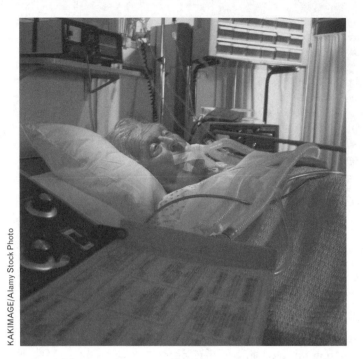

KAKIMAGE/Alamy Stock Photo

Although hospitals are well equipped to provide aggressive end-of-life care, such procedures may not be what the patient, or his or her family, wants.

they would communicate a more optimistic than realistic survival time 40.3% of the time (Lamont & Christakis, 2001). Similarly, a study of parents of children with cancer found that 10.6% of parents rated their child's prognosis as very good or excellent although their physicians had rated the child's prognosis as poor (Sung et al., 2009). Although doctors often report not wanting to give patients honest information about life expectancy due to a concern about "taking away hope," research actually demonstrates that patients continue to hope for a more positive outcome even after receiving such information; in fact, there are no differences in hope between patients with advanced cancer who are given such information and those who are not (Smith, Dow, Virago, Khatcheressian, Lyckholm, & Matsuyama, 2010).

The lack of realistic information provided by medical professionals to patients and their families about their condition deprives them of the opportunity to make informed health care decisions. For example, although medical techniques are often available to prolong people's lives, many people are not interested in having aggressive end-of-life care in cases in which such care is likely to be futile. Many people report they would prefer **palliative care**, meaning care focused on managing pain, when doctors determine that aggressive critical care would not be beneficial in saving their lives (Jacobs, Burns, & Bennett Jacobs, 2008). Unfortunately, most research suggests that relatively few terminally ill patients have the chance to discuss their preferences regarding end-of-life care. For example, researchers in one study examined 332 patients with advanced cancer and their caregivers from the time they were admitted to the hospital until they died (approximately four months later) (Wright et al., 2008). Only a bit over a third of patients—37.0%—reported having end-of-life discussions. However, patients who had such discussions experienced lower rates of aggressive medical care, such as ventilation and resuscitation. Sadly, more aggressive medical care was associated with worse patient quality of life as well as higher risk of major depressive disorder in bereaved caregivers. These findings suggest that discussions regarding end-of-life care lead to less aggressive medical care near death, which in turn is associated with better overall quality of life for the patient and better adjustment to bereavement for the caregiver.

Physicians may also ignore patients' reports of psychological difficulties, such as depression and anxiety, and focus instead on patients' physical state, in part because providing intense psychological care is time-consuming and emotionally draining. Researchers in one study examined conversations between patients with lung cancer and their doctors (Morse, Edwardsen, & Gordon, 2008). Although patients expressed numerous concerns about mortality, symptoms, and treatment, physicians provided little emotional support and instead tended to shift such concerns to biomedical questions (Morse, Edwardsen, & Gordon, 2008). In fact, physicians responded empathically to only 10% of the concerns raised by patients. Moreover, when empathy was provided, 50% of these statements occurred in the last third of the encounter, whereas patients' concerns were evenly raised throughout the encounter. Physicians rarely responded empathically to the concerns raised by patients with lung cancer, and empathic responses that did occur were more frequently in the last third of the encounter.

Holistic Approach

In contrast to the medical approach, which focuses entirely on people's physical state, the holistic approach to managing terminal illness focuses more broadly not only on providing physical care, but also psychological, social, cultural, and spiritual care. This interdisciplinary and holistic approach was created by Dr. Cicely Saunders in London in the late 1960s and was specifically designed to provide better care for terminally ill patients (Feifel, 1990; Kastenbaum, 1999). Specifically, she believed that dying people need pain relief and should be treated with dignity, compassion, and respect. This view directly contradicted the medical approach to managing terminal illness, which emphasized continuing to push for a cure (no matter what) and that medical professionals should not tell dying patients about their prognosis. Dr. Saunders is credited with founding the first **hospice**, which provided care for terminally ill patients and presented an alternative to dying in an impersonal institution such as a hospital or nursing home. Although hospice care was initially provided in a designated building, this type of care can also be provided in a particular unit or floor in a hospital or even at the patient's home. In fact, most hospice care is now provided in people's homes; this care can include visits from nurses, social workers, and chaplains. Hospice professionals also offer assistance to caregivers, including staying with patients while family members are out and helping families to understand and cope with the dying process.

Hospice care differs from hospital care in a number of ways (Kastenbaum, 1999). First, hospice care focuses primarily on treating the symptoms of terminal illness and minimizing the patient's discomfort and pain, not simply on helping patients recover or prolong their lives. Patients who choose hospice care typically have a limited amount of time to live—typically less than six months—and have illnesses or diseases, such as cancer, AIDS, or ALS (a progressive neurological condition often referred to as Lou Gehrig's disease) that cannot be cured. Second, hospice staff try to provide a sense of comfort and support for the patient and his or her family. They also encourage engaging in open discussions on death and dying and expressing feelings. Finally, when hospice care is provided outside the person's home, patients are allowed to personalize and control their surroundings much more than they could do in a hospital. They are not forced to cope with the rigid routines of hospital care, including constant monitoring by medical personnel, institutional meals provided on a set schedule, and limited visiting hours. Instead, patients can wear their own clothes, have visitors at any time, and even bring in special items from home, such as a quilt, family pictures, and special mementos.

Considerable research demonstrates the importance of addressing patients' broader needs, including not only physical but also social, psychological, and spiritual needs, in terms of improving the end-of-life illness experience (Lynn, 2001; Viney, Walker, Robertson, Lilley, & Ewan, 1994). Terminally ill people receiving hospice care, which provides this type of holistic care, report more enjoyment of life and better spiritual well-being as well as lower levels of anger, depression, and anxiety than those in a general hospital setting (Hinton, 1979; Kane, Wales, Bernstein, Leibowitz, & Kaplan, 1984; Miller, Chibnall, Videen, & Duckro, 2005). They also report greater satisfaction with the care they receive, more favorable interpersonal interactions, and lower levels of loneliness. As one man noted, "There's much more than the physical care. What they do comes from a place of very deep understanding of illness and so close to the end of life. I feel grateful. It's sort of like a big sigh of relief in the midst of all the anguish and upsetness" (Waldrop, Meeker, & Kutner, 2015, p. 11). In fact, patients who die in hospice settings are more satisfied with the emotional support they receive than those who die in a nursing home, hospital, or at home without hospice services (Teno et al., 2004).

Hospice care can also result in more peace of mind for family members, both during patients' illness and following their death. Specifically, family members of hospice patients tend to report more satisfaction and less anxiety than family members of patients in other settings (Kane et al., 1984; Lynn, 2001). Researchers in one study surveyed 1,500 family members of patients who had died about end-of-life outcomes (Teno et al., 2004). Seventy-one percent of family members of patients who received hospice care rated the care as "excellent" compared to fewer than 50% of those dying in a hospital, nursing home, or home without such care. Family members of patients who died in hospice units were also more likely to describe their loved ones as having had a "good death" than family members of those who had died on a general ward (Miyashita et al., 2008). The characteristics of a "good death" include environmental comfort, physical and psychological comfort, being respected as an individual, and having a "natural death." Moreover, these "good deaths" were more likely to include adequate pain medication and less likely to include aggressive treatments, such as chemotherapy in the last two weeks of life as well as treatments designed to prolong life.

What You'll Learn
12.1

Finally, people whose spouses use hospice care have lower rates of depression and mortality. Researchers in one study found that spouses of patients receiving hospice more frequently reported reduced depression symptoms compared to surviving spouses of patients who did not receive hospice (Ornstein et al., 2015). In another study, researchers compared life expectancy in nearly 60,000 widows and widowers whose spouses had used hospice care versus those whose spouses had not (Christakis & Iwashyna, 2003). Their findings revealed that for both men and women, survival rates 18 months after the loss of a spouse were higher in those who had used hospice care compared to those who had not. These findings suggest that both men and women may benefit in terms of their own life expectancy from having their spouse use hospice care, perhaps because such care focuses not only on treating the patient but also on providing care to his or her family.

Despite all the benefits of hospice care for patients and their families, this type of care is underutilized, in part due to misperceptions about its goals. Many people equate hospice care with "giving up" and assume they will die sooner as a result, which leads many patients, and their families, to resist hospice care. Doctors may also be reluctant to suggest hospice care for terminally ill patients (Feeg & Elebiary, 2005). However, palliative care can be provided alongside standard medical treatment, and as described in **Research in Action**, evidence suggests that hospice patients actually live longer than patients who receive standard hospital care. To examine whether educating terminally ill patients about the goals of hospice care would increase their preferences for receiving such services, researchers in one recent study randomly assigned some cancer patients to receive a summary of hospice care services (Hoerger, Perry, Gramling, Epstein, & Duberstein, 2017). Compared to those in the control condition, who received no information, people who received information about hospice care reported seeing such treatment as more effective in managing symptoms and side effects and as less scary and stressful. Most important, patients who received such information reported greater intentions to use such care in the future, if recommended by their doctor. People who have discussions involving end-of-life preferences are more likely to enroll in hospice care, and enroll earlier, which is associated with a better quality of life for the patient, which in turn leads to better quality of life for caregivers (Wright et al., 2008).

Terminal Illness in Children

Although medical advances have greatly reduced the number of childhood deaths, many children are still diagnosed with potentially life-threatening illnesses. In fact, cancer is the leading cause of disease-related death among children in the United States, with over 15,000 people under the age of 20 being diagnosed with cancer and nearly 2,000 dying of this disease each year (Ward, DeSantis, Robbins, Kohler, & Jemal, 2014). This section describes the distinct stages of death and dying in children, which vary as a function of age, and current perspectives on how medical professionals and parents should approach a child's terminal illness.

Stages of Death and Dying in Children

Fatally ill children have specialized needs, including the normal developmental needs of healthy children, the special needs of children who are sick and hospitalized, and the particular needs of children who are dying (Stevens, 1997). The specific concerns of terminally ill children, however, vary by age. The youngest children, ages three to five, worry primarily about separation from their parents, friends, and grandparents. They are worried that they will be left alone and are comforted by reassurance that their parents will never leave them. In contrast, children ages five to nine are concerned about the ending of their life and what will happen to their body.

Adolescents have their own particular concerns about death and dying and ironically seem to be more afraid of the process of dying than of death itself (Stevens & Dunsmore, 1996). Adolescents are very sensitive to body image issues; hence, the physical side effects of a terminal illness can be especially upsetting at this age. Adolescents are also very focused on separating from their parents and establishing peer relationships, which can be disrupted if they are forced to spend time away from school seeking treatment and are unable to participate in many normal social activities because of their illness. They may be particularly concerned about their inability to attract a boyfriend or girlfriend, and they may worry that their peers will reject them.

Extensive observation of hospitalized children by Myra Bluebond-Langner (1977) describes five stages that children pass through as they attempt to understand their illness. First, children are aware they have a serious illness and are concerned about feeling sick. They gradually become more sophisticated about the illness, learning names for medicines and side effects. In the second stage, they are still aware that they are ill but are optimistic about the outcome (e.g., "I am sick, but I'll get better"). In the third stage, they learn more about the procedures and their purposes and understand that this illness is long-term (e.g., "I'll always be sick, but I will get better"). This is followed by the fourth stage, which often comes after they have experienced several cycles of remissions and relapses. At this point they accept that they will never get better, that they will always have this illness. Finally, in the fifth state, their declining health and observation of other dying patients leads them to realize that they will die.

Current Perspectives

Health professionals generally believe that terminally ill children should be given honest information about their illness, in an age-appropriate way (Beale, Baile, & Aaron, 2005; Stillion & Wass, 1984). Although parents may fear that providing information about the nature of their illness will be upsetting, terminally ill children are often already aware of their condition, based on physiological changes in their bodies that indicate serious problems, observations of other children around them, and/or conversations they have overheard between family members and medical personnel. They may also sense from their parents' nonverbal behavior that their illness is more serious than they are being told, which creates considerable anxiety. This anxiety is exacerbated when children are not given accurate information on the disease and its impact, which creates feelings of uncertainty and a lack of control.

Although medical professionals and parents may worry that talking about death and dying will be upsetting to the child, the reality is that children feel more anxious and alone when they are not able to talk about their fears with the most trusted adults in their lives. Providing children with information allows them the opportunity to ask questions of parents and medical professionals. They may want to know whether they will experience pain or what will happen to their body after they die. This knowledge may also lead them to focus on more immediate future plans, such as their next birthday or a holiday, and not on longer-term plans. Parents therefore need to understand the benefits of giving children honest, even if very sad, information about their illness and prognosis, and that false reassurances are usually not helpful. One study found that no parents who had talked to their child about the fact that he or she was dying regretted having such a discussion, whereas some parents who did not have such discussions did have regrets about this decision (Kreicbergs, Valdimarsdóttir, Onelöv, Henter, & Steineck, 2004).

Unfortunately, even doctors who work regularly with terminally ill children may not have specific training in how to have such difficult conversations with children and/or their parents (Papadatou, 1997). Such conversations can be particularly difficult since parents may be struggling with accepting their child's terminal diagnosis and may not want accurate information given to their child. (Later in this chapter, you'll learn specific challenges parents face themselves regarding the death of a child.)

THE DEATH WITH DIGNITY MOVEMENT

LO 12.3

Explain the death with dignity movement

One of the most challenging ethical issues within the field of health psychology right now is that of whether a person should have a right to die—and if so, under what circumstances. This section describes assisted suicide and concerns about its use as well as the use of advanced care directives to help people gain some control over medical decision making at the end of their lives.

Understanding Assisted Suicide

The term *assisted suicide* refers to a death by suicide that is committed with help from another person. Proponents of assisted suicide believe that people who are in severe pain and who are terminally ill should have the right to end their suffering (Kastenbaum, 1999; Sears & Stanton, 2001). Some people with a terminal illness want the option of assisted suicide due to fear about losing physical and mental functioning and experiencing a very low quality of life, such as the inability to take care of oneself and engage in normal daily life activities (Ganzini, Goy, & Dobscha, 2009). In line with this view, advanced cancer patients who experience greater functional impairment, and in turn loss of autonomy, are more interested in speeding up their death (Villavicencio-Chávez et al., 2014). Terminally ill patients may also want to have the option of dying in order to maintain some control over their condition. As one patient with advanced cancer noted, "I am not afraid about death. I am only afraid of an agonizing death" (Pestinger et al., 2015, p. 715). In fact, wanting to control the circumstances of their death, and to die at home, was one of the most important reasons listed by those for expressing interest in assisted suicide (Ganzini et al., 2002, 2009).

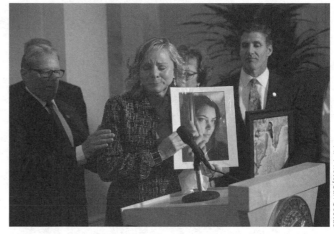

On November 1, 2014, Brittany Maynard, a 29-year-old woman with terminal brain cancer, ended her own life, using drugs prescribed by her doctor. Maynard had moved to Oregon given their Death With Dignity Law; at the time of her death, her home state, California, did not allow physician-assisted suicide.

In 1994, Oregon became the first state to pass a law (the Death With Dignity Act) allowing **physician-assisted suicide**, meaning that physicians can, at a patient's request, provide a lethal dose of medicine (typically through prescription drugs). The patient is then able, if he or she chooses, to take these lethal drugs. This type of suicide allows patients to die in a peaceful and nonviolent way and is a much less painful and faster way to die than simply refusing medical treatments (e.g., food, water, antibiotics). As of 2017, California, Colorado, Vermont, and Washington, as well as the District of Columbia, also allowed assisted suicide, and legislation is now pending in several other states. Most people who choose physician-assisted suicide have an advanced form of cancer (Emanuel, Onwuteaka-Philipsen, Urwin, & Cohen, 2016).

Although physician-assisted suicide is the only form of legal suicide in the United States, some other countries allow **euthanasia**. In this form of assisted suicide, a physician acts directly to end a person's life (such as by actually administering those drugs and not just prescribing them). Several countries allow some form of euthanasia, including Belgium, the Netherlands, and Luxembourg.

Most people in the United States are in favor of some form of physician-assisted suicide. According to a 2016 Gallup Poll, 69% of Americans believe people with a terminal illness should have the right to physician-assisted suicide (Gallup, 2016). Support for such laws is higher in people who are older, and presumably more concerned about terminal illness, and lower among those with strong religious beliefs (Periyakoil, Kraemer, & Neri, 2016; Stolz et al., 2015). However, and as shown in Figure 12.1, people tend to be more in favor of assisted suicide for people in general than for their own loved ones. Moreover, and as described in **Focus on Diversity**, people from different racial and ethnic backgrounds may differ in their beliefs about the circumstances under which assisted suicide is appropriate.

Concerns Regarding Assisted Suicide

Opponents of assisted suicide vehemently believe that this choice is wrong for several reasons (Kastenbaum, 1999; Van Norman, 2014). They believe that providing people with the means to commit suicide creates a slippery slope and that the potential for this procedure to be used

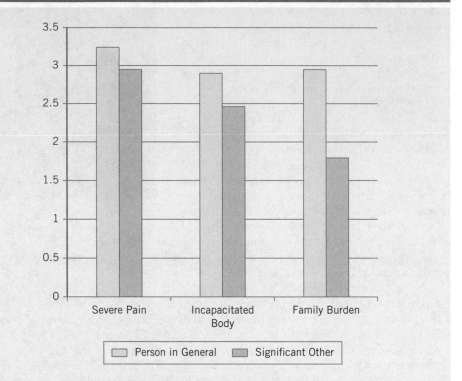

Figure 12.1 Data From Ho and Chantagul, 2015

Although people generally favor the right to assisted suicide, people are more in favor of this choice for people in general than for their significant others, including in cases in which the person is in severe pain, has a totally incapacitated body, and is a burden to his or her family.

Source: Data from Ho & Chantagul (2015).

wrongly is high. For example, people who are physically disabled or temporarily depressed, but not terminally ill, may want to end their lives, and such laws could also be used to provide that option. In fact, although in the United States, assisted suicide is limited to those with a terminal illness, in some other countries this option is available for those who have other illnesses, such as major depression, anxiety disorder, or dementia (Bolt, Snijdewind, Willems, Heide, & Onwuteaka-Philipsen, 2015; Kim, De Vries, & Peteet, 2016). Opponents also believe that the moral issues associated with assisted suicide, including the violation of the physician's oath "First, do no harm," should make assisted suicide illegal.

Some evidence suggests that terminally ill people who want to die often suffer from clinical depression or pain. For example, one study found that 58.8% of patients who wanted to die were depressed, as compared to only 7.7% of those who did not want to die (Chochinov et al., 1995). One study comparing terminally ill people who had pursued physician-assisted death with those who did not pursue this option found that those interested in dying had higher levels of depression and hopelessness (Smith, Harvath, Goy, & Ganzini, 2015). Similarly, while 76.5% of those in moderate or greater pain wanted to die, only 46.2% of those who did not want to die were in such severe pain (Chocinov et al., 1995). In turn, treating depression and managing pain could help improve the quality of life in terminally ill patients and thereby reduce the desire for assisted suicide.

FOCUS ON DIVERSITY

Cultural Perspectives on Assisted Suicide

One factor that influences people's perspectives about assisted suicide is their ethnic and cultural background. Researchers in one study interviewed Americans from different ethnic and cultural backgrounds regarding their beliefs about assisted suicide (Perkins, Cortez, & Hazuda, 2009). These participants included 26 Mexican Americans, 18 European Americans, and 14 African Americans. Although nearly all participants believed that God plays a role in determining when a person should die, the specific signals people relied on to judge whether assisted suicide was warranted varied by culture. For Mexican Americans and African Americans, the patient's suffering and dependence on artificial life support predicted belief in the appropriateness of assisted suicide. In contrast, for European Americans, the patient's acceptance of his or her own death predicted belief in the appropriateness of assisted suicide. These findings suggest that although Americans in general may share some beliefs about the right time to die, ethnicity also influences such beliefs in important ways.

Advanced Care Directives

Given people's general desire to have some control over end-of-life experiences, many people choose to specify what type of medical intervention they would or would not like. One approach to gaining some control over one's end-of-life experience is to create a **living will** (see Table 12.2). A living will provides very clear instructions to family members, friends, and medical personnel and thus allows people to specify their wishes about the type of care they would like to receive in the event they are incapacitated and therefore unable to make their own decisions (Kastenbaum, 1999). For example, a person may request to not be tube-fed while in a coma if there is no chance of emerging from that state. The use of living wills therefore allows people to express their medical directives in advance of having an illness; thus, they are able to maintain control over their lives even when they have lost the ability to speak for themselves.

Researchers in one study examined whether cancer patients with more deeply held religious beliefs would prefer more intensive lifesaving measures (Phelps et al., 2009). Patients reported how much they used religious coping, such as relying on God's love and support, to cope with their disease, and rated how much they wanted to receive specific types of end-of-life care, such as mechanical ventilation (being placed on a respiratory). Moreover, people who relied more on religious coping not only reported greater interest in such measures but also received more aggressive measures in their final week of life. Although this study did not examine the specific mechanisms explaining this association, patients who rely heavily on religious coping may believe such measures will help God heal them and/or that the use of such measures will provide time for God to perform a miracle.

What You'll Learn
12.2

As an alternative, other researchers suggest that people instead complete lists of "valued life activities" and then use these activities as a guide to determining whether or not to end someone's life (Ditto, Druley, Moore, Danks, & Smucker, 1996). For example, some people would choose to sustain their lives if they could still speak and think, even if they could not move (e.g., following a paralyzing physical injury); others might choose to end their lives if they could no longer recognize family and friends (e.g., following Alzheimer's disease).

Table 12.2 Sample Questions From a Living Will

These are my wishes for my future medical care if there ever comes a time when I can't make these decisions for myself.

A. These are my wishes if I have a terminal condition

Life-sustaining treatments

_____ I do not want life-sustaining treatment (including CPR) started. If life-sustaining treatments are started, I want them stopped.

_____ I want the life-sustaining treatments that my doctors think are best for me.

_____ Other wishes _____

Artificial nutrition and hydration

_____ I do not want artificial nutrition and hydration started if they would be the main treatments keeping me alive. If artificial nutrition and hydration are started, I want them stopped.

_____ I want artificial nutrition and hydration even if they are the main treatments keeping me alive.

_____ Other wishes _____

Comfort care

_____ I want to be kept as comfortable and free of pain as possible, even if such care prolongs my dying or shortens my life.

_____ Other wishes _____

B. These are my wishes if I am ever in a persistent vegetative state

Life-sustaining treatments

_____ I do not want life-sustaining treatments (including CPR) started. If life-sustaining treatments are started, I want them stopped.

_____ I want the life-sustaining treatments that my doctors think are best for me.

_____ Other wishes _____

Artificial nutrition and hydration

_____ I do not want artificial nutrition and hydration started if they would be the main treatments keeping me alive. If artificial nutrition and hydration are started, I want them stopped.

_____ I want artificial nutrition and hydration even if they are the main treatments keeping me alive.

_____ Other wishes _____

Comfort care

_____ I want to be kepl as comfortable and free of pain as possible, even if such care prolongs my dying or shortens my life.

_____ Other wishes _____

This is a sample living will. If you would like to register your own living will, go to www.uslivingwillregistry.com.

Source: Living Will Questions from American Academy of Family Physicians (AAFP).

These decisions are obviously very personal. Studies with both college students and elderly adults reveal that people's beliefs about whether various health impairments, such as being unable to communicate, being blind or deaf, or being confined to bed, would interfere with their ability to engage in valued life activities influence their preference for death. In other words, the more each disability is seen as interfering with their engagement in their most valued life activities, the more they would prefer death.

Although both living wills and valued life activity lists allow people to specify their preferences regarding end-of-life care, these approaches do have limitations (Annas, 1991). First, they require people to predict how they would feel, and what types of measures they would prefer, in a variety of different illness and injury situations. Moreover, living wills may require doctors to interpret patients' preferences, which may vary considerably depending on the specific medical situation they are facing.

An alternative approach to gaining some control over end-of-life measures is therefore to appoint a **health care proxy** (or durable power of attorney for health care). A health care proxy is a person who makes medical decisions on behalf of someone if they are unable to do so themselves. This person can then have discussions with medical personnel about treatment options, and ideally provide a more accurate sense of what types of procedures the patient would—or would not—want in different situations.

Advance directives can help patients receive the type of treatment they prefer (Silveira, Kim, & Langa, 2010). For example, one study found that patients who had prepared advance care directives were much more likely to receive care that was in line with their preferences. For example, 97% of patients who requested comfort care, meaning care designed to ease pain and suffering, in their advance care directive received it. Similarly, patients who requested all care possible were much more likely to receive such care than those who did not request it. These findings suggest that helping terminally ill patients think about the care they'd like to receive, and communicating such preferences to a health care proxy, is an effective strategy for improving the end-of-life experience.

UNDERSTANDING BEREAVEMENT

LO 12.4

Summarize the bereavement process

When people lose someone they care about, they experience a state of **bereavement**. This state is accompanied by both **grief**, meaning the feelings caused by this loss, and **mourning**, meaning the expression of these feelings. Grief and mourning are not signs of weakness or self-indulgence—they are a normal and natural human reaction to the loss of a significant person, which is intensified by our closeness to the person who has died (Berado, 1988; Feifel, 1990). In this section, you'll learn about the stages of bereavement, factors influencing the bereavement process, and the consequences of bereavement.

Stages of Mourning

Bereavement begins as soon as one learns that a loved one died, typically with an initial feeling of shock (Berado, 1988). During this *reaction stage*, survivors may feel numb and show little feeling. This period allows survivors to cope initially and to handle the necessary tasks, such as planning a funeral or memorial service, notifying friends and relatives, and handling legal arrangements. However, not all survivors will be able to handle such logistics and may therefore need considerable assistance from others. At this time, people may also try to make sense of the death, especially in cases in which the loss was unanticipated and inappropriate (e.g., the death of a child). They may experience anger and frustration with the person who died and others who could be seen as responsible in some way (e.g., doctors, God) as well as those who encourage them to accept the loss when they just aren't ready to do so. This anger may also be self-directed: survivors may wonder what they could have done differently to prevent this death.

After this initial period of numbness, survivors enter a stage of *yearning and searching* (Berado, 1988). This stage represents a desire to return things to how they once were. Survivors may search crowds hoping to see the lost one, may expect to see the person coming up the driveway, and may wake up in the morning wondering if the person is really dead. One man whose mother was killed when he was a child recalls coming home after school and calling, "Mom?" just hoping that she would answer. In this stage, people are still hoping things will return to how they were before the death and are not acknowledging or accepting the extent and finality of their loss.

After reality sets in, the survivor enters the stage of *disorganization and reorganization* (Berado, 1988), in which he or she is disappointed that the loss cannot be undone and may experience despair and depression. Survivors may have trouble enjoying old activities and hence have difficulty making plans and engaging in new activities. They may also struggle with forming a new identity, especially if they've lost a spouse or child—these types of deaths cause major role changes, since people have to give up their previous identity as wife, husband, or parent. The plans they had made are now ruined, and it can be difficult to know how to start a "new life." Survivors may become very dependent on those who provide care for them. Their feelings in this stage are often complicated and even conflicting—it can seem like a betrayal to the dead person to give up grieving and take joy in new activities.

Finally, people enter the *reorientation and recovery stage* (Berado, 1988), in which the bereaved person is able to take part in new activities and to "rejoin" the world. He or she has accepted the changes and is now able to get life back on track. In line with this model, bereaved people who have accepted the loss show lower levels of grieving (Davis, Deane, & Lyons, 2015). Survivors in this stage may also give the deceased a new identity, such as a place in heaven. They are still sad but are now able to move on with their own lives.

What You'll Learn
12.3

Although these stages of mourning are described as if they are a linear process, some bereaved people may have feelings of unresolved grief and never return to a normal pattern of living (Berado, 1988). This experience is known as **complicated grief**, meaning intense yearning, difficulty accepting the death, excessive bitterness, numbness, emptiness, feeling uneasy moving on, and a sense that the future is bleak. This more chronic and severe form of grief is more likely following a sudden and unexpected death and when survivors feel they have unresolved issues with the person who died (Klingspon, Holland, Neimeyer, & Lichtenthal, 2015). People who are generally pessimistic and/or depressed—even prior to the loss—are also more likely to experience complicated grief (Boelen, 2015; Bruinsma, Tiemeier, Heemst, Heide, & Rietjens, 2015; Thomas, Hudson, Trauer, Remedios, & Clarke, 2014; Tomarken et al., 2008).

Factors Influencing Bereavement

Bereavement is, understandably, difficult for all survivors. However, the circumstances of the loss and the nature of the person's relationship both influence the experience of bereavement in distinct ways.

Circumstances of the Loss

The specific circumstances surrounding the death are associated with very different reactions on the part of loved ones (Rainey, 1988). **Quick-trajectory deaths**, in which the loss is sudden and unexpected, are very hard on survivors (Berado, 1988; Bradach & Jordan, 1995). First, these deaths typically force survivors to cope with challenging practical issues. The deceased person typically has made no arrangements for his or her death, such as expressing wishes about funeral arrangements and burial preferences, writing a will, or taking care of financial issues (Becvar, 2001). Second, family members may feel a huge lack of closure—they've had no chance to say good-bye. People may feel tremendous guilt about unresolved conflicts or things left unsaid and may dwell on the final words they said to the person, particularly if those words were unkind. Survivors of quick-trajectory deaths also don't have the opportunity to prepare themselves for a loss; hence, they can experience disbelief and intense anxiety for some time. In turn, spouses whose partner was in excellent health immediately prior to his or her death show more depression following this loss, presumably because they were not able to prepare themselves for this reality (Sasson & Umberson, 2014).

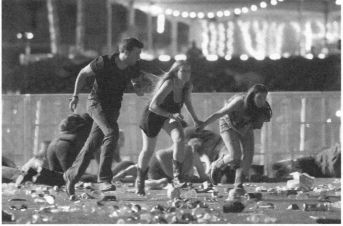

David Becker/Getty Images

Family members who lose loved ones unexpectedly and through violence, such as occurred with the terrorist attack in Las Vegas on October 1, 2017, often experience high levels of grief for some time.

Quick-trajectory deaths are particularly difficult if these deaths were caused by violence or suicide. Although bereaved parents have significantly worse health-related quality of life than nonbereaved parents, those whose child died in violent circumstances have especially low levels of health-related quality of life (Song, Floyd, Seltzer, Greenberg, & Hong, 2010) and are more likely to experience complicated grief symptoms (Keesee, Currier, & Neimeyer, 2008; Meert et al., 2010). Similarly, although children who experience the death of a parent show higher rates of depression and alcohol use than those who do not experience this loss, those who have lost a parent to suicide have particularly high rates of alcohol and substance abuse (Brent, Melhem, Donohue, & Walker, 2009). Adults who experience the death of a parent by suicide are also at increased risk of using antidepressants and being hospitalized for depression (Appel et al., 2016; Berg, Rostila, & Hjern, 2016).

On the other hand, people who have a chronic disease such as cancer, Parkinson's disease, multiple sclerosis, or Alzheimer's disease, typically experience **lingering-trajectory deaths**: the person is ill for a long time, and death comes after a period of gradually declining health. These are usually quiet deaths, in which efforts are made to help the person remain comfortable, and do not involve last-minute heroic attempts to save them. This type of open awareness—on the part of the patient and his or her family members—means that patients can make realistic plans. They may, for example, prepare a will, say good-bye to important people, make arrangements for their funeral and the custody of their children, and prepare psychologically for death (Rainey, 1988). Lingering-trajectory deaths are often easier for survivors to cope with—they allow people to prepare themselves for the loss of their loved one and to say their good-byes. Moreover, older people who have had to take care of their terminally ill spouse for some time may even feel some relief following the death (Schulz et al., 2001).

However, this type of progression toward death may also pose difficulties for survivors. First, loved ones may watch the patient go through long-term pain and suffering and experience the loss of physical bodily functions and of mental faculties. Friends and family members often engage in anticipatory grieving, namely, grieving small losses as they occur (e.g., loss of physical functioning, loss of ability to work); they are grieving the death, but also all that is lost in the process of dying. Lingering-trajectory deaths may be draining on the physical, emotional, and financial resources of family members.

Lingering-trajectory deaths can also be difficult on family members if they believe the patient experienced a difficult death or were themselves unprepared for the death. Family members who believe the person had not yet achieved a sense of completion regarding his or her life are more likely to experience prolonged bereavement (Miyajima et al., 2014). Caregivers who feel unprepared themselves for the patient's death, even if that death occurred following a lengthy illness, also have more difficulty coping with the loss (Nielsen, Neergaard, Jensen, Bro, & Guldin, 2016; Tsai et al., 2015).

Type of Relationship

A death in the family virtually always changes the types of interactions occurring in the family, and the reactions people have to death can differ depending on their relationship to the person who has died (Berado, 1988). This section examines how survivors react to different types of death.

LOSS OF A SPOUSE. Losing a spouse is particularly devastating for virtually any married person because it deprives people of the single relationship that they may have had for a lengthy period of time, which in turn means the loss of social support, plans and dreams, and even identity as a spouse (Field, Nichols, Holen, & Horowitz, 1999; Mclean, Gomes, & Higginson, 2017). Many people who experience the loss of a spouse feel lonely for some time, even if they have a generally strong and supportive social network (Lichtenstein, Gatz, Pederson, Berg, & McClearn, 1996). They may also experience a variety of physical symptoms, including believing they see, hear, or sense the presence of their spouse (Grimby, 1993; Lindstrom, 1995; LoConto, 1998).

What You'll Learn 12.4

Interestingly, men and women react to and cope with the loss of their spouses in strikingly different ways (Lamme, Dykstra, & Broese Van Groenou, 1996; Stroebe, Stroebe, & Abakoumkin, 1999). Men are more likely than women to remarry, in part because women tend to outlive men and because men tend to prefer slightly younger partners than women do; hence, there are simply more eligible partners for older men than there are for older women. However, women are more likely than men to form new social relationships, such as with neighbors and other casual friends. Men also tend to suffer a greater loss of social support following the death of a spouse, because they tend to rely primarily on their wives for considerable social support and, therefore, are particularly devastated when she dies. Women, on the other hand, tend to rely on a broader network of people for support, including family members and friends as well as their spouse; hence, they suffer less of a decline in social support when they are widowed. This gender gap in social support is one explanation for the greater mortality risk men who have lost their spouse face as compared to women. (You'll learn more about the health consequences of bereavement later in this chapter.)

The loss of a spouse is particularly difficult for younger people, perhaps in part because the death is less expected. People who are widowed at younger ages show more grief than those who are widowed at older ages (Sasson & Umberson, 2014). Similarly, people who lose a middle-aged person (age 40 to 59) to cancer experience higher levels of grief and depression than those who lose an older person (age 60 to 79) (Francis, Kypriotakis, O'Toole, & Rose, 2016). Younger widows may also receive lower levels of social support following such a loss, since fewer of their peers have likely experienced such a death, which can make coping with the death even harder.

Although most of the research on bereavement following the death of a spouse has examined heterosexual people, several recent studies have extended prior work by examining the loss of a romantic partner in same-sex relationships. These findings reveal some similarities to the pain and loss experienced following such a death by individuals in heterosexual relationships, but also several distinct differences (Bristowe, Marshall, & Harding, 2016). Some people experience rudeness and hostility on the part of health care professionals, presumably due to homophobia. Being excluded from end-of-life decision making and/or arrangements has also been reported by some. People in same-sex relationships are therefore more at risk of experienced disenfranchised grief, meaning grief that cannot be openly acknowledged or mourned, and thus may receive less support from others (Patlamazoglou, Simmonds, & Snell, 2017).

DEATH OF A PARENT. For adults, the death of a parent is the most common type of loss (Berado, 1988). Because these deaths are relatively common and not so unexpected, they tend to be less traumatic than the loss of a spouse or a child. Adult children are generally able to continue with their own occupational and family responsibilities following the death of a parent, in part because there is typically some distance (emotional and physical) between adult parents and adult children.

While adult children experience relatively little disruption following the death of a parent, the death of a parent is the most significant loss a young child can encounter (Stillion & Wass, 1984; Wass & Stillion, 1988). Children are likely to express the loss of a parent through actions, such as repeating play activities that they had engaged in with their parent, and may remember parents only in terms of a few salient images. They may blame themselves for the death, feel betrayed, and believe that if the parent had loved them enough, they would not have died. The loss of a parent may also trigger new worries for children, including a fear that they too will die, and anxiety about who will take care of them. Not surprisingly, bereaved children are quite likely to suffer from psychological problems and tend to be more submissive, dependent, and introverted. For example, one study found that children who lost a parent showed increases in depression, sadness, irritability, crying, and other difficulties (e.g., eating, bed-wetting, school performance, sleeping) (Van Eerdewegh, Bieri, Parilla, & Clayton, 1982). Unfortunately, the effects of losing a parent as a child are quite lasting, as described in **Focus on Development**.

DEATH OF A CHILD. Because parents expect that their children will outlive them, the death of a child is often seen as a particularly devastating type of loss—families literally can be torn apart dealing with this tragedy (Stillion & Wass, 1984). The intensity of grief following the death of a child is generally greater than that following the loss of a spouse or parent and may be quite long-lasting (Bass, Noelker, Townsend, & Deimling, 1990; Harvey & Hansen, 2000; Meert et al., 2010). For example, researchers in one study found that compared with parents who did not lose a child, parents who lost a child had an overall increased relative risk of a

FOCUS ON DEVELOPMENT

The Lasting Consequences of Death of a Parent

Experiencing the death of a parent during childhood is unfortunately associated with lasting psychological and physical consequences. Adults who have lost their parents during childhood are more likely to have problems with loneliness, depression, suicide, and physical disorders such as cardiovascular disease. For example, researchers in one study compared the long-term risk of suicide among people who experienced the loss of a parent before age 18 to those who had not (Guldin et al., 2015). Although suicide rates were, as expected, relatively low, individuals who had experienced the loss of a parent prior to age 18 were twice as likely to die from suicide as those had did not experienced this loss. Adults who have experienced the death of a parent are also more likely to use antidepressants (Appel et al., 2016). The longer-term effects of experiencing the death of a parent are particularly severe for children who lose their parents at a relatively young age (compared to during the teenage years; Berg, Rostila, & Hjern, 2016). These findings all point to the importance of providing children who experience such a loss with support and professional help to reduce the likelihood of long-term harmful consequences.

first psychiatric hospitalization for any disorder (Li, Laursen, Precht, Olsen, & Mortensen, 2005). Among mothers, the relative risk of being hospitalized for any psychiatric disorder was highest during the first year after the death of the child but remained significantly elevated five years or more after the death.

Parents who experience the death of their child show a range of emotions (Griffith, Davies, & Lavender, 2015). Anger is a very common first reaction to learning that a child is dying. Parents may lash out at doctors, nurses, and even God. Parents may also feel anxious about the upcoming separation from their child as well as their own eventual death (which is clearly brought home acutely in the case of a child's death). Guilt is another common reaction to learning that one's child is dying. Because parents see their role as protecting and nurturing their child, they can feel overwhelming guilt when they feel they have failed in this role. Parents often try to explain why the death happened and may feel that they are being punished (Downey, Silver, & Wortman, 1990). All of these emotions are particularly strong when the child was initially healthy and when the death is unexpected, as in cases of an accident or suicide. In fact, parents who lose children to suicide or accidents are 10 times more likely to experience anxiety or depression than those who don't experience the death of a child (Wilcox, Mittendorfer-Rutz, Kjeldgård, Alexanderson, & Runeson, 2015).

Another type of commonly experienced death of a child is that of the loss of a child in utero, during birth, or shortly after birth (Davis, 1991). These deaths, often called fetal deaths, include miscarriages, stillbirths, and perinatal deaths. For many years, it was assumed that such deaths caused relatively little grief to parents because they happened at such an early point in the new life. Grieving parents are often told, "You can always have another child," or "Thank goodness it happened before you really got attached to the child." But in most cases parents start planning for and anticipating the birth of a child even at the very early stages of pregnancy. They may choose a name; buy furniture, clothes, and toys; and start imagining their lives with this baby. The death of a child, even during pregnancy, therefore typically leads to very real grieving and a sense of loss. Compared to women who experienced a live birth, women who experienced perinatal loss were four times more likely to show signs of depression and seven times more likely to show signs of posttraumatic stress disorder nine months after the loss (Gold, Leon, Boggs, & Sen, 2016).

In recent years, programs have been developed in hospitals in which parents are encouraged to see and hold their dead baby. They may have the opportunity to take photographs of the child, to give it a name, and to take some type of memento (e.g., a lock of hair, a footprint, a hospital bracelet). These practices are thought to help parents acknowledge the depth of their loss and to validate their intense feelings of grief.

DEATH OF A SIBLING. Although considerable research has examined the impact on parents of losing a child, relatively little research has examined the impact of losing a child on his or her siblings. However, the sibling relationship is a very important and unique one; hence, siblings experience many of the same emotions parents do following a child's death, including shock, confusion, anxiety, depression, loneliness, and anger (Wass & Stillion, 1988). Children may feel guilty for surviving, anxious that they will die, and responsible for their sibling's death (e.g., if the sibling had wished in a moment of anger that the child would die). The surviving child must also cope with a changed family situation, including neglect from their parents, who are focusing attention on the dying or dead child. Children often try to deny their own grief and sometimes even avoid mentioning their sibling's name in an effort to avoid causing extreme pain to their parents. As one 12-year-old boy who recently lost a brother said, "My Dad doesn't talk about it, and my Mom cries a lot. I just stay in my room so I won't be a bother" (Wass & Stillion, 1988, p. 218). Finally, children can lose their own sense of identity if they have lost their only sibling and are now no longer a sister or brother.

To help children cope with the death of a sibling, try to make them feel included, if possible, during all stages of their sibling's illness (Stillion & Wass, 1984). They should be permitted to visit their sibling in the hospital and should be allowed to attend the funeral. Although parents may try to hide their grief in an effort to protect the surviving child, it is important for adults to acknowledge their own feelings as well as to encourage children to discuss their feelings. Siblings obviously should be reassured that their own thoughts were not responsible for their sibling's condition. Siblings' symptoms, including grief, depression, and PTSD, are strongly associated with how parents cope with this loss, so parents can help surviving children by making sure they are getting the help they need (Morris, Gabert-Quillen, Friebert, Carst, & Delahanty, 2016).

Consequences of Bereavement

Not surprisingly, bereavement is associated with numerous short- and long-term consequences for survivors. This section will describe the impact of bereavement on psychological, social, and physical problems, as well as some potential mechanisms explaining these associations.

Psychological Problems

Psychological problems, including depression, sadness, guilt, anger, and anxiety, are very common following the loss of a loved one (Kastenbaum, 1999; Li, Stroebe, Chan, & Chow, 2014; Moriarty, Maguire, O'Reilly, & McCann, 2015; Raphael & Dobson, 2000; Vable, Subramanian, Rist, & Glymour, 2015). People who are experiencing bereavement may feel sad and empty and may have trouble contemplating continuing on with their lives without the deceased person. One study with HIV-positive gay men found that those whose close friends or lovers had died from AIDS in the last year were more depressed and likely to think about suicide and more likely to use sedatives, such as sleeping pills and tranquilizers, than those who were HIV-positive and had not experienced this type of loss (Martin & Dean, 1993). Similarly, a study of caregivers of patients with advanced cancer found that 12.6% reported major depressive disorder or anxiety six months after the loss of the patient (Garrido & Prigerson, 2014).

Not surprisingly, these feelings of anxiety and depression occur even prior to the actual death. Caregivers for patients with cancer show increased anxiety and depression over the last year of the person's life, with 15% showing moderate to severe depression and 27% showing moderate to severe anxiety (Burridge, Barnett, & Clavarino, 2009).

Social Problems

Grief often leads to social problems, including loneliness and isolation (Berado, 1988; Harvey & Hansen, 2000). People who suffer the loss of a spouse or child may experience a decrease in available social networks. Widows may find that they are not invited to parties or other social gatherings at which other people are all part of a couple. Similarly, parents who've lost a child may lose the network of friends who have children of the same age. Even when bereaved people are included in social gatherings, they may have difficulty seeing other people's lives continuing normally while theirs is falling apart, which may lead them to withdraw from social situations.

Some people are at particular risk of experiencing social problems following bereavement. As described previously, younger widows feel more isolated socially than older widows, presumably because this type of loss is less common for younger people. Similarly, women who have lost a spouse tend to cope better than do men who have lost a spouse, again

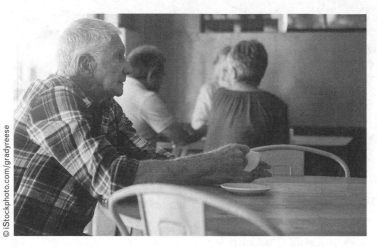

Some of the negative effects of bereavement are caused by a lack of social support, which is particularly common for older people, who may have experienced the death of not only a spouse but also friends and family members.

What You'll Learn 12.5

because the social support for widows tends to be greater than such support for widowers (Wisocki & Skowron, 2000).

Health Problems

People who are bereaved have increased rates of minor and major illnesses (Berado, 1988; Martikainen & Valkonen, 1996; Raphael & Dobson, 2000; Ray, 2004; Schaefer, Quesenberry, & Wi, 1995). They may experience a number of physical symptoms, such as emptiness in the abdomen, a sense of physical weakness, choking and shortness of breath, and a tightness in the chest. The death of a spouse is associated with a range of major cardiovascular events—myocardial infarction, stroke, pulmonary embolism—in the weeks and months immediately following (Carey et al., 2014). Similarly, parents who experience the death of a child have a slight increase in risk of mortality compared to nonbereaved parents, presumably due to the severe stress such a loss causes (Schorr et al., 2016).

Although losing a spouse in general is associated with poorer health and increased mortality, the cause of a spouse's death also influences one's own mortality. For example, researchers in one study found that for both men and women, the death of one's spouse was associated with an increase in mortality over the next nine years: 18% for men following the death of a wife and 16% for women following the death of a husband (Elwert & Christakis, 2008). However, different causes of deaths pose different levels of risk for the surviving spouse. Specifically, loss of a spouse from cancer (especially colon and lung cancer), cardiovascular disease or a stroke, or an accident are all associated with an increased risk of dying. In contrast, surviving spouses are not at increased risk of dying following the death of a spouse from Alzheimer's disease or Parkinson's. These findings suggest that experiencing the death of a spouse to chronic conditions that require considerable care and management (e.g., cancer, coronary heart disease) or acute events (e.g., accidents, infections) is associated with particularly great risks to one's own health, whereas experiencing the loss of a spouse to chronic conditions that do not require such extensive management is less detrimental to one's own mortality. Given the long-term nature of these conditions, spouses may have had considerable time to adjust to the reality of the expected loss of one's spouse, which may in turn buffer some of the negative effects of being widowed.

The death of a spouse is also particularly impactful for men's mortality (Martikainen & Valkonen, 1996; Stroebe & Stroebe, 1983). One large-scale study in Finland examined death rates in the period immediately following the death of a spouse (Martikainen & Valkonen, 1996). Compared to others their age, men were 17% more likely to die in this period, whereas women were only 6% more likely to die. Similarly, although female patients with lung cancer who lost their spouse did not have higher mortality rates than those who were married, male widowed patients with lung cancer had a higher mortality rate than male married patients (Saito-Nakaya et al., 2008). Perhaps most important, widowed men were at greater risk of dying from various causes, including infectious diseases, accidents, and suicide, than were men whose spouse was still living (65.3% versus 51.8%, respectively) (Helsing & Szklo, 1981). In contrast, there was no difference in death rates for women who were married as compared to those who were widowed (23.2% and 24.1%, respectively).

One reason women who experience the death of a spouse have not typically suffered from the same negative health consequences as men may be that women's generally larger social networks enable them to receive more social support following the death of their spouse. For example, women are likely to have more friends available to talk with about their loss, and this emotional support can lead to better health (Stroebe & Stroebe, 1983). Moreover, men generally rely on their wives for emotional support, but women are likely to rely on their children, friends, and other family members for support (Kohen, 1983). Married men may also have relied on their wives to maintain contact with friends and family members; hence, they may feel the loss of support not only from their wives but also from their lost contact with others. Finally, because women tend to live longer than men, women who lose a spouse are likely to find a much larger support group of similar others than are men (Stroebe & Stroebe, 1983). In fact, many community-based support groups for those who have lost a spouse are focused primarily on serving the needs of women.

UNDERSTANDING THE MECHANISM. One factor that may account for these increased rates of illness and death in bereaved people is that people who are bereaved are less likely to engage in health-promoting behavior and are more likely to engage in health-damaging behavior (Berado, 1988). For example, following the loss of a spouse, people may use alcohol to try to dull their grief or may forget to eat healthy foods. In line with this view, people who are bereaved tend to show increases in BMI (Oliveira, Rostila, Saarela, & Lopes, 2014). Similarly, bereaved people may have trouble sleeping and eating, which in turn can wear down their bodies. This explanation may work especially well to explain why men who lose their wives, who in many cases may have done most of the grocery shopping and cooking, are at such great risk of showing health problems. In line with this view, research reveals that people whose spouse has died are also three times as likely to enter long-term institutional care in the month following the spouse's death than they were prior to the death, presumably due to a loss of social and instrumental support (Nihtilä & Martikainen, 2008).

Another factor that may explain the link between bereavement and illness is that bereavement-related stress impairs the immune system, which thereby leads to higher susceptibility to infection and disease (Kemeny et al., 1995; Raphael & Dobson, 2000; Zisook, Schuchter, Sledge, & Judd, 1994). For example, one study of former caregivers of patients with Alzheimer's disease revealed that they experienced a significant decline in their natural

FOCUS ON NEUROSCIENCE

Why Bereavement Really Harms Older Adults

To help understand the effects of bereavement on the immune system, researchers in one study compared levels of stress hormones in bereaved and nonbereaved healthy adults (Vitlic, Khanfer, Lord, Carroll, & Phillips, 2014). In addition, half of the people in each group were young (mean age of 32) and half were older (mean age of 72). The participants completed measures of overall health, psychological states (anxiety and depression), and symptoms of bereavement, and also provided blood samples.

As expected, both older and younger bereaved people reported higher levels of depression and anxiety than the nonbereaved people and were showing symptoms of bereavement. However, while older bereaved people showed higher levels of stress hormones than the older nonbereaved people, there was no difference in stress hormone levels between the bereaved and nonbereaved younger people. These finding suggest that bereavement may be particularly harmful to health among older people.

killer cell function (a measure of the immune system's ability to respond to health threats; Esterling, Kiecolt-Glaser, Bodnar, & Glaser, 1994). (This link between stress and the immune system is discussed in more detail in *Chapter 4: Understanding Stress*.) As described in **Focus on Neuroscience**, bereavement has particularly harmful effects on older adults.

COPING WITH BEREAVEMENT

LO 12.5

Describe strategies for coping with bereavement

According to the **dual process model of coping with bereavement**, loss involves two distinct types of stressors: loss-oriented stressors and restoration-oriented stressors (see Figure 12.2; Stroebe & Schut, 1999). Loss-oriented stressors involve the inherent feelings of grief that we experience following the death of a loved one and include reflecting back on past times with that person, imagining what she or he would say or do if still alive, and yearning for additional time with that person. In contrast, restoration-oriented stressors are focused on accepting this person's death and moving on in various ways, such as by forming a new identity, taking care of tasks the person used to do, and building new relationships. This section will examine strategies people can use to cope with bereavement, including making sense and finding meaning, receiving social support, and seeking professional help.

Making Sense and Finding Meaning

Many bereaved people have a strong need to try to make sense of the loss and seek out any information related to the death (Raphael & Dobson, 2000; Toth, Stockton, & Browne, 2000).

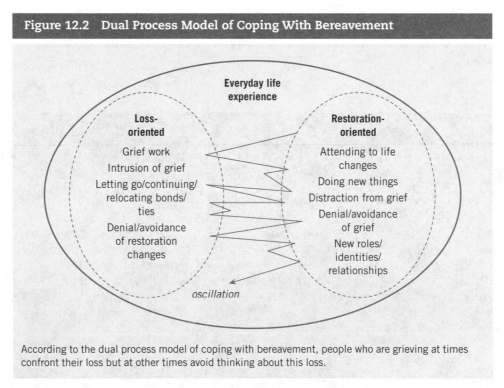

Figure 12.2 Dual Process Model of Coping With Bereavement

Everyday life experience

Loss-oriented
Grief work
Intrusion of grief
Letting go/continuing/relocating bonds/ties
Denial/avoidance of restoration changes

Restoration-oriented
Attending to life changes
Doing new things
Distraction from grief
Denial/avoidance of grief
New roles/identities/relationships

oscillation

According to the dual process model of coping with bereavement, people who are grieving at times confront their loss but at other times avoid thinking about this loss.

Source: Stroebe & Schut (1999, p. 213).

For example, they may go over and over the details surrounding the person's death, including the precise cause of death, the timing of the death, and whether the person experienced pain or fear. Even if these questions don't have answers, it can help the survivor recover to tell the story of their loss. Survivors have a particularly difficult time coping with deaths in which they don't have information, such as knowledge about how exactly the person died or whether their loved one suffered, and when they don't have the person's body.

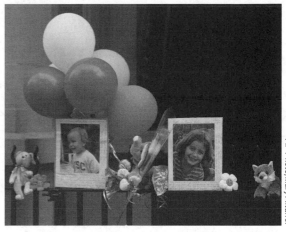

Bereaved people who are able to find some type of meaning show lower levels of grief and anger (Boyraz, Horne, & Waits, 2015; Harper, O'Connor, & O'Carroll, 2014; Kim, 2009). One study of parents who had experienced the death of their child found that making sense of the child's death was the strongest predictor of the severity of the grief, with parents who reported having made little to no sense of their child's death experiencing a greater intensity of grief (Keesee, Currier, & Neimeyer, 2008). Bereaved people may also benefit from taking some type of action in response to the loss, such as planting a tree, starting a scholarship fund in the person's name, or creating a scrapbook of the person's life.

After their two young children, Lulu (age 6) and Leo (20 months), were stabbed to death by their nanny in October 2012, Marina and Kevin Krim established the Lulu & Leo Fund to foster creativity and resilience through art for all children facing hardships.

Finding such meaning also predicts better physical health. For example, gay men who experienced the death of their partner to AIDS but found meaning in this loss—such as by appreciating and become closer to their friends, shifting their priorities, or increasing their faith—showed fewer signs of physical decline than those who were not able to find such "silver linings" (Bower, Kemeny, Taylor, & Fahey, 1998). In fact, only 3 of the 16 men who found meaning died during the follow-up period, whereas 12 of the 24 who did not find meaning died.

This type of thinking about and trying to make sense of the death can be a valuable and even necessary component of working through the loss (Bower et al., 1998; Folkman, Chesney, Cooke, Boccellari, & Collette, 1994; Folkman, Chesney, Collette, Boccellari, & Cooke, 1996; McIntosh, Silver, & Wortman, 1993; Stroebe & Stroebe, 1991). Some researchers even suggest that people who fail to engage in this type of "grief work" experience poorer psychological and physical well-being. For example, one study with parents who had experienced the sudden loss of their child found that those who thought frequently about the death of their child experienced more grief in the short term (three weeks following the death) but showed greater adjustment and less distress 18 months later than those who did not do this grief work (McIntosh et al., 1993). As discussed in **Chapter 4: Understanding Stress**, people who try to avoid thinking about difficult thoughts show increased physiological arousal, which may in turn lead to more health problems. In line with this view, men who tried to avoid thinking about the loss of their spouse by suppressing their feelings and distracting themselves from their grief showed more maladjustment two years later than those who didn't use those strategies (Stroebe & Stroebe, 1991). This research suggests that confronting the loss can be a helpful coping strategy.

However, keep in mind that persistently thinking—or ruminating—about the loss is not associated with adjustment and can even have harmful effects on psychological and physical well-being (Bonanno, Keltner, Holen, & Horowitz, 1995; Schut, van den Bout, De Keijser, & Stroebe, 1996; Stroebe & Stroebe, 1991). People who tend to ruminate more about the death of a loved one experience more stressors, receive less social support, and feel less optimistic about their expectations for the future, which leads, over time, to higher rates of depression (Nolen-Hoeksema, Parker, & Larson, 1994). In contrast, people who deliberately try to avoid thinking about the loss of their spouse and exposing themselves to reminders of the loss may experience better long-term adjustment.

What accounts for these differences in terms of the effects of different types of strategies of coping with death? One explanation is that these discrepancies are caused by the type of thinking (or not thinking) people do in response to loss. Certain types of thinking, such as reflecting on the positive aspects of the deceased person's life and the meaning of his or her death, are likely to be beneficial. It may, for example, be reassuring to bereaved parents to talk about their child and to find meaning in the child's death (e.g., "This is part of God's plan"; "Our child's organs helped other babies survive"). On the other hand, ruminating and dwelling on the depression associated with the loss is likely to be detrimental (Stroebe & Schut, 2001). Similarly, people may find it helpful at times to distract themselves from thinking about the loss, but actively trying to not think about the loss (e.g., thought suppression) may have undesirable effects. The decision to not talk about the loss should also come from the bereaved person and not from others: bereaved mothers who think frequently about their loss but believe their social environments would not be supportive of such disclosure experience high levels of depression (Lepore, Silver, Wortman, & Wayment, 1996). The most effective coping probably involves some moderate level of thinking about the loss, such as confronting memories when they arise but avoiding constant rumination about the deceased person.

Receiving Social Support

Survivors also have a strong need to express their reactions to the death, including their feelings of anger, guilt, anxiety, helplessness, and depression, and hence can really benefit from the presence of social support (Kastenbaum, 1999; Raphael & Dobson, 2000; Toth et al., 2000). These feelings may be strange and intense—survivors may be angry at their loved one for getting killed, even if such a thought is totally irrational. People may feel they are going crazy, and they appreciate hearing that their reactions are normal.

Simply talking to other people about the loss has both psychological and physical benefits. Greater satisfaction with social support received from family and friends is associated with lower levels of grief and depression in the first six months following the death of a spouse (de Vries, Utz, Caserta, & Lund, 2014). Similarly, following the death of their infant, parents who discuss difficulties with others who have endured similar circumstances and confide in relatives and/or friends show lower levels of grief and depression (Hawthorne, Youngblut, & Brooten, 2016). In contrast, people who don't feel it is socially acceptable to talk about loss show higher rates of depression and stress as well as worse physical health (Juth, Smyth, Carey, & Lepore, 2015). One study of people who had lost a spouse found that those who talked to friends about the death had a smaller increase in number of illnesses following the death, whereas those who continued to ruminate on their own about the death had more illnesses, including ulcers, headaches, and pneumonia (Pennebaker & O'Heeron, 1984).

Although some people stop participating in work and social activities while caring for a terminally ill loved one and while grieving following their death, maintaining some type of regular activities can be helpful. People who continue to pursue such activities get social support from friends and colleagues, which can help with coping (Roulston et al., 2016). In fact, the strongest predictors of resilience following the death of a spouse are engagement in regular daily life activities and social relationships as well as a belief that people will provide comfort if needed (Infurna & Luthar, 2017).

Survivors often find that friends and family are available to provide emotional and practical support immediately following the loss of a loved one, but this support typically declines over time. However, survivors often report experiencing intense pain for months, and even years, after the person's death. In fact, the intensity of a person's grief may not even be apparent immediately, when survivors must often cope with urgent matters, such as planning a funeral or memorial service, making plans for handling the body, and handling legal issues.

Many survivors also experience an anniversary reaction, namely, a reaction to the death again at a later date that has some special significance (Dlin, 1985), such as an anniversary (in months or years) of the person's death, holidays, the loved one's birthday, or other special occasions.

Both formal and informal grief support groups can provide valuable support for those who have experienced the loss of a loved one (Raphael & Dobson, 2000) (see Table 12.3). These support groups are particularly helpful because they allow people to affiliate with others in the same situation. For example, after the tragic shootings at Virginia Tech in 2007, several students started Facebook groups for students to share concerns, express grief, and post messages of support (Vicary & Fraley, 2010). Survivors can share their experiences, learn whether their reactions and experiences are normal, obtain guidance on coping, and discuss big questions (e.g., is life fair? is there a God?). Similarly, expressing grief via social media can help people receive comfort from others, keep the person's memory alive, and develop connections with others who also knew and cared about the loved one (Rossetto, Lannutti, & Strauman, 2015).

Many people find participating in a support group very helpful in terms of feeling understood by others and feeling less alone. Some evidence even suggests that group-based

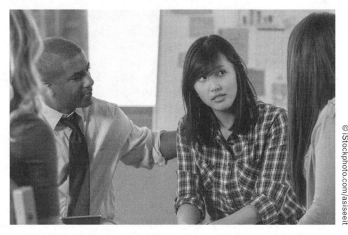

Social support groups with others who have experienced a similar loss can be a valuable resource for bereaved people.

Table 12.3 Survivor Support Groups	
Organization	**Description**
Infant Loss Resources (http://infantlossresources.org/)	This group provides information for people affected by sudden infant death syndrome.
Parents of Murdered Children (www.pomc.com)	This group provides information for parents whose children have died from homicide.
Widowed Persons Service (www.knology.net/~wpsemeraldcoast/)	This group provides information for people who are widowed.
Mothers Against Drunk Driving (www.madd.org)	This group provides information for people who have lost someone to a drunk-driving accident.
American Association of Suicidology (www.suicidology.org)	This group provides information for survivors of suicide.
Compassionate Friends (www.compassionatefriends.org)	This group provides information for those who have lost a child.

Support groups are especially helpful when they bring together people who have all suffered the same type of loss.

Source: Created by Catherine A. Sanderson.

interventions for bereaved people result in greater reductions in grief severity than does individual therapy (Sikkema et al., 2006). This type of support group may be particularly valuable for children and teenagers, who may have more difficulty finding peers who can relate to a loss (Juth et al., 2015). As one teenager who participated in such a group following the death of his father said, "You are not the only one who is young and fatherless" (Henoch, Berg, & Benkel, 2015, p. 4).

Seeking Professional Help

Professional help may aid survivors in coping with their loss (Neimeyer, 2000). Some people find guided imagery helpful as grief therapy (Aiken, 1985). In this technique, bereaved individuals are taken through exercises in which they relive aspects of their relationship with the deceased: they might recall their affection for the deceased person and then replay receiving news of the death, attending the funeral, and watching the person be buried. The bereaved person is told to describe these events out loud as if they are occurring at that moment. They may also share imaginary dialogues with the deceased person, ask the person's permission to start new relationships, and ultimately say good-bye. This technique is supposed to help people come to terms with their grief and to finally make peace with the loss.

Another technique for helping people manage grief following the death of a loved one is a **bereavement life review**. In this approach, a therapist interviews the bereaved person regarding both their own life experiences and those of the person who died. For example, a

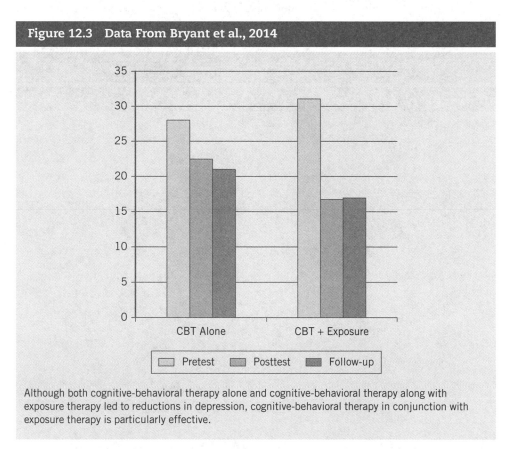

Figure 12.3 Data From Bryant et al., 2014

Although both cognitive-behavioral therapy alone and cognitive-behavioral therapy along with exposure therapy led to reductions in depression, cognitive-behavioral therapy in conjunction with exposure therapy is particularly effective.

Source: Data from Bryant, Kenny, Joscelyne, Rawson, Maccallum, Cahill, Hopwood, Aderka, & Nickerson (2014).

therapist might ask the person to describe the most important things in their own life and what they are proudest of, and also ask for their most vivid memory of the deceased person and how they grew through taking care of this person. People who undergo this type of bereavement life review show lower rates of depression as well as higher levels of spiritual well-being (Ando, Marquez-Wong, Simon, Kira, & Becker, 2015).

Interventions to assist family members who are experiencing bereavement may also help ease symptoms of grief. Researchers in one study randomly assigned family members of patients dying in ICUs to either typical care—meaning a conference about end-of-life options—or to an intervention designed to include more communication, including valuing what family members say, acknowledging their emotions, and eliciting questions (Lautrette et al., 2007). The family members in the enhanced-communication condition also received a brochure on bereavement. Participants in the enhanced-communication group had longer conferences than those in the control group (30 minutes vs. 20 minutes) and spent more of the time talking (14 minutes vs. 5 minutes). Moreover, three months after the patient's death, those in the intervention group had fewer symptoms of depression (29% versus 56%), anxiety (45% versus 67%), and PTSD (45% versus 69%). These findings reveal that providing family members of patients who are dying in the ICU with more communication at the time of end-of-life decision making, as well as a brochure on bereavement, may lead to long-term benefits in terms of coping with the loss. Similarly, and as shown in Figure 12.3, bereaved people who receive 10 weeks of exposure therapy along with cognitive-behavioral therapy show greater reductions in depression than those who receive only traditional cognitive-behavioral therapy (Bryant et al., 2014).

Table 12.4 Information YOU Can Use

- Although many people avoid talking about death, it is important to think about and talk about end-of-life preferences with your loved ones so that you know what they would—and would not—want if they were to become seriously ill or injured. And these conversations are easier to have prior to a crisis situation.

- Write your own living will so that those who would be asked to make decisions on your behalf know your preferences. Would you want to be tube-fed? Placed on a ventilator? These are important decisions and your loved ones should know what you would like in such a situation.

- If you, or a loved one, is diagnosed with a terminal illness, consider using hospice care in either a hospital or home setting. Hospice care does not require giving up other forms of treatment and leads to better psychological and physical well-being (and even longer life expectancy) for both patients and their caregivers.

- If you experience the loss of a loved one, understand that bereavement is a process; you will eventually feel better, but it will take time (especially if the loss was sudden, violent, and of a young person). Relying on others (either formally or informally) who have experienced a similar loss can be very helpful.

- If you have a friend who has suffered the loss of a loved one, try to support them in ways that are helpful: offer some concrete and practical help (such as preparing food for the bereaved person, assisting with funeral arrangements, or running errands), bring up the loved one's name in natural ways (people who have lost someone want the opportunity to talk about their memories of that person and often appreciate hearing stories about them), and signal your willingness to listen and help in any way (even simple statements, such as "I'm so sorry" and "Tell me how you're feeling" are appreciated).

Early Models of Death and Dying

- The best-known model for explaining how people cope with dying is the stages of death and dying developed by Dr. Elisabeth Kübler-Ross. According to this model, terminally ill people go through a series of five distinct stages: denial, anger, bargaining, depression, and acceptance.

- According to Charles Corr's task work model for coping with dying, people who are terminally ill focus on four distinct types of tasks: physical, psychological, social, and spiritual. Similarly, another model describes the phase-specific tasks that people with life-threatening illnesses encounter, including prediagnostic, acute, chronic, recovery, and terminal.

- Early models of death and dying have received some critiques. First, people may not go through these stages in a particular order. The model may also exclude some stages and fail to adequately describe others. These models also ignore the role of various factors, such as gender, age, and race/ethnicity, that could influence how people respond to a diagnosis of a terminal illness. Finally, these models ignore the distinct benefits that people who are close to death may experience.

Managing a Terminal Diagnosis

- The majority of people in the United States die in hospitals. The focus in hospitals is on curing patients, delivering technical skills and interventions, and preventing or delaying death. However, many people are not interested in having aggressive end-of-life care when such care is likely to be futile and would prefer to receive palliative care, meaning care focused on managing pain. People who are terminally ill are also viewed and treated in particular ways by medical professionals, who may not take into account their psychological concerns.

- The holistic, or hospice, approach to managing terminal illness focuses more broadly not only on providing physical care but also on psychological, social, cultural, and spiritual care. Hospice care focuses on treating the symptoms of terminal illness and minimizing the patient's discomfort and pain. This type of care improves the end-of-life illness experience for patients and their families; hospice patients even live longer than patients who receive standard hospital care.

- The specific concerns of fatally ill children vary by age. Terminally ill children also go through a series of distinct stages as they attempt to understand their illness. Health professionals generally believe that terminally ill children should be given honest information about their illness, in an age-appropriate way. Although parents and medical professionals may fear that providing such information will be upsetting, terminally ill children are often already aware of their condition. Providing children with information allows them the opportunity to ask questions and thereby reduces anxiety.

The Death With Dignity Movement

- Some people with a terminal illness want the option of assisted suicide due to fear about losing physical and mental functioning and experiencing a very low quality of life as well as a desire to maintain some control over their condition. Several states allow physician-assisted suicide, meaning that physicians can, at a patient's request, provide a lethal dose of medicine. Some other countries allow euthanasia, in which the physician acts directly to end a person's life. Although most people are in favor of some form of physician-assisted suicide, others believe that providing people with the means to commit suicide creates a slippery slope and that the moral issues associated with assisted suicide should make it illegal.

- One approach to gaining some control over one's end-of-life experience is to create a living will, which allows people to specify their wishes about the type of care they would like to receive in the event they are incapacitated and therefore unable to make their own decisions. People may also complete lists of "valued life activities" and then use these activities as a guide to determining whether or not to end someone's life. An alternative approach to gaining some control over end-of-life measures is therefore to appoint a health care proxy, who makes medical decisions on behalf of someone if they are unable to do so themselves. Advance directives can help patients receive the type of treatment they prefer.

Understanding Bereavement

- Bereavement typically proceeds through a series of stages, including reaction, yearning and searching, disorganization and reorganization, and reorientation and recovery. However, some bereaved people may have feelings of unresolved (or complicated) grief and never return to a normal pattern of living.

- Quick-trajectory deaths, in which the loss is sudden and unexpected, are very hard on survivors. Survivors must cope with practical issues (the funeral, burial preferences), lack a sense of closure, and have no opportunity to prepare themselves for the loss. In contrast, in the case of lingering-trajectory deaths, the death comes after a period of gradually declining health. Loved ones may watch the patient go through long-term pain and suffering and experience the loss of physical bodily functions and of mental faculties. Losing a spouse is particularly devastating, as is the death of a parent for young children. The death of a child is difficult for parents and siblings, who may experience shock, confusion, anxiety, depression, loneliness, anger, and guilt.

- Psychological problems, including depression, sadness, guilt, anger, and anxiety, are common following the loss of a loved one, as are social problems, such as loneliness and isolation. People who are bereaved have increased rates of minor and major illnesses and increased mortality; men are especially likely to experience higher rates of mortality following bereavement. Bereaved people are less likely to engage in health-promoting behavior and are more likely to engage in health-damaging behavior; bereavement-related stress also impairs the immune system, which leads to higher susceptibility to infection and disease.

Coping With Bereavement

- Many bereaved people want to make sense of the loss and seek out any information related to the death. Those who are able to find meaning show lower levels of grief and anger as well as better physical health. However, persistently thinking—or ruminating—about the loss is not associated with adjustment—and can even have harmful effects on psychological and physical well-being.

- Survivors also want to express their reactions to the death and benefit from the presence of social support. Simply talking to other people about the loss has both psychological and physical benefits. Although friends and family are available to provide support immediately following the loss of a loved one, this support typically declines over time. Both formal and informal grief support groups can provide valuable support for those who have experienced the loss of a loved one.

- Professional help may aid survivors in coping with their loss. This help can include guided imagery and/or a bereavement life review. Interventions to assist family members may also help ease symptoms of grief, including depression and anxiety.

13

MANAGING HEALTH CARE

Learning Objectives

13.1 Examine issues in health screening

13.2 Review factors that influence health care utilization

13.3 Summarize the experience of hospitalization

13.4 Compare different issues in health care interactions

13.5 Explain factors involved in measuring, predicting, and increasing adherence

What You'll Learn

13.1 How texting reminders about cancer screenings can save lives

13.2 How live plants in a hospital room speed up recovery from surgery

13.3 Why men have shorter life expectancies than women

13.4 Why electronic record keeping may lead to physician burnout

13.5 Why describing the effects of measles changes parents' attitudes toward vaccinations

Preview

One of the most essential components of staying healthy is seeking proper health care when needed. Yet a variety of personal and situational factors influence people's willingness to seek health care and to follow medical recommendations for managing illness. This chapter explores four key issues in managing health care, including screening for disease, utilizing health care, interacting with health care providers, and adhering to medical recommendations.

HEALTH SCREENING

LO 13.1

Examine issues in health screening

Screening to detect illness, or even an increased likelihood of developing illness, at an early stage can be an increasingly important part of health promotion. Screening behaviors, such as having your teeth cleaned to check for cavities, getting your blood pressure checked during a physical exam, and having a mammogram to check for signs of cancer, are secondary prevention strategies (see Table 13.1).

Advances in molecular genetics, including the mapping of disorders onto particular genes, has led to the ability to test for over 1,000 inherited disorders. In some cases, this testing can determine whether a person is at risk of developing a disease. For example, genetic tests are now available for breast, ovarian, and some types of colorectal cancer, as well as Huntington's disease and Alzheimer's disease. Genetic screening will increase as more genetic tests are developed. In other cases, genetic testing can determine whether a person carries a gene for a disorder, such as Tay-Sachs disease, cystic fibrosis, or sickle-cell anemia, which they could then transmit to their children. Couples may then use this information to determine whether they will have children or whether they might use in vitro fertilization with nongenetically related eggs or sperm to avoid passing this disease on to their children.

In still other cases, testing is used to evaluate whether a fetus has various genetic conditions, such as Down's syndrome. The vast majority of pregnant women in the United States undergo some kind of screening, such as blood tests, ultrasound, or amniocentesis, to help evaluate the health of the fetus. Based on the results, couples can then decide to continue the pregnancy or to terminate it in cases in which the baby would not survive more than a few days or would suffer extreme, and possibly life-threatening, disability.

Table 13.1 Recommended Cancer Screening Tests

Early Cancer Detection for Men and Women

- Colorectal cancer: Starting at age 50, both men and women should have one of the following four screening tests: flexible sigmoidoscopy every 5 years; double contrast barium enema every 5 years; colonoscopy every 10 years; or virtual colonoscopy every 5 years.

Early Cancer Detection for Men

- Prostate cancer: Starting at age 50 (or 45 for those at higher risk based on family history and demographics), men should discuss the pros and cons of prostate cancer screening to decide if testing is appropriate. Testing for prostate cancer includes the PSA blood test and digital rectal exam.

Early Cancer Detection for Women

- Cervical cancer: Women between the ages of 21 and 29 should have a Pap test every three years; women ages 30 to 65 should have a Pap test every five years.

- Breast cancer: Women ages 40 to 44 should have the choice to start having annual mammograms; women ages 45 to 54 should have annual mammograms; women ages 55 and older should have mammograms every other year.

These recommendations for screening were developed by the American Cancer Society. These tests are used to detect early stages of cancer before a person might be noticing symptoms.

Source: Data retrieved from the American Cancer Society.

Benefits and Costs of Screening

The decision to seek screening is a complex one for many people. Screening for medical conditions—and even genetic predispositions for particular medical conditions—has both potential advantages and disadvantages, as you'll learn in this section.

Benefits of Screening

Proponents of screening argue that this type of knowledge may help a person seek early treatment and/or engage in health-promoting behaviors (Baum, Friedman, & Zakowski, 1997; Patenaude, Guttmacher, & Collins, 2002). Learning that one has high blood pressure or elevated levels of cholesterol, for example, could motivate a person to make changes in diet or increase his or her rate of exercise in an attempt to prevent developing heart disease. In line with this view, people who learn they are HIV-positive often engage in better physical and psychological care for themselves and appear motivated to not spread this disease to others (Coates, Morin, & McKusick, 1987; Coates et al., 1988; Collins et al., 2001).

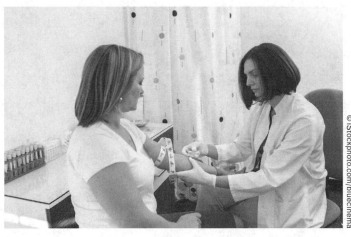

Individuals who test positive for HIV can begin undergoing highly active antiretroviral treatment (HAART), which changes what could be a fatal disease to a chronic disease.

Knowledge about one's genetic risk of developing a particular disease may also help reduce uncertainty and help people make realistic plans for their future. Knowing about one's genetic predisposition to a given disease can provide some peace of mind, especially for people who are already concerned they will develop such a disorder, perhaps based on family history, but do not know for sure (Baum et al., 1997). If testing results indicate a particular future health outcome, people then have the ability to plan accordingly. For example, a person who is aware that he or she is likely to develop Huntington's disease, which causes serious movement and cognitive disorders, could choose to forego a career that involves many years of education.

Moreover, in the case of diseases that progress over time, patients could be more vigilant for symptoms of the disease and, at least in some cases, take some steps to reduce their risk of developing the disease. For example, women who find out they have a genetic predisposition to breast cancer could be diligent about checking their own breasts, take the drug Tamoxifen to reduce their risk of developing breast cancer, or even undergo a mastectomy (Hartmann et al., 1999; Meijers-Heijboer et al., 2001). One study found that 68% of women who had learned they had the breast cancer gene had had a mammogram one year later as compared to 44% of those who learned they did not have this gene (Lerman et al., 2000).

Most important, by detecting a treatable disease or abnormality in its early stages, screening may enable the individual's life to be prolonged or enhanced (Harris, 1992). Early detection of cancer is particularly important, since cancer is much easier to treat when it is localized in a single part of the body and has not spread throughout. Researchers in one study compared rates of death from breast cancer among two groups of women: those who had not received an invitation to receive a mammogram and those who received such an invitation (Weedon-Fekjær, Romundstad, & Vatten, 2014). After researchers took into account other factors that could predict mortality, women who received the invitation to mammography screening were 28% less likely to die from breast cancer compared with those who did not receive this invitation. Similarly, and as described in **Focus on Neuroscience**, screening for ovarian cancer can have a substantial influence on life expectancy.

FOCUS ON NEUROSCIENCE

The Power of Genetic Screening for Ovarian Cancer

Researchers in one recent study examined the benefits of genetic screening for ovarian cancer on reducing cancer mortality (Jacobs et al., 2015). Ovarian cancer is a particular deadly cancer—with 60% of patients dying within five years of diagnosis—in part because most women are diagnosed at a relatively advanced stage of the disease. Researchers in this study recruited over 200,000 women ages 50 to 74 years old with no family history of ovarian cancer and randomly assigned women to either a control group (these women received no screening), a group receiving annual ultrasounds to check for early signs of cancer, or a group receiving ultrasounds as well as a blood test to check for early signs of cancer. Women in the two treatment groups received annual screenings for four years. The researchers then followed women in all three groups for the next 14 years to determine whether the two distinct types of screening methods would help doctors diagnose cancer at an earlier stage and thereby reduce mortality. Their findings provide substantial evidence for the benefits of screening, and in particular for the benefits of conducting two types of screening; compared to women who weren't screened, those who received only the ultrasound were 11% less likely to have died of ovarian cancer and those who received both the ultrasound and the blood test were 15% less likely to have died of ovarian cancer. The benefits of screening also became even more pronounced over time, as women aged. During the first seven years after screening, the reduction in death rates was only 8%, but in the following seven years, the mortality reduction climbed to 28%. These findings suggest that ovarian cancer screening can have a substantial impact on life expectancy

Costs of Screening

Despite the benefits of screening, this type of early detection also comes with significant potential costs. Individuals can experience psychological harm from a positive result (Marteau, Dundas, & Axworthy, 1997; Meissen et al., 1988; Tercyak et al., 2001; Tibben, Timman, Bannink, & Duivenvoorden, 1997). For example, people who test positive for Huntington's disease—an inherited disease that causes physical and cognitive impairments and eventually death—typically experience considerable anxiety, fear, and even depression. One study found that 33% of people reported they would consider suicide if they learned they tested positive for this disease (Bloch, Fahy, Fox, Hayden, & Reynolds, 1989). Because most people who learn that they are at risk of developing a serious illness experience negative reactions at least initially, crisis intervention should be available immediately to help people deal with anxiety and fear and work through issues related to stigma, sexuality, and intimacy. These responses are particularly severe when the diagnosis is unexpected (Croyle, Smith, Botkin, Baty, & Nash, 1997).

Although some studies suggest that the anxiety that follows a positive result lessens or even disappears over time, other research indicates that anxiety stays high, and can even increase (Jemmott, Sanderson, & Miller, 1995; Wiggins et al., 1992). One study of people who learned they were carriers for cystic fibrosis found that 44% reported having troubling thoughts even as long as three years after receiving the test results (Marteau et al., 1997). Similarly, people who learn they test positive for the gene for Huntington's disease show initial decreases in anxiety, but then anxiety increases again over time, presumably because they are getting closer to the age at which symptoms could be starting (Timman, Roos, Maat-Kievit, & Tibben, 2004). This research suggests that findings reporting relatively low long-term depression and anxiety following a negative test result may be underreporting the true impact of such a result, since negative emotions may actually increase over time.

Although many people choose to undergo screening in an attempt to reduce the anxiety of "not knowing," screening tests do not eliminate uncertainty (Lerman, 1997). The tests for breast, ovarian, and colon cancer, as well as Alzheimer's disease, all measure whether a person has an increased likelihood of developing the disease but do not predict whether a person will definitely get the disease. For example, in women who test positive for the gene indicating a predisposition for breast and ovarian cancer, the risk of developing breast cancer is between 56% and 85% and the risk of ovarian cancer is between 20% and 60% (Patenaude et al., 2002). However, additional genetic or environmental factors or both will determine whether the person develops the disease. Moreover, even in cases in which genetic testing reveals that the person will certainly develop the disease, it will not provide information about exactly when such symptoms will develop or about how the disease will progress. And because some types of diseases have no treatment (e.g., Huntington's disease), early detection only increases the amount of time the person knows about the problem before he or she begins to experience any symptoms (Wiggins et al., 1992).

Even screening to learn if one currently has a disease can in some cases provide people with information—and potentially thereby increase psychological distress—but have little or no benefit in terms of survival (Saquib, Saquib, & Ioannidis, 2015). For example, although some guidelines on early detection of prostate cancer recommend biopsy for those with a high prostate-specific antigen (PSA) score, this procedure has no impact on life expectancy (Vickers, Till, Tangen, Lilja, & Thompson, 2011). The American Cancer Society therefore does not currently recommend this type of testing, and instead recommends that men over 50 simply talk to their doctor about the advantages and disadvantages of testing for prostate cancer.

Similarly, for a long time, mammograms were seen as an important part of routine health care for women ages 50 years and over, with some experts believing mammograms should begin as early as age 40. However, in early 2002, a National Cancer Institute panel issued a startling statement: even for women over age 50, mammograms might make very little difference. Why? Some women have very slow-growing tumors, which are likely to be curable (by simply removing them) whenever a physician detects them during a manual exam. So, these women would not benefit from catching these tumors earlier than later, and very likely would experience a significant increase in anxiety for having to come in for follow-up mammograms (Heckman et al., 2004). Other women have very fast-growing, aggressive tumors, and, unfortunately, these tumors are so fast-growing that even when they are caught at a relatively early point, it is typically too late to make a difference in terms of survival. Therefore, these women would also not benefit from having regular mammograms. Women who have tumors that grow at a moderate rate benefit from regular mammograms because catching these tumors early is important. These women, however, represent only about 15% to 20% of breast cancer cases, meaning that the majority of women show no benefits from mammograms. These findings point to yet another tricky issue in terms of making decisions about screening.

When the results of a screening test indicate that a person does not have a particular disease, it can give a person peace of mind, but individuals can also experience psychological harm from a negative test result (Huggins et al., 1992; Lynch & Watson, 1992). A negative result may make people more comfortable with not getting screened again, perhaps because it decreases their feelings of vulnerability, or not taking adequate precautions (e.g., "I haven't gotten AIDS thus far, so why worry about condoms now?"). One study with patients at an urban STD clinic found that rates of gonorrhea decreased 29% six months after testing for those with a positive result but increased 106% for those who tested negative (Otten, Zaidi, Wroten, Witte, & Peterman, 1993). In other cases, people still feel susceptible to the disease, so receiving a negative test result does not even reduce uncertainty or distress (e.g., "I just haven't gotten AIDS yet"). Finally, receiving a negative test result can also make people feel guilty, especially if others in their family have tested positive (Biesecker et al., 1993). They may wonder why they were spared and feel guilty about showing their relief.

One of the most significant problems with screening is the possibility of receiving an inaccurate result, which can lead to substantial psychological and even physical consequences (Lerman & Rimer, 1995). Even a test that is 99% accurate will produce 1% false positives, meaning that in 1 of every 100 cases, the test will indicate that a person has the disease when he or she really does not (Sloand, Pitt, Chiarello, & Nemo, 1991). A false positive obviously can lead to psychological distress and anxiety, which in some cases may be maintained even after the patient receives accurate results (McCormick, 1989; Skrabanek, 1988). For example, one study found that 29% of women who received false-positive results from their mammogram continued to experience moderate anxiety even 18 months later as compared to 13% of those who received a negative result (Gram, Lund, & Slenker, 1990). A false positive can also lead to unwarranted medical procedures, including surgery. On the other hand, people who receive false-negative results, meaning the person has the disease but the test shows he or she doesn't, can experience a false sense of security (e.g., comfort with practicing unsafe sex).

Finally, some of the techniques used to screen people for medical conditions can actually cause physical harm (Henifin, 1993; Simon, 1977). For example, the use of mammography to detect breast cancer exposes women to radiation, which is itself linked to cancer. Amniocentesis, a procedure in which fluid is drawn from the sack surrounding a fetus to test for abnormalities, causes miscarriage in between 1 and 200 and 1 and 400 cases. Similarly, *chorionic villus sampling*, another type of prenatal testing, which can be done at 9 to 12 weeks of pregnancy, leads to miscarriage in 1 in 100 cases. Given these consequences, health professionals generally recommend that people undergo screening only in cases in which the risk of the disorder is greater than the risk of experiencing a negative outcome of the test. For example, it is recommended that women over age 35 years, who are at increased risk of having a baby with Down's syndrome, undergo amniocentesis, but this procedure is not generally recommended for younger women.

Conclusions

Although screening for diseases has the potential to save lives by allowing such diseases to be detected at an earlier stage, such screening also has the potential of some harm. Patients must therefore careful consider the pros and cons before deciding to undergo screening. Unfortunately, one recent study found that most cancer screening guidelines—including those for mammography screening for breast cancer, PSA testing for prostate cancer, colonoscopy for colon cancer, and HPV vaccination for cervical cancer—do not clearly spell out the benefits and harms of the recommended actions (Caverly et al., 2016). In fact, 69% of the guidelines produced by agencies such as the American Cancer Society and the National Comprehensive Cancer Network did not present the benefits and costs in comparable terms, and 55% presented the trade-offs unevenly, explaining the benefit but not the harm or presenting the numbers in different ways. This inaccurate presentation of harms relative to benefits can lead people to underestimate the risks of screening and to overestimate the benefits, which is especially concerning since patients are often very aware of the benefits of screening but may be less aware of the potential harms resulting from such tests (Sutkowi-Hemstreet et al., 2015).

Predictors of Screening

One consistent finding is that people with high levels of education are more likely to follow recommended screening guidelines (Jepson & Rimer, 1993; Pacelli et al., 2014). For example, 32% of those with only some high school education or less got screened for colorectal cancer as compared to 78% of those with a graduate school degree

(Manne et al., 2002). What explains this relationship? One explanation is that people with higher levels of education are more likely to have health insurance that pays for screening (Lee, Chen, Jung, Baezconde-Garbanati, & Juon, 2014; Rimer, Meissner, Breen, Legler, & Coyne, 2001).

Individual differences, such as self-efficacy, attitudes, and perceived vulnerability, also influence who screens (Shiloh, Ben-Sinai, & Keinan, 1999; Tiro et al., 2005). People who are conscientious and high in self-efficacy for carrying out screening behavior are more likely to have mammograms (Christensen & Smith, 1995; Siegler, Feaganes, & Rimer, 1995). Those with a family history of breast cancer, and hence feel more vulnerable to developing cancer, are more likely to seek screening for the genes linked to ovarian and breast cancer (Mellon et al., 2009). Not surprisingly, people who see more benefits of screening (e.g., it can lead to longer life expectancy) as well as those who see fewer costs (e.g., saves money, saves time, increases safety) are more likely to screen (Aiken, West, Woodward, & Reno, 1994; Schwartz, Peshkin, Tercyak, Taylor, & Valdimarsdottir, 2005; Shepperd, Solomon, Atkins, Foster, & Frankowski, 1990).

The link between anxiety about a particular health condition and screening behavior is complex. For example, while some research suggests that women who are concerned about developing breast cancer are more likely to engage in screening behavior than those with little concern about developing the disease (Diefenbach, Miller, & Daly, 1999; McCaul, Branstetter, Schroeder, & Glasgow, 1996; McCaul, Schroeder, & Reid, 1996), other research shows that people who worry about cancer are more likely to want to get screened for cancer but ironically are less likely to actually get tested. One study with over 8,000 people found that 89% of people who worried a lot about colon cancer intended to get screened, compared to only 79% of those who didn't worry about cancer (Vrinten, Waller, von Wagner, & Wardle, 2015). However, 68% of those who felt uncomfortable thinking about screening actually went for the screening, compared to 77% of those who did not. Similarly, women who are at high risk for developing breast cancer, such as those with a relative who had breast cancer, are actually less likely to attend mammogram screenings when they are high in anxiety (Lerman, Rimer, Trock, Balshem, & Engstrom, 1990; Lerman et al., 1993). In sum, a curvilinear relationship may best predict screening: people with moderate levels of anxiety engage in more screening than those with low or high anxiety.

Practitioners' beliefs also influence screening behavior in their patients (Grady, Lemkau, McVay, & Reisine, 1992; Jepson & Rimer, 1993; Manne et al., 2002; Schwartz et al., 2005). For example, rates of HIV testing at prenatal clinics vary from 3% to 82%, and rates of mammography screening vary across communities from 22% to 70%, suggesting that practitioners' attitudes about the tests may influence how they present it as an option to patients (Bergner, Allison, Diehr, Ford, & Feigl, 1990; Meadows, Jenkinson, Catalan, & Gazzard, 1990). Women with physician referrals for screening are more likely to have both clinical breast exams and mammograms. Similarly, one study found that 89% of those with a doctor recommendation got screened for colorectal cancer, as compared to only 44% of those without such a recommendation (Manne et al., 2002).

Strategies for Increasing Screening

Although screening can have significant benefits, many people do not follow screening recommendations. For example, although 80.8% of women ages 21 to 65 have had a Pap test (a screen for cervical cancer) in the last three years, only 58.6% of adults 50 and older have had a colorectal screening and only 51.3% of women ages 40 and over have had a mammogram in the last year (Fedewa, Sauer, Siegel, & Jemal, 2015). So, how can we increase screening?

First, some people simply are not aware of the need to screen; hence, one way of increasing screening is simply to provide education about its benefits (Jepson & Rimer, 1993).

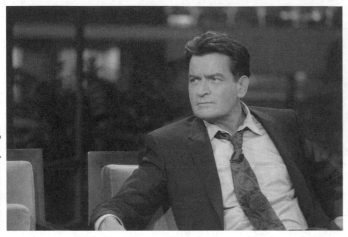

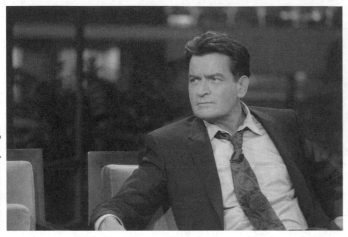

Paul Stacie McChesney/NBC/NBCU Photo Bank via Getty Images

After actor Charlie Sheen disclosed he was HIV-positive, Google searches for HIV testing increased substantially, which is a particularly important finding given that nearly one in eight people who are HIV-positive are unaware of their status (Centers for Disease Control and Prevention, 2017l).

What You'll Learn
13.1

Various interventions, including mass mailings, brochures, and mass media campaigns, have been somewhat successful in increasing screening behaviors (Rimer, 1994; Rimer et al., 2001). For example, women who receive information about the benefits of mammograms are four times as likely to have a mammogram than those who do not receive such information (Champion, 1994).

Celebrities exert a powerful influence on increasing awareness about the importance of screening. Researchers in one study examined Google searches for HIV testing the day of Charlie Sheen's announcement that he was HIV-positive (Ayers, Althouse, Dredze, Leas, & Noar, 2016). The highest number of HIV-related Google searches in the United States on a single day was recorded the day of his disclosure, with such searches being 417% more likely that day than expected. Moreover, sales of OraQuick, the only rapid in-home HIV test kit available in the United States, reached an all-time high the week of Sheen's disclosure, and remained higher than expected for the next three weeks (Allem et al., 2017). Similarly, and as described in *Chapter 3: Theories of Health Behavior*, Angelina Jolie's decision to announce she had tested positive for BRCA1, a gene associated with an increased risk of breast and ovarian cancers, and subsequently had a double mastectomy, led to increases in intentions to undergo genetic testing (Kosenko, Binder, & Hurley, 2015).

In other cases, people are aware of the need to screen but simply forget to do so; hence, providing reminders can be an effective way of increasing screening. For example, 72% of women who were sent a text message reminder attended their screening appointment, compared to 60% who were not (Kerrison, Shukla, Cunningham, Oyebode, & Friedman, 2015). Perhaps most important, these reminders were particularly effective for women from low-income areas, who were the least likely to attend a screening; these women were 28% more likely to attend an appointment if they received a text. Asking people to form their own specific plans about how, where, and when they will engage in screening behavior is an especially effective strategy for helping people follow through on screening intentions. In fact, 92% of those who formed an implementation intention attended a cervical cancer screening as compared to 69% of those who did not (Sheeran & Orbell, 2000).

Because the actual or perceived costs of screening, such as convenience, embarrassment, expense, and anxiety about pain, deter screening, removing these barriers is another effective way of increasing this type of health-promoting behavior (Aiken et al., 1994; Jepson & Rimer, 1993; Rimer et al., 2001). For example, using mobile vans, similar to bloodmobiles, leads to higher rates of mammograms (Rimer et al., 1992). Similarly, interventions that decrease the costs of mammography are quite effective at increasing screening, particularly among low-income people and those who do not have health insurance (Kiefe, McKay, Halevy, & Brody, 1994). For example, female patients at a health clinic for migrant workers who receive a voucher for a free mammogram are 47 times more likely to have a mammogram than women who do not receive such a voucher (Skaer, Robinson, Sclar, & Harding, 1996). Finally, because some people do not engage in screening because of fear of what they might find, it is important to try to reassure people that catching disease early is the best approach to maintaining health. One study revealed that giving women information on the logistics and outcomes of mammography—such as what to expect when having a mammogram and what to expect if called back for further testing—can lessen anxiety about screening, and thereby likely increase the likelihood that women will choose to have a mammogram (Lee, Hardesty, Kunzler, & Rosenkrantz, 2016).

HEALTH CARE UTILIZATION

LO 13.2

Review factors that influence health care utilization

People engage in different types of behaviors to manage illnesses and potential illnesses. **Illness behavior** is directed toward determining one's health status after experiencing symptoms (Kasl & Cobb, 1966a, 1966b). This could include talking to other people—family and friends as well as health professionals—monitoring symptoms yourself, and reading about your health problem. One of the most common illness behaviors is doing nothing and just waiting to see if the symptom will go away on its own! In contrast, **sick-role behavior** is directed at helping people who are ill return to good health (Parsons, 1951, 1975). The sick role has certain perks, including receiving sympathy and care from others and being exempt from daily responsibilities, such as chores, work, and classes. However, the person who is sick also has the responsibility to try to get better, which can include seeking medical attention and following medical recommendations. This section will describe factors that influence people's decision to seek medical care.

Seeking Medical Care

In many cases, receiving care for a medical problem is very important—sometimes even a matter of life or death. For example, cancers that are caught at an early stage can be treated directly and with less-invasive procedures, whereas cancer that has metastasized (spread to other parts of the body) is much more difficult to treat. Failing to seek medical care can also pose problems for other people, and for society at large; not seeking treatment can increase the likelihood that communicable diseases spread to others. So, what factors lead people to delay seeking medical care?

Individual Differences

First, people vary in how quickly they notice a physical experience. Some people pay more attention to their internal states than others and hence are more likely to notice symptoms (Pennebaker, 1982). For example, some people (*monitors*) tend to actively think about and focus on the physical sensations they are feeling, whereas others (*blunters*) tend to deny or ignore these sensations (Miller, Brody, & Summerton, 1988). One recently developed scale assesses the extent to which people are predisposed to seek medical care (see **Table 13.2: Test Yourself**; Scherer et al., 2016).

Certain people are particularly likely to seek health care. Specifically, people with *hypochondria* are very concerned about their health, pay careful attention to illness-related information, and interpret relatively benign symptoms as signs of more serious problems (Lecci & Cohen, 2002; Lecci, Karoly, Ruehlman, & Lanyon, 1996). For example, a person with hypochondria might interpret a headache as a sign of a brain tumor. In turn, these "worried well" people seek medical attention for a variety of minor problems (Wagner & Curran, 1984). Similarly, *somatizers* develop physical symptoms in response to psychological issues and hence seek medical treatment for problems, such as stomach pains, that have no specific physical cause (Miranda, Perez-Stable, Munoz, Hargreaves, & Henke, 1991). Several large-scale studies have shown that people who are high in neuroticism, anxiety, and/or depression report experiencing many health symptoms and may exaggerate the severity of these symptoms (Costa & McCrae, 1985, 1987; Ellington & Wiebe, 1999; Larson, 1992). People who are high in neuroticism or negative affect may also notice symptoms faster (Gramling, Clawson, & McDonald, 1996), as discussed in *Chapter 5: Managing Stress*.

Situational and Social Factors

Situational and social factors also influence how and even whether we perceive various symptoms (Pennebaker, 1982). In fact, people who are bored with their jobs and socially isolated

Table 13.2 Test Yourself: Are You a Medical Maximizer or Minimizer?

Please answer each of the following question on a scale of 1 to 7 (with 1 meaning disagree strongly and 7 meaning agree strongly).

1. It is important to treat disease even when it does not make a difference in survival.
2. It is important to treat disease even when it does not make a different in quality of life.
3. Doing everything to fight illness is always the right choice.
4. When it comes to health care, the only responsible thing to do is to actively seek medical care.
5. If I have a health issue, my preference is to wait and see if the problem gets better on its own before going to the doctor.
6. If I feel unhealthy, the first thing that I do is go to the doctor and get a prescription.
7. I often suggest that friends and family see their doctor.
8. When it comes to health care, watching and waiting is never an acceptable option.
9. If I have a medical problem, my preference is to go straight to a doctor and ask his or her opinion.
10. When it comes to medical treatment, more is usually better.

For item 5, give yourself 7 points for strongly disagree, 6 points for disagree, 5 points for disagree somewhat, 4 points for neutral or undecided, 3 points for agree somewhat, 2 points from agree, and 1 point for agree strongly. For all other items, give yourself 7 points for strongly agree, 6 points from agree, 5 points for agree somewhat, 4 points for neutral or undecided, 3 points for disagree somewhat, 2 points from disagree, and 1 point for disagree strongly. Then add up your scores on all 10 items. Higher scores indicate a greater tendency to seek medical care (e.g., medical maximizer).

Source: Scherer, Burke, Zikmund-Fisher, Caverly, Kullgren, Steinly, McCarthy, Roney, & Fagerlin (2016).

tend to notice symptoms more quickly, possibly because they have fewer distractions. In contrast, sometimes athletes suffer an injury during a game but do not notice the pain until the game is over. Similarly, the messages we get from friends, family members, and health professionals influence whether we notice as well as how we interpret health symptoms. You may have ignored an odd-shaped mole on your arm, for example, but may become concerned once a friend remarks that it could be a sign of cancer.

People's expectations about the symptoms they should experience may influence how intensely, and even whether, they feel various symptoms. For example, women who believe that most women experience severe physical symptoms prior to menstruation recall experiencing more symptoms themselves than they actually do (Marvan & Cortes-Iniestra, 2001). These expectations can be created very easily. Simply telling people that the inert substance they smelled was harmful led people to report more irritation and health symptoms than those who were told the odor was neutral or healthful (Dalton, 1999).

In some cases, these expectations can even cause various physical symptoms, such as rashes, nausea, and headaches, a phenomenon called *mass psychogenic illness*. When I teach the abnormal psychology section of my Introduction to Psychology course, an amazing thing happens each semester. As I describe the various clinical disorders (e.g., depression, schizophrenia), students all of a sudden recognize these relatively rare disorders in many of the people in their lives—their parents, siblings, friends, roommates, and sometimes even themselves all have abnormal psychological diseases. (This type of reaction is sometimes called "*medical student's disease*" because medical students, who study the symptoms of many serious [but rare] diseases, often come to believe that any relatively minor symptoms are a sign of more serious disorders [Mechanic, 1972].) This type of reaction, namely, hearing about a symptom and then suddenly seeing that symptom in everyone you know, can lead large numbers of people, typically in a relatively small and isolated group, to report experiencing particular symptoms. For example, students in a school may hear about a specific virus that is going around or a suspected case of food poisoning, and suddenly many will report experiencing related symptoms. Researchers believe that drawing people's attention to a particular type of symptom leads people to engage in careful (even too careful) monitoring of their bodies and to interpret various minor symptoms, such as a headache or nausea, as being caused by the suspected problem.

Illness Representations

Even after people notice a particular symptom, they do not necessarily decide that it requires medical attention. According to the self-regulatory model of illness behavior, people form *commonsense* **illness representations** about their symptoms, and these representations determine the steps the person must take, if any, to manage that illness (Leventhal, Meyer, & Nerenz, 1980). First, they try to *identify* the nature of their illness as well as its *cause*, based on the symptoms they are experiencing. If you are feeling pain in your stomach, you might interpret this as a stomach flu (a relatively mild condition) or appendicitis (a quite severe condition). People who experience a new and ambiguous symptom typically seek help relatively quickly, unless they are under conditions of stress, in which case they attribute the symptom to stress and delay seeking medical care (Cameron, Leventhal, & Leventhal, 1995). Third, they try to figure out the *timeline* of the illness, or how long it will last. People who believe their illness is acute, temporary, and likely to disappear soon are more likely to drop out of treatment than those who believe their illness is chronic, ongoing, and likely to continue (Meyer, Leventhal, & Gutmann, 1985). Fourth, they think about the *consequences* of their illness, including physical consequences (e.g., pain), social consequences (e.g., ability to go out with friends, play sports), and emotional consequences (e.g., loneliness, boredom). People tend to ignore symptoms that disrupt their daily lives little but are quite motivated to seek medical care for more disruptive symptoms. Finally, people think about whether the illness can be *treated and cured* and whether such treatment needs to be given by a doctor. If they believe that seeking a doctor won't help, they may not see a doctor or follow medical recommendations.

Stages of Delay

The **stages of delay model** describes the steps people go through when deciding to get help (Anderson, Cacioppo, & Roberts, 1995; Safer, Tharps, Jackson, & Leventhal, 1979) (see Figure 13.1). First, even after people experience—and notice—some type of symptoms, they often show a delay in deciding whether they are ill. This type of delay is called an **appraisal delay.** For example, you might notice a small lump under your armpit but decide it is just a clogged gland. Even after people decide they are sick, they may delay seeking professional help. **Illness delay** refers to the time between when people acknowledge they are sick and decide that help from a professional is required. People often believe that the symptoms will go away on their own and, hence, delay seeking medical care. For example, you may have a nagging sore throat for some time but decide that you should see a doctor only when it lasts more than a week. Even after people decide that medical care is required, they may delay making an appointment and actually going to a professional; this is called **utilization** or **behavioral delay. Scheduling delay** refers to the amount of time between scheduling the appointment and actually going to the appointment.

Figure 13.1   Stages of Delay Model

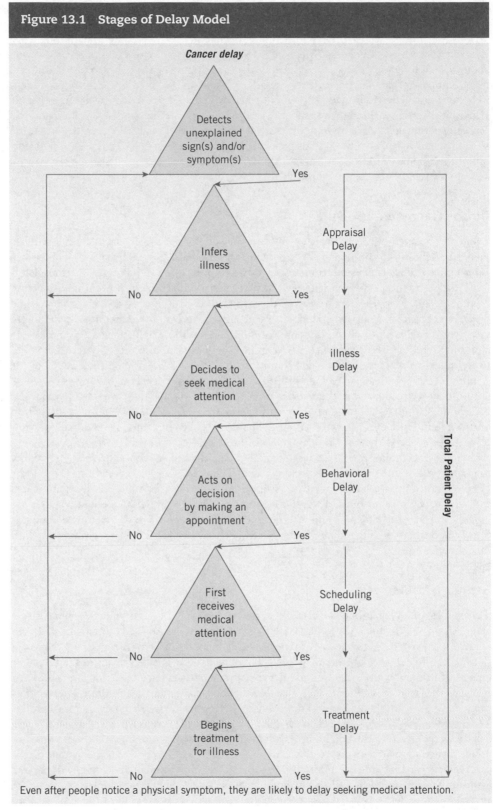

Even after people notice a physical symptom, they are likely to delay seeking medical attention.

Source: Anderson et al. (1995, p. 35).

(Ironically, one study of length of scheduling delay in seeing a dermatologist in a major metropolitan area found that the wait times for patients seeking a botulism injection—a cosmetic procedure—average only eight days, whereas the wait time for patients seeking an evaluation for a mole that appears to be changing—a symptom of skin cancer—average 26 days) (Resneck, Lipton, & Pletcher, 2007). Finally, **treatment delay** refers to the delay between receiving medical recommendations and acting on these recommendations.

What predicts when and how long people delay? The biggest predictor of length of delay during the appraisal phase is the nature of the symptoms—delay is short when people are experiencing very strong and clear signals that there is a problem, such as severe pain and bleeding (Eifert, Hodson, Tracey, Seville, & Gunawardan, 1996; Feng, Wang, Chai, Cheng, & Li, 2014; Safer et al., 1979). One study found that patients who were experiencing little or no severe pain waited an average of 7.5 days before seeking medical help, whereas those who were experiencing severe pain waited an average of 2.5 days. Similarly, patients who were bleeding delayed only 1.2 days compared to 4.8 days for those who were not bleeding. People also tend to seek help quickly for symptoms that involve a "vital organ," such as the heart, and when they experience visible, serious, and disruptive symptoms (Eifert et al., 1996; Prohaska, Keller, Leventhal, & Leventhal, 1987; Safer et al., 1979). On the other hand, people tend to delay seeking help for symptoms that are in private body parts, such as the genitals and anus (Klonoff & Landrine, 1993).

People's concern about the impact of the symptom can also influence the length of delay (Safer et al., 1979). For example, people who imagine severe negative consequences of being ill (e.g., can imagine themselves on the operating room table) wait an average of 1.9 days, whereas those without such imagery delay 4.4 days. One study with breast cancer patients found that 89% delayed seeking medical attention by more than three months after noticing symptoms of breast anomaly (Odongo, Makumbi, Kalungi, & Galukande, 2015). However, patients who perceived the symptoms as very serious were less likely to delay. People also show longer delays if they don't think the disease can be cured.

Because people don't like to experience pain, they tend to avoid—if at all possible—procedures and treatments that they believe will cause pain. For example, an estimated 12% to 15% of Americans never visit a dentist, in part because of fear of pain (Sokol, Sokol, & Sokol, 1985). One study found that 77% of women who indicated they would not undergo a future mammogram rated the experience of having a mammogram as "very uncomfortable" or "intolerable" (Jackson, Lex, & Smith, 1988).

Delay can also be caused by people's desire to seek information before resorting to the medical profession (Safer et al., 1979). People often rely on a **lay referral network** of friends and family to provide insight about health care symptoms and suggested treatment (Freidson, 1961). Similarly, people may choose to consult books or other information sources in an attempt to diagnose, and even treat, their health problem, and turn to health care professionals only if they believe medical treatment is necessary (Matthews, Kuller, Siegel, Thompson, & Varat, 1983).

The Impact of Demographic Factors

Demographic factors also influence people's willingness and interest in seeking health care (Baum & Grunberg, 1991). These include income, culture and religion, gender, and race/ethnicity.

INCOME. Not surprisingly, income influences how often, and where, people seek health care (Adler, Boyce, Chesney, Folkman, & Syme, 1993; Flack et al., 1995; Kaplan & Kiel, 1993). Although people in higher socioeconomic classes have fewer health symptoms than those with lower incomes, they seek health care more often. In contrast, those in lower socioeconomic

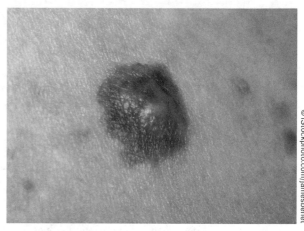

People's reluctance to seek help for symptoms that don't involve pain or disruption, such as a change in the color or size of a mole, can lead people to delay seeking help when they have a symptom of cancer.

classes are less likely to seek regular preventive care (e.g., prenatal care, regular checkups, and vaccinations), and when they do seek help, it is more likely to come from emergency rooms than private doctors' offices. This delay in seeking health care is in part due to concerns about the monetary cost of the treatment. In fact, patients who are very concerned about cost delay an average of 9.7 days, whereas those without such concern delay only 2.0 days (Safer et al., 1979). This delay unfortunately means that lower-income people are more likely to experience major illnesses that require intensive care (including hospitalization).

CULTURE AND RELIGION. Culture and religion influence how likely people are to utilize medical services (Bates, Edwards, & Anderson, 1993; Landrine & Klonoff, 1994; Sanders et al., 1992). First, people from different cultural backgrounds vary in their awareness of and attention to physical symptoms as well as in their willingness to express such symptoms (Burnam, Timbers, & Hough, 1984). For example, Americans tend to report much more pain and impairment from back pain than do people from other countries. Cultural factors may also influence people's beliefs in the efficacy of medicine in general. People from cultures that place a greater priority on using lay referral systems (e.g., family and friends) for advice about health problems may be reluctant to seek medical attention for such concerns. Similarly, people who practice certain religions, including Christian Scientists and Jehovah's Witnesses, reject the use of some or all medical treatments completely, including blood transfusions and antibiotics.

GENDER. Women are more likely than men to seek help and also have greater health knowledge (Addis & Mahalik, 2003; Beier & Ackerman, 2003). Pregnancy and childbirth, which typically involve frequent medical appointments, account for some of the difference, but not all. One possibility is that women are more focused on and aware of their physical states and hence are more likely than men to notice physical symptoms (Pennebaker, 1982). Another possibility is that women are simply more willing to admit they need help, whereas men may see expressing pain as a sign of weakness.

Similarly, research reveals consistent gender differences in the likelihood of receiving particular types of medical procedures. For example, a study examining all cases in which people were hospitalized for coronary heart disease in Massachusetts and Maryland in a particular year revealed that men were overall 15% to 45% more likely than women to receive these major diagnostic and therapeutic procedures (Ayanian & Epstein, 1991). Although women experienced symptoms that were even more disabling and severe than men's symptoms, their chest pains were addressed using less-sophisticated medical procedures for diagnosis and treatment. For example, 27.3% of men underwent cardiac catheterization compared to 15.4% of the women, and 12.7% of the men underwent coronary bypass surgery compared to 5.9% of the women (Steingart et al., 1991).

What causes these dramatic gender differences in receiving potentially lifesaving procedures? Physicians may be more likely to see women's physical symptoms, such as chest pain, as a sign of psychological problems, such as depression or anxiety. For example, medical school students who hear a patient complaining of symptoms typical of depression perceive the person as less seriously ill, less in need of lab tests and follow-up care, and more likely to require psychiatric evaluation when the patient is a woman than when the patient is a man (Hall, Epstein, DeCiantis, & McNeil, 1993). Similarly, the presence of stressful life events has no impact on the likelihood of diagnosing coronary heart disease or providing a referral to a cardiologist for men with symptoms of coronary heart disease, but women who report experiencing more stressful life events are much less likely to receive such a diagnosis or a referral (Chiaramonte & Friend, 2006).

RACE/ETHNICITY. Race and ethnicity also influence people's utilization of medical care in several ways. Although only 11.5% of Whites and 12.1% of Asians lack health insurance,

17.6% of Blacks and 34.1% of Latinos are without health insurance (Martinez, Ward, & Adams, 2015). In turn, people of color are less likely to receive preventive treatment (e.g., immunizations) and more likely to receive treatment for medical conditions at later—and less treatable—stages (Adler et al., 1993; Adler et al., 1994; Gornick et al., 1996). Black people may be more reluctant to seek treatment for health issues based on prior negative experiences with health care professionals. One focus group of Black patients with diabetes and/or hypertension found frequent reports of discrimination, including feeling they were treated with less courtesy and respect by office staff as well as with a lack of concern about their health issues by doctors (Cuevas, O'Brien, & Saha, 2016). As one patient noted about her experience in a waiting room, "I always feel like I'm getting skipped over. I do not know if it's a Black thing or not . . ." (p. 991). Race may also influence preference for different types of medical procedures. For example, Blacks have lower expectations about the benefits of knee replacements than do Whites and express a stronger preference for using natural remedies and avoiding surgery (Figaro, Russo, & Allegrante, 2004).

Perhaps most important, people of color receive less aggressive treatment for both diagnosing and treating serious illnesses, including coronary heart disease and cancer (Fiscella, Franks, Gold, & Clancy, 2000; Schulman et al., 1999). For example, 45.7% of White patients who were hospitalized for a heart attack received cardiac catheterization—which allows doctors to determine whether other treatments are required—within 60 days of the attack as compared to 38.4% of Black patients (Chen, Rathore, Radford, Wang, & Krumholz, 2001). Blacks are also less likely than White patients to be referred to a cardiologist following a report of heart symptoms or to receive angioplasty (repair of blood vessels by surgery) or bypass surgery (Crawford, McGraw, Smith, McKinlay, & Pierson, 1994; Whittle, Conigliaro, Good, & Lofgren, 1993). Similarly, only 64% of Black patients with lung cancer received surgery, whereas 76.7% of White patients received surgery (Bach, Cramer, Warren, & Begg, 1999). And sadly, this difference in rate of surgery was associated with survival rates five years later: 34.1% of Whites survived to this point as compared to 26.4% of Blacks.

Complementary and Alternative Medicine

Although this section has focused on factors influencing the use of traditional forms of medical care, many people use other approaches to managing their health, either instead of or in addition to conventional medical care (Clarke, Black, Stussman, Barnes, & Nahin, 2015). In fact, estimates are that about one third of all Americans use some form of complementary or alternative medicine (CAM), meaning a product or practice that falls outside traditional medicine, each year. CAM therapies may be used when traditional medical approaches have been unsuccessful in improving health, to manage symptoms or side effects of traditional medical treatments, and/or when the costs of medical treatment are very high. In this section, you'll learn about these different approaches and whether they are effective strategies for improving and maintaining health.

Types of Complementary and Alternative Medicine

The most common type of CAM treatment is dietary supplements, which help people meet—or exceed—the recommended daily allowance of particular substances (Clarke et al., 2015). For example, many older women take calcium supplements (to help bones stay strong), and many women of childbearing age take folic acid supplements (which helps reduce particular types of birth defects). Some people take extra amounts of vitamin C when they are feeling sick to try to ward off an impending cold. Eating particular types of diets, such as vegetarian or gluten-free, is also an example of a CAM treatment designed to promote health.

Other CAM approaches to improving health involve creating physical stimulation. As described in detail in *Chapter 9: Understanding and Managing Pain*, these methods are based in the principle that irritating body tissues can block the transmission of signals to the brain and thus can help ease pain (as described by the gate control theory of pain; Melzack & Wall, 1982). Acupuncture, massage therapy, and chiropractic therapy are all examples of such methods, and are often used to manage back pain, headaches, and arthritis.

Finally, CAM approaches may also focus on helping people relax their bodies and minds, which in turn should reduce anxiety and pain and thereby improve health. These methods include yoga, hypnosis, meditation, guided imagery, and relaxation. (Once again, these approaches are described in detail in *Chapter 9*.) Although these techniques vary considerably in their specific methods, they all focus on helping people change their reactions to and perceptions of pain, and their ability to manage that pain (Fernandez, 1986).

Evaluating CAM Approaches

Traditional medical drugs and treatments are evaluated through clinical trials to determine whether they are effective; they are also approved by the Food and Drug Administration (FDA) to ensure that they are safe. In contrast, many CAM drugs and treatments have not undergone such rigorous testing to demonstrate that they are in fact beneficial for improving health. People are often unwilling to participate in true randomized clinical trials (RCTs), in which some people are randomly assigned to receive no treatment. Ethical and practical constraints may also preclude this type of research; keeping both participants and researchers blind to condition is very difficult in the case of chiropractic therapy or acupuncture. Much of the research indicating that such treatments are effective is therefore based on case studies or surveys, which is not empirical proof for their effectiveness. Patients who spend considerable money and time undergoing a particular treatment may believe strongly that they have benefited, and practitioners are often convinced of the merits of the treatment they provide.

Moreover, even when empirical tests show CAM approaches are effective at reducing pain or symptoms, it may be unclear whether these effects are caused by specific aspects of the drug or treatment or whether they are due at least in part to the placebo effect. As described in *Chapter 9: Understanding and Managing Pain*, although there were no differences in migraine pain reduction for patients who received actual acupuncture versus sham acupuncture groups, people receiving either of these approaches reported greater pain reduction than those on a waiting-list control, suggesting that some of the beneficial effects of acupuncture may be caused by people's beliefs about the effectiveness of this treatment and not due to any specific physical properties of this treatment (Linde et al., 2005). Similarly, a meta-analysis examining the effects of different types of CAM treatments—such as relaxation, meditation, and biofeedback—revealed that they were more effective at reducing blood pressure in people with hypertension (Eisenberg et al., 1993). But these treatments were not more effective than a placebo, suggesting that people's expectations, and not specific aspects of the treatments, led to the improvement.

However, CAM approaches may help improve health precisely because they give people confidence that their symptoms will decrease. First, having confidence in the ability to control, or at least reduce, pain and symptoms may lead to lower levels of stress and anxiety, which in turn improves health outcomes. Such confidence may also lead to physiological changes that do improve health. Some forms of CAM, such as yoga, meditation, and massage, help reduce muscle tension, which can help reduce particular types of pain, such as headaches and back pain (Turner & Chapman, 1982). Moreover, belief that a particular treatment will work to reduce pain also leads to changes in the brain, and specifically to decreased brain activity in areas of the brain that respond to pain (Wager et al., 2004). In sum, although the specific mechanisms explaining their effects are not entirely clear, CAM treatments can indeed help people reduce pain and improve health.

THE EXPERIENCE OF HOSPITALIZATION

LO 13.3

Summarize the experience of hospitalization

Over 36.5 million people are admitted to the hospital each year in the United States, for an average stay of 4.5 days (Weiss & Elixhauser, 2014). This section examines negative effects of hospitalization as well as strategies for improving this experience.

Negative Effects of Hospitalization

Hospitalization poses a variety of challenges for patients, including a loss of control, loss of the opportunity to engage in rewarding activities, and loss of the ability to predict what will happen (Lorber, 1975; Taylor, 1979). People admitted to the hospital must live in an impersonal room (often with one or more roommates), are given typically bland food on a regimented schedule, and are subject to invasions of privacy when at virtually any moment hospital personnel may enter the room (to clean, provide food, deliver medicines, check patient's vital statistics, and so on). Patients are asked a series of very personal questions ("When did you last have a bowel movement?"), undergo a variety of unpleasant and sometimes painful tests, and often wear little clothing. They may also be forced to be dependent on health care professionals for assistance with many personal care tasks, including eating, dressing, and using the bathroom.

Another factor that negatively impacts the hospitalization experience is sleep disruption (Pilkington, 2013). Noise, lights, and various medical procedures (such as taking temperatures) can disrupt patients' normal sleep cycle; critically ill patients may experience as many as 60 disruptions per night (Freedman, Gazendam, Levan, Pack, & Schwab, 2001; Pilkington, 2013). Other factors that contribute to sleep difficulties in hospitalized patients include pain,

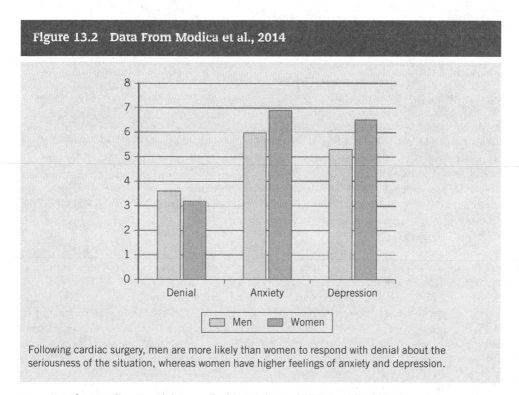

Figure 13.2   Data From Modica et al., 2014

Following cardiac surgery, men are more likely than women to respond with denial about the seriousness of the situation, whereas women have higher feelings of anxiety and depression.

Source: Data from Modica, Ferratini, Spezzaferri, De Maria, Previtali, & Castiglioni (2014).

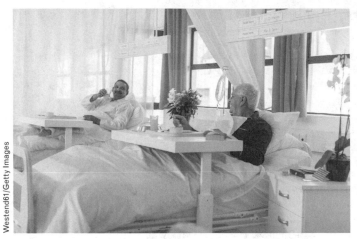

Patients who are given information about what to expect following recovery from surgery, either through hospital staff or a roommate who has experienced the same procedure, show lower levels of anxiety and a faster recovery time.

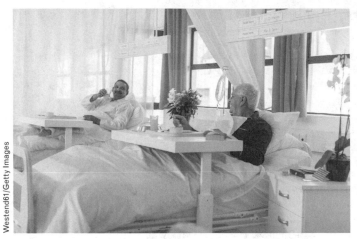

anxiety, and stress. Unfortunately, given the considerable evidence showing that sleep deprivation negatively impacts health in numerous ways, including weakening the immune system and increasing arousal, patients who experience such disruptions may impede recovery following medical procedures.

The hospital setting can also lead to considerable stress and anxiety, which in turn can inhibit recovery. One study found that 29% of pregnant women who had high blood pressure, an often dangerous condition during pregnancy, revealed such an increase only when they were measured in their doctor's office (a potentially anxiety-provoking situation), a condition described as "white-coat hypertension" (Bellomo et al., 1999). Moreover, women with white-coat hypertension were just as likely to undergo cesarean sections (45%) as those with true high blood pressure (41%) and much more likely to undergo this procedure than those without high blood pressure (12%). As shown in Figure 13.2, men and women also react in different ways following surgery, which in turn can impact recovery (Modica et al., 2014).

Improving the Hospital Experience

Fortunately, there are a number of relatively easy ways to improve the hospitalization experience and speed up recovery. Moreover, and as you'll read about in **Focus on Development**, children face particular challenges during hospitalization, but can also benefit from the use of specific strategies for improving this experience.

Provide Information

Simply giving patients information about what to expect during their surgery and recovery, as well as training in how to manage these experiences, leads them to require less pain medication and get released from the hospital earlier (Anderson, 1987; Johnston & Vogele, 1993; Ludwick-Rosenthal & Neufeld, 1993). For example, hip replacement surgery patients who saw a videotape of a patient who had been through that procedure showed less anxiety before surgery, lower blood pressure during surgery, and less use of pain medication after surgery (Doering et al., 2000). In fact, among 11 studies in which the amount of information provided was examined to predict post-surgery drug use and length of hospital stay, 10 of the studies showed that more information led to a faster recovery, with a mean decrease of two days in the hospital (Ley, 1982).

Other research reveals that patients scheduled for heart surgery who had a hospital roommate who had already undergone the same type of surgery reported feeling less anxiety, and they left the hospital sooner after surgery (Kulik, Mahler, & Moore, 1996). Those with an "experienced roommate" left the hospital more quickly after their own surgery than those whose roommate had had a different surgery—8.04 days as compared to 9.17 days, respectively. In this case, people may directly benefit from receiving support from people who have faced a similar situation. Similar others can provide a person with information about useful coping strategies as well as standards for judging one's own reaction (Thoits, 1986). Contact with similar others may also allow individuals to vent their feelings to those who are likely to understand, and who thus can provide important emotional support.

FOCUS ON DEVELOPMENT

The Difficulties of Hospitalization on Children

More than 2 million children under the age of 18 are hospitalized each year in the United States, which is difficult for both children and their families (Witt, Weiss, & Elixhauser, 2014). All of the aspects of the hospital environment that are anxiety-producing for adults are especially upsetting for children. The procedures and treatments, particularly if they are painful or restrict patients' movement, are very difficult, and children often have no understanding of why they must undergo these procedures. They may, for example, view hospitalization as a punishment for being bad or unloved by their families. For very young children, such as those under the age of five years, one of the most difficult aspects of hospitalization is separation from their families. Although older children are likely to have a better understanding of why they are in the hospital, they face new issues, including concern with a loss of personal control, disruption of peer relationships, embarrassment about showing their body to others, and worry about the consequences of their illness (e.g., dying).

So, what can parents and health professionals do to help children cope with hospitalization? First, children, like adults, benefit from knowing what to expect, and hospitals should provide children and their families with information about various hospital procedures and routines (Koetting O'Byrne, Peterson, & Saldana, 1997; Pinto & Hollandsworth,

1989). This information could include pamphlets, tours, books, videos, and even puppet shows (for very young children). The staff at Children's Medical Center in Boston, for example, worked with children's books author Margaret Rey to write the story *Curious George Goes to the Hospital*, which describes the experience of George during a brief hospitalization (Rey & Rey, 1966). One study with children who were about to undergo surgery found that those who watched a video describing the surgery experienced less anxiety and arousal than did children who did not watch this video (Pinto & Hollandsworth, 1989). Second, parents should try to spend as much time with the child as possible—some hospitals now offer parents the chance to "room in" with the child. Training parents in how to distract their children is also effective (Bush, Melamed, Sheras, & Greenbaum, 1986). Finally, children can be trained in how to cope with their own distress during hospitalization and surgery, which leads to reduced anxiety as well as fewer maladaptive behaviors (Jay, Elliott, Katz, & Siegel, 1987; Manne et al., 1992; Zastowny, Kirschenbaum, & Meng, 1986). Hospitals are putting this information to good use—one study of 123 pediatric hospitals in the United States found that 75% reported increasing their use of research in health psychology to assist children in coping with medical procedures (Koetting et al., 1997).

Train in Coping Strategies

In addition to giving patients knowledge about what to expect (i.e., informational control), other interventions focus on giving patients cognitive control (e.g., strategies for distracting/changing thoughts) or behavioral control (e.g., strategies for reducing discomfort, such as relaxation training) (Leventhal, Leventhal, Shacham, & Easterling, 1989). For example, abdominal surgery patients who received training in guided imagery had lower heart rates following surgery, had less pain, and requested less pain relief (Manyande et al., 1995). All of these approaches share one very important feature; they give patients a much-needed sense of control in a generally stressful environment.

Even relatively small manipulations that increase control and positive experiences have important benefits in terms of recovery from surgery. One way to enhance control is by allowing patients to control the amount and timing of pain medication they receive, as opposed to making them call for a nurse to deliver the medication or administering the medication on a set schedule (e.g., every four hours). But does this type of control encourage patients to overmedicate themselves? No—in fact, it does just the opposite. For example, one study with patients who were recovering from a bone marrow transplant revealed that those who received a device that directly provided pain relief intravenously, who were able to control the amount and timing of pain medication administration, reported lower levels of pain (and gave themselves less medicine) than those who had to ask the hospital staff for medicine (Zucker et al., 1998).

Change the Environment

What You'll Learn
13.2

Small changes to the hospital environment itself can also help improve psychological and physical well-being in patients. In one of the earliest demonstration of this effect, Roger Ulrich (1984) reviewed the records of patients who had gallbladder surgery in a Pennsylvania hospital during a period of about 10 years and noted whether the patient's room overlooked a group of trees or a brick wall. As predicted, patients who had a view of trees showed better improvement, including fewer requests of pain medication and fewer comments reflecting pain and difficulty coping recorded by the nurses on the patient's chart. Most important, patients whose hospital room had a view of trees recovered faster than those whose room looked out on a brick wall; patients in a room with a view stayed in the hospital for an average of 7.96 days, nearly one day shorter than those with a view of bricks (8.70 days). Even giving patients a live plant can facilitate recovery from surgery. Researchers in one study randomly assigned patients recovering from the same type of surgery to recover in either a standard hospital room or a room with a live plant (Park & Mattson, 2009). Patients in rooms with live plants showed a number of positive health outcomes during their recovery, including lower systolic blood pressure as well as lower ratings of pain, anxiety, and fatigue, compared to patients in the rooms without living plants.

HEALTH CARE INTERACTIONS

LO 13.4

Compare different issues in health care interactions

One of the particular challenges for both patients and medical professionals is that seeking and providing health care can involve difficult interactions. This section examines the challenges of patient–practitioner communication, strategies for improving such interactions, and the growing problem of burnout in health professionals.

Challenges in Patient–Practitioner Communication

Once a person has decided to see a health care professional for help with a medical condition, a variety of factors regarding the patient–practitioner relationship can influence the nature of that interaction. Communication is a crucial aspect of interaction between practitioner and patient: 75% of any doctor's diagnosis is made on the basis of the patient's history (Leitzell, 1977), and hence patients need to be able to clearly express their symptoms (Mentzer & Snyder, 1982). One recent study found that how patients report feeling is a better predictor of their health than more objective measures, such as blood tests (Murdock, Fagundes, Peek, Vohra, & Stowe, 2016). Moreover, patients who believe their doctor doesn't understand or accept them experience anger and distress, which in turn may cause physiological reactions that could worsen illness (Greville-Harris & Dieppe, 2015). Despite the importance of communication, health care providers and patients often have difficulty communicating effectively.

Patients Fail to Share Information

First, patients can be reluctant to share certain types of highly personal information, such as sexual problems and embarrassing symptoms (Julliard et al., 2008; Mentzer & Snyder, 1982).

This concern is most common when there are differences between the doctor and patient in terms of age, gender, social class, and ethnicity (Reiff, Zakut, & Weingarten, 1999). For example, health professionals typically call patients by their first names, regardless of whether the age of the patient is greater than that of the practitioner, and this is a sign of disrespect in the Black community; hence, Black patients may be less willing to provide information as well as to adhere to medical recommendations if so disrespected (Flack et al., 1995). Patients who believe they have very complex problems often aren't sure how to describe these symptoms to their doctors, and thus may not share important information (Peters et al., 2009). In other cases, patients may believe the doctor is able to discern their medical condition even without disclosing information. For example, they may believe that their symptoms will be evident throughout medical testing and that there is no need to describe them.

What You'll Learn
13.3

Patients may try to minimize how much pain they are experiencing—male patients, for example, report experiencing less pain to females than they do to males (Levine & DeSimone, 1991)! This reluctance to share medical symptoms can have serious consequences for health. For example, men who hold more traditional views about masculinity—such as believing that men should be tough, brave, and restrained in their expression of emotion—are particularly likely to prefer a male over a female doctor (Himmelstein & Sanchez, 2016). They are also more likely to ignore medical problems. Most important, men who hold such beliefs tend to be less open about their medical symptoms with their doctors, perhaps because they believe expressing health concerns is a sign of weakness. This lack of self-disclosure, however, makes it more difficult for doctors to diagnose a problem, and in turn leads to worse health outcomes.

Patients also may be reluctant to share their feelings, including anxiety and fear, with their physicians, which in turn impairs good communication (Peters et al., 2009). Even cancer patients are reluctant to share their feelings of emotional distress with their physicians, in part because they do not want to disturb their physicians or fear such a disclosure would have a negative impact (Okuyama et al., 2008).

Doctors Fail to Listen and Communicate

Doctors often fail to allow patients to provide information about their symptoms and to give patients adequate information about their diagnosis, prognosis, and recommended treatment (Ley, 1982; Waitzkin, 1985). For example, one study of 300 patient–practitioner interactions found that in 72% of cases, physicians interrupted the patient's description of his or her symptoms, and that on average, this interruption occurred after just 23 seconds (Marvel, Epstein, Flowers, & Beckman, 1999)! Another study revealed that patients received complete information, including regarding important medical decisions, with specific details about different treatment options available and their pros and cons, in only 9% of the cases (Braddock, Edwards, Hasenberg, Laidley, & Levinson, 1999). Instead, patients typically were told by their physician about the suggested choice (e.g., "I'd suggest you increase the dose of the atenolol you're already taking"). However, patients typically want as much information as possible about their illness, and those who get more information are more satisfied (Hall, Roter, & Katz, 1988; Mentzer & Snyder, 1982) (see Table 13.3).

Physicians may also overestimate the amount of information they provide, or that the patient understands and remembers. For example, a study examining how both physicians and their patients viewed the type of information provided and received regarding medical care in a hospital revealed several differences between how patients and physicians viewed such care (Olson & Windish, 2010). First, although 73% of patients thought they had one main physician, only 18% correctly named who that person was, whereas 67% of physicians thought the patients knew their name and that they were the primary physician. Second, although most physicians (77%) believed that their patients knew their diagnosis, in reality, only 57% of patients were aware of the diagnosis they had received. Finally, although almost

Table 13.3 How Much Information Would You Want? Would Your Doctor Agree?		
	Percentage Who Think Patients Should Be Informed	
Type of Information	Patients	Physicians
Name of drug	97	92
Common risks of normal use	89	85
Overdose information	86	76
Risks of using too little	80	52
Risks of not using at all	79	46
All possible risks of normal use	77	25
Other important uses	75	20

Patients generally want a lot of information, but physicians tend to underestimate this desire, which in turn leads to a gap between what patients want and what they get.

Source: Ley (1982).

all physicians (98%) reported sometimes discussing their patients' fears and anxieties, over half (54%) of patients reported that their physicians never discussed their fears and anxieties.

What factors influence how much information is given to patients? Physicians who earn less money—and hence see fewer patients per day—tend to give more information and involve their patients more in making diagnostic and treatment decisions (Kaplan, Greenfield, Gandek, Rogers, & Ware, 1996; Waitzkin, 1985). Compared to male physicians, female physicians have longer appointments, give more information, and ask more questions (Hall, Irish, Roter, Ehrlich, & Miller, 1994; Roter, Lipkin, & Korsgaard, 1991). One meta-analysis found that female physicians engage in more patient-centered behavior, including positive talk, emotionally focused talk, question asking, and counseling, than male physicians (Roter, Hall, & Aoki, 2002). Although female physicians generally spend more time with patients than do male physicians (on average about two additional minutes), they have especially long appointments when they are seeing female patients (Hall et al., 1988).

Patient characteristics also influence the amount of information that is given: patients who are White, female, college educated, and from an upper-middle-class background tend to get more information, ask more questions, and have longer appointments (Epstein, Taylor, & Seage, 1985; Hall et al., 1988; Waitzkin, 1985). One study revealed that high-socioeconomic-status patients received an average consultation of 7.3 minutes, compared to 6.3 minutes for those in the middle-status group and 5.8 minutes for those in the low-status group (Pendleton & Bochner, 1980). As described in **Focus on Diversity**, patients' ethnicity impacts the amount and type of information they receive. Finally, situational characteristics, including knowing the doctor for a longer period of time and having a serious illness, lead to getting more information.

Patient Errors

Even when doctors do convey information to their patients, much of this information may be forgotten or misunderstood (Ley, 1982). In fact, approximately 40% of what doctors say during a consultation is immediately forgotten. Although 90% of participants remembered their general cardiovascular risk pretty well a month after receiving the results, only 48% were accurate in remembering their cholesterol (Croyle et al., 2006). Not surprisingly, accuracy also declined over time. Moreover, although all participants generally remembered their health status as being better than it actually was, people at the highest level of cholesterol risk had the most optimistic recollections. Patients who are anxious are particularly susceptible to forgetting information (Charles, Goldsmith, Chambers, & Haynes, 1996).

Patients may also misinterpret the information they are given, especially if it includes complex medical jargon (Hadlow & Pitts, 1991). Patients may not understand a variety of terms commonly used by medical professionals, including *malignant*, *benign*, *void*, *sodium*, *migraine*, and *stroke*. Even telling a patient a test is positive or negative may be confusing to him or her—learning that the results of an HIV test is "positive" may seem like good news, but in reality it means the patient has contracted the disease. Although the use of medical jargon often is unintentional, in some cases physicians deliberately use confusing terms as a way of avoiding giving patients potentially upsetting information. For example, a physician may say, "We're worried about adreno-CA" to avoid directly mentioning the risk of lung cancer, or, "This is not an entirely benign procedure" to avoid describing the pain caused by a given procedure (Klass, 1987).

Models of Patient–Practitioner Interaction

Many of these problems in patient–practitioner interaction are caused by old-fashioned models of these relationships (Szasz & Hollender, 1956). The first model, *activity-passivity*, describes relationships in which the doctor is entirely in control and the patient is completely passive. This type of **doctor-centered model** is probably now best suited for describing situations in which the patient is unconscious (e.g., in surgery, in a coma), or when the patient is very young. However, this model was the common approach to medicine for much of the 1900s (Laine & Davidoff, 1996). The second model, *guidance-cooperation*, is probably still the most common model in medical practice today: the patient's thoughts and feelings are voiced, but the doctor still makes the major decisions. The third model, *mutual participation*, is favored by those who prefer a more active involvement in their own medical care in which both the patient and the practitioner share information and make decisions together.

This type of **patient-centered model** might be the most appropriate model for describing how people manage a chronic illness, for example.

Although most patients tend to prefer a more patient-centered style of interaction, others do prefer a more doctor-centered style, and, most important, patients are most satisfied when their physician uses the patient's preferred style. In one study, people read two doctor–patient scenarios and then rated how satisfied they would have been if they were the patient in each (Krupat et al., 2000). In one scenario, the physician exhibited a controlling, doctor-centered style: the physician focused on the biomedical meaning of the symptoms, used closed-ended questions, gave relatively little information, and maintained an air of neutrality. In the other, the physician exhibited a more open, patient-centered style: the physician used open-ended questions and showed warmth and personal interest in the patient. Although patient-centered physicians overall generated more satisfaction, people who preferred a patient-centered style (e.g., those who agreed with such statements as "the patient and doctor share responsibility for making a diagnosis") were more satisfied with a patient-oriented doctor, whereas those who preferred a more physician-centered style (e.g., those who agreed with such statements as "if doctors are truly skilled at diagnosis and treatment, the way they interact with patients is relatively unimportant") were more satisfied with doctor-centered physicians. This research suggests that physicians may need to adopt a congruent style with patient preferences in order to experience a good doctor–patient relationship. Training could focus on helping physicians recognize the orientations of their patients and being flexible in the interviewing style that they adopt.

Cultures also vary in the attitudes they hold about the preferred nature of the doctor–patient relationship (Alden et al., 2015). Although medical students in both the United States and Korea report similar levels of caring about patients, American students place a higher value on sharing information with patients than do students in Singapore (Lee, Seow, Luo, & Koh, 2008). These findings suggest that Americans may be more likely to view the doctor–patient relationship as a partnership, whereas those in Asian cultures may be more likely to prefer a doctor-centered decision-making process. This distinction may be a reflection of differences in cultural norms and expectations of doctor–patient interaction in different societies.

Strategies for Improving Patient-Practitioner Interaction

First, health care providers must pay attention not just to people's physical complaints, but also to their psychological concerns (Delbanco, 1992; Hall & Dornan, 1988a, 1988b). A man who is receiving treatment for prostate cancer, for example, may be more concerned about the potential side effect of impotence and its impact on his marriage than about his life expectancy. Basically, physicians must view patients as people, not just as a walking medical disease or condition. Second, health care providers must give straightforward explanations about the problem and its treatment in terms that are at the appropriate level—not too complex and not too simplistic (Mentzer & Snyder, 1982; Waitzkin, 1984).

Physicians must show better nonverbal behavior, such as maintaining eye contact, leaning toward the patient, and nodding their heads (Hall et al., 1988; LaCrosse, 1975). Physicians who engage in this type of verbal and nonverbal behavior are seen as warmer and friendlier, and in turn, their patients are more satisfied with their treatment—and are more likely to show up for future appointments (Feletti, Firman, & Sanson-Fisher, 1986; Yarnold, Michelson, Thompson, & Adams, 1998). For example, 86% of those who are pleased with their doctor's communication skills are satisfied with their medical care as compared to 25% of those who are not pleased with their doctor's communication skills (Mentzer & Snyder, 1982). They are also less likely to switch doctors—one study found that, when physicians engaged in high levels of interactive decision making with patients, only 15% of patients changed physicians within a year, as compared to 33% of those who were least interactive with their practitioners (Kaplan et al., 1996). Patients also give more information to physicians who engage in this type of verbal and nonverbal behavior, which in turn can help doctors make more accurate diagnoses more quickly (Hall et al., 1994; Marvel et al., 1999).

These findings all point to the importance of good physician–patient relationships for improving satisfaction with medical care. In fact, patients' trust in their physician is one of the largest predictors of their satisfaction with the outcome of their treatment (Janssen, Ommen, Ruppert, & Pfaff, 2008). Patients who believe they are treated respectfully by their doctor are also more willing to both confide information and follow the doctor's recommendations (Eggenberger Carroll, Smith, & Hillier, 2008). In sum, physicians who have an ability to build rapport with their patients can foster better communication, increase empathy and compassion, and lead to the establishment of trusting relationships in which disclosure is more likely. These characteristics may be particularly important when interacting with racial and ethnic minorities, who are more likely than Whites to have lower levels of trust and satisfaction with their physician (Hunt, Gaba, & Lavizzo-Mourey, 2005; Julliard et al., 2008).

Given the tremendous value of effective patient–practitioner communication, some hospitals have developed training programs that specifically focus on encouraging these types of skills (Tosteson, 1990). Researchers in one study randomly assigned physicians to one of four interventions: control, physician trained (physicians received a workshop on communication skills, adherence, interpersonal difficulties, etc.), patient trained (patients received a 20-minute audio CD about planning questions for physicians, asking questions, and making sure they had understanding), or both (Haskard et al., 2008). Physician training improved physicians' information giving, counseling, and communication, and increased patients' ratings of quality of care and willingness to recommend their physician to others (and this type of training was especially beneficial if both the physician and patient were trained). Encouragingly, medical students who were exposed to a communications curriculum show improvements on overall communication, relationship development and maintenance, organization and time management, patient assessment, and negotiation and shared decision making (Yedidia et al., 2003). These findings provide encouraging evidence that this type of training can lead to more satisfaction with medical care, and, in turn, better patient outcomes.

Patients also have a role in creating more effective doctor–patient interaction—those who take an active role in their medical care receive better care (Greenfield, Kaplan, Ware, Yano, & Frank, 1988). Patients who received a 20-minute "assertiveness training" session, which focused on how to convey honest and accurate information to their physician, were significantly better at both asking specific questions regarding medical care and eliciting information from their doctor (Greenfield & Kaplan, 1985). They also reported fewer health symptoms and missed fewer days of work, even four months later. Even having patients list the questions they have for their physician increases doctor–patient communication and patient satisfaction (Thompson, Nanni, & Schwankovsky, 1990).

Burnout in Health Care Professionals

Many people see doctors as having a relatively easy job—they are typically well paid, respected by society, and can have very flexible schedules (e.g., play golf on Wednesday afternoons). However, and as described in *Chapter 4: Understanding Stress*, doctors experience very high levels of stress caused by several factors, which can lead to **burnout**, a state of physical and emotional exhaustion (Maslach & Jackson, 1982; Shackelton et al., 2010). First, dealing with patients can be emotionally demanding. These demands can be especially difficult when the patient is in severe pain, has unsightly injuries, or has little chance of recovery. Doctors may also have to interact with the patient's family members, who may have time-consuming questions and be experiencing intense emotions. Moreover, no matter how good a doctor is, he or she will experience failure on a relatively consistent basis—all doctors have patients who die or who cannot be helped.

Another aspect of the job environment that leads to stress for doctors is their relative lack of control in a hectic and time-pressured environment. Doctors rarely get to choose exactly when they work, which patients they see, or how long they spend with a particular patient. Doctors are sometimes not even able to treat patients in their preferred way without seeking—and receiving—special permission from the patient's insurance company. One recent observational study of physicians found that physicians spent more than 49% of their time completing health records and other clerical work and only 27% of their total time on interacting with patients (Sinsky et al., 2016). Moreover, even when in the exam room, physicians spent almost 53% of their time directly interacting with the patient but 37% of their time on clerical tasks, such as updating records. Given prior research illustrating a link between increased time on recordkeeping as opposed to patient care (which tends to be more meaningful and thus linked with job satisfaction) and burnout, these findings suggest that burnout in health care professionals may become even more prevalent (Shanafelt et al., 2016).

How do health professionals react to this type of pressure? Sadly, sometimes they depersonalize the patients as a way of maintaining emotional distance (Maslach & Jackson, 1982; Parker & Kulik, 1995; Shinn, Rosario, Morch, & Chestnut, 1984). They may, for example, start thinking of patients in terms of their problems (e.g., "the fractured leg," "the liver cancer") as opposed to thinking of them as people; hence, they may treat patients in a cynical and callous way. One physician noted that when a patient's cancer did not respond to chemotherapy, she was described as "failing chemotherapy" (Klass, 1987). Unfortunately, burnout in medical professionals can have a dramatic impact on patient care: one study found that nurses who care for too many patients at one time experience a 23% increase in rate of burnout, which is in turn associated with a 7% increase in the rate of patient death (Aiken, Clarke, Sloan, Sochalski, & Silber, 2002).

Practitioners may also develop psychological and physical problems, including coronary heart disease, alcohol and drug abuse, and depression. For example, 12% of medical students show symptoms of depression, and these symptoms increase during the first two years of medical school (Clark & Zeldow, 1988). One study of 182 medical students found that 133 had cried at least once during their clinical rotations in the hospital, and another 30 reported being on the verge of crying (Angoff, 2001). One recent study found that medical students are twice as likely to report alcohol abuse or dependence as their peers not in medical school, especially if they are single (and potentially lacking in social support) and experiencing high debt (a substantial stressor) (Jackson, Shanafelt, Hasan, Satele, & Dyrbye, 2016). Not surprisingly, alcohol abuse is more common among those experiencing burnout, including emotional exhaustion and feelings of depersonalization.

Although some of the causes of burnout are largely unavoidable given the stressful nature of the medical profession, giving people the opportunity to express their feelings is one way to help ameliorate the effects of this environment (Angoff, 2001). Some hospitals have developed support groups for hospital personnel, which can provide much-needed emotional support and give people the opportunity to express their feelings of frustration, exhaustion, and grief. These groups also allow medical professionals to learn they are not alone in their feelings and to learn some strategies for coping with the difficult challenges of their profession. Moreover, physicians who are training medical students can encourage

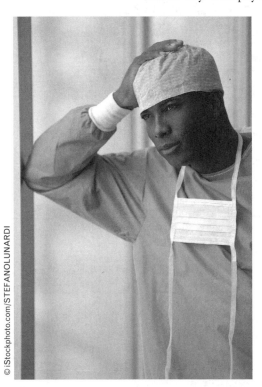

Doctors are at high risk of experiencing burnout, in part due to the emotional demands of their jobs coupled with a lack of control over their environment.

them to continue to express their feelings as opposed to denying them, as has often been the practice. One medical student described how wonderfully a physician handled the first death of a patient for a group of students:

> The whole team stayed outside the door while Doctor F and the intern went in to pronounce him. I was trying to fight back tears. Doctor F took us all into a room and handled it magnificently. He said let's take some time to talk about this, and said what a great guy the patient had been. He reminded us that when we had been in the patient's room, his mother looked out the window and said, "What a great day to go to God." I remember having a sense of peace. (Angoff, 2001, p. 1018)

Compare this experience to another report from a medical student:

> It was my first surgical rotation and the first patient I found out had cancer. The patient went down for a scan. My job was to not inform the patient of the results, but as the person who knew the patient best, she kept asking me. I was avoiding her. The resident saw me cry. She gave me a lecture to not be so weak, patients die, bad things happen. (Angoff, 2001, p. 1018)

In sum, hospital environments that provide support to doctors, nurses, and medical students and acknowledge the sometimes difficult emotions that come with these jobs can help prevent some of the problems associated with burnout.

ADHERENCE

LO 13.5

Explain factors involved in measuring, predicting, and increasing adherence

Although people invest a lot of time and energy in getting diagnosed and doctors invest considerable time in making diagnoses, many patients fail to show adherence to recommended medical regimens, such as taking antibiotics, making dietary changes, and having immunizations (DiMatteo, 1994). Rates of nonadherence range from 15% to 93% (depending on the regimen), with a mean of 30%; about 50% of people do not take prescribed medications on the recommended schedule, 20% to 40% of people do not receive the recommended immunizations, and 20% to 50% of people miss scheduled appointments for medical treatment. For example, one early study on adherence revealed that only 12% of patients who were instructed to take penicillin for 10 days were actually still taking this antibiotic by the 10th day—50% had stopped by the third day, 71% had stopped by the sixth day, and 82% had stopped by the ninth day (Bergman & Werner, 1963).

Nonadherence is associated with substantial costs to individuals and to society (Dunbar-Jabob, Burke, & Puczynski, 1995; Kirscht & Rosenstock, 1979). Not taking recommended medication typically leads to a continuation of symptoms; it can also cause the disease to persist or even get worse.

Individuals who do not adhere to medical recommendations show poorer outcomes, including a lower overall quality of life and higher mortality (Gallagher, Viscoli, & Horwitz, 1993; Horwitz et al., 1990; Irvin, Bowers, Dunn, & Wang, 1999; Saleh, Mumu, Ara, Hafez, & Ali, 2014). For example, hypertensive patients who fail to take their recommended medication are four times as likely to be hospitalized or die than those who adhere to the treatment (Psaty, Koepsell, Wagner, LoGerfo, & Inui, 1990). Nonadherence to medication regimens and the persistence of symptoms may then lead a health care professional to prescribe a larger dose of the drug—possibly causing an overdose—since he or she thinks the drug is having no effect at the lower dose. New diagnoses may be made based on patients' response to the treatment. Poor adherence also can lead to substantial societal costs, such as the development of drug-resistant strains of viruses (Catz, Kelly, Bogart, Benotsch, & McAuliffe, 2000; Dunbar-Jacob et al., 1995; Sumartojo, 1993) and widespread disease, with its attendant losses in productivity and quality of life.

Measuring Adherence

The most common method of measuring adherence is simply to ask the patient whether he or she has taken the required amount of medicine (Epstein & Cluss, 1982). This approach is easy, inexpensive, and sometimes the only option. However, this method has problems because patients will rarely admit that they are not complying and hence will typically report adherence even if it is not so. Patients may also forget whether they have complied, especially if they must report on their behavior over a long period of time, such as their diet and exercise behavior over the last month. Although some studies have tried using the reports of family members to judge adherence while avoiding problems of biased or forgetful reporting, family members often base their own estimates on what the patient reports to them!

Given the generally inaccurate findings from self-report measures, other studies measure adherence through pill or bottle counts, electronic monitoring, and/or pharmacy refills (Epstein & Cluss, 1982). For example, a physician could ask patients to bring in their pill bottles and could then measure whether the right number of pills is missing. As you might predict, patients' self-reported estimates of adherence are higher than those measured by electronic monitoring, which records the day, time, duration of bottle opening. Specifically, although patients in one study estimated they had adhered 90% of the time, electronic monitoring data revealed they had actually adhered only 67% of the time (Levine et al., 2006). Although these approaches may clarify whether the patient accurately understands the recommended dosage, obviously people can remove pills without actually ingesting them in order to appear compliant, or take the right number of pills, but on the wrong schedule. Perhaps because of the inaccuracies inherent in all of these measures of adherence, measuring pharmacy refills of medications is a better predictor of treatment outcome than patient self-reports or pill counts (Sangeda et al., 2014).

Therapeutic outcomes, such as whether the patient is getting better, are also used to judge adherence (DiNicola & DiMatteo, 1984; Epstein & Cluss, 1982). If the patient is showing signs of recovering, then he or she is assumed to be complying with medical recommendations. However, there is not a direct correspondence between adherence and recovery; people can show signs of recovery even when they are not complying, and people can show no signs of recovery even when they are complying (Hays et al., 1994). For example, 12% of people with hypertension are able to control the disease without complying with the regimen, and 34% comply faithfully, but the regimen is still ineffective in controlling the disease (Sackett, 1979).

Researchers have also tried to use more direct measures of testing adherence, including using blood, serum, or urine assays to test the concentration of the drug in the patient's body (Dunbar-Jacob et al., 1995; Epstein & Cluss, 1982). Although physiological methods are quite accurate, and they avoid the problems associated with self-report and pill counts, patients who are warned about these tests may take medication only immediately before the test. Physiological measures are also relatively impractical—they are not available for all drugs, are relatively expensive, and, given individual differences in rates of metabolism, may not be entirely accurate.

Causes of Nonadherence

Nonadherence may take a variety of forms and be caused by a variety of reasons (DiNicola & DiMatteo, 1984; Epstein & Cluss, 1982; Mo & Mak, 2009). In cases of **intentional nonadherence**, patients understand the practitioner's directions but modify the regimen in some way or ignore it completely because they are unwilling to follow the recommendations. In contrast, in the case of **unintentional nonadherence**, people intend to comply, and may even believe they are complying, but for some reason are not following instructions. Nonadherence may occur even in patients with serious, life-threatening conditions. For example, among patients who have experienced a heart attack, 15% show intentional nonadherence to medical regimens, and 53% show unintentional nonadherence, in the following months (Molloy et al., 2014). These distinct types of nonadherence have different causes.

Causes of Intentional Nonadherence

Intentional nonadherence may be caused by aspects of the treatment, including the condition being treated and the impact of the medication, as well as the patient's beliefs about the overall costs and benefits of adherence (DiNicola & DiMatteo, 1984; Schüz et al., 2011). People show high rates of adherence to medications and treatments that relieve painful and severe conditions (Brownlee-Duffeck et al., 1987). Most cancer patients, for example, undergo recommended chemotherapy and radiation treatments in the hope that these procedures will prolong their lives. People are also more likely to comply with short-term treatments than long-term treatments, particularly those that are complex, have unpleasant side effects, and provide few clear benefits (Catz et al., 2000; Christensen, Moran, & Wiebe, 1999; Robie, 1987). People who see more benefits derived from following a regimen (e.g., feel better, experience less pain) are more likely to adhere to medical treatments (Brock & Wartman, 1990; Sherbourne, Hays, Ordinay, DiMatteo, & Kravitz, 1992).

However, people often show lower levels of adherence to complex treatments. For example, the main treatment for HIV infection is *highly active antiretroviral therapy (HAART)*, which involves a complicated drug-taking schedule—sometimes as many as 16 pills must be taken each day at precise times and under precise conditions (e.g., some on an empty stomach, some an hour before eating, some an hour after eating). The HAART regimen can also lead to a variety of side effects, including mental confusion, headaches, and anemia. Adherence to this regimen therefore is particularly challenging, despite its benefits in terms of reducing AIDS-related symptoms and potentially delaying death. One study found that nonadherence is nine times more likely to occur on days in which people consume alcohol, presumably because impaired cognition makes adherence to such a complex regimen even more difficult (Parsons, Rosof, & Mustanski, 2008).

Individual differences, including self-efficacy and problem-solving style, can influence whether a person complies with medical recommendations (Christensen & Johnson, 2002). In some cases, people want to comply but lack the self-efficacy to successfully carry out the behavior (Catz et al., 2000; DiMatteo, 1994; Senecal, Nouwen, & White, 2000). For example, HIV-positive patients who adhere to treatment recommendations have higher self-efficacy, better overall mental health, and lower feelings of stigma compared to those who do not (Mo & Mak, 2009). People with more constructive problem-solving styles are also more likely to adhere, whereas those with more avoidant or destructive styles are less likely to adhere (Johnson, Eliot, Neilands, Morin, & Chesney, 2006; Mo & Mak, 2009).

As described in *Chapter 5: Managing Stress*, personality influences adherence to medical recommendations (Christensen & Johnson, 2002). People who are high on positive affect, optimism, and hope all show higher levels of treatment adherence, as do those who are conscientious (Christensen & Smith, 1995; Gonzalez et al., 2004; Nsamenang & Hirsch, 2015). In contrast, people who are high on pessimism, negative affect, and hostility show low levels of adherence, at least in part because being in a negative mood increases the use of maladaptive coping strategies (Chew, Hassan, & Sherina, 2015; Johnson, Heckman, Hansen, Kochman, & Sikkema, 2009; Weaver et al., 2005).

Interestingly, adherence is highest when patients' characteristics or coping styles correspond with the particular demands of the medical treatment they are undergoing

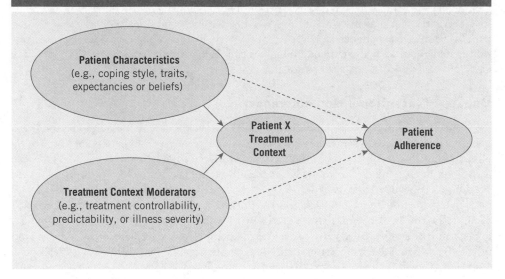

Figure 13.3   The Patient X Treatment Match Predicts Adherence

Patient Characteristics
(e.g., coping style, traits, expectancies or beliefs)

Treatment Context Moderators
(e.g., treatment controllability, predictability, or illness severity)

Patient X Treatment Context

Patient Adherence

Source: Christensen & Johnson (2002, p. 95).

(Christensen & Ehlers, 2002). Specifically, and as shown in Figure 13.3, individuals with more active and internally focused coping styles tend to show higher levels of adherence to treatments that emphasize self-control, whereas those with more avoidant styles of coping show higher levels of adherence when undergoing a treatment administered by a therapist in a hospital or clinic setting. For example, one study of hemodialysis patients revealed that those who preferred active involvement in their health care showed better dietary control and adherence to fluid-intake recommendations when they were given patient-controlled dialysis at home, whereas those who preferred low levels of involvement in their own care showed better dietary control and adherence to medical recommendations when they were given staff-controlled dialysis at a hospital or clinic (Christensen, 2000). What accounts for these effects? Patients who have an active and monitoring coping style might feel out of control when given a provider-directed type of treatment, and in turn may respond to this type of situation by trying to reassert control—by deliberately disobeying medical recommendations. Similarly, patients who are high in self-efficacy and conscientiousness might be more responsive to treatments that require independence and self-reliance because these treatments utilize their preferred coping styles and strategies. On the other hand, patients who are low in self-efficacy and high in agreeableness might prefer more passive, dependent, and possibly group-based treatments, which encourage more (much-needed) reliance on others as well as social support (Rosenbaum & Ben-Ari Smira, 1986; Smith & Williams, 1992).

Social support from family and friends leads to increased adherence to medical recommendations; in fact, adherence is 1.74 times higher in patients with cohesive families and 1.53 times lower in patients with families in conflict (Catz et al., 2000; DiMatteo, 2004; Gonzalez et al., 2004; Stanton, 1987; Weaver et al., 2005). One study of patients with tuberculosis found that 56% of those who regularly took their medication felt their families were supportive of their taking medication as compared to 28% of those who did not regularly take their medication (Barnhoorn & Adriaanse, 1992). Similarly, people who have more supportive interpersonal relationships show more adherence to diabetic regimens (Sherbourne et al., 1992), and people who have more supportive spouses are more likely to adhere to dietary changes than those without such spousal support (Bovbjerg et al., 1995).

Figure 13.4   Data From Hodeib et al., 2015

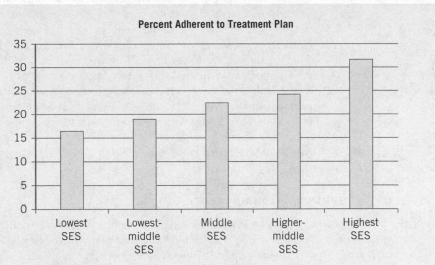

Percent Adherent to Treatment Plan

Researchers in this study examined whether women with ovarian cancer adhered to treatment guidelines. As shown in the figure, compared to patients in the highest socioeconomic quintile, those in the lowest quintile were much less likely to adhere to the recommended treatment plan. They were also less likely to receive surgery (27.3% vs. 47.9%) or chemotherapy (42.4% vs. 53.6%).

Source: Data from Hodeib, Chang, Liu, Ziogas, Dilley, Randall, . . . Bristow (2015).

Demographic and cultural factors may also influence adherence (Bovbjerg et al., 1995; Catz et al., 2000; Stanton, 1987). People who are older tend to show higher rates of adherence than people who are younger, perhaps because younger people tend to feel more invulnerable (Kang et al., 2015; Lynch et al., 1992; Monane et al., 1996; Sherbourne et al., 1992). People with higher levels of education are also more likely to adhere to medical regiments (Kirkman et al., 2015). There are few, if any, effects of gender on adherence.

Sadly, people with very low income may fail to comply simply because the recommended treatment is too costly (Cohen Castel, Keinan-Boker, Geyer, Milman, & Karkabi, 2014; Kirkman et al., 2015; Robie, 1987). Patients sometimes fail to adhere because they have run out of medication and may not have enough money to buy more (Hill-Briggs et al., 2005; Tucker et al., 2004). They may take medication less frequently than is recommended, skip follow-up appointments, or rely on nonprescription remedies as a way of saving money. For example, a study of patients with rheumatoid arthritis, a relatively common chronic condition, found that higher out-of-pocket expenses (meaning those not covered by health insurance) are associated with lower levels of adherence (De Vera, Mailman, & Galo, 2014). As shown in Figure 13.4, income is even associated with adherence to medical regiments for ovarian cancer, one of the five most deadly cancers in women.

Finally, because adherence depends in part on the patient's motivation to follow the doctor's recommendation, the quality of the relationship between the doctor and patient has a substantial impact on adherence (DiNicola & DiMatteo, 1984; Dunbar-Jacob et al., 1995; Goldring, Taylor, Kemeny, & Anton, 2002). Patients who are dissatisfied with interpersonal relationships with medical staff show higher levels of intentional nonadherence to chronic medication regimens (not unintentional nonadherence; Iihara et al., 2013). In contrast, patients who feel they are involved in decision making and goal setting and treated with respect show higher levels of adherence to medical recommendations

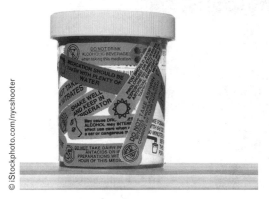

In some cases, nonadherence is caused by patients' misunderstanding of how exactly medication should be taken.

(Beach et al., 2005). In turn, practitioners who show warmth, encourage open communication, and address their patients' concerns have more satisfied patients, who in turn are more likely to follow recommendations. One study examined over 800 interactions between pediatricians and mothers who had brought their children in for some type of disorder (Korsch, Gozzi, & Francis, 1968). Although the majority (76%) were satisfied with the doctor's performance immediately after leaving the office, nearly 20% felt they did not receive a clear statement about their baby's problem, and almost 50% were left wondering what caused the baby's problem. Those who were satisfied with their interaction with their doctor were three times as likely to comply as those who were unsatisfied (53% for the highly satisfied versus 17% for the highly dissatisfied).

Causes of Unintentional Nonadherence

In the case of *unintentional nonadherence*, people intend to comply, and may even believe they are complying, but for some reason they are not following instructions. As described previously, physicians often give patients very little information about their diagnosis and treatment, which in turn can lead to nonadherence (Hall et al., 1988; Ley, 1982). Even when patients are given information about their condition, they may forget or misunderstand the instructions they are given (DiNicola & DiMatteo, 1984; Hill-Briggs et al., 2005). For example, one study found that patients failed to recall 56% of the instructions they had received and 48% of the treatment instructions even a short time after their appointments.

Moreover, instructions for medical regimens are often vague; hence, patients may legitimately misunderstand exactly what they are supposed to do. In one study, patients were told to take a drug "with meals," by which the practitioner meant to imply that patients should take the drug immediately after eating (Mazzullo, Lasagna, & Griner, 1974). However, 54% of the patients understood this to mean "take before meals," 33% thought it meant to "take during meals," and only 13% thought it meant to "take after meals." For example, when my son Andrew was an infant, he developed an ear infection, and I promptly took him to the doctor. The doctor carefully explained that he needed medicine and to give it twice a day for 10 days, and as I was leaving, he asked if I had any questions. I asked, "And I put the medication in his ear, right?" The doctor looked shocked, and quickly said, "No, the medication goes in his mouth!"

Strategies for Increasing Adherence

Nonadherence is clearly irrational, a waste of time for patients and health care professionals, and potentially dangerous for patients and for society. This section describes strategies for decreasing both intentional and unintentional nonadherence.

Decreasing Intentional Nonadherence

The strategies for decreasing intentional nonadherence are quite different, because in these cases, people understand the medical recommendations but are simply unmotivated or unable to follow them (Dunbar-Jacob et al., 1995; Ley, 1982). In cases in which people fail to comply because they have little concern about having or developing a particular disease, the use of fear warnings can be effective in increasing adherence (Higbee, 1969; Janis, 1967). In one study, mothers of obese children were randomly assigned to receive one of three communication messages—a control (no-information) message, a low-threat message, or a high-threat message (Becker, Maiman, Kirscht, Haefner, & Drachman, 1977). Children whose mothers had received either type of informational message had lost more weight than the controls at each of the four follow-up visits, and those whose mothers had received the high-threat message had lost the most weight.

Giving people information about the consequences of nonadherence is particularly important in the case of immunizations. As you may have heard, people's skepticism about the safety of vaccines can sometimes lead people to deliberately not adhere to recommended immunizations, such as those for measles, whooping cough, or chicken pox. (This skepticism is largely the result of a now widely discredited paper that appeared to show a link between vaccinations and the development of autism.) Failure to vaccinate can lead to serious health consequences, not only for the person who isn't vaccinated and therefore is at risk of developing a disorder, but also more broadly for society. Unfortunately, efforts to convince skeptical people about the safety of vaccines have largely been ineffective (in some cases, such efforts have even strengthened people's anti-vaccine attitudes). However, some recent research suggests that describing the symptoms of such disorders, which most people have never seen, may help change such attitudes (Horne, Powell, Hummel, & Holyoak, 2015). In this study, parents were randomly assigned to receive one of three types of messages: one type directly challenged anti-vaccination views; another gave specific information about the risks caused by measles, mumps, and rubella (including photographs and stories about children infected with such diseases); and a third group received no information about vaccines. Parents who received specific information about the risks of not getting vaccinated reported more positive attitudes toward vaccinations, including beliefs about the efficacy and safety of vaccines as well as intentions to vaccinate their children, than those in the other groups. This research provides valuable information about how to effectively change negative attitudes about vaccinations and thereby increase adherence to recommended vaccines.

What You'll Learn
13.5

Another strategy for increasing adherence is to give patients some type of incentive or reward for following medical recommendations (DiNicola & DiMatteo, 1984; Hegel, Ayllon, Thiel, & Oulton, 1992; Macharia et al., 1992). This approach is particularly effective if patients agree to a written contract, witnessed by others, that describes specific goals they intend to meet as well as the reward they will receive if the contract is specifically carried out. People who receive desirable—and self-chosen—rewards, such as attending a movie or purchasing a book, show better adherence to regimens for a variety of conditions, including arthritis, diabetes, asthma, and cardiovascular disease. For example, patients with high blood pressure who receive unexpected small gifts in the mail show higher levels of medical adherence than those who don't receive such gifts (Ogedegbe et al., 2012).

Intentional nonadherence can also be caused by patients' concern that following the medical recommendations will disrupt their lives in some way, such as by taking too much time or interfering with relationships (Kirscht & Rosenstock, 1979). Increasing the convenience of engaging in the recommended behavior, such as by making bottles easier to open (especially for older patients), lowering the cost, or improving the taste of medicine, can increase adherence (Robie, 1987). For example, patients who have to take one to three pills a day show an adherence rate of 77% to 88% as compared to 39% for those who have to take four pills a day (Cramer, Mattson, Prevey, Scheyer, & Ouelette, 1989). Simply helping patients make specific plans for how to adhere (when/where to take their medicine) and how to overcome barriers to adherence helps patients follow medical regiments (Pakpour et al., 2014).

Enlisting the support of family members or friends can increase adherence (Becker, 1985; DiNicola & DiMatteo, 1984; Kirscht, Kirscht, & Rosenstock, 1981). One program with hypertensive patients found that 53% of those who received an exit interview and family support complied with their medical regimen at two-year follow-up compared to only 40% off those in the control group (Morisky et al., 1983). Similarly, patients who regularly attend group social support sessions with others who share their health issue show greater adherence (Kirscht & Rosenstock, 1979).

Given the link between depression and nonadherence, reducing depression is another strategy that can help increase adherence. Depressed HIV-positive positive patients who received a cognitive-behavioral condition, which included information on both adherence and reducing depression, later show lower rates of depression as well as higher rates of adherence (Safren et al., 2009). Similarly, the use of antidepressants increases adherence in HIV-positive people (Walkup, Wei, Sambamoorthi, & Crystal, 2008).

Finally, and as described previously, patients are more likely to adhere to treatment recommendations when they like their doctor and when their doctor emphasizes the importance of adherence (Cohen Castel et al., 2014; DiMatteo et al., 1993; Sherbourne et al., 1992). For example, one study with over 1,000 chronic disease patients found that those who were satisfied with the interpersonal care they received from their physicians were more likely to adhere to medical recommendations (Sherbourne et al., 1992). Patients with physicians who make strong recommendations for adherence and provide realistic information about the importance of adherence also show higher rates of adherence (Goldring et al., 2002). Another important factor influencing patient satisfaction and adherence to medical recommendations is the physician's interactional style (Krantz, Baum, & Wideman, 1980; Laine & Davidoff, 1996). Specifically, physicians who use a patient-centered style encourage an interaction between the doctor and the patient to solve the problem and seek solutions, whereas those who use a doctor-centered style (the more traditional style) are more dominant and expect the patient largely to trust their expertise and defer to their judgment. One study demonstrated that overweight patients whose physicians used reflexive listening and a more collaborative style in discussing weight-loss techniques lost weight over the three-month follow-up, whereas those whose doctors lacked such a style either maintained or gained weight (Pollak et al., 2010).

Decreasing Unintentional Nonadherence

Many of the strategies for decreasing unintentional nonadherence focus on giving the patient correct information (Dunbar-Jacob et al., 1995; Ley, 1982). Simply providing clear and understandable information about the medication, its purposes, and its dosage reduce this type of nonadherence. For example, HIV-positive patients who receive tailored information about the importance of adherence, including setting adherence goals and developing self-monitoring strategies, show higher adherence over time than those who receive standard treatment (de Bruin et al., 2010). Practitioners should also ask patients directly whether they have any questions.

Moreover, because people sometimes forget or do not fully understand the information they receive from practitioners, providing easy-to-understand written materials, using illustrations to reinforce written materials, and even giving the patient an audio recording of the consultation can all be effective ways of increasing adherence (Ley, 1982). In fact, one study found that 91% of patients reported it was helpful to have a tape recording of their doctor visit, and patients claimed to have listened to the tape an average of 3.5 times (Butt, 1977). As described in **Research in Action**, redesigning medication packages can reduce medical errors and thereby increase adherence.

Because unintentional nonadherence can also be caused by forgetting to adhere, other strategies for increasing adherence simply focus on reminding people to engage in a particular behavior, such as taking their medication, measuring their blood pressure, and/or attending follow-up appointments (Kirscht & Rosenstock, 1979; Macharia, Leon, Rowe, Stephenson, & Haynes, 1992). For example, patients with hypertension who receive motivated interviewing and follow-up telephone calls by a pharmacist are more likely to adhere to medical recommendations than those who receive usual care instructions (79.7% versus 69.8%) (Hedegaard et al., 2015). Simply giving patients special reminders (e.g., a sticker for their refrigerator) doubles rates of adherence to medication regimens (Lima, Nazarian, Charney, & Lahti, 1976). More recently, text messages have been used to increase medical adherence, which can be quite effective (Thakkar et al., 2016). Pediatric liver transplant recipients who receive text messages reminding them to take their immunosuppressant medication are much less likely to reject their transplant than those who do not receive such reminders (Miloh et al., 2009).

Table 13.4   Information YOU Can Use

- Screening for diseases gives you valuable information that can increase your life expectancy, since early detection of diseases often increases treatment options. So, learn and follow recommended screenings.

- Make sure to adhere to medical regimens. Clarify any instructions about how to adhere, and develop strategies—such as creating reminders, incorporating treatment into your daily routine, and enlisting support from family and friends—that help you follow these recommendations.

- Given the importance of physician–patient interaction for increasing satisfaction with medical care as well as adherence to treatment recommendations, choose your medical care providers carefully. Try to find a doctor who shares your beliefs about patient–physician interaction, one with whom you feel comfortable sharing information.

- If you are hospitalized, take steps to improve your psychological and physical well-being. Try to bring your own clothes and a few items from home to personalize the space. Encourage family and friends to visit to provide support. Make sure to get information about the procedures you will undergo and what to expect during your recovery.

Health Screening

- Health screening to detect illness may help a person seek early treatment, engage in health-promoting behaviors, reduce uncertainty, and increase vigilance for symptoms of the disease. Most important, screening may enable the individual's life to be prolonged or enhanced. However, screening may cause psychological and/or physical harm and not truly eliminate uncertainty or increase life expectancy.

- People vary considerably in their screening behavior. People with high levels of education are more likely to follow recommended screening guidelines, whereas those who lack health insurance are less likely to have regular screenings. Individual difference factors, such as self-efficacy, attitudes, personality, and family history, all influence screening behavior, as do practitioners' beliefs about its value.

- Various strategies can increase screening behavior. These include providing education about its benefits, providing reminders, and removing potential costs of screening.

Health Care Utilization

- Researchers distinguish between illness behavior, meaning behavior that is directed toward determining one's health status after experiencing symptoms, and sick-role behavior, meaning behavior that is directed at helping people who are ill return to good health. In many cases, people delay seeking health care. Delay can be caused by not noticing a symptom, situational and social factors, and people's expectations. People's commonsense illness representations about their symptoms, and what they indicate, also impact how they choose to manage their illness.

- The stages of delay model describes the steps people go through when deciding to get help, including appraisal delay, illness delay, utilization or behavioral delay, scheduling delay, and treatment delay. Delay is influenced by the nature of the symptoms, including whether they clearly indicate a problem, are painful, and involve blood or a vital organ. People's concern about the impact of the symptom and the nature of the treatment may also influence delay. People often rely on a lay referral network of friends and family to provide insight about health care symptoms and suggested treatment.

- Demographic factors, including income, culture and religion, gender, and race/ethnicity, all influence how likely people are to utilize medical services. They may also impact the type of medical care they receive.

- Many people use some form of complementary or alternative medicine (CAM), meaning a product or practice that falls outside traditional medicine. CAM approaches include dietary supplements and diets, physical stimulation methods, and cognitive-behavioral strategies emphasizing relaxation. However, most CAM drugs and treatments have not undergone rigorous testing to demonstrate that they improve health. Although the specific mechanisms explaining the beneficial effects of some types of CAM approaches are not entirely clear, such treatments can at times help people reduce pain and improve health.

The Experience of Hospitalization

- The experience of hospitalization can be very difficult. Patients stay in unfamiliar environments with low levels of control and privacy, feel dependent on other people, and often experience anxiety-provoking procedures. Some people may become passive in such situations, whereas many experience anger and arousal in such circumstances.

- Patients who are given information about what to expect, as well as how to manage these experiences, demonstrate improved outcomes, including lower levels of anxiety and faster recovery. Patients also benefit from learning both cognitive and behavioral control strategies. Interestingly, patients with a view of nature also experience better outcomes.

Health Care Interactions

- Problems in patient–practitioner communication include patients' reluctance to share information and acknowledge pain, physicians' failure to allow patients to provide information and to give patients adequate information, and practitioners' overestimation of the amount of information they provide (and that the patient understands and remembers). Both physician and patient characteristics influence the amount of information given. Patients may also forget, misunderstand, or misinterpret the information they are given.

- Many of these problems in patient–practitioner interaction are caused by old-fashioned models of these relationships. The doctor-centered model describes relationships in which the doctor is in control and the patient is passive. In a second model, the patient's thoughts and feelings are voiced, but the doctor still makes the major decisions. The patient-centered model describes a mutual interaction, in which both the patient and the practitioner share information and they make decisions together. People vary in the type of model they prefer.

- First, health care providers must pay attention not just to people's physical complaints but also to their psychological concerns. Second, health care providers must give straightforward explanations about the problem and its treatment in terms that are at the appropriate level. Third, physicians must show good nonverbal behavior, such as maintaining eye contact, leaning toward the patient, and nodding their head. Having a good physician–patient relationship leads to greater satisfaction with medical care.

- Doctors experience very high levels of stress, which can lead to burnout. Factors that contribute to burnout include dealing with patients and their family members and a relative lack of control over their work environment. Doctors may respond by depersonalizing their patients and are at greater risk of developing psychological and physical problems. Giving people the opportunity to express their feelings is one way to help ameliorate the effects of this environment.

Adherence

- Many patients fail to show adherence to recommended medical regimens, which is associated with substantial costs to individuals and to society. Methods of measuring adherence include asking the patient whether he or she has taken the required amount of medicine; measuring pill or bottle counts, electronic monitors, and/or pharmacy refills; assessing therapeutic outcomes; and conducting direct tests of levels of a drug in the body. All of these methods have both strengths and weaknesses.

- Intentional nonadherence may be caused by aspects of the treatment, the patient's beliefs about the overall costs and benefits of adherence, and individual difference factors (personality, age, education, income). Social support from family and friends and the quality of the relationship between the doctor and patient both impact adherence. In the case of unintentional nonadherence, people intend to comply, and may even believe they are complying, but for some reason they are not following instructions. Patients may lack information about how to adhere to recommendations or may forget or misunderstand the instructions they are given.

- Strategies for decreasing unintentional nonadherence focus on giving the patient clear and correct information, including easy-to-understand written materials, illustrations, or an audio recording of the instructions, and reminding people to engage in a particular behavior. The strategies for decreasing intentional nonadherence include creating fear warnings to motivate behavior change, giving information about the consequences of nonadherence, providing some type of incentive or reward for following medical recommendations, increasing the ease and convenience of adhering, enlisting the support of family members and friends, reducing depression, and creating high-quality patient–practitioner relationships.

14

CONCLUSIONS AND FUTURE DIRECTIONS

Learning Objectives

14.1 Describe strategies for preventing health problems

14.2 Explain methods of reducing health care costs

14.3 Summarize the impact of demographic factors on health and health outcomes

14.4 Describe strategies for improving international health

14.5 Explain current challenges in making ethical medical decisions

What You'll Learn

14.1 How handgun laws prevent suicides

14.2 Why wellness programs reduce employer health costs

14.3 How stress reduces women's ability to conceive

14.4 Why breastfeeding reduces infant mortality

14.5 How a brief conversation increases organ donation

Preview

The field of health psychology has already made significant contributions to enhancing psychological and physical well-being, as you've learned throughout this book. In this final chapter, you'll learn about some of the crucial ways in which theory and research in health psychology can help solve problems we now face, and are currently under debate by researchers, politicians, and medical professionals.

PREVENTING HEALTH PROBLEMS

Describe strategies
for preventing
health problems

One major goal of health psychology is preventing the development of health problems, which is a much easier and cheaper way of increasing life expectancy and life quality than treating established medical problems (Sullivan, 1990). This is why many people take their car in for an oil change every 3,000 to 5,000 miles—they choose to pursue regular, brief, and inexpensive care for their car as a way of preventing the development of severe and costly problems. The difference between prevention and treatment is well illustrated by this example from physician John McKinlay:

> You know, sometimes it feels like this. There I am standing by the shore of a swiftly flowing river, and I hear the cry of a drowning man. So I jump into the river, put my arms around him, pull him to shore, and apply artificial respiration. Just as he begins to breathe, someone else cries for help. So I jump into the river again, reach him, pull him to shore, apply artificial respiration, and then, as he begins to breathe, there's another cry for help. So back into the river again, reaching, pulling, applying breathing, and then another yell. I'm so busy jumping in and pulling them to shore that I have no time to see who the [heck] . . . upstream is pushing them in. (McKinlay, 1975, p. 7. Reprinted with permission. © 1975 American Heart Association, Inc.)

Theories and principles of health psychology can be used to prevent health problems from developing in a variety of different ways. These include motivating behavior change, creating legislation, and increasing education.

Motivate Behavior Change

As we've discussed throughout this book, one way to increase the quality of life is through primary prevention, meaning preventing health problems from ever developing (see Table 14.1). Because people's behavioral choices and habits are responsible for most of the major causes of health problems today, some of the most important types of primary prevention strategies are avoiding smoking, eating a healthy diet, and engaging in regular exercise. Even very simple strategies, such as creating vegetable characters—Sammy Spinach, Oliver Onion, Suzy Sweet Pea—to increase children's interest in healthy eating, can lead to substantial benefits (Hanks, Just, & Brumberg, 2016). Moreover, since many health behaviors are established in late childhood and adolescence and then persist throughout adulthood, helping people make good health-related choices at a relatively young age should have a dramatic impact on preventing many future health problems (Smith, Orleans, & Jenkins, 2004).

Many health education campaigns, such as public service announcements, are designed to educate people about the risks of particular behaviors, with the goal of motivating people to take an active role in changing their health-related behavior. For example, and as described in *Chapter 7: Substance Use and Abuse*, cigarette smoking is the leading cause of preventable mortality in the United States and contributes to nearly half a million deaths per year (U.S. Department of Health and Human Services, 2014). In turn, efforts to reducing smoking could have a major impact on life expectancy. As described in **Focus on Neuroscience**, researchers are now using neuroscience techniques to determine which types of public health campaigns will be most effective in helping smokers quit.

Table 14.1 Timing of Prevention

Level	Primary	Secondary	Tertiary
Individual	Self-instruction guide on HIV prevention for noninfected lower-risk individuals	Screening and early intervention for hypertension	Designing a very low-fat vegetarian diet for an individual with heart disease
Group	Parents group to gain skills to communicate better with teens about risk behaviors	Supervised exercise program for lower-income individuals with higher risk of heart disease	Cardiac rehabilitation program for groups of heart disease patients
Organization	Worksite dietary change program focusing on altering vending machine and cafeteria offerings	Worksite incentive program to eliminate employee smoking	Extending leave benefits so employees can care for elderly/ill parent
Community	Focused media campaign to promote exercise in minority population segments	Developing support networks for recently widowed individuals	Providing better access for disabled individuals to all recreational facilities
Institution	Enforcing laws banning the sale of cigarettes to minors	Substantially increasing insurance premiums for smokers	Mandating a course of treatment to facilitate recovery of stroke victims

Prevention of health problems can occur at three different stages and can be provided at many different levels.

Source: Winett (1995).

The most effective types of primary prevention programs are multifaceted and community-based. An example of a widespread and quite successful health-promotion program occurred in San Francisco in the 1980s in response to the AIDS epidemic (Coates, 1990). This community-level HIV risk reduction program included giving out information about risky behavior, increasing feelings of vulnerability, and modeling skills to prevent such

FOCUS ON NEUROSCIENCE

How Studying Brain Activity Improves Anti-Smoking Messages

To examine how neuroscience techniques can help reduce smoking, researchers in one study recorded brain activity in smokers as they viewed 40 different anti-smoking images (Falk, O'Donnell, Tompson, et al., 2015). They were particularly interested in which types of images provoked the largest response in the medial prefrontal cortex (MPFC), a part of the brain that helps us decide what type of information is personally relevant to us. Specifically, if smokers find particular types of images self-relevant, those might be the most effective ones to use in anti-smoking campaigns. They

then sent an anti-smoking email that contained one of the 40 images to 800,000 smokers who had signed up through a smokers' quit line. Each email contained one of the images, along with the message "Quit smoking. Start living," as well as a link to online quit-smoking resources. Their findings revealed that the anti-smoking images that created the most activity in the MPFC were also the most effective at leading people to reach out for help to quit after receiving the email. This type of research can therefore be used to design the most effective health-promotion campaigns.

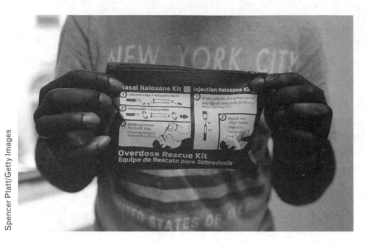

Many police officers carry the drug Narcan, which can reverse the effects of opioid overdose and thus, if administered in time, save lives. This is an example of a tertiary prevention strategy.

behavior (e.g., using condoms, saying "no") and was presented through multiple organizations, including schools, churches, worksites, the health care system, and community agencies as well as the media. This program was very successful—although before the program 60% of the gay and bisexual men in the sample engaged in high-risk behavior, only 30% reported such behavior three to four years later. A similar communitywide approach to fighting the problem of unplanned teenage pregnancy was implemented in South Carolina (Vincent, Clearie, & Schluchter, 1987). This program included school-based sex education for children in all grades with the participation of parents and church leaders in various educational programs and communitywide events as well as media coverage to raise awareness of the problem. Once again, this approach was highly successful: the pregnancy rate among teenage girls ages 14 to 17 years dropped from 5.4% to 2.5%—a 23.3% decrease in pregnancy rate—over the course of this intervention, whereas it remained unchanged in surrounding communities that did not use this type of widespread prevention technique.

Although primary prevention strategies, which prevent health problems from ever developing, are the best way to improve health, other types of prevention strategies can also be useful (see Table 14.1). Secondary prevention strategies, which help people identify and thus treat problems at an early point in the disease's progression, help increase quality of life as well as life expectancy. For example, a recent report by the American Cancer Society reveals that the overall death rate from cancer has decreased by 25% over the last 15 years, meaning more than 2 million cancer deaths were prevented (Siegel et al., 2017). This decline in cancer deaths is attributed in part to changes in behavior, such as fewer people smoking, but also to increases in the ability to detect and treat cancer at early stages. Similarly, people who test positive for HIV are able to start antiretroviral therapy (ART), which reduces the level of virus in the blood, and the earlier this drug is started after HIV infection, the better the outcome. Finally, tertiary prevention strategies, which focus on helping people manage or control the effects of an already-developed illness or disease, can lead to improved psychological and physical well-being. These could include social support groups for people with cancer or broad lifestyle intervention programs for people with diabetes.

Create Legislation

Another effective strategy for preventing health problems is to enact laws and regulation that either incentivize or deter particular types of behavior (Burris et al., 2010). For example, taxing particular products (tobacco, soda, alcohol, etc.) increases their cost and should thereby discourage their use. As described in **Chapter 7: Substance Use and Abuse**, raising the price of cigarettes decreases smoking; in fact, estimates are that a 10% increase in price decreased the odds of teenagers' starting smoking by as much as 10% (Ross, Powell, Tauras, & Chaloupka, 2005). Moreover, this may be particularly true for teenagers, who typically have relatively little money to spend. Similarly, a recent meta-analysis found that lowering the cost of healthy foods, and increasing the cost of unhealthy foods, would lead to significantly healthier eating patterns (Afshin et al., 2017). Specifically, each 10% decrease in the price of fruits and vegetables increases their consumption by 14%, whereas each 10% increase in the price of sugar-sweetened beverages and fast foods decreases their consumption by 7% and 3%, respectively.

Laws have already been used effectively to reduce injuries and injury-related deaths. As described in *Chapter 6: Injury and Injury Prevention*, efforts to increase motor vehicle safety, through requiring seat belt use, restricting cell phone use and texting while driving, and requiring child safety seats, have led to major reductions in unintentional injuries, which are the leading cause of death for people ages 1 to 44. Laws that provide immediate punishments are especially effective in reducing risky health behavior. For example, laws that require the immediate suspension of a person's driver's license following a DUI arrest have a dramatic impact on drunk driving, saving an estimated 800 lives a year (Wagenaar & Maldonado-Molina, 2007). Perhaps most important, laws that ban particular types of risky health behaviors can also lead to reductions in other types of risky behaviors. For example, laws restricting alcohol sales are associated with reductions in rates of cardiovascular disease, and, as described in **Research in Action**, more severe penalties for drunk driving are associated with reductions in domestic-violence arrests (Dukes et al., 2016; Kilmer, Nicosia, Heaton, & Midgette, 2013).

Researchers in one study examined whether state laws regarding access to handguns would be associated with rates of suicides (Anestis et al., 2015). To test this question, researchers compared rates of suicide in states with various laws regarding purchasing a handgun, such as required background checks, restrictions on open carry, and mandated gun locks, to rates in states without such laws. As predicted, states with more restrictive gun laws had lower rates of suicide. Specifically, compared to states without such laws, those with background checks have a 53% lower gun suicide rate, those with gun locks have a 68% lower gun suicide rate, and those with restrictions on open carry have a 42% lower gun suicide rate. Their findings also revealed that states with such laws had lower suicide rates overall, not just lower rates of suicides caused by guns, which indicates that the presence of such laws may lead to overall fewer suicide attempts and/or fewer completed suicides (meaning people who attempt suicide are using less lethal means).

What You'll Learn
14.1

RESEARCH IN ACTION

How Laws Restricting Alcohol Use Reduce Domestic Violence

Researchers in this study examined the effects of an innovative program in South Dakota designed to reduce drunk driving (Kilmer et al., 2013). This program, called the 24/7 Sobriety Project, required anyone arrested for a second alcohol-related offense to either undergo Breathalyzer tests twice a day or continuously wear an alcohol monitoring bracelet. Because refraining from any alcohol use was a requirement for those arrested a second time for an alcohol-related offense, anyone who was found to be drinking alcohol during these tests was immediately sent to jail for a day or two. The researchers then compared differences between counties that instituted this program to those that did not in various health-related measures, including arrests for driving under the influence, traffic crashes, and domestic violence arrests. Although evidence for the effects of this program on rate of traffic crashes was mixed, this program led to strong reductions in arrests for both repeat DUIs and domestic violence. Specifically, repeat DUI arrests declined 12% and domestic violence arrests declined 9%. This study provides powerful evidence that frequent alcohol testing, with immediate consequences for its use, can lead to a variety of positive health outcomes.

Laws can also be implemented that require changes not in people's behavior, but in products and/or the environment in some way. For example, data showing that airbags reduced injuries and deaths caused by car accidents led to a congressional mandate requiring all cars to have airbags. Similarly, one recent study demonstrated that requiring cars to have alcohol ignition interlocks, which connect a breath-testing unit to the ignition and won't start if the person's breath contains alcohol above a certain level, would reduce crashes caused by drunk driving more than 80%, and thus dramatically reduce injuries and fatalities caused by such accidents (Carter, Flannagan, Bingham, Cunningham, & Rupp, 2015).

Increase Education

Another crucial strategy for preventing health problems is to improve education. Higher levels of education are consistently associated with better health, even when researchers take into account other factors, such as income (Peters, Baker, Dieckmann, Leon, & Collins, 2010). People with higher levels of education practice more health-protective behaviors, in part because education informs people about the risks of particular behavior and equips them with the skills needed to think about long-term consequences of their actions. For example, 34% of American adults with a GED smoke, compared to 7.4% of those with a college degree and only 3.6% of those with a graduate degree (Jamal et al., 2016). Moreover, compared to people who have completed college, those with lower levels of education, meaning a high school degree or less, have higher rates of a protein in the body that is associated with the development of chronic diseases, including cardiovascular disease, osteoporosis, and Alzheimer's disease (Morozink, Friedman, Coe, & Ryff, 2010). This link remains even when researchers consider the effects of other variables associated with such diseases, such as age, gender, and health behaviors. Although the specific mechanisms explaining this association are unclear, all of these findings suggest that increasing education is a good strategy for preventing chronic diseases.

REDUCING HEALTH CARE COSTS

LO 14.2

Explain methods of reducing health care costs

One of the hottest topics in health psychology is the rapidly increasing costs of health care in the United States and how these costs can be controlled. Nearly 18% of the gross domestic product is spent on health care each year, with a total cost of over $3 trillion (National Center for Health Statistics, 2016). Strategies for reducing the high cost of health care are reducing spending on administrative costs, decreasing reliance on medical technology, and conducting cost/benefit analyses.

Reduce Administrative Costs

A number of factors contribute to the higher rate of administrative costs in the United States than in other countries. One reason costs are so much higher is that physicians and hospitals in the United States spend much more on administrative costs, including advertising to recruit patients, filing for reimbursement from insurance companies, and obtaining permission to do various procedures (Woolhandler & Himmelstein, 1991). For example, the average physician's office in the United States spends about one hour on each insurance claim, which is 20 times as long as time spent in Canada.

These administrative costs are largely due to the complexity of different ways in which people in the United States receive health insurance, depending on their employer, income, and age. In many countries, including Canada and most European countries, health care is viewed as a guaranteed consumer good or service and is funded at least in part by the government. Patients can typically choose any doctor they want, and all citizens' medical bills, including prescription drugs and mental health services, are covered by taxes. In contrast, people in the United States pay for health coverage in very different ways; employers may offer different types of managed care systems (such as health maintenance organizations, or HMOs; preferred provider organizations, or PPPs; or high-deductible health plans, or HDHPs), people 65 and older receive government coverage (Medicare), people with limited income receive government coverage (Medicaid), and other people opt for traditional (and most costly) fee-for-service care. These different types of health care options contribute to the higher cost of health care in the United States compared to that in other countries, as shown in Figure 14.1.

Other factors also contribute to the high administrative costs of health care in the United States. Physicians in the United States spend more money than do physicians in other countries on "amenities" for their offices, including renting desirable office space, buying attractive furniture, and paying for interior decorating perhaps as a way of attracting patients. Given the litigious nature of U.S. society, physicians in the United States often carry expensive malpractice insurance (the cost naturally is passed on to patients) and often practice "defensive medicine" in which they order every test and do every procedure to protect themselves from lawsuits (Butter, 1993). Physicians in the United States also rely more on technology and use more medically advanced procedures than physicians in other countries; however, and as you'll learn in the next section, the use of more technology does not necessarily lead to better health outcomes (Kaplan, 1989).

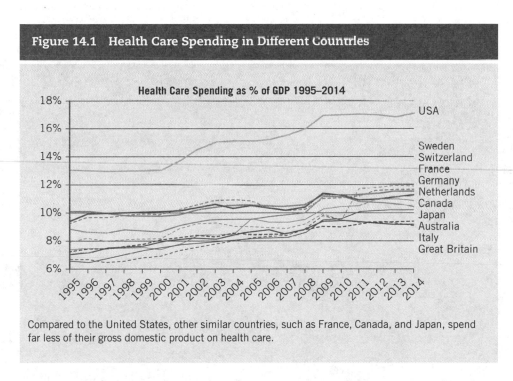

Figure 14.1   Health Care Spending in Different Countries

Compared to the United States, other similar countries, such as France, Canada, and Japan, spend far less of their gross domestic product on health care.

Source: Data from Mother Jones (http://www.motherjones.com/kevin-drum/2017/06/chart-day-health-care-spending-percentage-gdp/).

Following the 2016 United States presidential election, there has been considerable debate about the best government strategies for reducing health care costs. The Affordable Care Act (ACA), which is sometimes referred to as "Obamacare," was adopted in 2010 with the goal of making health care more generally affordable to all Americans and increasing access to health care for lower-income adults. Although the debate is ongoing about whether the ACA succeeded in these broad goals and some efforts continue to attempt to repeal parts of this law, this law did result in expanded health coverage to people of color, as described in **Focus on Diversity**.

Decrease Reliance on Technology

Another factor contributing to the high cost of health care is the increasing reliance on medical technology. State-of-the-art treatment is often seen as superior to low-tech options (Butter, 1993). Technology use is also profitable for hospitals (who can charge for the equipment) and physicians (who can charge for their specialized services). In fact, rates of cesarean section are lower among women who are uninsured or are covered by Medicaid (a government program that pays health care costs for poor people) than those who are using private insurance (Gould, Davey, & Stafford, 1989; Placek, Taffel, & Moien, 1988).

Unfortunately, this infatuation with technology has led to an overreliance on it in some cases. Some surgeries, such as coronary bypass surgery and cesarean section, are clearly beneficial to some patients, but they are often overused for patients who might benefit the same or more from other less expensive procedures. In fact, one study suggested that about 20% of the pacemakers implanted in people were unwarranted (Greenspan et al., 1988). To test whether patients benefit in terms of survival from more aggressive care, researchers compared the effectiveness of two different treatments for coronary artery disease: percutaneous

FOCUS ON DIVERSITY

Why Increased Health Care Access Reduces Racial Disparities in Health

Researchers in one study analyzed data on health care access and utilization following the adoption of the Affordable Care Act (ACA), which went into effect in 2014 (Chen, Vargas-Bustamante, Mortensen, & Ortega, 2016). Specifically, they compared answers on the National Health Interview Survey, a national survey of American adults, from 2011 to 2014, to questions about health care access and utilization.

Their findings revealed that following the adoption of the ACA, people overall were more likely to have health insurance, seek medical care without delay, and see a doctor within the past year. However, health care access and utilization was influenced more by the passage of this law for people of color than for Whites. For example, the percentage of Whites who were uninsured was reduced by only 3%, compared to a 7% reduction in the rates of uninsured Blacks and Latinos and a 5% reduction for people in other racial/ethnic groups. Compared to Whites, people of color also reported greater increases in having seen a doctor in the last year and seeking health care without delay after ACA coverage began.

Given the substantial racial and ethnic disparities in health access, which contribute to such disparities in overall health, these findings suggest that people of color particularly benefit from the increase in insurance options made available by the adoption of the ACA.

coronary intervention versus a conservative treatment in which patients were not given any intervention (Katritsis & Ioannidis, 2005). Findings revealed no differences between patients treated in these different ways in terms of hearts attacks or morality, suggesting that the more aggressive approach may in fact not lead to any benefits. Similarly, researchers in another study examined whether implantable cardioverter-defibrillators reduced mortality in women with advanced heart failure (Ghanbari et al., 2009). Once again, there were no statistically significant decreases in mortality in women with heart failure who received implantable cardioverter-defibrillators.

Although the research described thus far has focused on treatment for heart problems, which represent a very serious and potentially fatal disease, more aggressive treatment is also used for less serious medical conditions. For example, childbirth is usually straightforward and certainly can occur with relatively little technological intervention: historically women gave birth at home, often with only the assistance of a midwife. Now childbirth often includes the use of many different types of technology, including ultrasounds, epidural pain relief, and electronic fetal monitoring (Butter, 1993). This means that women today typically have more "technologically advanced" births, but not necessarily "better" births.

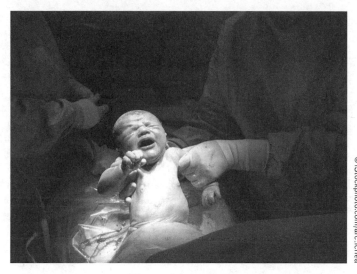

An estimated 32% of all births in the United States occur through cesarean section, which many obstetricians believe is far too high.

Finally, technology is expensive, and therefore when money is spent on technology, it takes money away from other types of health care (Butter, 1993). Health professionals must therefore decide when to use technology. For example, in 1987, the legislature of the state of Oregon had to make a decision about how to use its limited health care budget, and specifically to choose between funding organ transplantation surgery and prenatal care. This choice is really between providing a very large effect for a small number of people (only about 30 people each year in Oregon will need an organ transplant, but for those who do, this surgery literally saves their lives) and providing a relatively small effect for a large number of people (over 1,500 women in Oregon become pregnant and need prenatal care each year, and providing such care decreases infant mortality and birth defects). Similarly, and as discussed in *Chapter 12: Terminal Illness and Bereavement*, because we now have the capacity to keep people alive using technological means, medical professionals are forced to examine when such technology should be used and when individuals and/or their families should have the right to refuse this type of treatment. Very expensive technologies are often used to keep people alive for very short periods of time—hours or days—and sometimes in an unconscious state (Kaplan, 1991). One researcher describes this phenomenon as turning "inexpensive dying into prolonged living, usually through expensive means" (McGregor, 1989, p. 119).

Conduct Cost/Benefit Analyses

Given the skyrocketing costs of health care, health psychologists are increasingly asked about the costs of health-promotion interventions, specifically, whether these costs justify the programs (Friedman, Sobel, Myers, Caudill, & Benson, 1995; Johnson & Millstein, 2003; Kaplan, 1989; Kaplan & Groessl, 2002; Nation et al., 2003). In many cases, the costs of health-promotion programs are quite low, given their potential benefits. For example, the Stanford

What You'll Learn 14.2

Five City Project provided five years of intensive education and training, including television and radio spots, brochures, classes, and contests, to two small cities in northern California in an effort to decrease coronary heart disease (Farquhar et al., 1990). Although the overall effects of this intervention were relatively small, the cost was only about $4 per person per year. In this case, the benefits (even if small) would probably outweigh the costs (also quite small). Similarly, a 12-session, small-group HIV-prevention intervention for gay men cost about $470 per person, yet the medical cost savings of this program were substantial (Holtgrave & Kelly, 1996). Other studies indicate that giving people information about detrimental health behavior (e.g., problem drinking, smoking) and providing advice about home remedies for common health problems are quite inexpensive and lead to a substantial overall savings (Fries et al., 1993; Windsor et al., 1993).

Even relatively expensive lifestyle interventions can be cost-effective, if they reduce costly medical procedures or reliance on expensive drugs (e.g., lifestyle programs to reduce the risk of diabetes, which focus on increasing physical activity and reducing weight, are more effective than drug treatment) (Knowler et al., 2002; Ornish et al., 1990). For example, companies may prefer to pay the considerable costs of a lifestyle-change program that includes diet, exercise, meditation, and so on than the cost of a coronary artery bypass surgery. Researchers in one study examined the impact of people's lifestyle choices on their employers' health care costs (O'Donnell, Schultz, & Yen, 2015). Specifically, this study gathered data from over 200,000 people working in different industries on the health-related costs associated with various behaviors that people could modify in some way, such as smoking, exercise, and seat belt use. Their findings revealed that 25% of all health care costs employers pay are linked to unhealthy lifestyle choices. The most common, and expensive, health-related behavior was obesity, followed by stress and use of drugs. Employers clearly benefit from having healthy employees; the average health care cost for healthy employees in this study was less than $3,000 a year, compared to over $10,000 a year for employees with at least one medical condition. In sum, employee wellness programs, which both increase awareness about the link between behavioral choices and health outcomes and help people build skills to change these health-related behaviors, could lead to substantial cost savings for both employees and businesses.

However, in other cases the benefits of a program in terms of health may not justify its costs (White, Urban, & Taylor, 1993). Screening programs, for example, are often found not to be as cost-effective because they involve testing many people who would never develop the disease (Moum, 1995). For example, requiring yearly mammograms is more expensive (in general and per cancer prevented) than biannual or even screenings once every five years, yet is more effective in reducing cancer deaths. Screening programs are also more cost-effective when they focus on those at greatest risk for the disease (Kaplan, 2000). Mammograms cost about $21,400 to produce a single year of life when used with women ages 50 to 64 years, but $105,000 per quality year lived when used in women ages 40 to 49 years. Similarly, a mass prenatal screening for cystic fibrosis could detect whether children have this disease. However, given the tremendous costs associated with this screening, including genetic counseling, public education, and the tests themselves, it is estimated that more than $1 million would be spent to avoid a single cystic fibrosis birth (Wilfond & Fost, 1990). Because this is five times the cost of caring for a person with cystic fibrosis, this type of screening is clearly cost-ineffective. Finally, screening is especially cost-inefficient when it is used for relatively old people, who will not benefit from increased life expectancy as dramatically as younger people, and in cases in which the treatment for the condition detected leads to lower quality of life (Kaplan, 2000). For example, screening 70-year-old men for prostate cancer extends life expectancy less than five hours, and the treatment for prostate cancer often significantly reduces their overall enjoyment of life (Krahn et al., 1994). Once again, screening is not always the right approach to enhancing health.

UNDERSTANDING THE IMPACT OF DEMOGRAPHIC FACTORS ON HEALTH

Many of the predictors of health are consistent across the lifespan, for people from different racial/ethnic and socioeconomic backgrounds, and for both men and women. Cigarette smoking, for example, is a consistent predictor of poor health outcomes, as are obesity and substance abuse. However, demographic factors do impact health in a variety of ways, including the prevalence of particular health-related behaviors, the nature of health concerns, and access to health care. This section examines the impact of race/ethnicity, socioeconomic status, age, and gender on health.

LO 14.3

Summarize the impact of demographic factors on health and health outcomes

Race/Ethnicity

Although overall life expectancy has climbed dramatically in the United States over the last 100 years, the average life span differs considerably for people in different ethnic groups. Specifically, Asian people have the longest life expectancies (86.3 years), followed by Latinos (82 years), and Whites (78.7 years), with Blacks overall having the lowest life expectancy at 75.1 years (Acciai, Noah, & Firebaugh, 2015). This gap in life expectancy starts very early in life; as shown in Figure 14.2, rates of infant mortality are highest in Black babies. Moreover, compared to people in other ethnic and racial groups, as adults, Black Americans have higher rates of death caused by homicide, cancer, and cardiovascular disease and a higher mortality

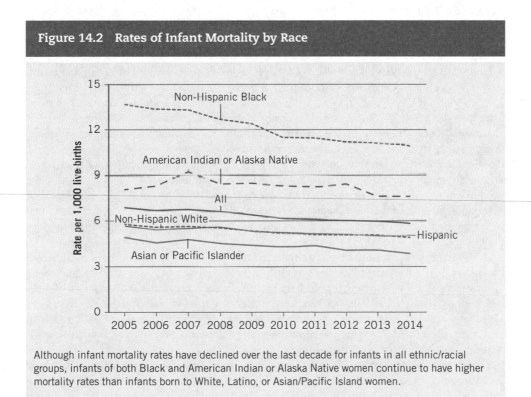

Figure 14.2   Rates of Infant Mortality by Race

Although infant mortality rates have declined over the last decade for infants in all ethnic/racial groups, infants of both Black and American Indian or Alaska Native women continue to have higher mortality rates than infants born to White, Latino, or Asian/Pacific Island women.

Source: Mathews & Driscoll (2017).

rate at every age category (Masters et al., 2014). They are also more likely to experience chronic diseases, such as asthma, diabetes, and HIV. For example, although Blacks make up only 12% of the total United States population, 45% of people living with HIV are Black (Centers for Disease Control and Prevention, 2017j).

One factor contributing to these differences in health as a function of race/ethnicity is the prevalence of particular health behaviors. For example, rates of obesity are higher in Blacks (48.1%) and Latinos (42.5%) than in Whites (34.5%) and Asians (11.7%) (Ogden, Carroll, Kit, & Flegal, 2014). Although overall smoking rates are relatively similar for Whites and Blacks, the patterning of smoking differs. Specifically, Whites tend to start smoking earlier but are also more likely to quit in adulthood than Blacks (Holford, Levy, & Meza, 2016). Because many of the health conditions caused by smoking, such as lung cancer and chronic obstructive pulmonary disease, occur later in life, Blacks' higher rate of smoking during older adulthood is particularly problematic. As you learned in *Chapter 6: Injury and Injury Prevention*, Blacks are also more likely than Whites to die of homicide at every age.

Another factor contributing to racial/ethnic differences in health is the availability of regular, preventive health care. People of color are much less likely than Whites to engage in regular, preventive health care, in part because they have higher rates of unemployment and are more likely to hold low-paying jobs that do not provide health insurance (Fiscella, Franks, Gold, & Clancy, 2000; Flack et al., 1995; Johnson et al., 1995). In turn, this lack of regular health care increases people's risk of developing major health problems, because they do not use preventive measures or catch health problems at earlier, treatable, stages (Adler et al., 1994; Adler, Boyce, Chesney, Folkman, & Syme, 1993; Gornick et al., 1996). Similarly, although White women are more likely to get breast cancer than Black women, more Black women die from breast cancer than women from any other racial or ethnic group (Centers for Disease Control and Prevention, 2016a).

Moreover, people of color are less likely than Whites to rely on medical professionals for health care even when they have health insurance (Fiscella et al., 2000). Both Latinos and Asians sometimes avoid seeking health care because of a lack of comfort with speaking English as well as a cultural preference for both relying primarily on family members and friends for advice about physical symptoms and using alternative medical treatments (e.g., acupuncture, herbs). As described in *Chapter 13: Managing Health Care*, Blacks have lower expectations about the benefits of knee replacements than do Whites and express a stronger preference for using natural remedies and avoiding surgery (Figaro, Williams-Russo, & Allegrante, 2005). People of color may also have a general distrust of the medical community, based in part on prior experiments in which minority group members were used—without their knowledge or consent—in medical experiments (Jemmott & Jones, 1993; Marin & Marin, 1991). For example, and as described in *Chapter 2: Research Methods*, in the 1930s some Black men with syphilis were left untreated so that researchers could measure the long-term effects of the disease.

Eliminating racial and ethnic differences in health is a difficult task, but an extremely important goal. One step toward accomplishing this goal would be to provide some type of universal health care, which would help increase access to health care services to Blacks and Latinos, who are less likely to have health insurance than Whites and Asians (Barnett & Vornovitsky, 2016). As described in the prior section, racial/ethnic differences in access to health care decreased following the adoption of the Affordable Care Act, and further expansions of health care for all Americans would go a long way toward reducing such disparities. Focusing on prevention is another strategy for decreasing these differences, particularly because members of minority groups often engage in high rates of health-compromising behaviors. Strategies for this type of prevention could include emphasizing the importance of eating a healthy diet and engaging in regular exercise as well as avoiding smoking. As shown in Figure 14.3, Black adolescent girls who receive brief telephone counseling sessions every couple of months to remind them of the importance of engaging in HIV/STD-preventive

Figure 14.3   Data From DiClemente et al., 2014

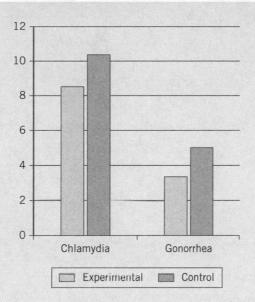

At the 3-year follow-up, girls who received brief phone calls every other month reminding them of the importance of engaging in STD/HIV-preventive behavior reported using condoms more frequently during sex and engaging in sex while under the influence of alcohol and/or drugs less often compared to those who did not receive such calls. Most important, girls who received the phone calls were also less likely to become infected with chlamydia or gonorrhea.

Source: Data from DiClemente, Wingood, Sales, Brown, Rose, Davis, . . . Hardin (2014).

behavior are less likely to have an STD at the three-year follow-up (DiClemente et al., 2014). Most important, reducing the drastic rate of poverty in some parts of the United States, especially in inner cities, is probably the most important means of improving health in people of color. Improving the overall standard of living, by encouraging people to continue their education, providing low-cost housing and job training, and decreasing poverty, would go a long way toward reducing many of the ethnic and racial differences in health. (The link between poverty and health will be described in detail in the next section.)

Socioeconomic

Although life expectancy has increased dramatically in the United States over the last century, substantial gaps continue to exist as a function of income. As shown in Figure 14.4, the very wealthiest people in the United States—the top 1%—live on average 14.6 more years (for men) and 10.1 more years (for women) than the very poorest (those in the bottom 1% of income) (Chetty et al., 2016). People who are low in socioeconomic status also have a higher rate of chronic diseases, such as diabetes, arthritis, and cardiovascular disease (Gallo & Matthews, 2003; Matthews, Raikkonen, Gallo, & Kuller, 2008). Moreover, many of the ethnic/racial differences in health described in the prior section are caused, at least in part, by differences in income; data from the most recent U.S. Census reveals that only 9.1% of

Figure 14.4 Life Expectancy by Gender and Income

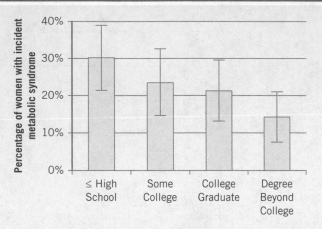

Although women at all income levels have a greater life expectancy than men, life expectancy increases dramatically with income for both men and women.

Source: Matthews et al. (2008).

Whites and 11.4% of Asians are living in poverty, compared to 21.4% of Latinos and 24.1% of Blacks (Proctor, Semega, & Kollar, 2016). Sadly, and as described in **Focus on Development**, poverty during childhood has lasting effects on health.

FOCUS ON DEVELOPMENT

Why Poverty Really Hurts Kids' Health

Children who grow up in poverty are at greater risk of both engaging in behaviors that are detrimental to health, such as being obese and not being physically active, and experiencing numerous negative health outcomes, such as unintentional injuries and homicide (Emerson, 2009). Moreover, poverty in childhood is associated with a greater likelihood of developing life-threatening health conditions in adulthood, including diabetes, stroke, coronary heart disease, and certain types of cancer. Although the specific mechanisms explaining this link between childhood poverty and adult health outcomes isn't entirely clear, one possibility is that exposure to poverty early in life has a lasting impact on individuals' physiological response to stress (Boylan, Jennings, & Matthews, 2016). For example, a longitudinal study examining the link between duration of exposure to poverty and psychological stress in children from birth through age 13 revealed that the more years a child had spent living in poverty, the more elevated were the child's stress reactions (e.g., cortisol levels, cardiovascular reactivity to stress) (Evans & Kim, 2007). Encouragingly, however, even children who grow up in poverty may be able to overcome this disadvantage if given adequate social resources. Specifically, although adolescents who grow up in low-income households smoke more and have more body fat than those who grow up in more affluent environments, children who live at the poverty line but feel support and connections with their community do not show these detrimental health behaviors (Evans & Kutcher, 2011). Moreover, children whose family income increases during their childhood and adolescence are not more likely to experience poor physical health as adults (Cundiff, Boylan, Pardini, & Matthews, 2017).

One of the most important factors explaining the link between income and life expectancy is that people who are living below the poverty line are less likely to have access to regular medical care. In line with this explanation, in 2015, 85.2% of people with household incomes less than $25,000 had health insurance, compared to 92.7% of people with incomes of $75,000 to $99,999 and 95.5% of those with incomes of $100,000 or more (Barnett & Vornovitsky, 2016). People without health insurance have a higher risk of acquiring preventable diseases. For example, over 75% of children living above the poverty line are fully vaccinated, compared to 66% of those living below the poverty line, placing low-income children at greater risk of acquiring serious and even life-threatening illnesses that are largely preventable (National Center for Health Statistics, 2017). People without health insurance are also less likely to catch diseases at an early, and more treatable, stage. One study of women with annual household incomes below $15,000 found that 90% did not obtain regular mammograms and more than 33% had never even heard of mammography (Mickey, Durski, Worden, & Danigelis, 1995).

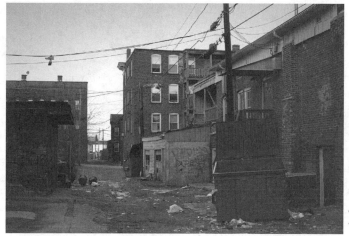

One explanation for the link between lower socioeconomic status and poor health is that low-income families face a variety of stressors, including overcrowded housing, pollution, and neighborhood crime, all of which can have negative effects on health.

Although lack of access to regular health care is one explanation for the link between low income and poor health, even in countries with universal free health care, people with low income are less healthy than those with more income (Adler et al., 1993). This finding indicates that factors other than the ability to pay for health care must also contribute to the link between low income and poor health. One explanation is that poor people tend to engage in more destructive health-related behaviors, including smoking, alcohol consumption, failure to exercise, and obesity (Adler et al., 1994; Anderson & Armstead, 1995; Stunkard & Sorensen, 1993; Wardle, Waller, & Jarvis, 2002). For example, 26.1% of those living below the poverty line smoke, compared to only 13.9% of those living at or above the poverty time (Jamal et al., 2016).

Another explanation is that people in low socioeconomic groups experience higher levels of stress, such as overcrowded housing, homelessness, pollution, and neighborhood crime (Anderson & Armstead, 1995; Chen & Paterson, 2006; Jackson, Knight, & Rafferty, 2010; Myers, Kagawa-Singer, Kumanyika, Lex, & Markides, 1995; Yee et al., 1995). As described in *Chapter 4: Understanding Stress*, stress can have both direct and indirect effects on health. Relatedly, people with low socioeconomic resources may have limited ability to cope with stressful life events, which in turn further heightens feelings of stress (Gallo, de los Monteros, & Shivpuri, 2009). According to the **reserve capacity model**, people with low SES experience more frequent stressful situations—by living in more crowded, noisy, and dangerous environments—and have a smaller supply of resources—tangible, interpersonal, intrapersonal—to manage stressful events. A family with little disposable income, for example, may experience a variety of negative life events as more stressful, such as needing to have a car repaired, losing a job, or having a child with a chronic medical condition. They may also have fewer resources available to cope with such stressors; they may be less able to borrow money from a friend for emergencies or take time off of work for a personal emergency. In line with this view, people who are low in SES show lower levels of optimism, self-esteem, and social support, which in turn is associated with worse health outcomes (Matthews et al., 2008). People who are low in SES also have more difficulty quitting smoking, in part because they live in more stressful environments and receive lower levels of social support (Businelle et al., 2010).

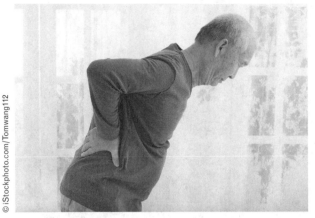

©iStockphoto.com/Tomwang112

Chronic health problems, such as Alzheimer's disease, osteoporosis, and arthritis, can severely decrease a person's overall quality of life.

The most effective strategy for reducing socioeconomic disparities in health is to increase affordable access to health care to people at relatively low-income levels. As described previously, the adoption of the ACA in 2014 expanded health insurance coverage throughout the United States. This expansion was particularly helpful to low-income people who lived just above the poverty line, and thus were previously unable to receive coverage through Medicaid, because it allowed states to provide health insurance at low cost to additional low-income families. In turn, the percentage of poor and near-poor people who had health insurance increased from 2013 to 2015, as did the percentage who had seen a health professional in the last year (Martinez & Ward, 2016).

Age

One of the dramatic changes over the last 100 years is the increase in life expectancy. In the early 1900s, people lived to an average age of 47.3 years, whereas the mean life expectancy today is nearly 79 years (Crimmins, 2015). This increase, in turn, has led to a growing number of older adults. In fact, estimates are that the number of Americans who are ages 65 and older will reach over 98 million by 2060 (compared to about 46 million today) and will then make up almost 25% of the total population (compared to only 15% today) (Mather, Jacobsen, & Pollard, 2015).

But this increase in the number of people living into their 80s, 90s, and even 100s, also poses particular challenges. One major goal of health psychology is to help people live higher-quality lives, meaning lives that are free from pain and major disability. However, the increase in life expectancy has led to an increase in the number of people suffering from chronic, disabling conditions. Many diseases, such as cancer, coronary heart disease, and Alzheimer's disease, are much more prevalent with age; hence, as people live longer, they are more likely to develop such problems. Other diseases are not life-threatening but also increase in incidence with age and can decrease people's overall quality of life. For example, osteoporosis, arthritis, hearing loss, and vision problems caused by glaucoma and cataracts are all more prevalent in older people and can severely hamper a person's ability to engage in various activities. However, the ultimate goal is to allow people to maintain very good psychological and physical well-being for a long time and then experience a relatively short period of pain and disability immediately prior to death (a compression of mortality).

This focus on quality of life, not just quantity of life, has led researchers to measure people's disability-adjusted life expectancy (Kaplan & Bush, 1982). This measure calculates the number of years a person can spend free from disease and disability—their well years or health expectancy. Some researchers even propose that people should rate the quality of their overall life, based on the symptoms they are experiencing as well as the length of time they will spend experiencing these symptoms, to determine their **quality-adjusted life years (QALY)** (Kaplan, 1991). The quality is determined both by the severity of the symptoms (e.g., being confined to a wheelchair or experiencing considerable pain that is more severe than experiencing a mild headache or spraining an ankle) and their duration (e.g., even a very painful bout of food poisoning lasts a few days at most, whereas severe cancer pain could last for years).

People's rating of their QALYs can have a substantial impact on their decisions regarding health care. For example, many people would choose to have surgery to remove a cancerous tumor, in part because this surgery can lengthen life expectancy dramatically and is associated only with a relatively brief period of low life quality during the recovery from surgery. However, many people might choose to not undergo a treatment that provides only a small increase in life expectancy and puts one in a very dependent state (e.g., being tube-fed and on a respirator). Since doctors' estimates of their patients' preferences regarding living in various health states are not particularly accurate, it is extremely important for patients to communicate their preferences regarding such states to both their families and medical professionals (Elstein, Chapman, & Knight, 2005).

Unfortunately, and as described in *Chapter 12: Terminal Illness and Bereavement*, many people, even those who are terminally ill, don't complete living wills or share their preferences with loved ones. Patients may be optimistic about the likelihood of recovery, and thus not see expressing such preferences as important. Patients and their families may also find discussing end-of-life scenarios distressing, and thus avoid the topic completely. Moreover, even when a person has completed a living will and/or shared their preferences with family members, it can be difficult for loved ones to interpret and/or follow through on such wishes. Family members may therefore push for more aggressive care, even if this is not the expressed preference of the patient. Health psychologists are currently exploring ways to help people communicate their end-of-life preferences to loved ones, which should help make sure patients' preferences are honored (Ditto & Hawkins, 2005; Fried, Bradley, Towle, & Allore, 2002).

Gender

For many years, research in psychology in general and health psychology in particular was based largely on samples of men (and typically samples of young, White, upper-class men who were in college) (Matthews et al., 1997). This focus was caused in part by the easy access of this type of population—many researchers worked in college and university settings (and many prestigious schools did not even admit women until relatively recently) and hence often used students who were readily available. Women may also be excluded from medical studies because of concern about the influence of hormonal changes across the menstrual cycle as well as the potential dangers to fetuses (Wenger, Speroff, & Packard, 1993). However, this exclusion of women severely limits our knowledge about the factors that influence women's health and how women respond to various psychological and medical treatments. In fact, women are even excluded from many studies of drugs that are primarily used by women, such as weight-loss pills and antidepressants (Rodin & Ickovics, 1990).

One explanation for the greater focus on men's health is that because women have a longer life expectancy than men, research on women's health is less essential. However, the gender gap in life expectancy is narrowing, in part because women are now engaging in health-compromising behaviors at higher rates (Rodin & Ickovics, 1990). For example, at all ages a higher percentage of women are overweight and obese than men (Ogden, Carroll, Kit, & Flegal, 2014). Although more men than women smoke, rates of both smoking and lung cancer are declining faster in men than women (Henley et al., 2014; Jamal et al., 2016). Moreover, and as described in *Chapter 13: Managing Health Care*, women are less likely than men to receive a number of major diagnostic and therapeutic procedures, even when they are experiencing symptoms that are as severe as men's, in part because physicians are more likely to see women's physical symptoms as signs of psychological problems (Ayanian & Epstein, 1991; Fiscella et al., 2000; Rathore et al., 2001; Schulman et al., 1999; Steingart et al., 1991).

Women also have unique health issues and concerns (Rodin & Ickovics, 1990; Stanton, Lobel, Sears, & DeLuca, 2002). First, reproductive issues and technology, including pregnancy, infertility, abortion, contraception, prenatal screening, cesarean sections, and in vitro fertilization, impact women more directly than they do men. Researchers in one study

What You'll Learn
14.3

examined the link between women's level of stress and ability to get pregnant (Akhter, Marcus, Kerber, Kong, & Taylor, 2016). Sexually active women completed daily measures that reported their stress level (1 meaning low, 4 meaning high) as well as other factors that could impact fertility, such as age, BMI, alcohol use, smoking, and sexual activity. Women who reported feeling more stressed during the days in which they were ovulating were 40% less likely to conceive during that month compared to other months. Moreover, women who generally reported feeling stressed were about 45% less likely to conceive than other women. This link between stress and difficult conceiving held true even when researchers took into account the other factors that could impact conception. These findings suggest that women who are trying to conceive take deliberate steps to reduce stress, such as exercising, meditating, and talking with a therapist. In fact, the impact of stress on fertility may be as important as other factors known to influence fertility, such as smoking, alcohol use, and obesity.

Women also face unique challenges related to the experience of menstruation and menopause. Many women take the hormone estrogen, often as part of oral contraceptives prior to menopause and as hormone replacement therapy following menopause. Although for some time researchers thought that taking these hormones was an effective way of preventing some of the side effects of menopause, a study by the National Institutes of Health revealed that women who take estrogen and progestin to minimize the effects of menopause are at risk of experiencing major health problems (Writing Group for the Women's Health Initiative Investigators, 2002). Specifically, compared to women in the control group who received a placebo, those who took these hormones experienced a 41% increase in strokes, a 29% increase in heart attacks, and a 26% increase in breast cancer. Finally, other diseases, such as osteoporosis and Alzheimer's disease, can occur in men and women, but are much more common in women, in part because they tend to live longer. In sum, women face particular health issues and challenges, and research must focus on examining how best to promote women's health. As described by Andrew Baum and Neil Grunberg (1991):

> Research on health and behavior should consider men and women—not because it is discriminatory not to do so—but because it is good science. The study of women and men, of young and old, of African Americans and Caucasians, Asians, Latinos, and American Indians will all help to reveal psychosocial and biological mechanisms that are critical to understanding mortality, morbidity, and quality of life. (p. 84)

IMPROVING INTERNATIONAL HEALTH

LO 14.4

Describe strategies for improving international health

Although this book has focused largely on strategies for improving health within the United States and other Western, industrialized, nations, a major focus of the future in health psychology must be on improving health worldwide. As shown in Figure 14.5, life expectancy rates vary substantially around the world; in fact, the average life expectancy in Europe is more than 16 years greater than that in Africa. Chronic diseases, such as coronary heart disease, cancer, stroke, and diabetes, are the leading causes of death in the United States and throughout the world, largely because risk factors, such as rates of smoking and obesity, continue to escalate. But in Africa, an estimated 56% of deaths are caused by communicable diseases (tuberculosis, malaria, HIV), starvation, and complications to mothers and/or infants during childbirth (World Health Organization, 2018), and many of these deaths are preventable. This section examines how theories and research in health psychology could be used to improve global health.

Figure 14.5   Life Expectancy by Country

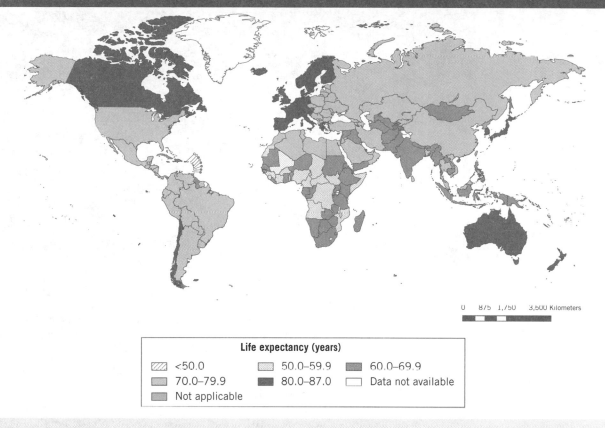

Life expectancy (years)

- ▨ <50.0
- ▨ 50.0–59.9
- ■ 60.0–69.9
- ■ 70.0–79.9
- ■ 80.0–87.0
- ▢ Data not available
- ■ Not applicable

Babies born in 2015 have a life expectancy of 71.4 years (73.8 years for girls, 69.1 years for boys). However, life expectancy varies considerably throughout the world, from a high of 76.8 years for babies born in parts of Europe to a low of 60.0 years for babies born in Africa.

Source: Courtesy of the World Health Organization (2016). http://gamapserver.who.int/mapLibrary/Files/Maps/Global_LifeExpectancy_bothsexes_2015.png

Reduce Rates of Smoking

One of the biggest health problems facing the world is the prevalence of tobacco use. More than 1 billion people worldwide smoke, and smoking contributes to many chronic and life-threatening illnesses, including cancer, stroke, and heart disease (World Health Organization, 2017b). Moreover, smoking kills an estimated 7 million people each year. Although most of these deaths are the result of people's own tobacco use, nearly one in seven are caused by exposure to secondhand smoke. Smoking is a leading cause of illness and death throughout the world but is especially common among men living in Western Pacific countries, such as China, Japan, Thailand, and Korea (see Table 14.2).

As you learned in ***Chapter 7: Substance Use and Abuse***, theories and research in health psychology can be used to both prevent people from starting to smoke and to help smokers quit. However, countries vary tremendously in the steps they have taken to reduce tobacco use. Only 42 countries, which include less than 20% of the world's population, require pictorial warnings that cover at least half of the front and back of cigarette packs, which have been shown to reduce rates of smoking (Noar et al., 2016). (The United States is among those

Table 14.2　Prevalence of Smoking Around the World

	% Men	% Women
Africa	24.2	2.4
Americas	22.8	13.3
Southeast Asia	32.1	2.6
Europe	39	19.3
Eastern Mediterranean	36.2	2.9
Western Pacific	48.5	3.4

Although an estimated 36.1% of men and 6.8% of women worldwide smokes, rates of smoking vary considerably by region.

Source: Courtesy of the World Health Organization (2015). http://apps.who.int/gho/data/view.sdg.3-a-data-reg?lang=en.

that do not have this requirement.) Only 29 countries have banned all forms of tobacco advertising, promotion, and sponsorship, and only 33 countries have implemented sizable taxes on tobacco to dramatically increase the cost of cigarettes. These steps would go a long way toward reducing smoking, and in turn, smoking-related illnesses and deaths.

Decrease the Spread of HIV

Overall, the number of people dying of AIDS worldwide is decreasing; over a million people died from HIV in 2015 compared to a peak of 1.8 million in 2005. However, the rate of new HIV infections continues to increase in some countries, including Egypt, Pakistan, Cambodia, Mexico, and Russia (Wang et al., 2016). The number of people living with HIV worldwide also continues to increase, largely due to the development, and greater availability, of antiretroviral therapy (ART). In 2015, 41% of the people living with HIV were using ART as compared to less than 2% in 2000.

Although the spread of HIV infection is a worldwide problem, the region most impacted by HIV infection is sub-Saharan Africa (see Table 14.3). Nearly 70% of people with HIV worldwide live in Africa, and 4.4% of adults in sub-Saharan Africa are HIV-positive. A number of factors contribute to the high rate of prevalence in this region of the world, including HIV-related stigma, poverty, and a relative lack of power for women.

Interventions are clearly needed to decrease the spread of HIV infection in Africa, and both theory and research suggest a number of strategies that may, particularly in combination, help reduce this epidemic (Jones et al., 2014; Kharsany & Karim, 2016). These include primary prevention strategies—such as increasing awareness about HIV, access to condoms, and rates of male circumcision—as well as secondary and tertiary strategies—such as increasing HIV testing and access to ART. Encouragingly, some evidence suggests that both types of strategies may be effective. For example, a sexual risk-reduction intervention based in social cognitive theory led to increases in consistent condom use in men living in South Africa (Jemmott et al., 2014). Similarly, a community-based intervention for young adults in three countries led to substantial increases in rates of HIV testing (Sweat et al., 2011). These findings provide some hope that with sustained and multifaceted efforts, the spread of HIV in Africa will eventually slow.

Table 14.3	Prevalence of AIDS Around the World
Region	**Adults and children estimated to be living with HIV**
Africa	25,600,000
Americas	3,300,000
Southeast Asia	3,500,000
Europe	2,400,000
Eastern Mediterranean	360,000
Western Pacific	1,500,000

Although the spread of HIV is a concern throughout the world, the region most impacted by AIDS so far is Africa.

Source: Courtesy of the World Health Organization (2017). http://apps.who.int/gho/data/view.main .22100WHO?lang=en.

Improve Maternal Health

Another factor that could have a dramatic impact on increasing life expectancy, especially in developing countries, is to improve maternal health, meaning women's health during pregnancy, childbirth, and the postpartum period. More than 275,000 women worldwide die in pregnancy or childbirth each year, and over half of these deaths occur in Africa (Canudas-Romo, Liu, Zimmerman, Ahmed, & Tsui, 2014). Women who have experienced multiple pregnancies are at greater risk of developing complications during pregnancy, as are those with anemia (which is more prevalent in Africa). Improving maternal health also leads to reductions in infant mortality. Although worldwide rates of deaths to children under the age of five have reduced dramatically, largely due to decreases in infectious diseases such as malaria and measles, some countries in Africa still have very high rates of child mortality. Most of these deaths are caused by birth complications, including premature birth and birth asphyxia (meaning babies don't receive enough oxygen during birth).

Although some of the factors contributing to poor maternal health are difficult to overcome in parts of Africa, such as ready access to soap and water for washing hands and availability of health facilities, other factors that improve maternal health are more feasible to implement. For example, one study in a rural part of Ethiopia found that the single biggest predictor of infant survival was breastfeeding (Biks, Berhane, Worku, & Gete, 2015). Breastfeeding reduces the infant's risk of developing various infectious diseases, such as diarrhea, respiratory infections, and pneumonia, as well as malnutrition (Victora et al., 2016). Another strategy is to increase the use of contraceptives, which helps reduce the number of pregnancies and allows for better family spacing, both of which are associated with better maternal health. Babies that are born to mothers who have given birth less than 18 months before are more likely to be born premature and have higher rates of infant mortality (Kozuki et al., 2013). Increasing contraceptive use would also help reduce family size, and in turn decrease deaths caused by starvation and malnutrition. According to the United Nations, nearly 800 million people worldwide, meaning one in nine, suffer from chronic undernourishment each year; most of these people live in developing countries, as shown in Table 14.4. Finally, helping adolescent girls delay their first pregnancy can also help improve maternal and infant health, since

What You'll Learn
14.4

Table 14.4	Percent of People Suffering From Starvation
Developed Regions	Less than 5
Developing Regions	12.9
Africa	20.0
Asia	12.1
Latin America & Caribbean	5.5
Oceana	14.2
Rates of food insecurity vary substantially by region of the world.	

Source: Food and Agriculture Organization (2015).

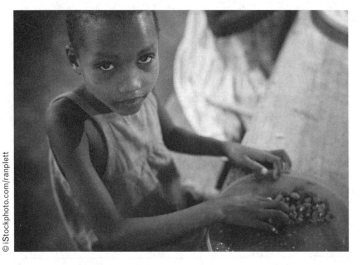
© iStockphoto.com/ranplett

Sadly, global warming may make increasing life expectancy in Africa more difficult. Global warming leads to more places in which disease-carrying insects can live and reproduce, which can cause outbreaks of infectious diseases such as yellow fever, malaria, and West Nile disease. Global warming also causes major weather events, such as droughts and floods, which can ruin farmers' crops and thus cause food shortages.

adolescent girls who become pregnant are at greater risk of experiencing complications themselves, as are their babies.

Theories in health psychology can be used to help implement all of these changes. For example, a radio-based soap opera that featured popular characters communicating about the importance of using contraceptives and planning for small families led to increased conversations between spouses about family planning (Rogers et al., 1999). Similarly, exposure to mass media messages about family planning are associated with increased use of contraceptives among young women in Nigeria (Bajoga, Atagame, & Okigbo, 2015). Interventions that include men as well as women are particularly effective at increasing contraceptive use, since men are often the primary decision makers regarding family size and contraceptive use in African countries (Shattuck et al., 2011; Tilahun, Coene, Temmerman, & Degomme, 2015).

MAKING ETHICAL MEDICAL DECISIONS

LO 14.5

Explain current challenges in making ethical medical decisions

One of the major advances in health care over the last 20 years is clearly the development of new medical technology, such as organ transplantation, chemotherapy, and artificial hearts. Although the growing number of technological advances in health and medicine have had a major impact on life expectancy by allowing some people to live who would certainly have died, these advances lead to some tricky ethical decisions for medical professionals, patients, and families. Health psychologists are examining how doctors can best make such decisions and how to help patients and families cope with these most challenging ethical dilemmas.

Use of Reproductive Technology

Growing advances in reproductive technology have enabled many couples who were previously considered infertile to have biological children. For example, researchers are now able, at least in some cases, to extract an egg from a woman and sperm from a man, combine the egg and sperm, and then implant the resulting embryo into the woman's uterus, thereby allowing many couples to have children who were previously considered infertile. Physicians can also screen these embryos prior to implantation and then choose to implant only those that meet some specified set of criteria. A couple who is at risk of having a child with cystic fibrosis, for example, might choose to implant only those embryos that do not carry this gene, and most people would probably think this selection is morally appropriate.

But the availability of technology that allows for this type of genetic selection also raises serious ethical issues. Would it be morally acceptable for a couple to implant only those embryos that would produce babies with perfect eyesight, or who would be right-handed, or a boy? Some experts are concerned that advancing reproductive technology will lead to an unending quest for "better babies."

Even when the couple is choosing to implant embryos only to avoid having a baby with a life-threatening disease or disability, ethical issues can still emerge. For example, in one case a woman with a rare genetic mutation that would almost certainly lead her to develop Alzheimer's disease by age 40 sought help from fertility experts in creating a child who would not share her dismal fate. Doctors extracted eggs from the woman, fertilized those without the mutation, and then replanted these eggs into the woman's uterus. Although this child will not develop early-onset Alzheimer's, she will suffer from the loss of her mother at a relatively early age.

Genetic Screening

The increasing use of genetic screening is another example of a technological advance that leads to challenging ethical issues (Moum, 1995; Saab et al., 2004). Researchers with the Human Genome Project are now working to map the location and precise role of every gene in the human body (Watson, 1990). This information will provide health professionals with new ways to prevent, diagnosis, and treat illness and disease but will also raise numerous complex ethical, moral, and legal issues. Some types of screening, such as for HIV infection and cholesterol levels, are already commonly used by insurance companies to set premium rates, and genetic screening could be next. Genetic screening could also determine whether a person has a "preexisting condition," which is typically excluded from insurance.

Screening can lead to discrimination in hiring and in securing health insurance. Employers obviously want healthy workers who are absent less, more productive, and less likely to quit work and/or need disability (Faden & Kass, 1993). Employers also pay less for health insurance if they hire healthy workers; hence, they are motivated to hire people who don't use a lot of health care. Would a company want to hire a worker who was certain to develop Huntington's disease within a few years? Would an insurance company charge higher rates to women with the "breast cancer gene"? How about a worker who is a carrier for a life-threatening disease, such as cystic fibrosis, and who may then have a child who needs expensive medical care (which would be covered by the employer)? Would you want to hire a diabetic or someone with a genetic predisposition for alcoholism?

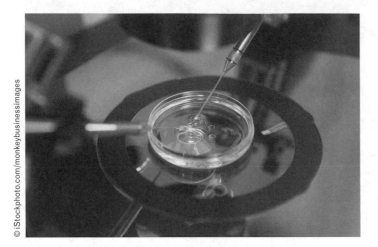

Advances in genetic screening can in some cases be used to prevent or treat diseases but have also created numerous challenging ethical issues for families and medical professionals.

Organ Transplants

Advances in medical technology have led to remarkable success in transplanting organs from one person to another, yet have also led to multiple ethical dilemmas. Because the demand for organs far exceeds the number of usable organs available, health professionals must decide who receives each available organ (Jennings, 1993; Saab et al., 2004). These decisions are particularly tricky since patients who are in need of an organ, but do not receive one in time, may likely die.

Organ transplant networks use a number of different criteria in determining how to allocate organs. These decisions are made in part based on the patient's ability to cope with the stress of such a major procedure and their ability to follow the complex medical procedures necessary to help their body accept the new organ (Olbrisch, 1996; Olbrisch, Benedict, Ashe, & Levenson, 2002). Some people believe that patients who are sickest, and therefore do not have time to wait for a subsequent organ, should receive priority for transplants. Other people believe that younger, healthier people should receive priority over older, sicker patients. The goal of this policy is to maximize the number of years saved for each organ donation: obviously a person who receives a transplant at age 18 is likely to live longer than someone who receives one at age 65. However, this policy would mean that older people, who might well continue to live for 20 or more years, would almost certainly die waiting for an organ.

Ethical considerations such as fairness and justice may also influence how organs are allocated. When baseball great Mickey Mantle received a liver transplant in 1995, following the destruction of his own liver through years of alcohol abuse, some people questioned whether he was "deserving" of this organ and whether his celebrity status had shortened his waiting time. In line with these concerns, one study found that people were much more likely to offer heart transplant to someone who had never smoked than to someone who was either a current or former smoker (Sears, Marhefka, Rodrigue, & Campbell, 2000).

Because many more people need organs each year than organs are available, there is considerable interest in increasing the number of usable organs for transplant. But various strategies for accomplishing such a goal also raise serious ethical concerns. One potential strategy would be to automatically allow for usable organs to be transplanted following a person's death, as typically occurs in some other countries (see Figure 14.6). However, some people have concerns about organ donation, such as the belief that doctors will work less diligently to save someone's life if they know he or she is willing to donate their organs (O'Carroll, Foster, McGeechan, Sandford, & Ferguson, 2011). Another strategy is to allow people to sell one of their own kidneys, which could provide a benefit to the donor as well as the recipient (people have two kidneys and need only one to survive). However, one study examining the impact of selling kidneys in India (where this is a legal practice) revealed that there are few lasting benefits to most donors: in fact, 86% of those who sold a kidney experienced a deterioration of their health, 75% continued to live in poverty, and 79% would not recommend selling a kidney to others (Goyal, Mehta, Schneiderman, & Sehgal, 2002).

Some medical ethicists have proposed that family members should receive some type of incentive for donating a loved one's organs in order to increase the number of organs available for transplantation. If the person had expressed his or her intention to donate organs and the family chose to follow the person's wishes, family members would receive a $10,000 federal income tax credit to apply to the deceased person's estate. This type of

Figure 14.6   Data From Johnson and Goldstein, 2003

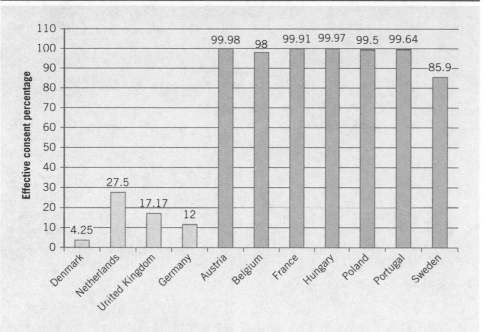

Countries in which people are assumed to consent to organ donation unless they have specifically opted out show a significantly higher rate of organ donation than those in which people must specifically opt in to donate their organs.

Source: Johnson & Goldstein (2003, p. 1338).

program would also bring publicity to the organ donation program and thereby encourage discussion of people's wishes.

Others are firmly opposed to this proposal for a variety of reasons. First, the majority of people who can successfully donate viable organs die in relatively unusual situations, namely, accidents while they are relatively young. These people are unlikely to have thought about or expressed their wishes about organ donation; hence, this incentive program would be unsuccessful in reaching them. Second, some people believe this type of incentive could encourage family members to hasten deaths, and potentially make people less willing to sign an organ donor card or express their wishes to family members. Finally, some people believe this type of incentive would devalue the altruism demonstrated by the person and his or her family in donating an organ, thereby making it less likely that people would choose to donate. You can test your own attitudes about organ donation using **Table 14.5: Test Yourself.**

Theories and research from health psychology can help increase organ donation rates, and thereby save lives. For example, increasing awareness about the need for organs—and the number of people who die waiting for an organ—is one effective strategy for persuading people to join an organ donation registry. Changing common misperceptions about organ donation, such as a belief that doctors won't try as hard to save potential organ donors and that being an organ donor eliminates the option for an open-casket funeral, also helps increase people's willingness to become organ donors. This type of education program is particularly effective at increasing rates of organ donations among people of color, who are less likely to register as donors, to more than double (Callender & Miles, 2010).

Table 14.5 Test Yourself: How Do You Feel About Organ Donation?

Answer the following questions using a scale of 1 (strongly disagree) to 5 (strongly agree).

1. Donating organs to another person after your death is humane.

2. Organ transplantation saves lives.

3. If we donate organs after our death, we will prolong the life of another person.

4. Organ transplantation improves life in the community.

5. Organ donation insults human rights.

6. A dead person is ruined by organ transplantation.

7. If we decide to donate organs, it is like we are ready to die.

8. Organ donation insults human dignity.

First, reverse-score your answers to items 5 to 8, meaning you give yourself a 1 if you put 5, 2 if you put 4, 3 if you put 3, 4 if you put 2, and 5 if you put 1. Then, add up your original scores on the first four items and the new scores on items 5 to 8 to measure your attitudes toward organ donation. Higher scores indicate greater agreement.

Source: Topic, Brkljacic, & Grahovac (2006).

What You'll Learn 14.5

Researchers in one study randomly assigned some clerks at the Department of Motor Vehicles to receive training on talking to people about organ and tissue donation (Degenholtz, Resnick, Tang, Razdan, & Enos, 2015). (This setting was chosen since people are asked specifically about whether they would like to be listed as an organ donor when they get a driver's license.) This training provided general information about the organ donor registry and answers to common misperceptions about agreeing to be an organ donor. They then tracked whether customers who interacted with these clerks were more likely to register as organ donors than those who interacted with clerks who did not receive this training. Their findings revealed that customers who interacted with clerks who received the training were 7.5% more likely to register as organ donors, suggesting that even a very brief conversation can be effective at increasing organ donation rates.

IN CONCLUSION

Now that you are at the end of this book—and perhaps at the end of your health psychology course—you should be asking yourself, "What exactly have I learned?" I hope that, most of all, you have a clear understanding of the diverse ways in which psychological factors influence physical well-being: our thoughts about various daily life situations influence whether we experience arousal; the amount and type of our social support influences how long we live; our feelings of vulnerability influence our health-promoting behavior; and our need for information can influence how we respond to surgical procedures, to name a few instances. I also hope you've learned some things in this book that you will use in your everyday life, regardless of whether your career path takes you to a health-related field. Perhaps information you've learned in this book will motivate you to always wear your seat belt, start an exercise program, or even teach your children healthy eating behaviors. One of the reasons I love teaching health psychology—why I've enjoyed writing this book—is because this is a field that truly matters to us all. Good health also matters to our society. As Marc Lalonde (1974), the Canadian minister of national health and welfare in the 1970s, describes,

> Good health is the bedrock on which social progress is built. A nation of healthy people can do those things that make life worthwhile, and as the level of health increases so does the potential for happiness. The Governments of the Provinces and of Canada have long recognized that good physical and mental health are necessary for the quality of life to which everyone aspires. (p. 5)

I hope this book helps you to have a life that is long in quantity and high in quality, including physical, mental, and psychological health.

SUMMARY

Preventing Health Problems

- One way to increase the quality of life is through primary prevention. Many health education campaigns are designed to educate people about the risks of particular behaviors, with the goal of motivating people to take an active role in changing their health-related behavior. Secondary and tertiary prevention strategies also help improve psychological and physical well-being.

- Enacting laws and regulation that either incentivize or deter particular types of behavior can help reduce health problems. Laws have already been used effectively to reduce injuries and injury-related deaths, and are particularly effective when they provide immediate punishments. These laws can also lead to reductions in other types of risky behaviors. Laws can also be implemented that require changes not in people's behavior, but in products and/or the environment in some way.

- Another crucial strategy for preventing health problems is to improve education. Higher levels of education are consistently associated with better health, even when researchers take into account other factors, such as income. People with higher levels of education practice more health-protective behaviors, in part because education informs people about the risks of particular behavior and equips them with the skills needed to think about long-term consequences of their actions.

Reducing Health Care Costs

- One reason costs are so much higher in the United States is that physicians and hospitals spend much more on administrative costs. These costs are largely due to the complexity of different ways in which people receive health insurance, depending on their employer, income, and age. Other factors that contribute to these costs include use of amenities for doctors' offices, expensive malpractice insurance, and greater use of technology and advanced procedures.

- Another factor contributing to the high cost of health care is the increasing reliance on medical technology, which is seen as superior and is also more profitable. However, in some cases there is an overreliance on such technology. More aggressive treatment is often used even for less serious medical conditions, with little evidence that this leads to better health outcomes. Technology is also expensive, and therefore, when money is spent on technology, it takes money away from other types of health care.

- Health psychologists are increasingly asked about the costs of health-promotion interventions, and specifically whether these costs justify the programs. In many cases, the costs of health-promotion programs are quite low, given their potential benefits. Even relatively expensive lifestyle interventions can be cost-effective, if they reduce costly medical procedures or reliance on expensive drugs. However, in some cases, the health benefits of a program do not justify its costs; this is especially true for screening programs.

Understanding the Impact of Demographic Factors on Health

- The average life span differs considerably as a function of race/ethnicity; Blacks have the lowest life expectancy and higher rates of chronic diseases. Factors that contribute to these differences include the prevalence of particular health behaviors, the availability of preventive health care, and feelings of trust in and comfort with medical professionals. Strategies for reducing such disparities include increasing access to health care, focusing on prevention, and reducing poverty.

- Substantial gaps in life expectancy and rates of chronic diseases exist as a function of income. Factors that contribute to this link include access to regular medical care, the prevalence of health-related behaviors, and the experience of stress. The most effective strategy for reducing socioeconomic disparities in health is to increase access to health care to people with low income.

- Increases in life expectancy have led to corresponding increases in both the number of older adults and the number of people with chronic, disabling conditions. This change has led to a focus on people's disability-adjusted life expectancy as well as their quality-adjusted life years (QALY). People's rating of these measures can have a substantial impact on their decisions regarding health care.

- Research is needed on the factors that influence women's health and how women respond to various psychological and medical treatments. Women also have unique health issues and concerns, including reproductive issues and technology, the experience of menstruation and menopause, and the greater prevalence of particular diseases.

Improving International Health

- One of the biggest health problems facing the world is the prevalence of tobacco use. Smoking contributes to many chronic and life-threatening illnesses and kills an estimated 7 million people each year. Theories and research in health psychology can be used to both prevent people from starting to smoke and to help smokers quit. However, countries vary tremendously in the steps they have taken to reduce tobacco use.

- Although the number of people dying of AIDS worldwide is decreasing, the rate of new HIV infections continues to increase in some countries. The number of people living with HIV worldwide also continues to increase, largely due to use of antiretroviral therapy (ART). The region most impacted by HIV infection by far is sub-Saharan Africa. Interventions are needed to decrease the spread of HIV infection, and both theory and research suggest a number of strategies that may help reduce this epidemic.

- Another factor that could have a dramatic impact on increasing life expectancy is improved maternal health. More than 275,000 women worldwide die in pregnancy or childbirth each year. Improving maternal health also leads to reductions in infant mortality. Many factors can help improve maternal health, including breastfeeding, spacing out pregnancies, and delaying the first pregnancy. Theories in health psychology can be used to help lead to such changes.

Making Ethical Medical Decisions

- Growing advances in reproductive technology have enabled many couples who were previously considered infertile to have biological children. But the availability of technology that allows for this type of genetic selection also raises serious ethical issues, including questions about selecting for particular characteristics.

- The increasing use of genetic screening is another example of a technological advance that leads to challenging ethical issues. Screening can lead to discrimination in hiring and in securing health insurance.

- Advances in medical technology have led to remarkable success in transplanting organs from one person to another yet have also led to multiple ethical dilemmas. Because the demand for organs far exceeds the number of usable organs available, health professionals must decide who receives each available organ using various criteria. Because many more people need organs each year than organs are available, there is considerable interest in increasing the number of usable organs for transplant. But various strategies for accomplishing such a goal also raise serious ethical concerns. Theories and research from health psychology can help increase organ donation rates and thereby save lives.

GLOSSARY

acquired immunodeficiency syndrome (AIDS): A set of symptoms and illnesses caused by the human immunodeficiency virus (HIV), which results in a weakened immune system

active strategies: Approaches to injury prevention that require engaging in some type of deliberate action to prevent health problems

acupuncture: A technique in which needles are inserted at specific points on the skin to reduce pain

acute disease: A type of disease that develops quickly and lasts only a relatively short time

acute pain: Intense but time-limited pain that is generally the result of tissue damage or disease

addiction: A condition in which a person has a physical and psychological dependence on a given substance

adherence: A person's ability and willingness to follow recommended health practices

affect-regulation model: A model proposing that people smoke to attain positive affect or avoid (or reduce) negative affect

alarm stage: A stage in the General Adaptation Syndrome (GAS) in which the body mobilizes to fight off a threat

alcohol myopia: A state in which individuals under the influence of alcohol make decisions focused on short-term consequences and ignore longer-term consequences of their behavior

alcohol use disorder (AUD): A medical condition that is characterized by both alcohol abuse and dependence and occurs when drinking causes a person distress or harm

Alcoholics Anonymous: The most widely known and widely used self-help program for alcohol abuse, which is based on the belief that people who abuse alcohol are (and will always be) alcoholics and should therefore abstain from all alcohol

allostatic load: A physiological response to long-term stress that impacts multiple systems, including cardiovascular, neuroendocrine, and immune

Alzheimer's disease: A brain disorder that damages and destroys brain cells, causing serious problems with memory, thinking, language, and behavior

angina: A feeling of pain and tightness in the chest as the heart is deprived of oxygen

anorexia nervosa: An eating disorder characterized by weight loss, difficulties maintaining an appropriate body weight for height and age, and often a distorted body image

appraisal delay: The delay between when people first experience—and notice—some type of symptoms and when they decide they are ill

approach (vigilant) coping: Changing how one thinks about the problem or venting about the problem to others

archival research: A study design in which researchers use already-recorded behavior.

arteriosclerosis: A condition in which the arteries become thick and stiff, making it difficult for them to expand and contract with the blood pressure and thus leading to a decrease in blood flow to organs and tissues

arthritis: A term referring to over 100 different rheumatic diseases and conditions that affect the joints, the tissues that surround the joints, and other connective tissue

atherosclerosis: A condition in which buildup of fatty substances in the arteries occurs, causing decreases in blood flow and increasing the likelihood of a blood clot

attitudes: A person's positive or negative feelings about engaging in a particular behavior

aversion strategies: Strategies designed to reduce substance abuse by pairing the use of a particular drug with some type of negative stimulus, such as electric shocks, nausea, or unpleasant images

avoidance (minimizing) coping: Denying or avoiding the problem

behavioral genetics: A field that examines the relative impact of genetic factors versus environmental factors on health and behavior

behavioral health: A subdiscipline of behavioral medicine that emphasizes enhancing health and preventing disease in currently healthy people

behavioral medicine: An interdisciplinary field that focuses on the integration of behavioral and biomedical sciences

benefit finding: An ability to find beneficial aspects of an adverse situation

bereavement: A state experienced following the loss of a loved one

bereavement life review: A procedure in which a therapist interviews the bereaved person regarding both their own life experiences and those of the person who died

binge eating disorder: An eating disorder characterized by recurrent episodes of eating large quantities of food (often very quickly and to the point of discomfort), coupled with feeling a loss of control during the binge and experiencing shame, distress, and/or guilt afterward

biobehavioral model: A model proposing that both psychological and physiological factors lead people to continue to smoke

biofeedback: A technique in which people are trained, using electric monitors, to monitor and change selected physiological functions, such as their heart rate, finger temperature, muscle activity, and brain wave patterns

biomedical model: A model proposing that health problems are rooted in physical causes, such as viruses, bacteria, injuries, and biochemical imbalances

biopsychosocial model: A model that views health and illness as the consequences of the complex interplay between biological factors (e.g., genetics, physiology), psychological factors (e.g., personality, cognition), and social factors (e.g., culture, community, family)

body mass index (BMI): A measure of obesity calculated by dividing a person's weight (in kilograms) by the person's height (in meters) and squaring the sum

broaden-and-build theory: A theory that positive emotions broaden people's attention and cognition, which in turn leads to increases in physical, intellectual, social, and psychological resources

buffering hypothesis: A hypothesis proposing that social support provides a buffer from the daily life stress that people experience, which in turn protects them against illness

bulimia nervosa: An eating disorder characterized by repeated cycles of bingeing (eating very large quantities of food) coupled with behaviors to compensate for such eating

burnout: A state of physical and emotional exhaustion

cancer: A disease caused by an uncontrolled division of abnormal cells in a part of the body

carcinogen: Any substance capable of converting normal cells into cancerous ones

cardiovascular disease: Disease that involve the heart and blood vessels

cardiovascular system: A network of body systems that work to transport oxygen to and remove carbon dioxide from each cell and organ in the body; this work is accomplished through the beating of the heart, which generates the necessary force in the bloodstream.

case study: A research technique that relies on studying one or more individuals in great depth to determine the causes of the person's behavior and to predict behavior in others who are similar

central nervous system: A system consisting of the brain and spinal cord

chiropractic therapy: A technique that focuses on manipulating the bones, muscles, and joints to improve body alignment

chronic disease: A disease that persists over time and generally cannot be prevented by vaccines or cured by medication

chronic pain: A type of pain that begins in response to a specific injury or disease) but does not go away after a minimum of six months

classical conditioning: A type of learning that occurs when a previously neutral stimulus comes to evoke the same response as another stimulus with which it is paired.

cognitive dissonance theory: A theory stating that when people's thoughts are inconsistent with their behavior, or two thoughts are in conflict, they experience unpleasant physiological arousal, and in turn will change their behavior or thoughts to restore consistency

complementary or alternative medicine (CAM): A health-promoting product or practice that falls outside traditional medicine

complicated grief: An intense experience of grief, which includes deep yearning, difficulty accepting the death, excessive bitterness, numbness, emptiness, feeling uneasy moving on, and a sense that the future is bleak

conscientiousness: A personality trait in which people are hardworking, motivated, and persistent

contingency-contracting: An operant conditioning–based approach in which people receive some type of a reward for successfully engaging in a behavior

coping: Efforts to manage the stressful demands of a specific situation

coronary heart disease (CHD): A disease in which a waxy substance called plaque builds up inside the coronary arteries

correlation coefficient: A number ranging from −1.00 to +1.00 that indicates the direction and strength of the relationship between two variables

cross-sectional study: A study in which researchers compare people of different ages at the same point in time

dependent variable: The measured outcome of a study

depressants: Drugs that act on the central nervous system to slow down normal bodily activity, causing increases in relaxation and drowsiness

descriptive research: Research in which behavior and/or thoughts are systematically observed (but not manipulated)

detoxification: The process in which a person withdraws completely from the drug he or she is abusing

diabetes: A disorder in which the body is unable to properly convert glucose (sugar) into usable energy

direct effects hypothesis: A hypothesis proposing that having high levels of social support is always advantageous to health

disease model: A model proposing that addiction is caused primarily by internal physiological forces, such as cravings, urges, and compulsions

doctor-centered model: A model of health care decision making in which the doctor is entirely in control and the patient is completely passive

double-blind: A study in which neither the participants nor the experimenter knows which participants are in which condition

dual process model of coping with bereavement: A model proposing that loss involves two distinct types of stressors: loss-oriented stressors (the inherent feelings of grief following the death of a loved one) and restoration-oriented stressors (the acceptance of this person's death)

emotion-focused coping: An approach that focuses on managing one's reaction to stress

endocrine system: A body system that regulates a number of physiological processes in the body (including physical growth, sexual arousal, metabolism, and the stress response) by releasing hormones

epidemiology: A branch of medicine that studies and analyzes the patterns, causes, and effects of health and disease

epigenetics: The study of how non-genetic factors influence whether genes are expressed

euthanasia: A procedure in which a physician acts directly to end a person's life, such as by administering drugs to the patient

exhaustion stage: A stage in the General Adaptation Syndrome (GAS) in which the body's resources are depleted and thus it becomes very susceptible to physiological damage and disease

experiment: A research technique in which participants are randomly assigned to receive one or more independent variables and then measure the impact of these variables on one or more dependent variables

external validity: The degree to which researchers have reasonable confidence that the same results may be obtained using the same experiment for other people and in other situations

fear-based appeals: Messages that use negative stimuli to create the threat of impending danger or harm caused by either engaging in particular types of behavior or failing to engage in other types of behavior

fight-or-flight response: A physiological response to any stressor, characterized by activation of the sympathetic nervous system, that prepares the body to fight or flee

gain-framed messages: Messages that focus on the positive outcomes that can be attained—or the negative outcomes that can be avoided—by adopting a particular type of health-related behavior

gate control theory of pain: A theory describing the experience of pain that states that when body tissues are injured, pain impulses may travel to the brain (and then be experienced as pain) or be stopped by a "gate" (which then reduces the experience of pain)

General Adaptation Syndrome: A model to describe how stress can lead to negative health consequences over time

gratitude: A tendency to appreciate the positive aspects of one's life

grief: Feelings caused by the loss of a loved one

grit: A trait measuring passion and motivation to achieve a longer-term goal

guided imagery: A technique that pairs deep muscle relaxation with a specific pleasant image that serves to focus a patient's mind on something other than the pain

hallucinogens: Drugs that distort perception in some way, creating feelings of relaxation and heightened sensations and causing people to see and hear things that are not really there

hardiness: A personality trait in which people are committed to goals and activities, show a sense of control over what happened to them, and view stressful events as challenging rather than threatening

health: A state of complete physical, mental, and social well-being, and not merely the absence of disease and illness

health action process approach: A stage model predicting that people making changes in their behavior undergo a motivation stage, in which they form an intention to change their behavior, followed by a volition phase, in which they make specific plans to carry out these intentions

health belief model: A model predicting that the likelihood of a person engaging in a behavior is a function of five factors: susceptibility, severity, barriers, benefits, and cues to action

health care proxy: A person who makes medical decisions on behalf of someone if she or he is unable to do so for herself/himself.

health psychology: A field that examines how biological, social, and psychological factors influence health and illness

hospice: A type of care for terminally ill patients that includes medical services, emotional support, and spiritual resources

hostility/disagreeableness: A personality trait characterized by the belief that others are motivated by selfish concerns and will deliberately try to hurt them

human immunodeficiency virus (HIV): A virus spread through body fluids that attacks the body's immune system

hypertension: A condition in which blood pressure is at a consistently high level, increasing the risk of developing CHD

hypnosis: An altered state of consciousness, leading to increased responsiveness, that individuals can experience under the guidance of a trained therapist

hypothalamic-pituitary-adrenal (HPA) axis: A part of the endocrine system that responds during times of stress

hypothesis: A testable prediction about the conditions under which an event will occur

illness behavior: Behavior directed toward determining one's health status after experiencing symptoms

illness delay: The delay between when people acknowledge they are sick and when they decide that help from a professional is required

illness representations: People's beliefs about their illness, including its nature and cause, timeline, consequences, and treatment

immune system: The body system that is the major line of defense against infection, illness, and disease; the immune system works to eliminate foreign ("nonself") materials, such as bacteria, viruses, and parasites, that contact or enter the body

implementation intentions: Specific plans of how, where, and when to perform a behavior

incidence: The frequency of new cases of a disease

independent variable: The factor that is studied to see if and how it will influence attitudes and/or behavior

intentional injuries: Injuries that deliberately harm one's self or someone else

intentional nonadherence: A type of nonadherence in which patients understand the practitioner's directions but modify the regimen in some way or ignore it completely because they are unwilling to follow the recommendations

internal-external hypothesis: A hypothesis proposing that people often fail to listen to internal cues for eating, such as hunger, and instead rely on external cues, such as food taste, smell, and variety

internal locus of control: A personality trait in which people believe that their decisions and behaviors impact their outcomes

internal validity: The degree to which researchers have reasonable confidence that the effects on the dependent variable were caused by the independent variable

intimate partner violence (IPV): Physical, sexual, or psychological aggression that is committed by a current or former romantic partner

lay referral network: A network of friends and family that people rely on to provide insight about health care symptoms and suggested treatment

learning theories: Theories describing behavior as influenced by basic learning processes, such as association, reinforcement, and modeling

leptin: A hormone that decreases appetite and increases energy expenditure

lingering-trajectory deaths: Deaths that occur after a person is ill for a long time and has gradually declining health

living will: An advanced care directive that provides instructions to family members, friends, and medical personnel regarding a person's wishes about the type of care he or she would like to receive in the event of incapacitation and therefore inability to make his or her own decisions

longitudinal study: A study in which a single group of people is followed over time

loss-framed messages: Messages that focus on the negative outcomes that may occur from failing to adopt a particular type of health-related behavior

massage therapy: A technique in which people receive deep-tissue manipulation by a trained therapist

matching hypothesis: A hypothesis proposing that people benefit most from receiving the type of social support that fits their particular problem

medical anthropology: A field that examines the differences in how health and illness are viewed by people in different cultures

medical sociology: A field that examines how social relationships influence illness, cultural and societal reactions to illness, and the organization of health care services

meditation: A technique in which people relax their bodies and focus attention on a single thought, sometimes while verbalizing a single word or thought

meta-analysis: A type of statistical procedure in which researchers combine data from multiple studies to determine overall trends

metabolism: The rate the body uses energy to carry out basic physiological processes, such as respiration, digestion, and blood pressure

mindfulness: A state of concentrated awareness of what is happening in the present moment

morbidity: The number of cases of a specific disease, illness, or health condition

mortality: The number of deaths resulting from a specific cause

mourning: The expression of feelings caused by grief

multiple regulation model: A model proposing that a combination of physiological and psychological factors leads to addiction

myocardial infarction: A complete blockage of the coronary arteries, meaning the heart is deprived of oxygen (also known as a heart attack)

narcotics: Drugs that bind to opioid receptors, reducing feelings of pain and producing feelings of pleasure or euphoria

natural experiments: A method of research in which researchers compare people in two (or more) conditions but have not been able to randomly assign people to those conditions

naturalistic (participant) observation: A study in which researchers observe and record people's behavior in everyday situations and interactions and then systematically measure that behavior in some way

nervous system: The body system responsible for transmitting information between the body and the brain; the nervous system consists of the central nervous system and the peripheral nervous system

neuromatrix theory: A theory positing that a network of neurons is distributed throughout the brain, which processes the information that flows through it, and can process experiences even in the absence of sensations

neurons: Specialized cells that transmit information to and from the brain

neuroticism (negative affect): A personality trait characterized by the tendency to frequently experience negative emotions, such as distress, anxiety, nervousness, fear, shame, anger, and guilt

neurotransmitters: Chemicals that transmit information from one neuron to another neuron

nicotine fixed-effect model: A model proposing that nicotine stimulates reward-inducing centers in the nervous system

nicotine regulation model: A model proposing that smoking is rewarding only when the level of nicotine is above a certain "set point" in the body nicotine replacement

nicotine-replacement therapy: A pharmacological treatment for quitting

smoking that involves providing nicotine in some other way

nonsuicidal self-injury: The deliberate, self-inflicted destruction of body tissue resulting in immediate damage, without suicidal intent and for purposes not culturally sanctioned

obesity: A weight greater than what is generally considered healthy for a given height, which is calculated in terms of having a BMI greater than 30 (about 40% over ideal weight)

operant conditioning: A theory of learning proposing that behaviors can be increased or decreased as a function of the consequences of engaging in them

optimism: A personality trait characterized by the expectation that good things will happen in the future and bad things will not

outcome expectancies: Beliefs about the consequences of engaging in a particular behavior

overweight: A weight greater than what is generally considered healthy for a given height, which is calculated in terms of having a BMI of 25 to 29.9 (about 15% to 30% over ideal weight)

pain: An unpleasant sensory and emotional experience caused by actual or potential tissue damage

palliative care: Care focused on managing pain

passive strategies: Approaches to injury prevention that change people's environment.

patient-centered model: A model of health care decision making in which both the patient and the practitioner share information and make decisions together.

pattern theory: A theory that describes pain as resulting from the type of stimulation received by the nerve endings

perceived behavioral control: The extent to which a person believes that he or she can successfully enact a behavior

peripheral nervous system: A part of the nervous system consisting of the neural pathways that bring information to and from the brain; the peripheral nervous system includes the somatic nervous system and the autonomic nervous system

personality: Basic characteristics of the person that are relatively stable across situations and over time

physical stimulation (counterirritation): A technique involving irritating body tissue to ease pain

physician-assisted suicide: A procedure in which a physician provides a person with the means to die (typically through prescription drugs)

placebo: A neutral treatment added to a research study as a way of controlling for the effects caused by a person's expectations

placebo: A treatment that affects someone even though it contains no specific medical or physical properties relevant to the condition it is supposedly treating

poison: Any substance that can be harmful to your health if too much of that substance is taken into your body via any mechanism

positive psychology: A field that examines how psychological factors influence positive human functioning and flourishing

positive states: Conditions in which people experience positive emotions, such as happiness, joy, enthusiasm, and contentment

posttraumatic growth: Experiencing significant positive changes after struggling with a major life crisis

posttraumatic stress disorder (PTSD): A type of anxiety disorder caused by experiencing extreme stressors, such as war, natural disasters, and assault

precaution adoption process model: A model proposing that people go through a series of seven stages when attempting to change a behavior

prevalence: The proportion of a population that has a particular disease

primary appraisal: The first stage of the transactional model, in which people assess the situation and what it will mean for them

primary prevention: Behavior that involves preventing or diminishing the severity of illnesses and diseases

problem-focused coping: An approach that focuses on dealing directly with the source of the stress and trying to reduce its impact

progressive muscle relaxation: A technique for managing stress in which people focus on consciously tensing and then releasing each part of their body (hands, shoulders, legs, etc.) one at a time

prospective study: A study in which researchers compare people with a given characteristic to those without it to see whether these groups differ in their development of a disease

psychoneuroimmunology: A field examining the connection between psychosocial factors, such as stress, and different body systems, including the nervous, cardiovascular, endocrine, and immune systems

psychosomatic medicine: A field that studies how emotional, social, and psychological factors influence the development and progression of illness

qualitative research: A method of research that focuses on understanding and interpreting behavior in a natural setting,

quality-adjusted life years (QALY): A measure of the quality of a person's life as determined both by the severity of their symptoms and their duration

quasi-experiment: A study in which there are distinct groups of people in different conditions, but unlike in true experiments, the people were not randomly assigned to the groups

quick-trajectory deaths: Deaths in which the loss was sudden and unanticipated

random assignment: A research technique in which every participant has an equal chance of being subjected to either of the conditions

randomized controlled trial (RCT): A research technique designed to test the effectiveness of different drugs or treatments; uses random assignment to conditions

relapse: Returning to an unwanted behavior after beginning to change it

religiosity: A formal link to religious organizations

reserve capacity model: A model proposing that people living in lower socioeconomic circumstances experience more frequent stressful situations and have a smaller supply of resources to manage these situations

resilience: A character strength that allows an individual to grow and even thrive in the face of adversity

resistance stage: The second stage of the General Adaptation Syndrome (GAS) in which the body continues to respond to the threat

response substitution: A strategy in which people choose another way to handle situations that lead them to want to engage in substance use

restraint theory: A theory stating that when people ignore internal physiological signals for hunger and instead use cognitive rules to limit their caloric intake, if self-control processes are undermined in some way, overeating may occur

retrospective study: A study in which researchers examine differences in a group after a disease has occurred and attempt to look back over time to examine what factors might have led to the development of the disease

scheduling delay: The delay between when people schedule an appointment and actually go to the appointment

scientific method: A method researchers use to describe a phenomenon, make predictions about it, and explain why it happens

screening: Tests that look for signs of disease before symptoms have developed

secondary appraisal: The second stage of the transactional model in which people assess the resources available for coping with the situation

secondary prevention: Behavior that involves detecting illness at an early stage as a way of reducing the illness's potential effects

self-compassion: A tendency to treat oneself with kindness and compassion

self-efficacy: A person's confidence that he or she can effectively engage in a behavior

set-point theory: A theory that each person's body has a certain weight that it strives to maintain; thus, when a person eats fewer calories, his or her metabolism slows to maintain weight at the same level

sick-role behavior: Behavior that is directed at helping people who are ill return to good health

social cognitive theory: A theory describing how people's behavior is influenced by observing other people engaging in such behavior and seeing the outcomes these people experience from such behavior, as well as by their own confidence that they could engage in that behavior

social learning theory: A theory that children learn attitudes and behaviors by watching others, including their parents, siblings, and peers

social support: General help that people may receive, or perceive they receive, from others

specificity theory: A theory positing that specific sensory receptors process different types of sensations, such as pain, warmth, touch, and pressure.

spirituality: A personal orientation toward religious beliefs

stages of death and dying: A model proposing that terminally ill people go through a series of five distinct stages: denial, anger, bargaining, depression, acceptance

stages of delay model: A model describing the steps people go through when deciding to get help

stimulants: Drugs that create physiological arousal, leading to increases in energy and alertness

stimulus control: A strategy in which people avoid situations that lead them to want to engage in substance use

stress: The process by which we perceive and respond to stressors.

stress management: Behavioral and cognitive strategies for reducing reactions to stress

stress reactivity hypothesis: A hypothesis proposing that people who recover more quickly from stress are less at risk of developing a stress-related illness than those who take longer to recover

stressor: Any type of physically or psychologically challenging event or situation

stroke: A condition in which a blood vessel that carries oxygen and nutrients to the brain is either blocked by a clot or bursts (or ruptures), which deprives the brain of blood and oxygen

subjective norms: Individuals' beliefs about whether other people would support them in engaging in a new behavior and whether they are motivated to follow the beliefs of these salient others

suicide contagion: Increases in suicide attempts resulting from exposure to suicide or suicidal behaviors within one's family, one's peer group, or through the media

survey: A research technique in which people are asked about their thoughts, feelings, desires, and actions and their answers are recorded

sympathetic adrenomedullary (SAM) system: A part of the nervous system that responds during times of stress

systematic desensitization: A technique in which a person describes the specific source of his or her anxiety, and then creates a hierarchy of different stimuli (which cause increasing levels of arousal) associated with that anxiety

task work approach: A model proposing that people who are terminally ill focus on four distinct types of tasks (physical, psychological, social, spiritual)

tend-and-befriend: A pattern in which the response to stress is to affiliate with other people

tension-reduction theory: A theory positing that people drink alcohol to cope with or regulate negative moods, including feelings of tension, anxiety, and nervousness

tertiary prevention: Behavior taken to minimize or slow the damage caused by an illness or disease

theory: An organized set of principles used to explain observed phenomena

theory of planned behavior: A theory describing the role of attitudes, subjective norms, and perceived behavioral control in leading to intentions, which in turn lead to behavior

theory of reasoned action: A theory describing the role of attitudes and subjective norms in leading to intentions, which in turn lead to behavior

tolerance: A state in which one's body no longer responds at the same level to a particular dose of a substance but rather needs larger and larger doses to experience the same effects

transactional (relational) model: A model predicting that the meaning a particular event has for a person is a more important predictor of the experience of stress than the actual event

transcutaneous electrical nerve stimulation (TENS): A technique of pain reduction involving placing electrodes on the skin and administering continuous electrical stimulation

transtheoretical (stages of change) model: A model describing the five stages (precontemplation, contemplation, preparation, action, maintenance) that people go through as they attempt to change a behavior

treatment delay: The delay between receiving medical recommendations and acting on these recommendations

Type A behavior: A behavior pattern characterized by time urgency, competitive drive, anger, and hostility

unintentional injuries: Injuries that people do not mean to occur

unintentional nonadherence: A type of nonadherence in which people intend to comply, and may even believe they are complying, but for some reason are not following instructions

utilization (behavioral) delay: The delay between when people decide that medical care is required and when they make an appointment to see a professional

withdrawal: Undesirable symptoms that occur when a person discontinues use of a particular substance

REFERENCES

Abar, B. W., Turrisi, R., Hillhouse, J., Loken, E., Stapleton, J., & Gunn, H. (2010). Preventing skin cancer in college females: Heterogeneous effects over time. *Health Psychology, 29*(6), 574–582. **doi:10.1037/a0021236**

Abbasi, A., Juszczyk, D., Jaarsveld, C. H., & Gulliford, M. C. (2017). Body mass index and incident type 1 and type 2 diabetes in children and young adults: A retrospective cohort study. *Journal of the Endocrine Society, 1*(5), 524–537. **doi:10.1210/js.2017-00044**

Abel, E. L., & Kruger, M. L. (2010). Smile intensity in photographs predicts longevity. *Psychological Science, 21*(4), 542–544. **doi:10.1177/0956797610363775**

Aboa-Éboulé, C., Brisson, C., Maunsell, E., Mâsse, B., Bourbonnais, R., Vézina, M., . . . Dagenais, G. R. (2007). Job strain and risk of acute recurrent coronary heart disease events. *Journal of the American Medical Association, 298*(14), 1652–1660. **https://doi.org/10.1001/jama.298.14.1652**

Abraham, C., & Sheeran, P. (2015). The health belief model. In M. Conner & P. Norman (Eds.), *Predicting health behavior* (3rd ed., pp. 30–69). New York, NY: McGraw-Hill.

Abraído-Lanza, A. F., Chao, M. T., & Flórez, K. R. (2005). Do healthy behaviors decline with greater acculturation?: Implications for the Latino mortality paradox. *Social Science & Medicine (1982), 61*(6), 1243–1255.

Abraído-Lanza, A. F., & Revenson, T. A. (1996). Coping and social support resources among Latinas with arthritis. *Arthritis & Rheumatism, 9*, 501–508. **doi:10.1002/art.1790090612**

Abramson, L. Y., Metalsky, G. I., & Alloy, L. B. (1989). Hopelessness depression: A theory-based subtype of depression. *Psychological Review, 96*(2), 358–372.

Acciai, F., Noah, A. J., & Firebaugh, G. (2015). Pinpointing the sources of the Asian mortality advantage in the United States. *Journal of Epidemiology and Community Health, 69*(10), 1006–1011. **http://doi.org/10.1136/jech-2015-205623**

Accurso, E. C., Fitzsimmons-Craft, E. E., Ciao, A., Cao, L., Crosby, R. D., Smith, T. L., . . . Peterson, C. B. (2015). Therapeutic alliance in a randomized clinical trial for bulimia nervosa. *Journal of Consulting and Clinical Psychology, 83*(3), 637–642.

Accurso, E. C., Wonderlich, S. A., Crosby, R. D., Smith, T. L., Klein, M. H., Mitchell, J. E., . . . Peterson, C. B. (2016). Predictors and moderators of treatment outcome in a randomized clinical trial for adults with symptoms of bulimia nervosa. *Journal of Consulting and Clinical Psychology, 84*(2), 178–184.

Adams, K. B. (2008). Specific effects of caring for a spouse with dementia: Differences in depressive symptoms between caregiver and non-caregiver spouses. *International Psychogeriatrics, 20*(3), 508–520. **doi:10.1017/s1041610207006278**

Adams, S. S., Eberhard-Gran, M., & Eskild, A. (2012). Fear of childbirth and duration of labour: A study of 2206 women with intended vaginal delivery. *BJOG: An International Journal of Obstetrics & Gynaecology, 119*(10), 1238–1246.

Addis, M. E., & Mahalik, J. R. (2003). Men, masculinity, and the contexts of help seeking. *American Psychologist, 58*(1), 5–14.

Adelman, H. S., & Taylor, L. (2003). Creating school and community partnerships for substance abuse prevention programs. *The Journal of Primary Prevention, 23*(3), 329–369. **doi:10.1023/A:1021345808902**

Ader, R., & Cohen, N. (1975). Behaviorally conditioned immunosuppression. *Psychosomatic Medicine, 37*(4), 333–340.

Ader, R., & Cohen, N. (1985). CNS–immune system interactions: Conditioning phenomena. *Behavioral and Brain Sciences, 8*(3), 379–395.

Ader, R., & Robert, A. (1996). Psychoneuroimmunology: Animal models of disease. *Psychosomatic Medicine, 58*(6), 546–558.

Adler, N. E., Boyce, T., Chesney, M. A., Cohen, S., Folkman, S., Kahn, R. L., & Syme, S. L. (1994). Socioeconomic status and health: The challenge of the gradient. *American Psychologist, 49*(1), 15–24.

Adler, N. E., Boyce, W. T., Chesney, M. A., Folkman, S., & Syme, S. L. (1993). Socioeconomic inequalities in health: No easy solution. *Journal of the American Medical Association, 269*(24), 3140–3145.

Adler, N. E., & Stone, G. C. (1979). Social science perspectives on the health system. In G. C. Stone, F. Cohen, & N. E. Adler (Eds.), *Health psychology: A handbook* (pp. 19–46). San Francisco, CA: Jossey-Bass.

Adler, N., & Matthews, K. (1994). Health psychology: Why do some people get sick and some stay well? *Annual Review of Psychology, 45*(1), 229–259.

Adler, R. (2001). Psychoneuroimmunology. *Current Directions in Psychological Science, 10*, 94–98.

Adriaanse, M. A., de Ridder, D. T., & de Wit, J. B. (2009). Finding the critical cue: Implementation intentions to change one's diet work best when tailored to personally relevant reasons for unhealthy eating. *Personality and Social Psychology Bulletin, 35*(1), 60–71.

Affleck, G., Tennen, H., Urrows, S., & Higgins, P. (1992). Neuroticism and the pain-mood relation in rheumatoid arthritis: Insights from a prospective daily study. *Journal of Consulting and Clinical Psychology, 60*(1), 119–126.

Afshin, A., Peñalvo, J. L., Del Gobbo, L., Silva, J., Michaelson, M., O'Flaherty, M., . . . Mozaffarian, D. (2017). The prospective impact of food pricing on improving dietary consumption: A systematic review and meta-analysis. *PLOS ONE, 12*(3), e0172277.

Agras, W. S. (1993) Short-term psychological treatments for binge eating. In C. G. Fairburn & G. T. Wilson (Eds.), *Binge eating* (pp. 270–286). London, UK: Guilford Press.

Agras, W. S., Taylor, C. B., Kraemer, H. C., Southam, M. A., & Schneider, J. A. (1987). Relaxation training for essential hypertension at the worksite: II. The poorly controlled hypertensive. *Psychosomatic Medicine, 49*(3), 264–273.

Ai, A. L., Park, C. L., Huang, B., Rodgers, W., & Tice, T. N. (2007). Psychosocial mediation of religious coping styles: A study of short-term psychological distress following cardiac surgery. *Personality & Social Psychology Bulletin, 33*(6), 867–882.

Aiken, L. H., Clarke, S. P., Sloane, D. M., Sochalski, J., & Silber, J. H. (2002). Hospital nurse staffing and patient mortality, nurse burnout, and job dissatisfaction. *Journal of the American Medical Association, 288*, 1987–1993.

Aiken, L. R. (1985). *Dying, death, and bereavement*. Boston, MA: Allyn and Bacon.

Aiken, L. S., West, S. G., Woodward, C. K., & Reno, R. R. (1994). Health beliefs and compliance with mammography-screening recommendations in asymptomatic women. *Health Psychology, 13*(2), 122–129.

Aizer, A. A., Chen, M.-H., McCarthy, E. P., Mendu, M. L., Koo, S., Wilhite, T. J., . . . Nguyen, P. L. (2013). Marital status and survival in patients with cancer. *Journal of Clinical Oncology, 31*(31), 3869–3876. **https://doi .org/10.1200/JCO.2013.49.6489**

Ajzen, I. (1985). From intentions to actions: A theory of planned behavior. In J. Kuhl & J. Beckman (Eds.), *Action control: From cognition to behavior* (pp. 11–39). Berlin, DE: Springer.

Ajzen, I. (1991). The theory of planned behavior. *Organizational Behavior and Human Decision Processes, 50*(2), 179–211.

Akhter, S., Marcus, M., Kerber, R. A., Kong, M., & Taylor, K. C. (2016). The impact of periconceptional maternal stress on fecundability. *Annals of Epidemiology, 26*(10), 710–716.

Al Khatib, H. K., Harding, S. V., Darzi, J., & Pot, G. K. (2017). The effects of partial sleep deprivation on energy balance: A systematic review and meta-analysis. *European Journal of Clinical Nutrition, 71*(5), 614–624.

Alabas, O. A., Hall, M., Dondo, T. B., Rutherford, M. J., Timmis, A. D., Batin, P. D., . . . Gale, C. P. (2016). Long-term excess mortality associated with diabetes following acute myocardial infarction: A population-based cohort study. *Journal of Epidemiology and Community Health, 71*(1), 25–32. **doi:10.1136/jech-2016-207402**

Albarracín, D., Johnson, B. T., Fishbein, M., & Muellerleile, P. A. (2001). Theories of reasoned action and planned behavior as models of condom use: A meta-analysis. *Psychological Bulletin, 127*(1), 142–161.

Albert, C. M., Hennekens, C. H., O'Donnell, C. J., Ajani, U. A., Carey, V. J., Willett, W. C., . . . Manson, J. E. (1998). Fish consumption and risk of sudden cardiac death. *Journal of the American Medical Association, 279*, 23–28.

Albuquerque, D., Manco, L., & Nóbrega, C. (2016). Genetics of human obesity. In S. Ahmad & S. Imam (Eds.), *Obesity: A practical guide* (pp. 87–106). Cham: Springer. **doi:10.1007/978-3-319-19821-7_7**

Albuquerque, D., Stice, E., Rodriguez-Lopez, R., Manco, L., & Nobrega, C. (2015). Current review of genetics of human obesity: From molecular mechanisms to an evolutionary perspective. *Molecular Genetics and Genomics, 290*(4), 1191–1221.

Alcoholics Anonymous World Services. (1977). *Alcoholics anonymous: The twelve steps and twelve traditions* (3rd ed.). New York, NY: Author.

Alden, D. L., Friend, J. M., Lee, A. Y., de Vries, M., Osawa, R., & Chen, Q. (2015). Culture and medical decision making: Healthcare consumer perspectives in Japan and the United States. *Health Psychology, 34*(12), 1133–1144. **doi:10.1037/hea0000229**

Aldwin, C. M., Jeong, Y., Igarashi, H., Choun, S., & Spiro, I. A. (2014). Do hassles mediate between life events and mortality in older men? Longitudinal findings from the VA Normative Aging Study. *Experimental Gerontology, 59*(Special Issue: Stress and Aging), 74–80. **doi:10.1016/j .exger.2014.06.019**

Aldwin, C. M., Park, C. L., Jeong, Y. J., & Nath, R. (2014). Differing pathways between religiousness, spirituality, and health: A self-regulation perspective. *Psychology of Religion and Spirituality, 6*(1), 9–21.

Alegria, M., Woo, M., Cao, Z., Torres, M., Meng, X., & Striegel-Moore, R. (2007). Prevalence and correlates of eating disorders in Latinos in the U.S. *The International Journal of Eating Disorders, 40*(Suppl), S15–S21. **http:// doi.org/10.1002/eat.20406**

Alferi, S. M., Carver, C. S., Antoni, M. H., Weiss, S., & Duran, R. E. (2001). An exploratory study of social support, distress, and life disruption among low-income Hispanic women under treatment for early stage breast cancer. *Health Psychology, 20*, 41–46.

Alford, D. P., German, J. S., Samet, J. H., Cheng, D. M., Lloyd-Travaglini, C. A., & Saitz, R. (2016). Primary care patients with drug use report chronic pain and self-medicate with alcohol and other drugs. *Journal of General Internal Medicine, 31*(5), 486–491. **https://doi.org/10.1007/s11606-016-3586-5**

Allem, J. P., Leas, E. C., Caputi, T. L., Dredze, M., Althouse, B. M., Noar, S. M., & Ayers, J. W. (2017). The Charlie Sheen effect on rapid in-home human immunodeficiency virus test sales. *Prevention Science, 18*(5), 541–544. **https://doi.org/10.1007/s11121-017-0792-2**

Allen, A. B., & Leary, M. R. (2010). Self-compassion, stress, and coping. *Social and Personality Psychology Compass, 4*(2), 107–118. **http://doi.org/10.1111/j.1751-9004.2009.00246.x**

Allen, J. P., Uchino, B. N., & Hafen, C. A. (2015). Running with the pack: Teen peer-relationship qualities as predictors of adult physical health. *Psychological Science, 26*(10), 1574–1583.

Allen, K., Blascovich, J., & Mendes, W. B. (2002). Cardiovascular reactivity and the presence of pets, friends, and spouses: The truth about cats and dogs. *Psychosomatic Medicine, 64*(5), 727–739.

Allen, K. L., Byrne, S. M., & Crosby, R. D. (2014). Distinguishing between risk factors for bulimia nervosa, binge eating disorder, and purging disorder. *Journal of Youth and Adolescence, 44*(8), 1580–1591.

Allen, N. E., Beral, V., Casabonne, D., Kan, S. W., Reeves, G. K., Brown, A., & Green, J. (2009). Moderate alcohol intake and cancer incidence in women. *Journal of the National Cancer Institute, 101*(5), 296–305. **https://doi.org/10.1093/jnci/djn514**

Allison, D. B., & Faith, M. S. (1997). Issues in mapping genes for eating disorders. *Psychopharmacology Bulletin, 33*(3), 359–368.

Aloise-Young, P. A., Hennigan, K. M., & Graham, J. W. (1996). Role of the self-image and smoker stereotype in smoking onset during early adolescence: A longitudinal study. *Health Psychology, 15*(6), 494–497.

Alonzo, D., Thompson, R. G., Stohl, M., & Hasin, D. (2014). The influence of parental divorce and alcohol abuse on adult offspring risk of lifetime suicide attempt in the United States. *American Journal of Orthopsychiatry, 84*(3), 316–320.

Alvanzo, A. A., Wand, G. S., Kuwabara, H., Wong, D. F., Xu, X., & McCaul, M. E. (2015). Family history of alcoholism is related to increased D2/D3 receptor binding potential: A marker of resilience or risk? *Addiction Biology, 22*(1), 218–228.

Alzheimer's Association. (2016). 2016 Alzheimer's disease facts and figures. *Alzheimer's & Dementia, 12*(4), 459–509.

Amaro, H. (1995). Love, sex, and power: Considering women's realities in HIV prevention. *American Psychologist, 50*(6), 437–447.

American Foundation for Suicide Prevention. (2017). Suicide statistics. Retrieved from **https://afsp.org/about-suicide/suicide-statistics/**

American Psychiatric Association. (2013). *Diagnostic and statistical manual of mental disorders* (5th ed.). Arlington, VA: American Psychiatric Publishing.

American Psychological Association. (2017). *Stress in America: Coping with change. Stress in America™ Survey.* Washington, DC: American Psychological Association.

American Psychological Association, Task Force on Health Research. (1976). Contributions of psychology to health research: Patterns, problems, and potentials. *American Psychologist, 31*, 263–274.

Ameringer, K. J., Chou, C. P., & Leventhal, A. M. (2015). Shared versus specific features of psychological symptoms and cigarettes per day: Structural relations and mediation by negative- and positive-reinforcement smoking. *Journal of Behavioral Medicine, 38*(2), 224–236.

Anand, K. J., & Craig, K. D. (1996). New perspectives on the definition of pain. *Pain, 67*, 3–6.

Anand, P., Kunnumakara, A. B., Sundaram, C., Harikumar, K. B., Tharakan, S. T., Lai, O. S., . . . Aggarwal, B. B. (2008). Cancer is a preventable disease that requires major lifestyle changes. *Pharmaceutical Research, 25*(9), 2097–2116. **https://doi.org/10.1007/s11095-008-9661-9**

Anda, R. F., Williamson, D. F., Escobedo, L. G., Mast, E. E., Giovino, G. A., & Remington, P. L. (1990). Depression and the dynamics of smoking: A national perspective. *Journal of the American Medical Association, 264*(12), 1541–1545.

Andersen, A. E., & DiDomenico, L. (1992). Diet vs. shape content of popular male and female magazines: A dose-response relationship to the incidence of eating disorders? *International Journal of Eating Disorders, 11*(3), 283–287.

Andersen, B. L., Cacioppo, J. T., & Roberts, D. C. (1995). Delay in seeking a cancer diagnosis: Delay stages and psychophysiological comparison processes. *British Journal of Social Psychology, 34*(1), 33–52.

Andersen, B. L., Thornton, L. M., Shapiro, C. L., Farrar, W. B., Mundy, B. L., Yang, H.-C., & Carson, W. E. (2010). Biobehavioral, immune, and health benefits following recurrence for psychological intervention participants. *Clinical Cancer Research: An Official Journal of the American Association for Cancer Research, 16*(12), 3270–3278. **http://doi.org/10.1158/1078-0432.CCR-10-0278**

Andersen, B. L., Yang, H.-C., Farrar, W. B., Golden-Kreutz, D. M., Emery, C. F., Thornton, L. M., . . . Carson, W. E. (2008). Psychologic intervention improves survival for breast cancer patients. *Cancer, 113*(12), 3450–3458. **https://doi.org/10.1002/cncr.23969**

Andersen, M. R., Bowen, D. J., Morea, J., Stein, K. D., & Baker, F. (2009). Involvement in decision-making and breast cancer survivor quality of life. *Health Psychology, 28*(1), 29–37. **doi:10.1037/0278-6133.28.1.29**

Andersen, R. E., Crespo, C. J., Bartlett, S. J., Cheskin, L. J., & Pratt, M. (1998). Relationship of physical activity and television watching with body weight and level of fatness among children: Results from the Third National Health and Nutrition Examination Survey. *Journal of the American Medical Association, 279*(12), 938–942.

Andersen, R. E., Franckowiak, S. C., Snyder, J., Bartlett, S. J., & Fontaine, K. R. (1998). Can inexpensive signs encourage the use of stairs? Results from a community intervention. *Annals of Internal Medicine, 129*(5), 363–369.

Andersen, R. E., Wadden, T. A., Bartlett, S. J., Zemel, B., Verde, T. J., & Franckowiak, S. C. (1999). Effects of lifestyle activity vs structured aerobic exercise in obese women: A randomized trial. *Journal of the American Medical Association, 281*(4), 335–340.

Anderson, E. A. (1987). Preoperative preparation for cardiac surgery facilitates recovery, reduces psychological distress, and reduces the incidence of acute postoperative hypertension. *Journal of Consulting and Clinical Psychology, 55,* 513–520.

Anderson, E. S., Wojcik, J. R., Winett, R. A., & Williams, D. M. (2006). Social-cognitive determinants of physical activity: The influence of social support, self-efficacy, outcome expectations, and self-regulation among participants in a church-based health promotion study. *Health Psychology, 25*(4), 510–520.

Anderson, J. L., Crawford, C. B., Nadeau, J., & Lindberg, T. (1992). Was the Duchess of Windsor right? A cross-cultural review of the socioecology of ideals of female body shape. *Ethology and Sociobiology, 13*(3), 197–227.

Anderson, N. B., & Armstead, C. A. (1995). Toward understanding the association of socioeconomic status and health: A new challenge for the biopsychosocial approach. *Psychosomatic Medicine, 57*(3), 213–225.

Anderson, S. E., Andridge, R., & Whitaker, R. C. (2016). Bedtime in preschool-aged children and risk for adolescent obesity. *The Journal of Pediatrics, 176,* 17–22.

Ando, M., Marquez-Wong, F., Simon, G. B., Kira, H., & Becker, C. (2015). Bereavement life review improves spiritual well-being and ameliorates depression among American caregivers. *Palliative and Supportive Care, 13*(2), 319–325. **https://doi.org/10.1017/S1478951514000030**

Anestis, M. D., Khazem, L. R., Law, K. C., Houtsma, C., LeTard, R., Moberg, F., & Martin, R. (2015). The association between state laws regulating handgun ownership and statewide suicide rates. *American Journal of Public Health, 105*(10), 2059–2067.

Angoff, N. R. (2001). Crying in the curriculum. *Journal of the American Medical Association, 286,* 1017–1018.

Annas, G. J. (1991). The health care proxy and the living will. *New England Journal of Medicine, 324,* 1210–1213. **doi:10.1056/NEJM199104253241711**

Antoni, M. H., Cruess, D. G., Cruess, S., Lutgendorf, S., Kumar, M., Ironson, G., . . . Schneiderman, N. (2000). Cognitive-behavioral stress management intervention effects on anxiety, 24-hr urinary norepinephrine output, and T-cytotoxic/suppressor cells over time among symptomatic HIV-infected gay men. *Journal of Consulting and Clinical Psychology, 68*(1), 31–45.

Antoni, M. H., Lehman, J. M., Kilbourn, K. M., Boyers, A. E., Culver, J. L., Alferi, S. M., . . . Carver, C. S. (2001). Cognitive-behavioral stress management intervention decreases the prevalence of depression and enhances benefit finding among women under treatment for early-stage breast cancer. *Health Psychology, 20,* 20–32.

Antoni, M. H., & Lutgendorf, S. (2007). Psychosocial factors and disease progression in cancer. *Current Directions in Psychological Science, 16*(1), 42–46.

Antonovsky, A. (1987). *Unraveling the mystery of health: How people manage stress and stay well.* San Francisco, CA: Jossey-Bass.

Apovian, C. M., Aronne, L. J., Bessesen, D. H., McDonnell, M. E., Murad, M. H., Pagotto, U., . . . Still, C. D. (2015). Pharmacological management of obesity: An Endocrine Society clinical practice guideline. *The Journal of Clinical Endocrinology & Metabolism, 100*(2), 342–362.

Appel, C. W., Johansen, C., Christensen, J., Frederiksen, K., Hjalgrim, H., Dalton, S. O., . . . Dyregrov, A. (2016). Risk of use of antidepressants among children and young adults exposed to the death of a parent. *Epidemiology, 27*(4), 578–585. **https://doi.org/doi:10.1097/EDE.0000000000000481**

Arena, J. G., & Blanchard, E. B. (1996). Biofeedback and relaxation therapy for chronic pain disorders. In R. J. Gatchel & D. C. Turk (Eds.), *Psychological approaches to pain management: A practitioner's handbook* (pp. 179–230). New York, NY: Guilford.

Armitage, C. J. (2004). Evidence that implementation intentions reduce dietary fat intake: A randomized trial. *Health Psychology, 23*(3), 319–323.

Armitage, C. J. (2009). Effectiveness of experimenter-provided and self-generated implementation intentions to reduce alcohol consumption in a sample of the general population: A randomized exploratory trial. *Health Psychology, 28*(5), 545–553.

Armitage, C. J. (2015). Randomized test of a brief psychological intervention to reduce and prevent emotional eating in a community sample. *Journal of Public Health, 37*(3), 438–444.

Armitage, C. J., & Arden, M. A. (2008). How useful are the stages of change for targeting interventions? Randomized test of a brief intervention to reduce smoking. *Health Psychology, 27*(6), 789–798. **doi:10.1037/0278-6133.27.6.789**

Arnow, B., Kenardy, J., & Agras, W. S. (1995). The Emotional Eating Scale: The development of a measure to assess coping with negative affect by eating. *International Journal of Eating Disorders*, *18*(1), 79–90.

Aronoff, G. M., Wagner, J. M., & Spangler, A. S. (1986). Chemical interventions for pain. *Journal of Consulting and Clinical Psychology*, *54*, 769–775.

Arsenault-Lapierre, G., Kim, C., & Turecki, G. (2004). Psychiatric diagnoses in 3275 suicides: A meta-analysis. *BMC Psychiatry*, *4*(1), 37.

Ary, D. V., & Biglan, A. (1988). Longitudinal changes in adolescent cigarette smoking behavior: Onset and cessation. *Journal of Behavioral Medicine*, *11*(4), 361–382.

Aseltine, R. H., Jr., & DeMartino, R. (2004). An outcome evaluation of the SOS suicide prevention program. *American Journal of Public Health*, *94*(3), 446–451.

Ashley, M. J., & Rankin, J. G. (1988). A public health approach to the prevention of alcohol-related health problems. *Annual Review of Public Health*, *9*(1), 233–271.

Ashton, E., Vosvick, M., Chesney, M., Gore-Felton, C., Koopman, C., O'shea, K., . . . Spiegel, D. (2005). Social support and maladaptive coping as predictors of the change in physical health symptoms among persons living with HIV/AIDS. *AIDS Patient Care & STDs*, *19*(9), 587–598.

Aspinwall, L. G., & Taylor, S. E. (1997). A stitch in time: Self-regulation and proactive coping. *Psychological Bulletin*, *121*(3), 417–436.

Atkins, C. J., Kaplan, R. M., Timms, R. M., Reinsch, S., & Lofback, K. (1984). Behavioral exercise programs in the management of chronic obstructive pulmonary disease. *Journal of Consulting and Clinical Psychology*, *52*(4), 591–603.

Audrain-McGovern, J., Rodriguez, D., Patel, V., Faith, M. S., Rodgers, K., &

Cuevas, J. (2006). How do psychological factors influence adolescent smoking progression? The evidence for indirect effects through tobacco advertising receptivity. *Pediatrics*, *117*(4), 1216–1225.

Ayanian, J. Z., & Epstein, A. M. (1991). Differences in the use of procedures between women and men hospitalized for coronary heart disease. *New England Journal of Medicine*, *325*(4), 221–225.

Ayers, J. W., Althouse, B. M., Dredze, M., Leas, E. C., & Noar, S. M. (2016). News and internet searches about human immunodeficiency virus after Charlie Sheen's disclosure. *JAMA Internal Medicine*, *176*(4), 552–554.

Baams, L., Grossman, A. H., & Russell, S. T. (2015). Minority stress and mechanisms of risk for depression and suicidal ideation among lesbian, gay, and bisexual youth. *Developmental Psychology*, *51*(5), 688–696.

Baan, R., Straif, K., Grosse, Y., Secretan, B., El Ghissassi, F., Bouvard, V., . . . Cogliano, V. (2007). Carcinogenicity of alcoholic beverages. *Lancet Oncology*, *8*(4), 292–293.

Babb, S., Malarcher, A., Schauer, G., Asman, K., & Jamal, A. (2017). Quitting smoking among adults—United States, 2000–2015. *Morbidity and Mortality Weekly Report*, *65*, 1457–1464. http://dx.doi.org/10.15585/mmwr.mm6552a1

Bąbel, P. (2016). Memory of pain induced by physical exercise. *Memory*, *24*(4), 548–559. https://doi.org/10.1080/09658211.2015.1023809

Bach, P. B., Cramer, L. D., Warren, J. L., & Begg, C. B. (1999). Racial differences in the treatment of early-stage lung cancer. *New England Journal of Medicine*, *341*(16), 1198–1205.

Bachiocco, V., Scesi, M., Morselli, A. M., & Carli, G. (1993). Individual pain history and familial pain tolerance models: Relationships to postsurgical pain. *Clinical Journal of Pain*, *9*, 266–271.

Badr, H., Carmack, C. L., Kashy, D. A., Cristofanilli, M., & Revenson, T. A. (2010). Dyadic coping in metastatic breast cancer. *Health Psychology*, *29*(2), 169–180.

Badr, H., & Carmack Taylor, C. L. (2009). Sexual dysfunction and spousal communication in couples coping with prostate cancer. *Psycho-Oncology*, *18*(7), 735–746. https://doi.org/10.1002/pon.1449

Badr, H., & Taylor, C. L. C. (2008). Effects of relationship maintenance on psychological distress and dyadic adjustment among couples coping with lung cancer. *Health Psychology*, *27*(5), 616–627. doi:10.1037/0278-6133.27.5.616

Baek, R. N., Tanenbaum, M. L., & Gonzalez, J. S. (2014). Diabetes burden and diabetes distress: The buffering effect of social support. *Annals of Behavioral Medicine*, *48*(2), 145–155.

Baer, J. S., & Carney, M. M. (1993). Biases in the perceptions of the consequences of alcohol use among college students. *Journal of Studies on Alcohol*, *54*(1), 54–60.

Baer, J. S., Stacy, A., & Larimer, M. (1991). Biases in the perception of drinking norms among college students. *Journal of Studies on Alcohol*, *52*(6), 580–586.

Bailey, J. E., Kellermann, A. L., Somes, G. W., Banton, J. G., Rivara, F. P., & Rushforth, N. P. (1997). Risk factors for violent death of women in the home. *Archives of Internal Medicine*, *157*(7), 777–782.

Bajoga, U. A., Atagame, K. L., & Okigbo, C. C. (2015). Media influence on sexual activity and contraceptive use: A cross sectional survey among young women in urban Nigeria. *African Journal of Reproductive Health*, *19*(3), 100–110.

Baker, C. W., Whisman, M. A., & Brownell, K. D. (2000). Studying intergenerational transmission of eating attitudes and behaviors: Methodological and conceptual questions. *Health Psychology*, *19*(4), 376–381.

Baker, E. A., Schootman, M., Barnidge, E., & Kelly, C. (2006). The role of race and poverty in access to foods that enable individuals to adhere to dietary guidelines. *Preventing Chronic Disease, 3*(3), A76.

Baker, T. B., Piper, M. E., Stein, J. H., Smith, S. S., Bolt, D. M., Fraser, D. L., & Fiore, M. C. (2016). Effects of nicotine patch vs varenicline vs combination nicotine replacement therapy on smoking cessation at 26 weeks: A randomized clinical trial. *Journal of the American Medical Association, 315*(4), 371–379.

Baldwin, A. S., Rothman, A. J., Hertel, A. W., Linde, J. A., Jeffery, R. W., Finch, E. A., & Lando, H. A. (2006). Specifying the determinants of the initiation and maintenance of behavior change: An examination of self-efficacy, satisfaction, and smoking cessation. *Health Psychology, 25*(5), 626–634.

Banaji, M. R., & Steele, C. M. (1989). Alcohol and self-evaluation: Is a social cognition approach beneficial? *Social Cognition, 7*(2), 137–151.

Bandiera, F. C., Atem, F., Ma, P., Businelle, M. S., & Kendzor, D. E. (2016). Post-quit stress mediates the relation between social support and smoking cessation among socioeconomically disadvantaged adults. *Drug and Alcohol Dependence, 163*, 71–76.

Bandura, A. (1969). *Principles of behavior modification.* New York, NY: Holt, Rinehart & Winston.

Bandura, A. (1977). Self-efficacy: Toward a unifying theory of behavioral change. *Psychological Review, 84*, 191–215.

Bandura, A. (1986). *Social foundations of thought and action: A social cognitive theory.* Englewood Cliffs, NJ: Prentice Hall.

Bandura, A. (1994). Social cognitive theory and exercise of control over HIV infection. In R. J. DiClemente & J. L. Peterson (Eds.), *Preventing AIDS: Theories and methods of behavioral interventions* (pp. 25–59). New York, NY: Plenum.

Bandura, A. (1998). Health promotion from the perspective of social cognitive theory. *Psychology and Health, 13*, 623–649.

Bandura, A., O'Leary, A., Taylor, C. B., Gauthier, J., & Gossard, D. (1987). Perceived self-efficacy and pain control: Opioid and nonopioid mechanisms. *Journal of Personality and Social Psychology, 53*, 563–571.

Bandura, A., & Simon, K. M. (1977). The role of proximal intentions in self-regulation of refractory behavior. *Cognitive Therapy and Research, 1*(3), 177–193.

Bandura, A., Taylor, C. B., Williams, S. L., Mefford, I. N., & Barchas, J. D. (1985). Catecholamine secretion as a function of perceived coping self-efficacy. *Journal of Consulting and Clinical Psychology, 53*(3), 406–414. **doi:10.1037/0022-006X.53.3.406**

Banks, K., Newman, E., & Saleem, J. (2015). An overview of the research on mindfulness-based interventions for treating symptoms of posttraumatic stress disorder: A systematic review. *Journal of Clinical Psychology, 71*(10), 935–963.

Banks, S. M., Salovey, P., Greener, S., Rothman, A. J., Moyer, A., Beauvais, J., & Epel, E. (1995). The effects of message framing on mammography utilization. *Health Psychology, 14*(2), 178–184.

Barakat, L. P., & Wodka, E. L. (2006). Posttraumatic stress symptoms in college students with a chronic illness. *Social Behavior and Personality: An International Journal, 34*(8), 999–1006.

Barber, J. (1998). When hypnosis causes trouble. *International Journal of Clinical & Experimental Hypnosis, 46*, 157–170.

Barbour, K. E., Helmick, C. G., Boring, M., & Brady, T. J. (2017). Vital signs: Prevalence of doctor-diagnosed arthritis and arthritis-attributable activity limitation — United States, 2013–2015. *Morbidity and Mortality Weekly Report, 66*(9), 246–253. **doi:10.15585/mmwr.mm6609e1**

Barbour, K. E., Helmick, C. G., Boring, M., Qin, J., Pan, L., & Hootman, J. M. (2017). Obesity trends among US adults with doctor-diagnosed arthritis 2009–2014. *Arthritis Care & Research, 69*(3), 376–383.

Barefoot, J. C., Dahlstrom, G. W., & Williams, R. B., Jr. (1983). Hostility, CHD incidence, and total mortality: A 25-year follow-up study of 255 physicians. *Psychosomatic Medicine, 45*(1), 59–63.

Barefoot, J. C., Dodge, K. A., Peterson, B. L., Dahlstrom, W. G., & Williams, R. B., Jr. (1989). The Cook-Medley hostility scale: Item content and ability to predict survival. *Psychosomatic Medicine, 51*(1), 46–57.

Bárez, M., Blasco, T., Fernández-Castro, J., & Viladrich, C. (2009). Perceived control and psychological distress in women with breast cancer: A longitudinal study. *Journal of Behavioral Medicine, 32*(2), 187–196.

Barnes, D., Gatchel, R. J., Mayer, T. G., & Barnett, J. (1990). Changes in MMPI profiles of chronic low back pain patients following successful treatment. *Journal of Spinal Disorders, 3*, 353–355.

Barnes, V. A., Kapuku, G. K., & Treiber, F. A. (2012). Impact of transcendental meditation on left ventricular mass in African American adolescents. *Evidence-Based Complementary and Alternative Medicine: eCAM, 2012*, 923153. **http://doi.org/10.1155/2012/923153**

Barnett, J. C., & Vornovitsky, M. S. (2016). *Current population reports: Health insurance coverage in the United States, 2015.* Washington, DC: U.S. Department of Commerce.

Barnett, R. C., Gareis, K. C., & Brennan, R. T. (1999). Fit as a mediator of the relationship between work hours and burnout. *Journal of Occupational Health Psychology, 4*(4), 307–317.

Barnhoorn, F., & Adriaanse, H. (1992). In search of factors responsible for noncompliance among tuberculosis patients in Wardha District, India. *Social Science & Medicine, 34*, 291–306.

Barrera, M., Chassin, L., & Rogosch, F. (1993). Effects of social support and conflict on adolescent children of alcoholic and nonalcoholic fathers. *Journal of Personality and Social Psychology, 64*(4), 602–612.

Bass, D. M., Noelker, L. S., Townsend, A. L., & Deimling, G. T. (1990). Losing an aged relative: Perceptual differences between spouses and adult children. *OMEGA – Journal of Death and Dying, 21*(1), 21–40. https://doi.org/10.2190/PKJM-MXCV-YRQU-Q577

Bateganya, M., Amanyeiwe, U., Roxo, U., & Dong, M. (2015). The impact of support groups for people living with HIV on clinical outcomes: A systematic review of the literature. *Journal of Acquired Immune Deficiency Syndromes (1999), 68*(3), S368.

Bates, M. E., & Labouvie, E. W. (1995). Personality, environment constellations and alcohol use: A process-oriented study of intraindividual change during adolescence. *Psychology of Addictive Behaviors, 9*(1), 23–35.

Bates, M. S., Edwards, W. T., & Anderson, K. O. (1993). Ethnocultural influences on variation in chronic pain perception. *Pain, 52*(1), 101–112.

Baucom, D. H., & Aiken, P. A. (1981). Effect of depressed mood on eating among obese and nonobese dieting and nondieting persons. *Journal of Personality and Social Psychology, 41*(3), 577–585.

Baum, A., Friedman, A. L., & Zakowski, S. G. (1997). Stress and genetic testing for disease risk. *Health Psychology, 16*(1), 8–19.

Baum, A., & Grunberg, N. E. (1991). Gender, stress, and health. *Health Psychology, 10*(2), 80–85.

Baum, A., Grunberg, N. E., & Singer, J. E. (1982). The use of psychological and neuroendocrinological measurements in the study of stress. *Health Psychology, 1*(3), 217–236. doi:10.1037/0278-6133.1.3.217

Bazargan-Hejazi, S., Teruya, S., Pan, D., Lin, J., Gordon, D., Krochalk, P. C., & Bazargan, M. (2017). The theory of planned behavior (TPB) and texting while driving behavior in college students. *Traffic Injury Prevention, 18*(1), 56–62.

Beach, M. C., Sugarman, J., Johnson, R. L., Arbelaez, J. J., Duggan, P. S., & Cooper, L. A. (2005). Do patients treated with dignity report higher satisfaction, adherence, and receipt of preventive care? *Annals of Family Medicine, 3*(4), 331–338. http://doi.org/10.1370/afm.328

Beale, E. A., Baile, W. F., & Aaron, J. (2005). Silence is not golden. Communicating with children dying from cancer. *Journal of Clinical Oncology, 23*(15), 3629–3631. https://doi.org/10.1200/JCO.2005.11.015

Becker, A. E., Grinspoon, S. K., Klibanski, A., & Herzog, D. B. (1999). Current concepts: Eating disorders. *New England Journal of Medicine, 340*(14), 1092–1098. doi:10.1056/NEJM199904083401407

Becker, C. B., Bull, S., Schaumberg, K., Cauble, A., & Franco, A. (2008). Effectiveness of peer-led eating disorders prevention. A replication trial. *Journal of Consulting and Clinical Psychology, 76*(2), 347–354.

Becker, M. H. (1985). Patient adherence to prescribed therapies. *Medical Care, 23*, 539–555.

Becker, M. H., Maiman, L. A., Kirscht, J. P., Haefner, D. P., & Drachman, R. H. (1977). The health belief model and prediction of dietary compliance: A field experiment. *Journal of Health and Social Behavior, 18*, 348–366.

Beckjord, E. B., Glinder, J., Langrock, A., & Compas, B. E. (2009). Measuring multiple dimensions of perceived control in women with newly diagnosed breast cancer. *Psychology & Health, 24*(4), 423–438. https://doi.org/10.1080/08870440701832634

Becvar, D. S. (2001). *In the presence of grief: Helping family members resolve death,*

dying, and bereavement issues. New York, NY: Guilford.

Beecher, H. K. (1955). The powerful placebo. *Journal of the American Medical Association, 159*, 1602–1606.

Beecher, H. K. (1959). *Measurement of subjective responses.* New York, NY: Oxford University Press.

Beesdo, K., Jacobi, F., Hoyer, J., Low, N. C. P., Höfler, M., & Wittchen, H.-U. (2010). Pain associated with specific anxiety and depressive disorders in a nationally representative population sample. *Social Psychiatry and Psychiatric Epidemiology, 45*(1), 89–104. https://doi.org/10.1007/s00127-009-0045-1

Bègue, L., Bushman, B. J., Giancola, P. R., Subra, B., & Rosset, E. (2010). "There is no such thing as an accident," especially when people are drunk. *Personality & Social Psychology Bulletin, 36*(10), 1301–1304.

Beier, M. E., & Ackerman, P. L. (2003). Determinants of health knowledge: An investigation of age, gender, abilities, personality, and interests. *Journal of Personality and Social Psychology, 84*(2), 439–448.

Belar, C. D. (1997). Clinical health psychology: A specialty for the 21st century. *Health Psychology, 16*(5), 411–416.

Bell, D. R., Post, E. G., Trigsted, S. M., Hetzel, S., McGuine, T. A., & Brooks, M. A. (2016). Prevalence of sport specialization in high school athletics: A 1-year observational study. *The American Journal of Sports Medicine, 44*(6), 1469–1474.

Bellomo, G., Narducci, P. L., Rondoni, F., Pastorelli, G., Stangoni, G., Angeli, G., & Verdecchia, P. (1999). Prognostic value of 24-hour blood pressure in pregnancy. *Obstetrical & Gynecological Survey, 55*(4), 196–198.

Bender, R., Trautner, C., Spraul, M., & Berger, M. (1998). Assessment of excess mortality in obesity. *American Journal of Epidemiology, 147*(1), 42–48.

Benedetti, F., & Amanzio, M. (1997). The neuro-biology of placebo analgesia:

From endogenous opioids to cholecystokini. *Progress in Neurobiology*, *52*, 109–125.

Benedikt, R., Wertheim, E. H., & Love, A. (1998). Eating attitudes and weight-loss attempts in female adolescents and their mothers. *Journal of Youth and Adolescence*, *27*(1), 43–57.

Ben-Eliyahu, S., Yirmiya, R., Liebeskind, J., Taylor, A., & Gale, R. (1991). Stress increases metastatic spread of a mammary tumor in rats: Evidence for mediation by the immune system. *Brain Behavior and Immunity*, *5*(2), 193–205. **doi:10.1016/0889-1591(91)90016-4**

Benjamins, M. R. (2006). Religious influences on preventive health care use in a nationally representative sample of middle-age women. *Journal of Behavioral Medicine*, *29*(1), 1–16.

Benoliel, J. Q. (1988). Institutional dying: A convergence of cultural values, technology, and social organization. In H. Wass, F. M. Berado, & R. A. Neimeyer (Eds.), *Dying: Facing the facts* (2nd ed., pp. 159–184). New York, NY: Hemisphere.

Berado, D. H. (1988). Bereavement and mourning. In H. Wass, F. M., Berado, & R. A. Neimeyer (Eds.), *Dying: Facing the facts* (2nd ed., pp. 279–300). New York, NY: Hemisphere.

Berg, L., Rostila, M., & Hjern, A. (2016). Parental death during childhood and depression in young adults – a national cohort study. *Journal of Child Psychology and Psychiatry*, *57*(9), 1092–1098. **https://doi.org/10.1111/jcpp.12560**

Bergen, G., Stevens, M. R., & Burns, E. R. (2016). Falls and fall injuries among adults aged ≥65 years – United States, 2014. *Morbidity and Mortality Weekly Report*, *65*(37), 993–998. **doi:10.15585/mmwr.mm6537a2**

Berger, J., Heinrichs, M., Von Dawans, B., Way, B. M., & Chen, F. S. (2016). Cortisol modulates men's affiliative responses to acute social stress. *Psychoneuroendocrinology*, *63*, 1–10. **doi:10.1016/j.psyneuen.2015.09.004**

Berger, L. M. (2005). Income, family characteristics, and physical violence toward children. *Child Abuse & Neglect*, *29*(2), 107–133.

Bergin, A. E., Masters, K. S., & Richards, P. S. (1987). Religiousness and mental health reconsidered: A study of an intrinsically religious sample. *Journal of Counseling Psychology*, *34*(2), 197–204.

Bergman, A. B., Rivara, F. P., Richards, D. D., & Rogers, L. W. (1990). The Seattle children's bicycle helmet campaign. *American Journal of Diseases of Children*, *144*(6), 727–731.

Bergman, A. B., & Werner, R. J. (1963). Failure of children to receive penicillin by mouth. *New England Journal of Medicine*, *268*, 1334–1338.

Bergman, K., Given, B., Fabiano, R., Schutte, D., Von Eye, A., & Davidson, S. (2013). Symptoms associated with mild traumatic brain injury/concussion: The role of bother. *Journal of Neuroscience Nursing*, *45*(3), 124–132.

Bergner, M., Allison, C. J., Diehr, P., Ford, L. G., & Feigl, P. (1990). Early detection and control of cancer in clinical practice. *Archives of Internal Medicine*, *150*(2), 431–436.

Berkman, E. T., Dickenson, J., Falk, E. B., & Lieberman, M. D. (2011). Using SMS text messaging to assess moderators of smoking reduction: Validating a new tool for ecological measurement of health behaviors. *Health Psychology*, *30*(2), 186–194.

Berkman, L. F. (1985). The relationship of social networks and social support to morbidity and mortality. In S. Cohen & S. L. Syme (Eds.), *Social support and health* (pp. 241–262). San Diego, CA: Academic Press.

Berkman, L. F., Leo-Summers, L., & Horwitz, R. I. (1992). Emotional support and survival after myocardial infarction. *Annals of Internal Medicine*, *117*(12), 1003–1009.

Berkman, L. F., & Syme, S. L. (1979). Social networks, host resistance, and mortality: A nine-year follow-up study of Alameda County residents. *American Journal of Epidemiology*, *109*(2), 186–204.

Bernstein, L., Henderson, B. E., Hanisch, R., Sullivan-Halley, J., & Ross, R. K. (1994). Physical exercise and reduced risk of breast cancer in young women. *Journal of the National Cancer Institute*, *86*, 1403–1408.

Best, J. A., Flay, B. R., Towson, S. M., Ryan, K. B., Perry, C. L., Brown, K. S., . . . d'Avernas, J. R. (1984). Smoking prevention and the concept of risk. *Journal of Applied Social Psychology*, *14*(3), 257–273.

Beyer, K. M., Kaltenbach, A., Szabo, A., Bogar, S., Nieto, F. J., & Malecki, K. M. (2014). Exposure to neighborhood green space and mental health: Evidence from the survey of the health of Wisconsin. *International Journal of Environmental Research and Public Health*, *11*(3), 3453–3472.

Biener, L., & Heaton, A. (1995). Women dieters of normal weight: Their motives, goals, and risks. *American Journal of Public Health*, *85*(5), 714–717.

Biesecker, B. B., Boehnke, M., Calzone, K., Markel, D. S., Garber, J. E., Collins, F. S., & Weber, B. L. (1993). Genetic counseling for families with inherited susceptibility to breast and ovarian cancer. *Journal of the American Medical Association*, *269*(15), 1970–1974.

Biks, G. A., Berhane, Y., Worku, A., & Gete, Y. K. (2015). Exclusive breast feeding is the strongest predictor of infant survival in Northwest Ethiopia: A longitudinal study. *Journal of Health, Population, and Nutrition*, *34*, 9. **http://doi.org/10.1186/s41043-015-0007-z**

Birken, C. S., & MacArthur, C. (2004). Socioeconomic status and injury risk in children. *Journal of Paediatrics and Child Health*, *9*(5), 323–325.

Biron, P., Mongeau, J. G., & Bertrand, D. (1977). Familial resemblance of body weight and weight/height in 374 homes with adopted children. *Journal of Pediatrics*, *91*(4), 555–558.

Bishop, D. B., Roesler, J. S., Zimmerman, B. R., & Ballard, D. J. (1993). Diabetes. In R. C. Brownson, P. L., Remington, & J. R. Davis (Eds.), *Chronic disease epidemiology and control* (pp. 221–240). Washington, DC: American Public Health Association.

Bishop, S. R., Lau, M., Shapiro, S., Carlson, L., Anderson, N. D., Carmody, J., . . . Devins, G. (2004). Mindfulness: A proposed operational definition. *Clinical Psychology: Science and Practice, 11*(3), 230–241. https://doi.org/10.1093/clipsy.bph077

Biswas, A., Oh, P. I., Faulkner, G. E., Bajaj, R. R., Silver, M. A., Mitchell, M. S., & Alter, D. A. (2015). Sedentary time and its association with risk for disease incidence, mortality, and hospitalization in adults: A systematic review and meta-analysis. *Annals of Internal Medicine, 162*(2), 123–132. doi:10.7326/M14-1651

Biswas, D., Szocs, C., Chacko, R., & Wansink, B. (2017). Shining light on atmospherics: How ambient light influences food choices. *Journal of Marketing Research, 54*(1), 111–123.

Black, D. R., Gleser, L. J., & Kooyers, K. J. (1990). A meta-analytic evaluation of couples weight-loss programs. *Health Psychology, 9*(3), 330–347.

Black, M. C., Basile, K. C., Breiding, M. J., Smith, S. G., Walters, M. L., Merrick, M. T., . . . Stevens, M. R. (2011). *The national intimate partner and sexual violence survey (NISVS): 2010 summary report.* Atlanta, GA: National Center for Injury Prevention and Control, Centers for Disease Control and Prevention.

Blalock, D. V., Young, K. C., & Kleiman, E. M. (2015). Stability amidst turmoil: Grit buffers the effects of negative life events on suicidal ideation. *Psychiatry Research, 228*(3), 781–784. https://doi.org/10.1016/j.psychres.2015.04.041

Blalock, S. J., DeVellis, R. F., Giorgino, K. B., DeVellis, B. M., Gold, D. T.,

Dooley, M. A., . . . Smith, S. L. (1996). Osteoporosis prevention in premenopausal women: Using a stage model approach to examine the predictors of behavior. *Health Psychology, 15*(2), 84–93.

Blanchard, E. B., Appelbaum, K. A., Guarnieri, P., Morrill, B., & Dentinger, M. P. (1987). Five year prospective follow-up on the treatment of chronic headache with biofeedback and/or relaxation. *Headache, 27,* 580–583.

Blanc-Lapierre, A., Rousseau, M.-C., Weiss, D., El-Zein, M., Siemiatycki, J., & Parent, M.-É. (2017). Lifetime report of perceived stress at work and cancer among men: A case-control study in Montreal, Canada. *Preventive Medicine, 96,* 28–35. https://doi.org/10.1016/j.ypmed.2016.12.004

Bland, S. H., Krogh, V., Winkelstein, W., & Trevisan, M. (1991). Social network and blood pressure: A population study. *Psychosomatic Medicine, 53*(6), 598–607.

Blanton, H., Snyder, L. B., Strauts, E., & Larson, J. G. (2014). Effect of graphic cigarette warnings on smoking intentions in young adults. *PLOS ONE, 9*(5).

Blatt, S. J. (1995). The destructiveness of perfectionism: Implications for the treatment of depression. *American Psychologist, 50*(12), 1003–1020.

Bloch, M., Fahy, M., Fox, S., Hayden, M. R., & Reynolds, J. F. (1989). Predictive testing for Huntington disease: II. Demographic characteristics, life-style patterns, attitudes, and psychosocial assessments of the first fifty-one test candidates. *American Journal of Medical Genetics Part A, 32*(2), 217–224.

Block, A. R., Kremer, E. F., & Gaylor, M. (1980). Behavioral treatment of chronic pain: The spouse as a discriminative cue for pain behavior. *Pain, 9,* 243–252.

Block, J. P., He, Y., Zaslavsky, A. M., Ding, L., & Ayanian, J. Z. (2009). Psychosocial stress and change in weight among US adults. *American Journal of Epidemiology, 170*(2), 181–192.

Blond, K., Jensen, M. K., Rasmussen, M. G., Overvad, K., Tjønneland, A., Østergaard, L., & Grøntved, A. (2016). Prospective study of bicycling and risk of coronary heart disease in Danish men and women. *Circulation, 134*(18), 1409–1411. https://doi.org/10.1161/CIRCULATIONAHA.116.024651

Blount, R. L., Corbin, S. M., Sturges, J. W., Wolfe, V. V., Prater, J. M., & James, L. D. (1989). The relationship between adults' behavior and child coping and distress during BMA/LP procedures: A sequential analysis. *Behavior Therapy, 20,* 585–601.

Bluebond-Langner, M. (1977). Meanings of death to children. In H. Feifel (Ed.), *New meanings of death* (pp. 47–66). New York, NY: McGraw-Hill.

Blumenthal, J. A., Babyak, M., Wei, J., O'Connor, C., Waugh, R., Eisenstein, E., . . . Reed, G. (2002). Usefulness of psychosocial treatment of mental stress-induced myocardial ischemia in men. *American Journal of Cardiology, 89,* 164–168.

Blumenthal, J. A., Burg, M. M., Barefoot, J., Williams, R. B., Haney, T., & Zimet, G. (1987). Social support, type A behavior, and coronary artery disease. *Psychosomatic Medicine, 49*(4), 331–340.

Bly, J. L., Jones, R. C., & Richardson, J. E. (1986). Impact of worksite health promotion on health care costs and utilization: Evaluation of Johnson & Johnson's Live for Life program. *Journal of the American Medical Association, 256*(23), 3235–3240.

Boehm, J. K., & Kubzansky, L. D. (2012). The heart's content: The association between positive psychological well-being and cardiovascular health. *Psychological Bulletin, 138*(4), 655–691.

Boelen, P. A. (2015). Optimism in prolonged grief and depression following loss: A three-wave longitudinal study. *Psychiatry Research, 227*(2), 313–317. https://doi.org/10.1016/j.psychres.2015.03.009

Boffetta, P., & Hashibe, M. (2006). Alcohol and cancer. *The Lancet Oncology*, *7*(2), 149–156. https://doi.org/10.1016/S1470-2045(06)70577-0

Bogart, L. M., Walt, L. C., Pavlovic, J. D., Ober, A. J., Brown, N., & Kalichman, S. C. (2007). Cognitive strategies affecting recall of sexual behavior among high-risk men and women. *Health Psychology*, *26*(6), 787–793.

Bogg, T., & Roberts, B. W. (2004). Conscientiousness and health-related behaviors: A meta-analysis of the leading behavioral contributors to mortality. *Psychological Bulletin*, *130*(6), 887–919.

Bolger, N., Delongis, A., Kessler, R., & Schilling, E. (1989). Effects of daily stress on negative mood. *Journal of Personality and Social Psychology*, *57*(5), 808–818.

Bolinder, G., Alfredsson, L., Englund, A., & De Faire, U. (1994). Smokeless tobacco use and increased cardiovascular mortality among Swedish construction workers. *American Journal of Public Health*, *84*(3), 399–404.

Bollinger, B., Leslie, P., & Sorensen, A. (2011). Calorie posting in chain restaurants. *American Economic Journal: Economic Policy*, *3*(1), 91–128.

Bolt, E. E., Snijdewind, M. C., Willems, D. L., van der Heide, A., & Onwuteaka-Philipsen, B. D. (2015). Can physicians conceive of performing euthanasia in case of psychiatric disease, dementia or being tired of living? *Journal of Medical Ethics*, *41*(8), 592–598. https://doi.org/10.1136/medethics-2014-102150

Bonanno, G. A., Keltner, D., Holen, A., & Horowitz, M. J. (1995). When avoiding unpleasant emotions might not be such a bad thing: Verbal-autonomic response dissociation and midlife conjugal bereavement. *Journal of Personality and Social Psychology*, *69*, 975–989.

Boop, S., Axente, M., Weatherford, B., & Klimo, P., Jr. (2016). Abusive head trauma: An epidemiological and cost analysis. *Journal of Neurosurgery: Pediatrics*, *18*(5), 542–549.

Booth-Kewley, S., & Vickers, R. R. (1994). Associations between major domains of personality and health behavior. *Journal of Personality*, *62*(3), 281–298.

Boothroyd, L. G., Jucker, J. L., Thornborrow, T., Jamieson, M. A., Burt, D. M., Barton, R. A., . . . Tovee, M. J. (2016). Television exposure predicts body size ideals in rural Nicaragua. *British Journal of Psychology*, *107*(4), 752–767.

Boots, E. A., Schultz, S. A., Clark, L. R., Racine, A. M., Darst, B. F., Koscik, R. L., . . . Okonkwo, O. C. (2017). BDNF Val66Met predicts cognitive decline in the Wisconsin Registry for Alzheimers Prevention. *Neurology*, *88*(22), 2098–2106. doi:10.1212/wnl.0000000000003980

Borawski, E. A., Ievers-Landis, C. E., Lovegreen, L. D., & Trapl, E. S. (2003). Parental monitoring, negotiated unsupervised time, and parental trust: The role of perceived parenting practices in adolescent health risk behaviors. *Journal of Adolescent Health*, *33*(2), 60–70.

Borderías, L., Duarte, R., Escario, J. J., & Molina, J. A. (2015). Addiction and other reasons adolescent smokers give to justify smoking. *Substance Use and Misuse*, *50*(12), 1552–1559.

Borrelli, B., McQuaid, E. L., Novak, S. P., Hammond, S. K., & Becker, B. (2010). Motivating Latino caregivers of children with asthma to quit smoking: A randomized trial. *Journal of Consulting and Clinical Psychology*, *78*(1), 34–43. doi:10.1037/a0016932

Bosma, H., Marmot, M. G., Hemingway, H., Nicholson, A. C., Brunner, E., & Stansfeld, S. A. (1997). Low job control and risk of coronary heart disease in Whitehall II (prospective cohort) study. *British Medical Journal*, *314*, 558–565.

Bosma, H., Stansfeld, S. A., & Marmot, M. G. (1998). Job control, personal characteristics, and heart disease. *Journal of Occupational Health Psychology*, *3*, 402–409.

Bostwick, J. M., Pabbati, C., Geske, J. R., & McKean, A. J. (2016). Suicide attempt as a risk factor for completed suicide: Even more lethal than we knew. *American Journal of Psychiatry*, *173*(11), 1094–1100.

Botvin, G. J., Baker, E., Renick, N. L., Filazzola, A. D., & Botvin, E. M. (1984). A cognitive-behavioral approach to substance abuse prevention. *Addictive Behaviors*, *9*(2), 137–147.

Bouchard, C. (1991). Current understanding of the etiology of obesity: Genetic and nongenetic factors. *The American Journal of Clinical Nutrition*, *53*(6), 1561–1565.

Bould, H., De Stavola, B., Magnusson, C., Micali, N., Dal, H., Evans, J., . . . Lewis, G. (2016). The influence of school on whether girls develop eating disorders. *International Journal of Epidemiology*, *45*(2), 480–488.

Boutelle, K. N., Kirschenbaum, D. S., Baker, R. C., & Mitchell, M. E. (1999). How can obese weight controllers minimize weight gain during the high risk holiday season? By self-monitoring very consistently. *Health Psychology*, *18*(4), 364–368.

Bovbjerg, V. E., McCann, B. S., Brief, D. J., Follette, W. C., Retzlaff, B. H., Dowdy, A. A., . . . Knopp, R. H. (1995). Spouse support and long-term adherence to lipid-lowering diets. *American Journal of Epidemiology*, *141*, 451–460.

Bowen, S., Witkiewitz, K., Clifasefi, S. L., Grow, J., Chawla, N., Hsu, S. H., . . . Larimer, M. E. (2014). Relative efficacy of mindfulness-based relapse prevention, standard relapse prevention, and treatment as usual for substance use disorders: A randomized clinical trial. *JAMA Psychiatry*, *71*(5), 547–556.

Bower, J. E., Kemeny, M. E., Taylor, S. E., & Fahey, J. L. (1998). Cognitive processing, discovery of meaning, CD4 decline, and AIDS-related mortality among bereaved HIV-seropositive men. *Journal of Consulting and Clinical Psychology*, *66*(6), 979–986.

Boylan, J. M., Jennings, J. R., & Matthews, K. A. (2016). Childhood socioeconomic status and cardiovascular reactivity and recovery among Black and White men: Mitigating effects of psychological resources. *Health Psychology*, 35(9), 957–966.

Boyraz, G., Horne, S. G., & Waits, J. B. (2015). Accepting death as part of life: Meaning in life as a means for dealing with loss among bereaved individuals. *Death Studies*, 39(1), 1–11. https://doi.org/10.1080/07481187.2013.878767

Bradach, K. M., & Jordan, J. R. (1995). Long-term effects of a family history of traumatic death on adolescent individuation. *Death Studies*, 19, 315–336.

Bradburn, N. M., & Sudman, S. (1988). *Polls & surveys: Understanding what they tell us.* San Francisco, CA: Jossey-Bass.

Braddock, C. H., III, Edwards, K. A., Hasenberg, N. M., Laidley, T. L., & Levinson, W. (1999). Informed decision making in outpatient practice: Time to get back to basics. *Journal of the American Medical Association*, 282, 2313–2320.

Braden, B. B., Pipe, T. B., Smith, R., Glaspy, T. K., Deatherage, B. R., & Baxter, L. C. (2016). Brain and behavior changes associated with an abbreviated 4-week mindfulness-based stress reduction course in back pain patients. *Brain and Behavior*, 6(3), e00443. http://doi.org/10.1002/brb3.443

Brafford, L. J., & Beck, K. H. (1991). Development and validation of a condom self-efficacy scale for college students. *Journal of American College Health*, 39(5), 219–225.

Braga, A. A., Kennedy, D. M., Waring, E. J., & Piehl, A. M. (2001). Problem-oriented policing, deterrence, and youth violence: An evaluation of Boston's Operation Ceasefire. *Journal of Research in Crime and Delinquency*, 38(3), 195–225.

Brandon, T. H., Copeland, A. L., & Saper, Z. L. (1995). Programmed therapeutic messages as a smoking treatment adjunct: Reducing the impact of negative affect. *Health Psychology*, 14(1), 41–47.

Brattberg, G. (1983). Acupuncture therapy for tennis elbow. *Pain, 16*, 285–288

Brault, M. W., Hootman, J., Helmick, C. G., Theis, K. A., & Armour, B. S. (2009). Prevalence and most common causes of disability among adults—United States, 2005. *Morbidity and Mortality Weekly Report*, 58(16), 421–426.

Bray, G. A. (1992). Pathophysiology of obesity. *The American Journal of Clinical Nutrition*, 55(2), 488S–494S.

Bray, G. A. & Gray, D. S. (1988). Obesity, Part I, Pathogenesis. *Western Journal of Medicine, 149*, 429 441.

Brent, D. A., Kerr, M. M., Goldstein, C., Bozigar, J., Wartella, M., & Allan, M. J. (1989). An outbreak of suicide and suicidal behavior in a high school. *Journal of the American Academy of Child & Adolescent Psychiatry*, 28(6), 918–924.

Brent, D., Melhem, N., Donohoe, M. B., & Walker, M. (2009). The incidence and course of depression in bereaved youth 21 months after the loss of a parent to suicide, accident, or sudden natural death. *The American Journal of Psychiatry*, 166(7), 786–794. https://doi.org/10.1176/appi.ajp.2009.08081244

Brewer, N. T., Hall, M. G., Noar, S. M., Parada, H., Stein-Seroussi, A., Bach, L. E., . . . Ribisl, K. M. (2016). Effect of pictorial cigarette pack warnings on changes in smoking behavior: A randomized clinical trial. *JAMA Internal Medicine*, 176(7), 905–912.

Bril, V., England, J., Franklin, G. M., Backonja, M., Cohen, J., Del Toro, D., . . . Zochodne, D. (2011). Evidence-based guideline: Treatment of painful diabetic neuropathy. *PM&R*, 3(4), 345–352.e21. https://doi.org/10.1016/j.pmrj.2011.03.008

Bristowe, K., Marshall, S., & Harding, R. (2016). The bereavement experiences of lesbian, gay, bisexual and/or trans* people who have lost a partner: A systematic review, thematic synthesis and modelling of the literature. *Palliative Medicine*, 30(8), 730–744. https://doi.org/10.1177/0269216316634601

Broadstock, M., Borland, R., & Gason, R. (1992). Effects of suntan on judgements of healthiness and attractiveness by adolescents. *Journal of Applied Social Psychology*, 22(2), 157–172.

Brock, D. W., & Wartman, S. A. (1990). When competent patients make irrational choices. *New England Journal of Medicine*, 322, 1595–1599.

Brody, G. H., Kogan, S. M., Murry, V. M., Chen, Y. F., & Brown, A. C. (2008). Psychological functioning, support for self-management, and glycemic control among rural African American adults with diabetes mellitus type 2. *Health Psychology*, 27(1), 83–90.

Brody, J. E. (2001, May 15). A conversation with: Dan Shapiro; A doctor's story of hope, humor, and deadly cancer. *The New York Times*. Retrieved from http://www.nytimes.com/2001/05/15/health/a-conversation-with-dan-shapiro-a-doctor-s-story-of-hope-humor-and-deadly-cancer.html

Brook, D. W., Brook, J. S., Zhang, C., Whiteman, M., Cohen, P., & Finch, S. J. (2008). Developmental trajectories of cigarette smoking from adolescence to the early thirties: Personality and behavioral risk factors. *Nicotine & Tobacco Research*, 10(8), 1283–1291.

Brooks, R. A., Etzel, M. A., Hinojos, E., Henry, C. L., & Perez, M. (2005). Preventing HIV among Latino and African American gay and bisexual men in a context of HIV-related stigma, discrimination, and homophobia: Perspectives of providers. *AIDS Patient Care and STDs*, 19(11), 737–744. doi:10.1089/apc.2005.19.737

Brown, G. K., Wallston, K. A., & Nicassio, P. M. (1989). Social support and depression in rheumatoid arthritis: A one-year prospective study. *Journal of Applied Social Psychology, 19*(14), 1164–1181.

Brown, J. D. (1991). Staying fit and staying well: Physical fitness as a moderator of life stress. *Journal of Personality and Social Psychology*, *60*(4), 555–561.

Brown, K. W., & Ryan, R. M. (2003). The benefits of being present: Mindfulness and its role in psychological well-being. *Journal of Personality and Social Psychology*, *84*(4), 822–848.

Brown, S. C., Lombard, J., Wang, K., Byrne, M. M., Toro, M., Plater-Zyberk, E., . . . Szapocznik, J. (2016). Neighborhood greenness and chronic health conditions in Medicare beneficiaries. *American Journal of Preventive Medicine*, *51*(1), 78–89. doi:10.1016/j.amepre.2016.02.008

Brown, S. L., Nesse, R. M., Vinokur, A. D., & Smith, D. M. (2003). Providing social support may be more beneficial than receiving it: Results from a prospective study of mortality. *Psychological Science*, *14*(4), 320–327.

Brown, S. S. (1985). Can low birth weight be prevented? *Family Planning Perspectives*, *17*(3), 112–118.

Brownell, K. D., & Fairburn, C. G. (1995). *Eating disorders and obesity: A comprehensive handbook*. New York, NY: Guilford.

Brownell, K. D., Stunkard, A. J., & Albaum, J. M. (1980). Evaluation and modification of exercise patterns in the natural environment. *The American Journal of Psychiatry*, *137*(12), 1540–1545.

Brownlee-Duffeck, M., Peterson, L., Simonds, J. F., Goldstein, D., Kilo, C., & Hoette, S. (1987). The role of health beliefs in the regimen adherence and metabolic control of adolescents and adults with diabetes mellitus. *Journal of Consulting and Clinical Psychology*, *55*, 139–144.

Brownson, R. C., Reif, J. S., Alavanja, M. C. R., & Bal, D. G. (1993). Cancer. In R. C. Brownson, P. L. Remington, & J. R. Davis (Eds.), *Chronic disease epidemiology and control* (pp. 137–167). Washington, DC: American Public Health Association.

Brudey, C., Park, J., Wiaderkiewicz, J., Kobayashi, I., Mellman, T. A., &

Marvar, P. J. (2015). Autonomic and inflammatory consequences of post-traumatic stress disorder and the link to cardiovascular disease. *American Journal of Physiology-Regulatory, Integrative and Comparative Physiology*, *309*(4), 315–321.

Brug, J., Steenhuis, I., van Assema, P., & de Vries, H. (1996). The impact of a computer-tailored nutrition intervention. *Preventive Medicine*, *25*(3), 236–242.

Bruinsma, S. M., Tiemeier, H. W., Heemst, J. V., van der Heide, A., & Rietjens, J. A. (2015). Risk factors for complicated grief in older adults. *Journal of Palliative Medicine*, *18*(5), 438–446.

Brunner, E., White, I., Thorogood, M., Bristow, A., Curle, D., & Marmot, M. (1997). Can dietary interventions change diet and cardiovascular risk factors? A meta-analysis of randomized controlled trials. *American Journal of Public Health*, *87*, 1415–1422.

Bryant, R. A., Kenny, L., Joscelyne, A., Rawson, N., Maccallum, F., Cahill, C., . . . Nickerson, A. (2014). Treating prolonged grief disorder: A randomized clinical trial. *JAMA Psychiatry*, *71*(12), 1332–1339.

Buchbinder, R., Osborne, R. H., Ebeling, P. R., Wark, J. D., Mitchell, P., Wriedt, C., . . . Murph, B. (2009). A randomized trial of vertebroplasty for painful osteoporotic vertebral fractures. *New England Journal of Medicine*, *361*, 557–568. https://doi.org/10.1001/jamapsychiatry.2014.1600

Bucholz, E. M., Strait, K., M., Dreyer, R. P., Geda, M., Spatz, E. S., Bueno, H., . . . Krumholz, H. M. (2014). Effect of low perceived social support on health outcomes in young patients with acute myocardial infarction: Results from the variation in recovery: Role of gender on outcomes of young AMI patients (VIRGO) study. *Journal of the American Heart Association*, *3*(5), e001252. https://doi.org/10.1161/JAHA.114.001252

Buckelew, S. P., Baumstark, K. E., Frank, R. G., & Hewett, J. E. (1990).

Adjustment following spinal cord injury. *Rehabilitation Psychology*, *35*(2), 101–109.

Bunketorp, L., Lindh, M., Carlsson, J., & Stener-Victorin, E. (2006). The perception of pain and pain-related cognitions in subacute whiplash-associated disorders: Its influence on prolonged disability. *Disability and Rehabilitation*, *28*(5), 271–279. https://doi.org/10.1080/09638280500158323

Burch, R. C., Loder, S., Loder, E., & Smitherman, T. A. (2015). The prevalence and burden of migraine and severe headache in the United States: Updated statistics from government health surveillance studies. *Headache: The Journal of Head and Face Pain*, *55*(1), 21–34. https://doi.org/10.1111/head.12482

Burgio, E., Lopomo, A., & Migliore, L. (2014). Obesity and diabetes: From genetics to epigenetics. *Molecular Biology Reports*, *42*(4), 799–818.

Burish, T. G., & Bradley, L. A. (1983). Coping with chronic disease: Definitions and issues. In T. G. Burish & L. A. Bradley (Eds.), *Coping with chronic disease: Research and applications* (pp. 3–12). New York, NY: Academic Press.

Burish, T. G., Snyder, S. L., & Jenkins, R. A. (1991). Preparing patients for cancer chemotherapy: Effect of coping preparation and relaxation interventions. *Journal of Consulting and Clinical Psychology*, *59*, 518–525.

Burnam, M. A., Timbers, D. M., & Hough, R. L. (1984). Two measures of psychological distress among Mexican Americans, Mexicans and Anglos. *Journal of Health and Social Behavior*, *25*(1), 24–33.

Burns, J. W., Quartana, P. J., & Bruehl, S. (2007). Anger management style moderates effects of emotion suppression during initial stress on pain and cardiovascular responses during subsequent pain-induction. *Annals of Behavioral Medicine*, *34*(2), 154–165. https://doi.org/10.1007/BF02872670

Burridge, L. H., Barnett, A. G., & Clavarino, A. M. (2009). The impact of perceived stage of cancer on carers' anxiety and depression during the patients' final year of life. *Psycho-Oncology, 18*(6), 615–623. https://doi.org/10.1002/pon.1435

Burris, S., Wagenaar, A. C., Swanson, J., Ibrahim, J. K., Wood, J., & Mello, M. M. (2010). Making the case for laws that improve health: A framework for public health law research. *The Milbank Quarterly, 88*(2), 169–210.

Burt, R. D., Dinh, K. T., Peterson, A. V., & Sarason, I. G. (2000). Predicting adolescent smoking: A prospective study of personality variables. *Preventive Medicine, 30*(2), 115–125.

Burton, C. L., Hatzenbuehler, M. L., & Bonanno, G. A. (2014). Familial social support predicts a reduced cortisol response to stress in sexual minority young adults. *Psychoneuroendocrinology, 47*, 241–245.

Bush, C., Ditto, B., & Feurestein, M. (1985). A controlled evaluation of paraspinal EMG biofeedback in the treatment of chronic low back pain. *Health Psychology, 4*, 307–321.

Bush, J. P., Melamed, B. G., Sheras, P. L., & Greenbaum, P. E. (1986). Mother–child patterns of coping with anticipatory medical stress. *Health Psychology, 5*(2), 137–157.

Bushman, B. J. (1997). Effects of alcohol on human aggression: Validity of proposed explanations. *Recent Developments in Alcoholism, 13*, 227–243.

Bushman, B. J., Newman, K., Calvert, S. L., Downey, G., Dredze, M., Gottfredson, M., . . . Webster, D. W. (2016). Youth violence: What we know and what we need to know. *American Psychologist, 71*(1), 17–39. doi:10.1037/a0039687

Businelle, M. S., Kendzor, D. E., Reitzel, L. R., Costello, T. J., Cofta-Woerpel, L., Li, Y., . . . Wetter, D. W. (2010). Mechanisms linking socioeconomic status to smoking cessation: A structural equation modeling approach. *Health Psychology, 29*(3), 262–273.

Buss, A. H., & Durkee, A. (1957). An inventory for assessing different kinds of hostility. *Journal of Consulting Psychology, 21*(4), 343–349.

Butt, H. R. (1977). A method for better physician–patient communication. *Annals of Internal Medicine, 86*, 478–480.

Butter, I. H. (1993). Premature adoption and routinization of medical technology: Illustrations from childbirth technology. *Journal of Social Issues, 49*(2), 11–34.

Butterworth, P., Leach, L. S., Strazdins, L., Olesen, S. C., Rodgers, B., & Broom, D. H. (2011). The psychosocial quality of work determines whether employment has benefits for mental health: Results from a longitudinal national household panel survey. *Occupational and Environmental Medicine, 68*(11), 806–812. doi:10.1136/oem.2010.059030

Byrnes, D. M., Antoni, M. H., Goodkin, K., Efantis-Potter, J., Asthana, D., Simon, T., . . . Fletcher, M. A. (1998). Stressful events, pessimism, natural killer cell cytotoxicity, and cytotoxic/suppressor T cells in HIV+ Black women at risk for cervical cancer. *Psychosomatic Medicine, 60*(6), 714–722.

Cachelin, F. M., Phinney, J. S., Schug, R. A., & Striegel-Moore, R. H. (2006). Acculturation and eating disorders in a Mexican American community sample. *Psychology of Women Quarterly, 30*(4), 340–347. doi:10.1111/j.1471-6402.2006.00309.x

Calle, E. E., Miracle-McMahill, H. L., Thun, M. J., & Heath, C. W. (1994). Cigarette smoking and risk of fatal breast cancer. *American Journal of Epidemiology, 139*, 1001–1007.

Callender, C. O., & Miles, P. V. (2010). Minority organ donation: The power of an educated community. *Journal of the American College of Surgeons, 210*(5), 708–715.

Camargo, C. A., Hennekens, C. H., Gaziano, J. M., Glynn, R. J., Manson, J. E., & Stampfer, M. J. (1997). Prospective study of moderate alcohol consumption and mortality in US male physicians. *Archives of Internal Medicine, 157*(1), 79–85.

Cameron, C. L., Cella, D., Herndon, J. E., II, Kornblith, A. B., Zukerman, E., Henderson, E., . . . Canellos, G. P. (2001). Persistent symptoms among survivors of Hodgkin's disease: An explanatory model based on classical conditioning. *Health Psychology, 20*(1), 71–75.

Cameron, L., Leventhal, E. A., & Leventhal, H. (1995). Seeking medical care in response to symptoms and life stress. *Psychosomatic Medicine, 57*(1), 37–47.

Campbell, M. K., Carbone, E., Honess-Morreale, L., Heisler-MacKinnon, J., Demissie, S., & Farrell, D. (2004). Randomized trial of a tailored nutrition education CD-ROM program for women receiving food assistance. *Journal of Nutrition Education and Behavior, 36*(2), 58–66.

Campbell, M. K., DeVellis, B. M., Strecher, V. J., Ammerman, A. S., DeVellis, R. F., & Sandler, R. S. (1994). Improving dietary behavior: The effectiveness of tailored messages in primary care settings. *American Journal of Public Health, 84*(5), 783–787.

Cannon, W. B. (1932). *The wisdom of the body*. New York, NY: W.W. Norton & Company, Inc.

Cantrell, J., Vallone, D. M., Thrasher, J. F., Nagler, R. H., Feirman, S. P., Muenz, L. R., . . . Viswanath, K. (2013). Impact of tobacco-related health warning labels across socioeconomic, race and ethnic groups: Results from a randomized web-based experiment. *PLOS ONE, 8*(1).

Canudas-Romo, V., Liu, L., Zimmerman, L., Ahmed, S., & Tsui, A. (2014). Potential gains in reproductive-aged life expectancy by eliminating maternal mortality: A demographic bonus of achieving MDG 5. *PLOS ONE, 9*(2), e86694. http://doi.org/10.1371/journal.pone.0086694

Capaldi, D. M., Knoble, N. B., Shortt, J. W., & Kim, H. K. (2012). A systematic review of risk factors for intimate partner violence. *Partner Abuse*, *3*(2), 231–280. http://doi.org/10.1891/1946-6560.3.2.231

Carey, I. M., Shah, S. M., DeWilde, S., Harris, T., Victor, C. R., & Cook, D. G. (2014). Increased risk of acute cardiovascular events after partner bereavement: A matched cohort study. *JAMA Internal Medicine*, *174*(4), 598–605. https://doi.org/10.1001/jamainternmed.2013.14558

Carey, M. P., & Burish, T. G. (1988). Etiology and treatment of the psychological side effects associated with cancer chemotherapy: A critical review and discussion. *Psychological Bulletin, 104*, 307–325.

Carlson, C. R., & Hoyle, R. H. (1993). Efficacy of abbreviated muscle relaxation training: A quantitative review of behavior medicine research. *Journal of Consulting and Clinical Psychology, 61*, 1059–1067.

Carlsson, E., Frostell, A., Ludvigsson, J., & Faresjö, M. (2014). Psychological stress in children may alter the immune response. *Journal of Immunology, 192*(5), 2071–2081. doi:10.4049/jimmunol.1301713

Carney, M. A., Armeli, S., Tennen, H., Affleck, G., & O'Neil, T. P. (2000). Positive and negative daily events, perceived stress, and alcohol use: A diary study. *Journal of Consulting and Clinical Psychology, 68*(5), 788–798.

Carpenter, D. J., Gatchel, R. J., & Hasegawa, T. (1994). Effectiveness of a videotaped behavioral intervention for dental anxiety: The role of gender and the need for information. *Behavioral Medicine, 20*(3), 123–132.

Carpentier, M. Y., Mullins, L. L., & Van Pelt, J. C. (2007). Psychological, academic, and work functioning in college students with childhood-onset asthma. *Journal of Asthma, 44*(2), 119–124.

Carskadon, M. A., Wolfson, A. R., Acebo, C., Tzischinsky, O., & Seifer, R. (1998). Adolescent sleep patterns, circadian timing, and sleepiness at a transition to early school days. *Sleep, 21*(8), 871–881.

Carson, J. W., Keefe, F. J., Lynch, T. R., Carson, K. M., Goli, V., Fras, A. M., & Thorp, S. R. (2005). Loving-kindness meditation for chronic low back pain. *Journal of Holistic Nursing, 23*(3), 287–304. https://doi.org/10.1177/0898010105277651

Carter, P. M., Buckley, L., Flannagan, C. A., Cicchino, J. B., Hemmila, M., Bowman, P. J., . . . Bingham, C. R. (2017). The impact of Michigan's partial repeal of the universal motorcycle helmet law on helmet use, fatalities, and head injuries. *American Journal of Public Health, 107*(1), 166–172.

Carter, P. M., Flannagan, C. A., Bingham, C. R., Cunningham, R. M., & Rupp, J. D. (2015). Modeling the injury prevention impact of mandatory alcohol ignition interlock installation in all new US vehicles. *American Journal of Public Health, 105*(5), 1028–1035.

Carvalho, C., Caetano, J. M., Cunha, L., Rebouta, P., Kaptchuk, T. J., & Kirsch, I. (2016). Open-label placebo treatment in chronic low back pain: A randomized controlled trial. *Pain, 157*(12), 2766–2772. https://doi.org/10.1097/j.pain.0000000000000700

Carver, C. S., & Antoni, M. H. (2004). Finding benefit in breast cancer during the year after diagnosis predicts better adjustment 5 to 8 years after diagnosis. *Health Psychology, 23*(6), 595–598.

Carver, C. S., Pozo, C., Harris, S. D., Noriega, V., Scheier, M. F., Robinson, D. S., . . . Clark, K. C. (1993). How coping mediates the effect of optimism on distress: A study of women with early stage breast cancer. *Journal of Personality and Social Psychology, 65*(2), 375–390.

Carver, C. S., Pozo-Kaderman, C., Price, A. A., Noriega, V., Harris, S. D., Dehagopion, R. P., . . . Moffatt, F. L., Jr. (1998). Concern about aspects of body image and adjustment to early stage breast cancer. *Psychosomatic Medicine, 60*, 168–174.

Carver, C. S., Scheier, M. F., & Weintraub, J. K. (1989). Assessing coping strategies: A theoretically based approach. *Journal of Personality and Social Psychology, 56*(2), 267–283.

Case, A., & Deaton, A. (2015). Rising morbidity and mortality in midlife among White non-Hispanic Americans in the 21st century. *Proceedings of the National Academy of Sciences of the United States of America, 112*(49), 15078–15083.

Caspi, A., Begg, D. J., Dickson, N., Harrington, H., Langley, J. D., Moffitt, T. E., & Silva, P. A. (1997). Personality differences predict health-risk behaviors in young adulthood: Evidence from a longitudinal study. *Journal of Personality and Social Psychology, 73*(5), 1052–1063.

Caspi, A., Moffitt, T. E., Silva, P. A., Stouthamer-Loeber, M., Krueger, R. F., & Schmutte, P. S. (1994). Are some people crime-prone? Replications of the personality-crime relationship across countries, genders, races, and methods. *Criminology, 32*(2), 163–196.

Cassileth, B. R., Lusk, E. J., Strouse, T. B., Miller, D. S., Brown, L. L., Cross, P. A., & Tenaglia, A. N. (1984). Psychosocial status in chronic illness: A comparative analysis of six diagnostic groups. *New England Journal of Medicine, 311*(8), 506–511.

Castonguay, A. L., Wrosch, C., & Sabiston, C. M. (2017). The roles of negative affect and goal adjustment capacities in breast cancer survivors: Associations with physical activity and diurnal cortisol secretion. *Health Psychology, 36*(4), 320–331. doi:10.1037/hea0000477

Catz, S. L., Kelly, J. A., Bogart, L. M., Benotsch, E. G., & McAuliffe, T. L. (2000). Patterns, correlates, and barriers to medication adherence among persons prescribed new treatments for HIV disease. *Health Psychology, 19*, 124–133.

Cavanagh, J. T., Carson, A. J., Sharpe, M., & Lawrie, S. M. (2003). Psychological autopsy studies of suicide: A systematic review. *Psychological Medicine, 33*(3), 395–405.

Caverly, T. J., Hayward, R. A., Reamer, E., Zikmund-Fisher, B. J., Connochie, D., Heisler, M., & Fagerlin, A. (2016). Presentation of benefits and harms in US cancer screening and prevention guidelines: Systematic review. *Journal of the National Cancer Institute, 108*(6), djv436. http://doi.org/10.1093/jnci/djv436

Centers for Disease Control and Prevention. (2014). *National diabetes statistics report: estimates of diabetes and its burden in the United States, 2014.* Atlanta, GA: U.S. Department of Health and Human Services.

Centers for Disease Control and Prevention. (2016a). Breast cancer rates by race and ethnicity. Retrieved from https://www.cdc.gov/cancer/breast/statistics/race.htm

Centers for Disease Control and Prevention. (2016b). Costs of injuries and violence in the United States. Retrieved from https://www.cdc.gov/injury/wisqars/overview/cost_of_injury.html

Centers for Disease Control and Prevention. (2016c). Fact sheets: Alcohol use and your health. Retrieved from https://www.cdc.gov/alcohol/fact-sheets/alcohol-use.htm

Centers for Disease Control and Prevention. (2016d). *HIV surveillance report, 2015, vol. 27.* Retrieved from https://www.cdc.gov/hiv/pdf/library/reports/surveillance/cdc-hiv-surveillance-report-2015-vol-27.pdf

Centers for Disease Control and Prevention. (2016e). Key injury and violence data. Retrieved from https://www.cdc.gov/injury/wisqars/overview/key_data.html

Centers for Disease Control and Prevention. (2016f). Motor vehicle crash deaths: How is the US doing? *CDC vitalsigns.* Atlanta, GA: Centers for Disease Control and Prevention.

Retrieved from https://www.cdc.gov/vitalsigns/pdf/2016-07-vitalsigns.pdf

Centers for Disease Control and Prevention. (2016g). Smokeless tobacco use in the United States. Retrieved from https://www.cdc.gov/tobacco/data_statistics/fact_sheets/smokeless/use_us/index.htm

Centers for Disease Control and Prevention. (2016h). Unintentional drowning: Get the facts. Retrieved from https://www.cdc.gov/homeandrecreationalsafety/water-safety/waterinjuries-factsheet.html

Centers for Disease Control and Prevention. (2017a). About diabetes. Retrieved from https://www.cdc.gov/diabetes/basics/diabetes.html

Centers for Disease Control and Prevention. (2017b). Adult obesity causes & consequences. Retrieved from https://www.cdc.gov/obesity/adult/causes.html

Centers for Disease Control and Prevention. (2017c). Alzheimer's disease. Retrieved from https://www.cdc.gov/chronicdisease/resources/publications/aag/alzheimers.htm

Centers for Disease Control and Prevention. (2017d). Burden of tobacco use in the US. Retrieved from https://www.cdc.gov/tobacco/campaign/tips/resources/data/cigarette-smoking-in-united-states.html

Centers for Disease Control and Prevention. (2017e). Chronic disease overview. Retrieved from https://www.cdc.gov/chronicdisease/overview/index.htm

Centers for Disease Control and Prevention. (2017f). Diabetes quick facts. Retrieved from https://www.cdc.gov/diabetes/basics/quick-facts.html

Centers for Disease Control and Prevention. (2017g). Exercise or physical activity. Retrieved from https://www.cdc.gov/nchs/fastats/exercise.htm

Centers for Disease Control and Prevention. (2017h). Health expenditures.

Retrieved from https://www.cdc.gov/nchs/fastats/health-expenditures.htm

Centers for Disease Control and Prevention. (2017i). Heart attack. Retrieved from https://www.cdc.gov/heartdisease/heart_attack.htm

Centers for Disease Control and Prevention. (2017j). HIV among African Americans. Retrieved from https://www.cdc.gov/hiv/group/racialethnic/africanamericans/index.html

Centers for Disease Control and Prevention. (2017k). HIV among gay and bisexual men. Retrieved from https://www.cdc.gov/hiv/group/msm/index.html

Centers for Disease Control and Prevention. (2017l). HIV in the United States: *At a glance.* Retrieved from https://www.cdc.gov/hiv/statistics/overview/ataglance.html

Centers for Disease Control and Prevention. (2017m). Illegal drug use. Retrieved from https://www.cdc.gov/nchs/fastats/drug-use-illegal.htm

Centers for Disease Control and Prevention. (2017n). Intimate partner violence. Retrieved from https://www.cdc.gov/violenceprevention/intimatepartnerviolence/index.html

Centers for Disease Control and Prevention. (2017o). Most recent asthma data. Retrieved from https://www.cdc.gov/asthma/most_recent_data.htm

Centers for Disease Control and Prevention. (2017p). National statistics. Retrieved from https://www.cdc.gov/arthritis/data_statistics/national-statistics.html

Centers for Disease Control and Prevention. (2017q). New CDC report: More than 100 million Americans have diabetes or prediabetes. Retrieved from https://www.cdc.gov/media/releases/2017/p0718-diabetes-report.html

Centers for Disease Control and Prevention. (2017r). Prescription opioid overdose data. Retrieved from https://www.cdc.gov/drugoverdose/data/overdose.html

Centers for Disease Control and Prevention. (2017s). Provisional counts of drug overdose deaths, as of 8/6/2017. Retrieved from https://www.cdc.gov/nchs/data/health_policy/monthly-drug-overdose-death-estimates.pdf

Centers for Disease Control and Prevention. (2017t). Racial and ethnic approaches to community health. Retrieved from https://www.cdc.gov/nccdphp/dnpao/state-local-programs/reach/

Centers for Disease Control and Prevention. (2017u). Suicide and self-inflicted injury. Retrieved from https://www.cdc.gov/nchs/fastats/suicide.htm

Centers for Disease Control and Prevention. (2017v). Ten leading causes of deaths and injury. Retrieved from https://www.cdc.gov/injury/wisqars/leadingcauses.html

Centers for Disease Control and Prevention. (2017w). Today's heroin epidemic. Retrieved from https://www.cdc.gov/drugoverdose/opioids/heroin.html

Centers for Disease Control and Prevention. (2017x). Understanding the epidemic. Retrieved from https://www.cdc.gov/drugoverdose/epidemic/index.html

Centers for Disease Control and Prevention. (2017y). Youth violence: Consequences. Retrieved from https://www.cdc.gov/violenceprevention/youthviolence/consequences.html

Centers for Disease Control and Prevention. (n.d.). HIV surveillance reports. Retrieved from https://www.cdc.gov/hiv/library/reports/hiv-surveillance.html

Cerdá, M., Wall, M., Feng, T., Keyes, K. M., Sarvet, A., Schulenberg, J., . . . Hasin, D. S. (2017). Association of state recreational marijuana laws with adolescent marijuana use. *JAMA Pediatrics*, *171*(2), 142–149.

Cesaroni, G., Forastiere, F., Agabiti, N., Valente, P., Zuccaro, P., & Perucci, C. A. (2008). Effect of the Italian smoking ban on population rates of acute coronary events. *Circulation*, *117*(9), 1183–1188. https://doi.org/10.1161/CIRCULATIONAHA.107.729889

Chaiken, S. (1987). The heuristic model of persuasion. In M. P. Zanna, J. M. Olson, & C. P. Herman (Eds.), *Social influence: The Ontario symposium* (Vol. 5, pp. 3–39). Hillsdale, NJ: Erlbaum.

Chaiton, M., Diemert, L., Cohen, J. E., Bondy, S. J., Selby, P., Philipneri, A., & Schwartz, R. (2016). Estimating the number of quit attempts it takes to quit smoking successfully in a longitudinal cohort of smokers. *BMJ Open*, *6*(6), e011045.

Chajut, E., Caspi, A., Chen, R., Hod, M., & Ariely, D. (2014). In pain thou shalt bring forth children. *Psychological Science*, *25*(12), 2266–2271. https://doi.org/10.1177/0956797614551004

Champion, V. L. (1994). Strategies to increase mammography utilization. *Medical Care*, *32*(2), 118–129.

Chan, C. S., Lowe, S. R., Weber, E., & Rhodes, J. E. (2015). The contribution of pre and post disaster social support to short and long term mental health after Hurricanes Katrina: A longitudinal study of low-income survivors. *Social Science & Medicine*, *138*, 38–43.

Chandwani, K. D., Perkins, G., Nagendra, H. R., Raghuram, N. V., Spelman, A., Nagarathna, R., . . . Cohen, L. (2014). Randomized, controlled trial of yoga in women with breast cancer undergoing radiotherapy. *Journal of Clinical Oncology*, *32*(10), 1058–1065. https://doi.org/10.1200/JCO.2012.48.2752

Chang, P. H., Chiang, C. H., Ho, W. C., Wu, P. Z., Tsai, J. S., & Guo, F. R. (2015). Combination therapy of varenicline with nicotine replacement therapy is better than varenicline alone: A systematic review and meta-analysis of randomized controlled trials. *BMC Public Health*, *15*(1), 689.

Chapman, C. R., Casey, K. L., Dubner, R., Foley, K. M., Gracely, R. H., & Reading, A. E. (1985). Pain measurement: An overview. *Pain*, *22*, 1–31.

Charette, S., Fiola, J. L., Charest, M.-C., Villeneuve, E., Théroux, J., Joncas, J., . . . Le May, S. (2015). Guided imagery for adolescent post-spinal fusion pain management: A pilot study. *Pain Management Nursing*, *16*(3), 211–220. https://doi.org/10.1016/j.pmn.2014.06.004

Charles, C., Goldsmith, L. J., Chambers, L., & Haynes, R. B. (1996). Provider-patient communication among elderly and nonelderly patients in Canadian hospitals: A national survey. *Health Communication*, *8*, 281–302.

Charles, S. T., Gatz, M., Kato, K., & Pedersen, N. L. (2008). Physical health 25 years later: The predictive ability of neuroticism. *Health Psychology*, *27*(3), 369–378.

Charney, E., Goodman, H. C., McBride, M., Lyon, B., Pratt, R., Breese, B., . . . Marx, K. (1976). Childhood antecedents of adult obesity: Do chubby infants become obese adults? *New England Journal of Medicine*, *295*(1), 6–9.

Chassin, L., Presson, C. C., Rose, J. S., & Sherman, S. J. (1996). The natural history of cigarette smoking from adolescence to adulthood: Demographic predictors of continuity and change. *Health Psychology*, *15*(6), 478–484.

Chassin, L., Presson, C. C., Sherman, S. J., Corty, E., & Olshavsky, R. W. (1981). Self-images and cigarette smoking in adolescence. *Personality and Social Psychology Bulletin*, *7*(4), 670–676.

Chassin, L., Presson, C. C., Todd, M., Rose, J. S., & Sherman, S. J. (1998). Maternal socialization of adolescent smoking. *Developmental Psychology*, *34*(6), 1189–1201.

Chassin, L., Presson, C., Seo, D. C., Sherman, S. J., Macy, J., Wirth, R. J., & Curran, P. (2008). Multiple trajectories of cigarette smoking and the intergenerational transmission of smoking: A multigenerational, longitudinal study of a Midwestern community sample. *Health Psychology, 27*(6), 819–828.

Chaudhary, N. K., Connolly, J., Tison, J., Solomon, M., & Elliott, K. (2015). *Evaluation of the NHTSA distracted driving high-visibility enforcement demonstration projects in California and Delaware* (Report No. DOT HS 812 108). Washington, DC: National Highway Traffic Safety Administration.

Chaves, J. F. (1994). Recent advances in the application of hypnosis to pain management. *American Journal of Clinical Hypnosis, 37*, 117–129.

Chein, J., Albert, D., O'Brien, L., Uckert, K., & Steinberg, L. (2011). Peers increase adolescent risk taking by enhancing activity in the brain's reward circuitry. *Developmental Science, 14*(2), 1–10.

Chen, E., & Paterson, L. Q. (2006). Neighborhood, family, and subjective socioeconomic status: How do they relate to adolescent health? *Health Psychology, 25*(6), 704–714.

Chen, E. Y., Weissman, J. A., Zeffiro, T. A., Yiu, A., Eneva, K. T., Arlt, J. M., & Swantek, M. J. (2016). Family-based therapy for young adults with anorexia nervosa restores weight. *International Journal of Eating Disorders, 49*(7), 701–707.

Chen, J., Rathore, S. S., Radford, M. J., Wang, Y., & Krumholz, H. M. (2001). Racial differences in the use of cardiac catheterization after acute myocardial infarction. *New England Journal of Medicine, 344*(19), 1443–1449.

Chen, J., Vargas-Bustamante, A., Mortensen, K., & Ortega, A. N. (2016). Racial and ethnic disparities in health care access and utilization under the Affordable Care Act. *Medical Care, 54*(2), 140–146. doi:10.1097/MLR.0000000000000467

Chen, M. H., Pan, T. L., Li, C. T., Lin, W. C., Chen, Y. S., Lee, Y. C., . . . Bai, Y. M. (2015). Risk of stroke among patients with post-traumatic stress disorder: Nationwide longitudinal study. *The British Journal of Psychiatry, 206*(4), 302–307.

Cheney, A. M., Booth, B. M., Borders, T. F., & Curran, G. M. (2016). The role of social capital in African Americans' attempts to reduce and quit cocaine use. *Substance Use & Misuse, 51*(6), 777–787.

Cherkin, D. C., Sherman, K. J., Balderson, B. H., Cook, A. J., Anderson, M. L., Hawkes, R. J., . . . Turner, J. A. (2016). Effect of mindfulness-based stress reduction vs cognitive behavioral therapy or usual care on back pain and functional limitations in adults with chronic low back pain: A randomized clinical trial. *Journal of the American Medical Association, 315*(12), 1240–1249. https://doi.org/10.1001/jama.2016.2323

Chetty, R., Stepner, M., Abraham, S., Lin, S., Scuderi, B., Turner, N., . . . Cutler, D. (2016). The association between income and life expectancy in the United States, 2001-2014. *Journal of the American Medical Association, 315*(16), 1750–1766.

Chew, B.-H., Hassan, N.-H., & Sherina, M.-S. (2015). Determinants of medication adherence among adults with type 2 diabetes mellitus in three Malaysian public health clinics: A cross-sectional study. *Patient Preference and Adherence, 9*, 639–648. http://doi.org/10.2147/PPA.S81612

Chiaramonte, G. R., & Friend, R. (2006). Medical students' and residents' gender bias in the diagnosis, treatment, and interpretation of coronary heart disease symptoms. *Health Psychology, 25*(3), 255–266.

Chida, Y., & Steptoe, A. (2009). The association of anger and hostility with future coronary heart disease. *Journal of the American College of Cardiology, 53*(11), 936–946. https://doi.org/10.1016/j.jacc.2008.11.044

Ching, P. L., Willett, W. C., Rimm, E. B., Colditz, G. A., Gortmaker, S. L., & Stampfer, M. J. (1996). Activity level and risk of overweight in male health professionals. *American Journal of Public Health, 86*(1), 25–30.

Chirles, T. J., Reiter, K., Weiss, L. R., Alfini, A. J., Nielson, K. A., & Smith, J. C. (2017). Exercise training and functional connectivity changes in mild cognitive impairment and healthy elders. *Journal of Alzheimer's Disease, 57*(3), 845–856. doi:10.3233/JAD-161151

Chochinov, H. M., Wilson, K. G., Enns, M. W., & Mowchun, N. (1995). Desire for death in the terminally ill. *American Journal of Psychiatry, 152*(8), 1185–1191. https://doi.org/10.1176/ajp.152.8.1185

Chopik, W. J., & O'Brian, E. (2016). Happy you, healthy me? Having a happy partner is independently associated with better health in oneself. *Health Psychology, 36*(1), 21–30.

Christakis, N. A., & Fowler, J. H. (2007). The spread of obesity in a large social network over 32 years. *New England Journal of Medicine, 357*, 370–379.

Christakis, N. A., & Iwashyna, T. J. (2003). The health impact of health care on families: A matched cohort study of hospice use by decedents and mortality outcomes in surviving, widowed spouses. *Social Science & Medicine, 57*(3), 465–475. https://doi.org/10.1016/S0277-9536(02)00370-2

Christenfeld, N., Glynn, L. M., Phillips, D. P., & Shrira, I. (1999). Exposure to New York City as a risk factor for heart attack mortality. *Psychosomatic Medicine, 61*, 740–743.

Christensen, A. J. (2000). Patient-by-treatment context interaction in chronic disease: A conceptual framework for the study of patient adherence. *Psychosomatic Medicine, 62*, 435–443.

Christensen, A. J., & Ehlers, S. L. (2002). Psychological factors in end-stage renal disease: An emerging context for behavioral medicine research. *Journal* of *Consulting and Clinical Psychology, 70*, 712–724.

Christensen, A. J., & Johnson, J. A. (2002). Patient adherence with medical treatment regimens: An interactive approach. *Current Directions in Psychological Science, 11*, 94–97.

Christensen, A. J., Moran, P. J., & Wiebe, J. S. (1999). Assessment of irrational health beliefs: Relation to health practices and medical regimen adherence. *Health Psychology, 18*, 169–176.

Christensen, A. J., & Smith, T. W. (1995). Personality and patient adherence: Correlates of the five-factor model in renal dialysis. *Journal of Behavioral Medicine, 18*(3), 305–313.

Christensen, A. J., Smith, T. W., Turner, C. W., Holman, J. M., Gregory, M. C., & Rich, M. A. (1992). Family support, physical impairment, and adherence in hemodialysis: An investigation of main and buffering effects. *Journal of Behavioral Medicine, 15*(4), 313–325.

Christie, K. M., Meyerowitz, B. E., Giedzinska-Simons, A., Gross, M., & Agus, D. B. (2009). Predictors of affect following treatment decision-making for prostate cancer: Conversations, cognitive processing, and coping. *Psycho-Oncology, 18*(5), 508–514. **https://doi.org/10.1002/pon.1420**

Christine, P. J., Auchincloss, A. H., Bertoni, A. G., Carnethon, M. R., Sánchez, B. N., Moore, K., . . . Roux, A. V. (2015). Longitudinal associations between neighborhood physical and social environments and incident Type 2 diabetes mellitus. *JAMA Internal Medicine, 175*(8), 1311.

Christophi, C. A., Pampaka, D., Paisi, M., Ioannou, S., & DiFranza, J. R. (2016). Levels of physical dependence on tobacco among adolescent smokers in Cyprus. *Addictive Behaviors, 60*, 148–153.

Chrousos, G. P. (1998). Stressors, stress, and neuroendocrine integration of the adaptive response: The 1997 Hans Selye Memorial Lecture. *Annals of the New York Academy of Sciences, 851*(1), 311–335.

Chrousos, G. P., & Gold, P. W. (1992). The concepts of stress and stress system disorders: Overview of physical and behavioral homeostasis. *Journal of the American Medical Association, 267*(9), 1244–1253.

Chu, Y. L., Farmer, A., Fung, C., Kuhle, S., Storey, K. E., & Veugelers, P. J. (2013). Involvement in home meal preparation is associated with food preference and self-efficacy among Canadian children. *Public Health Nutrition, 16*(1), 108–112.

Cicero, V., Lo Coco, G., Gullo, S., & Lo Verso, G. (2009). The role of attachment dimensions and perceived social support in predicting adjustment to cancer. *Psycho-Oncology, 18*(10), 1045–1052. **https://doi.org/10.1002/pon.1390**

Cinciripini, P. M., Lapitsky, L., Seay, S., Wallfisch, A., Kitchens, K., & Van Vunakis, H. (1995). The effects of smoking schedules on cessation outcome: Can we improve on common methods of gradual and abrupt nicotine withdrawal? *Journal of Consulting and Clinical Psychology, 63*(3), 388–399.

Clark, D. C., & Zeldow, P. B. (1988). Vicissitudes of depressed mood during four years of medical school. *Journal of the American Medical Association, 260*, 2521–2528.

Clark, R., Anderson, N. B., Clark, V. R., & Williams, D. R. (1999). Racism as a stressor for African Americans: A biopsychosocial model. *American Psychologist, 54*(10), 805–816.

Clarke, T. C., Black, L. I., Stussman, B. J., Barnes, P. M., & Nahin, R. L. (2015). Trends in the use of complementary health approaches among adults: United States, 2002–2012. *National Health Statistics Reports, *(79), 1–16.

Clarke, T. C., Norris, T., & Schiller, J. S. (2017). *Early release of selected estimates based on data from 2016 National Health Interview Survey*. Atlanta, GA: National Center for Health Statistics.

Classen, C., Koopman, C., Angell, K., & Spiegel, D. (1996). Coping styles associated with psychological adjustment to

advanced breast cancer. *Health Psychology, 15*(6), 434–437.

Claus, E. B., Risch, N., & Thompson, W. D. (1993). Autosomal dominant inheritance of early onset breast cancer: Implications for risk prediction. *Cancer, 73*, 643–651.

Cleeland, C. S., Gonin, R., Hatfield, A. K., Edmonson, J. H., Blum, R. H., Stewart, J. A., & Pandya, K. J. (1994). Pain and its treatment in outpatients with metastatic cancer. *New England Journal of Medicine, 330*, 592–596.

Clemow, L., Costanza, M. E., Haddad, W. P., Luckmann, R., White, M. J., Klaus, D., & Stoddard, A. M. (2000). Underutilizers of mammography screening today: Characteristics of women planning, undecided about, and not planning a mammogram. *Annals of Behavioral Medicine, 22*(1), 80–88.

Cloninger, C. R. (1991). D2 dopamine receptor gene is associated but not linked with alcoholism. *Journal of the American Medical Association, 266*(13), 1833–1834.

Coates, T. J. (1990). Strategies for modifying sexual behavior for primary and secondary prevention of HIV disease. *Journal of Consulting and Clinical Psychology, 58*(1), 57–69.

Coates, T. J., Morin, S. F., & McKusick, L. (1987). Behavioral consequences of AIDS antibody testing among gay men. *Journal of the American Medical Association, 258*(14), 1889–1889.

Coates, T. J., Stall, R. D., Kegeles, S. M., Lo, B., Morin, S. F., & McKusick, L. (1988). AIDS antibody testing: Will it stop the AIDS epidemic? Will it help people infected with HIV? *American Psychologist, 43*(11), 859–864.

Cobb, L. A., Thomas, G. I., Dillard, D. H., Merendino, K. A., & Bruce, R. A. (1959). An evaluation of internal mammary artery ligation by double blind technique. *New England Journal of Medicine, 260*, 1115–1118.

Cochran, S. D., & Mays, V. M. (1993). Applying social psychological models to predicting HIV-related sexual risk behaviors among African Americans. *Journal of Black Psychology, 19,* 142–154.

Cogan, R., Cogan, D., Waltz, W., & McCue, M. (1987). Effects of laughter and relaxation on discomfort thresholds. *Journal of Behavioral Medicine, 10,* 139–144.

Cohen, D., Nisbett, R. E., Bowdle, B. F., & Schwarz, N. (1996). Insult, aggression, and the southern culture of honor: An "experimental ethnography." *Journal of Personality and Social Psychology, 70*(5), 945–959.

Cohen, L. (2002). Reducing infant immunization distress through distraction. *Health Psychology, 21,* 207–211.

Cohen, L., Blount, R. L., Cohen, R. J., Schaen, E. R., & Zaff, J. F. (1999). Comparative study of distraction versus topical anesthesia for pediatric pain management during immunizations. *Health Psychology, 18,* 591–598.

Cohen, S. (1988). Psychosocial models of the role of social support in the etiology of physical disease. *Health Psychology, 7*(3), 269–297.

Cohen, S., Alper, C. M., Doyle, W. J., Treanor, J. J., & Turner, R. B. (2006). Positive emotional style predicts resistance to illness after experimental exposure to rhinovirus or influenza A virus. *Psychosomatic Medicine, 68*(6), 809–815.

Cohen, S., Doyle, W. J., Alper, C. M., Janicki-Deverts, D., & Turner, R. B. (2009). Sleep habits and susceptibility to the common cold. *Archives of Internal Medicine, 169*(1), 62–67.

Cohen, S., Doyle, W. J., Skoner, D. P., Fireman, P., Gwaltney, J. M., Jr., & Newsom, J. T. (1995). State and trait negative affect as predictors of objective and subjective symptoms of respiratory viral infections. *Journal of Personality and Social Psychology, 68*(1), 159–169.

Cohen, S., Doyle, W. J., Skoner, D. P., Rabin, B. S., & Gwaltney, J. M. (1997). Social ties and susceptibility to the common cold. *Journal of the American Medical Association, 277*(24), 1940–1944.

Cohen, S., Frank, E., Doyle, W. J., Skoner, D. P., Rabin, B. S., & Gwaltney, J. M., Jr. (1998). Types of stressors that increase susceptibility to the common cold in healthy adults. *Health Psychology, 17*(3), 214–223.

Cohen, S., Gianaros, P. J., & Manuck, S. B. (2016). A stage model of stress and disease. *Perspectives on Psychological Science, 11*(4), 456–463. **doi:10.1177/1745691616646305**

Cohen, S., & Herbert, T. B. (1996). Health psychology: Psychological factors and physical disease from the perspective of human psychoneuroimmunology. *Annual Review of Psychology, 47*(1), 113–142.

Cohen, S., Janicki-Deverts, D., Doyle, W. J., Miller, G. E., Frank, E., Rabin, B. S., & Turner, R. B. (2012). Chronic stress, glucocorticoid receptor resistance, inflammation, and disease risk. *Proceedings of the National Academy of Sciences of the United States of America, 109*(16), 5995–5999.

Cohen, S., Janicki-Deverts, D., & Miller, G. E. (2007). Psychological stress and disease. *Journal of the American Medical Association, 298*(14), 1685–1687.

Cohen, S., Janicki-Deverts, D., Turner, R. B., & Doyle, W. J. (2015). Does hugging provide stress-buffering social support? A study of susceptibility to upper respiratory infection and illness. *Psychological Science, 26*(2), 135–147.

Cohen, S., Kamarck, T., & Mermelstein, R. (1983). A global measure of perceived stress. *Journal of Health and Social Behavior, 24*(4), 385–396.

Cohen, S., & Lemay, E. P. (2007). Why would social networks be linked to affect and health practices? *Health Psychology, 26*(4), 410–417.

Cohen, S., & Lichtenstein, E. (1990). Partner behaviors that support quitting smoking. *Journal of Consulting and Clinical Psychology, 58*(3), 304–309.

Cohen, S., Mermelstein, R., Karmarck, T., & Hoberman, H. M. (1985). Measuring the functional components of social support. In I. G. Sarason & B. R. Sarason (Eds.), *Social support: Theory, research, and applications* (pp. 73–94). The Hague, NL: Martinus Nijhoff.

Cohen, S., Tyrrell, D. A., & Smith, A. P. (1991). Psychological stress and susceptibility to the common cold. *New England Journal of Medicine, 325*(9), 606–612.

Cohen, S., & Wills, T. A. (1985). Stress, social support, and the buffering hypothesis. *Psychological Bulletin, 98*(2), 310–357.

Cohen Castel, O., Keinan-Boker, L., Geyer, O., Milman, U., & Karkabi, K. (2014). Factors associated with adherence to glaucoma pharmacotherapy in the primary care setting. *Family Practice, 31*(4), 453–461. **http://doi.org/10.1093/fampra/cmu031**

Cohen-Gilbert, J. E., Sneider, J. T., Crowley, D. J., Rosso, I. M., Jensen, J. E., & Silveri, M. M. (2015). Impact of family history of alcoholism on glutamine/glutamate ratio in anterior cingulate cortex in substance-naive adolescents. *Developmental Cognitive Neuroscience, 16,* 147–154.

Colditz, G. A., Willett, W. C., Hunter, D. J., Stampfer, M. J., Manson, J. E., Hennekens, C. H., & Rosner, B. A. (1993). Family history, age, and risk of breast cancer: Prospective data from the Nurses' Health Study. *Journal of the American Medical Association, 270,* 338–343.

Cole, S. W., Kemeny, M. E., Taylor, S. E., Visscher, B. R., & Fahey, J. L. (1996). Accelerated course of human immunodeficiency virus infection in gay men who conceal their homosexual identity. *Psychosomatic Medicine, 58*(3), 219–231.

Colerick, E. J. (1985). Stamina in later life. *Social Science & Medicine, 21*(9), 997–1006.

Collaborative Group on Hormonal Factors in Breast Cancer. (2002).

Alcohol, tobacco and breast cancer—collaborative reanalysis of individual data from 53 epidemiological studies, including 58515 women with breast cancer and 95067 women without the disease. *British Journal of Cancer*, 87(11), 1234–1245. https://doi.org/10.1038/sj.bjc.6600596

Collins, R. L., Ellickson, P. L., McCaffrey, D., & Hambarsoomians, K. (2007). Early adolescent exposure to alcohol advertising and its relationship to underage drinking. *Journal of Adolescent Health*, 40(6), 527–534.

Collins, R. L., Kanouse, D. E., Gifford, A. L., Senterfitt, J. W., Schuster, M. A., Mccaffrey, D. F., . . . Wenger, N. S. (2001). Changes in health-promoting behavior following diagnosis with HIV: Prevalence and correlates in a national probability sample. *Health Psychology*, 20(5), 351–360.

Collins, R. L., Taylor, S. E., & Skokan, L. A. (1990). A better world or a shattered vision? Changes in life perspectives following victimization. *Social Cognition*, 8(3), 263–285. https://doi.org/10.1521/soco.1990.8.3.263

Comerci, G. D. (1990). Medical complications of anorexia nervosa and bulimia nervosa. *Medical Clinics of North America*, 74(5), 1293–1310.

Compare, A., & Tasca, A. G. (2014). The rate and shape of change in binge eating episodes and weight: An effectiveness trial of emotionally focused group therapy for binge-eating disorder. *Clinical Psychology & Psychotherapy*, 23(1), 24–34.

Compas, B. E., Haaga, D. A., Keefe, F. J., Leitenberg, H., & Williams, D. A. (1998). Sampling of empirically supported psychological treatments from health psychology: Smoking, chronic pain, cancer, and bulimia nervosa. *Journal of Consulting and Clinical Psychology*, 66, 89–112.

Comuzzie, A. G., & Allison, D. B. (1998). The search for human obesity genes. *Science*, 280(5368), 1374–1377.

Connor, J. (2017). Alcohol consumption as a cause of cancer. *Addiction*, 112(2), 222–228. https://doi.org/10.1111/add.13477

Conti, G., & Heckman, J. J. (2010). Understanding the early origins of the education–health gradient: A framework that can also be applied to analyze gene–environment interactions. *Perspectives on Psychological Science*, 5(5), 585–605.

Contrada, R. J. (1989). Type A behavior, personality hardiness, and cardiovascular responses to stress. *Journal of Personality and Social Psychology*, 57(5), 895–903.

Contrada, R. J., Goyal, T. M., Cather, C., Rafalson, L., Idler, E. L., & Krause, T. J. (2004). Psychosocial factors in outcomes of heart surgery: The impact of religious involvement and depressive symptoms. *Health Psychology*, 23(3), 227–238.

Conway, T. L., Vickers, R. R., Jr., Ward, H. W., & Rahe, R. H. (1981). Occupational stress and variation in cigarette, coffee, and alcohol consumption. *Journal of Health and Social Behavior*, 22(2), 155–165.

Cook, W. W., & Medley, D. M. (1954). Proposed hostility and pharisaic-virtue scales for the MMPI. *Journal of Applied Psychology*, 38(6), 414–418.

Coon, K. A., Goldberg, J., Rogers, B. L., & Tucker, K. L. (2001). Relationships between use of television during meals and children's food consumption patterns. *Pediatrics*, 7(1), e7. doi:10.1542/peds.107.1.e7

Cooper, J., Borland, R., McKee, S. A., Yong, H. H., & Dugué, P. A. (2016). Depression motivates quit attempts but predicts relapse: Differential findings for gender from the International Tobacco Control Study. *Addiction*, 111(8), 1438–1447.

Cooper, M. L., Frone, M. R., Russell, M., & Mudar, P. (1995). Drinking to regulate positive and negative emotions: A motivational model of alcohol use. *Journal of Personality and Social Psychology*, 69(5), 990–1005.

Cooper, M. L., Russell, M., Skinner, J. B., Frone, M. R., & Mudar, P. (1992). Stress and alcohol use: Moderating effects of gender, coping, and alcohol expectancies. *Journal of Abnormal Psychology*, 101(1), 139–152.

Cooperman, N. A., & Simoni, J. M. (2005). Suicidal ideation and attempted suicide among women living with HIV/AIDS. *Journal of Behavioral Medicine*, 28(2), 149–156.

Corathers, S. D., Kichler, J. C., Fino, N. F., Lang, W., Lawrence, J. M., Raymond, J. K., . . . Seid, M. (2017). High health satisfaction among emerging adults with diabetes: Factors predicting resilience. *Health Psychology*, 36(3), 206–214. doi:10.1037/hea0000419

Corbin, W. R., Iwamoto, D. K., & Fromme, K. (2011). Broad social motives, alcohol use, and related problems: Mechanisms of risk from high school through college. *Addictive Behaviors*, 36(3), 222–230.

Cornil, Y., & Chandon, P. (2013). From fan to fat? Vicarious losing increases unhealthy eating, but self-affirmation is an effective remedy. *Psychological Science*, 24(10), 1936–1946.

Corr, C. A. (1992). A task-based approach to coping with dying. *OMEGA – Journal of Death and Dying*, 24(2), 81–94. https://doi.org/10.2190/CNNF-CX1P-BFXU-GGN4

Coskun, B., Coskun, B. N., Atis, G., Ergenekon, E., & Dilek, K. (2014). Evaluation of sexual function in women with rheumatoid arthritis. *Urology Journal*, 10(4), 1081–1087.

Costa, P. T., & McCrae, R. R. (1980). Influence of extraversion and neuroticism on subjective well-being: Happy and unhappy people. *Journal of Personality and Social Psychology*, 38(4), 668–678.

Costa, P. T., & McCrae, R. R. (1985). Hypochondriasis, neuroticism, and aging: When are somatic complaints unfounded? *American Psychologist*, 40(1), 19–28.

Costa, P. T., & McCrae, R. R. (1987). Neuroticism, somatic complaints, and disease: Is the bark worse than the bite? *Journal of Personality*, *55*(2), 299–316.

Costa, P. T., & McCrae, R. R. (1992). Normal personality assessment in clinical practice: The NEO Personality Inventory. *Psychological Assessment*, *4*(1), 5–13.

Costello, D. M., Dierker, L. C., Jones, B. L., & Rose, J. S. (2008). Trajectories of smoking from adolescence to early adulthood and their psychosocial risk factors. *Health Psychology*, *27*(6), 811–818.

Cotton, S., Puchalski, C. M., Sherman, S. N., Mrus, J. M., Peterman, A. H., Feinberg, J., . . . Tsevat, J. (2006). Spirituality and religion in patients with HIV/AIDS. *Journal of General Internal Medicine*, *21*(Suppl 5), S5–S13. http://doi.org/10.1111/j.1525-1497.2006.00642.x

Cotton, S., Tsevat, J., Szaflarski, M., Kudel, I., Sherman, S. N., Feinberg, J., . . . Holmes, W. C. (2006). Changes in religiousness and spirituality attributed to HIV/AIDS: Are there sex and race differences? *Journal of General Internal Medicine*, *21*(Suppl 5), S14–S20. http://doi.org/10.1111/j.1525-1497.2006.00641.x

Council, J. R., Ahern, D. K., Follick, M. J., & Kline, C. L. (1988). Expectancies and functional impairment in chronic low back pain. *Pain*, *33*, 323–331.

Coyne, J. C., Rohrbaugh, M. J., Shoham, V., Sonnega, J. S., Nicklas, J. M., & Cranford, J. A. (2001). Prognostic importance of marital quality for survival of congestive heart failure. *American Journal of Cardiology*, *88*, 526–529.

Craig, K. D., Prkachin, K. M., & Grunau, R. V. E. (1992). The facial expression of pain. In D. C. Turk & R. Melzack (Eds.), *Handbook of pain assessment* (pp. 257–276). New York, NY: Guilford.

Cramer, J. A., Mattson, R. H., Prevey, M. L., Scheyer, R. D., & Ouellette, V. L. (1989). How often is medication taken as prescribed? *Journal of the American Medical Association*, *261*, 3273–3277.

Crandall, C. S. (1988). Social contagion of binge eating. *Journal of Personality and Social Psychology*, *55*(4), 588–598.

Crawford, M. A., Knight, R. G., & Alsop, B. L. (2007). Speed of word retrieval in postconcussion syndrome. *Journal of the International Neuropsychological Society*, *13*(1), 178–182.

Crawford, S. L., McGraw, S. A., Smith, K. W., McKinlay, J. B., & Pierson, J. E. (1994). Do Blacks and Whites differ in their use of health care for symptoms of coronary heart disease? *American Journal of Public Health*, *84*(6), 957–964.

Creatore, M. I., Glazier, R. H., Moineddin, R., Fazli, G. S., Johns, A., Gozdyra, P., . . . Booth, G. L. (2016). Association of neighborhood walkability with change in overweight, obesity, and diabetes. *Journal of the American Medical Association*, *315*(20), 2211–2220.

Crepaz, N., Passin, W. F., Herbst, J. H., Rama, S. M., Malow, R. M., Purcell, D. W., & Wolitski, R. J. (2008). Meta-analysis of cognitive-behavioral interventions on HIV-positive persons' mental health and immune functioning. *Health Psychology*, *27*(1), 4–14. doi:10.1037/0278-6133.27.1.4

Creswell, J. D., Taren, A. A., Lindsay, E. K., Greco, C. M., Gianaros, P. J., Fairgrieve, A., . . . Ferris, J. L. (2016). Alterations in resting-state functional connectivity link mindfulness meditation with reduced interleukin-6: A randomized controlled trial. *Biological Psychiatry*, *80*(1), 53–61.

Creswell, K. G., Cheng, Y., & Levine, M. D. (2015). A test of the stress-buffering model of social support in smoking cessation: Is the relationship between social support and time to relapse mediated by reduced withdrawal symptoms? *Nicotine & Tobacco Research: Official Journal of the Society for Research on Nicotine and Tobacco*, *17*(5), 566–571. doi:10.1093/ntr/ntu192

Crews, F. T., & Vetreno, R. P. (2016). Mechanisms of neuroimmune gene induction in alcoholism. *Psychopharmacology*, *233*(9), 1543–1557.

Crifasi, C. K., Meyers, J. S., Vernick, J. S., & Webster, D. W. (2015). Effects of changes in permit-to-purchase handgun laws in Connecticut and Missouri on suicide rates. *Preventive Medicine*, *79*, 43–49.

Crimmins, E. M. (2015). Lifespan and healthspan: Past, present, and promise. *The Gerontologist*, *55*(6), 901–911.

Crow, S. J., Peterson, C. B., Swanson, S. A., Raymond, N. C., Specker, S., Eckert, E. D., & Mitchell, J. E. (2009). Increased mortality in bulimia nervosa and other eating disorders. *American Journal of Psychiatry*, *166*(12), 1342–1346.

Crow, S. J., Swanson, S. A., le Grange, D., Feig, E. H., & Merikangas, K. R. (2014). Suicidal behavior in adolescents and adults with bulimia nervosa. *Comprehensive Psychiatry*, *55*(7), 1534–1539.

Croyle, R. T., Loftus, E. F., Barger, S. D., Sun Y. C., Hart M., & Gettig J. (2006). How well do people recall risk factor test results? Accuracy and bias among cholesterol screening participants. *Health Psychology*, *25*(3), 425–432.

Croyle, R. T., Smith, K. R., Botkin, J. R., Baty, B., & Nash, J. (1997). Psychological responses to BRCA1 mutation testing: Preliminary findings. *Health Psychology*, *16*(1), 63–72.

Croyle, R. T., Sun, Y. C., & Louie, D. H. (1993). Psychological minimization of cholesterol test results: Moderators of appraisal in college students and community residents. *Health Psychology*, *12*(6), 503–507.

Cruess, D. G., Antoni, M. H., McGregor, B. A., Kilbourn, K. M., Boyers, A. E., Alferi, S. M., . . . Kumar, M. (2000). Cognitive-behavioral stress management reduces serum cortisol by enhancing benefit finding among women being treated for early stage breast cancer. *Psychosomatic Medicine*, *62*(3), 304–308.

Crum, A., & Langer, E. (2007). Mindset matters: Exercise as a placebo. *Psychological Science*, *18*(2), 165–171.

Cservenka, A. (2016). Neurobiological phenotypes associated with a family history of alcoholism. *Drug and Alcohol Dependence*, *158*, 8–21.

Cservenka, A., Alarcón, G., Jones, S. A., & Nagel, B. J. (2015). Advances in human neuroconnectivity research: Applications for understanding familial history risk for alcoholism. *Alcohol Research: Current Reviews*, *37*(1), 89–95.

Cuevas, A. G., O'Brien, K., & Saha, S. (2016). African American experiences in healthcare: "I always feel like I'm getting skipped over." *Health Psychology*, *35*(9), 987–995.

Cui, J., Matsushima, E., Aso, K., Masuda, A., & Makita, K. (2009). Psychological features and coping styles in patients with chronic pain. *Psychiatry and Clinical Neurosciences*, *63*(2), 147–152. https://doi.org/10.1111/j.1440-1819.2009.01934.x

Culyba, A. J., Jacoby, S. F., Richmond, T. S., Fein, J. A., Hohl, B. C., & Branas, C. C. (2016). Modifiable neighborhood features associated with adolescent homicide. *JAMA Pediatrics*, *170*(5), 473–480.

Cundiff, J. M., Birmingham, W. C., Uchino, B. N., & Smith, T. W. (2016). Marital quality buffers the association between socioeconomic status and ambulatory blood pressure. *Annals of Behavioral Medicine*, *50*(2), 330–335.

Cundiff, J. M., Boylan, J. M., Pardini, D. A., & Matthews, K. A. (2017). Moving up matters: Socioeconomic mobility prospectively predicts better physical health. *Health Psychology*, *36*(6), 609–617. doi:10.1037/hea0000473

Cunningham-Myrie, C. A., Theall, K. P., Younger, N. O., Mabile, E. A., Tulloch-Reid, M. K., Francis, D. K., . . . Wilks, R. J. (2015). Associations between neighborhood effects and physical activity, obesity, and diabetes: The Jamaica Health and Lifestyle Survey 2008. *Journal of Clinical Epidemiology*, *68*(9), 970–978.

Curb, J. D., & Marcus, E. B. (1991). Body fat and obesity in Japanese Americans. *The American Journal of Clinical Nutrition*, *53*(6), 1552–1555.

Curry, A. E., Mirman, J. H., Kallan, M. J., Winston, F. K., & Durbin, D. R. (2012). Peer passengers: How do they affect teen crashes? *Journal of Adolescent Health*, *50*(6), 588–594.

Curry, S. J., & McBride, C. M. (1994). Relapse prevention for smoking cessation: Review and evaluation of concepts and interventions. *Annual Review of Public Health*, *15*(1), 345–366.

Curry, S., Marlatt, G. A., & Gordon, J. R. (1987). Abstinence violation effect: Validation of an attributional construct with smoking cessation. *Journal of Consulting and Clinical Psychology*, *55*(2), 145–149.

Curtin, S. C., Warner, M., & Hedegaard, H. (2016). Increase in suicide in the United States, 1999–2014. *National Center for Health Statistics Data Brief*, (241), 1–8.

Cutrona, C. E., & Russell, D. W. (1990). Type of social support and specific stress: Toward a theory of optimal matching. In B. R. Sarason, I. G. Sarason, & G. R. Pierce (Eds.), *Social support: An interactional view* (pp. 319–366). New York, NY: Wiley.

Dager, A. D., McKay, D. R., Kent, J. W., Jr., Curran, J. E., Knowles, E., Sprooten, E., . . . Glahn, D. C. (2015). Shared genetic factors influence amygdala volumes and risk for alcoholism. *Neuropsychopharmacology*, *40*(2), 412–420.

Dahlen, E. R., Martin, R. C., Ragan, K., & Kuhlman, M. M. (2005). Driving anger, sensation seeking, impulsiveness, and boredom proneness in the prediction of unsafe driving. *Accident Analysis & Prevention*, *37*(2), 341–348.

Dahlquist, L. M., McKenna, K. D., Jones, K. K., Dillinger, L., Weiss, K. E., & Ackerman, C. S. (2007). Active and passive distraction using a head-mounted display helmet: Effects on cold pressor pain in children. *Health Psychology*, *26*(6), 794–801.

Dahne, J., Hise, L., Brenner, M., Lejuez, C. W., & MacPherson, L. (2015). An experimental investigation of the functional relationship between social phobia and cigarette smoking. *Addictive Behaviors*, *43*, 66–71.

Dakof, G. A., & Taylor, S. E. (1990). Victims' perceptions of social support: What is helpful from whom? *Journal of Personality and Social Psychology*, *58*(1), 80–89.

Dal Cin, S., MacDonald, T. K., Fong, G. T., Zanna, M. P., & Elton-Marshall, T. E. (2006). Remembering the message: The use of a reminder cue to increase condom use following a safer sex intervention. *Health Psychology*, *25*(3), 438–443.

Dalgaard, K., Landgraf, K., Heyne, S., Lempradl, A., Longinotto, J., Gossens, K., . . . Ruf, M., (2016). Trim28 haploinsufficiency triggers bi-stable epigenetic obesity. *Cell*, *164*(3), 353–364.

Dalton, M. A., Sargent, J. D., Beach, M. L., Titus-Ernstoff, L., Gibson, J. J., Ahrens, M. B., . . . Heatherton, T. F. (2003). Effect of viewing smoking in movies on adolescent smoking initiation: A cohort study. *The Lancet*, *362*(9380), 281–285.

Dalton, P. (1999). Cognitive influences on health symptoms from acute chemical exposure. *Health Psychology*, *18*(6), 579–590.

Daly, M., Egan, M., Quigley, J., Delaney, L., & Baumeister, R. F. (2016). Childhood self-control predicts smoking throughout life: Evidence from 21,000 cohort study participants. *Health Psychology*, *35*(11), 1254–1263.

D'Amico, E. J., & Fromme, K. (1997). Health risk behaviors of adolescent and young adult siblings. *Health Psychology*, *16*(5), 426–432.

Danhauer, S. C., Crawford, S. L., Farmer, D. F., & Avis, N. E. (2009). A longitudinal investigation of coping strategies and quality of life among younger women with breast cancer. *Journal of Behavioral Medicine*, *32*(4), 371–379. https://doi.org/10.1007/s10865-009-9211-x

Dannenberg, A. L., Gielen, A. C., Beilenson, P. L., Wilson, M. H., & Joffe, A. (1993). Bicycle helmet laws and educational campaigns: An evaluation of strategies to increase children's helmet use. *American Journal of Public Health*, *83*(5), 667–674.

Darbes, L. A., & Lewis, M. A. (2005). HIV-specific social support predicts less sexual risk behavior in gay male couples. *Health Psychology*, *24*(6), 617–622.

Dar-Nimrod, I., Cheung, B. Y., Ruby, M. B., & Heine, S. J. (2014). Can merely learning about obesity genes affect eating behavior? *Appetite*, *81*, 269–276.

Dattore, P. J., Shontz, F. C., & Coyne, L. (1980). Premorbid personality differentiation of cancer and non-cancer groups: A list of the hypotheses of cancer proneness. *Journal of Consulting and Clinical Psychology*, *48*, 388–394.

Davidson, K. W., Gidron, Y., Mostofsky, E., & Trudeau, K. J. (2007). Hospitalization cost offset of a hostility intervention for coronary heart disease patients. *Journal of Consulting and Clinical Psychology*, *75*(4), 657–662.

Davidson, L. L., Durkin, M. S., Kuhn, L., O'Connor, P., Barlow, B., & Heagarty, M. C. (1994). The impact of the Safe Kids/Healthy Neighborhoods Injury Prevention Program in Harlem, 1988 through 1991. *American Journal of Public Health*, *84*(4), 580–586.

Davies, J. E., Gibson, T., & Tester, L. (1979). The value of exercises in the treatment of low back pain. *Rheumatology and Rehabilitation*, *18*, 243–247.

Davis, C. (2015). The epidemiology and genetics of binge eating disorder (BED). *CNS Spectrums*, *20*(6), 522–529.

Davis, C. G., Nolen-Hoeksema, S., & Larson, J. (1998). Making sense of loss and benefiting from the experience: Two construals of meaning. *Journal of Personality and Social Psychology*, *75*(2), 561–574.

Davis, D. L. (1991). *Empty cradle, broken heart: Surviving the death of your baby*. Golden, CO: Fulcrum.

Davis, E. L., Deane, F. P., & Lyons, G. C. B. (2015). Acceptance and valued living as critical appraisal and coping strengths for caregivers dealing with terminal illness and bereavement. *Palliative and Supportive Care*, *13*(2), 359–368. **https://doi.org/10.1017/S1478951514000431**

Davis, M. C., & Swan, P. D. (1999). Association of negative and positive social ties with fibrinogen levels in young women. *Health Psychology*, *18*(2), 131–139.

de Bruin, M., Hospers, H. J., van Breukelen, G. J. P., Kok, G. J., Koevoets, W. M., & Prins, J. M. (2010). Electronic monitoring-based counseling to enhance adherence among HIV-infected patients: A randomized controlled trial. *Health Psycho-Oncology*, *29*, 421–428. **doi:10.1037/a0020335**

de Castro, J. M. (1994). Family and friends produce greater social facilitation of food intake than other companions. *Physiology & Behavior*, *56*(3), 445–455.

de Castro, J. M., & de Castro, E. S. (1989). Spontaneous meal patterns of humans: Influence of the presence of other people. *The American Journal of Clinical Nutrition*, *50*(2), 237–247.

De Choudhury, M., Sharma, S., & Kiciman, E. (2016). Characterizing dietary choices, nutrition, and language in food deserts via social media. In *Proceedings of the 19th ACM Conference on Computer-Supported Cooperative Work & Social Computing* (pp. 1157–1170). New York, NY: ACM.

de Moor, J. S., de Moor, C. A., Basen-Engquist, K., Kudelka, A., Bevers, M. W., & Cohen, L. (2006). Optimism, distress, health-related quality of life, and change in cancer antigen 125 among patients with ovarian cancer undergoing chemotherapy. *Psychosomatic Medicine*, *68*(4), 555–562.

De Tommaso, M., Sardaro, M., & Livrea, P. (2008). Aesthetic value of paintings affects pain thresholds. *Consciousness and Cognition*, *17*(4), 1152–1162.

De Vera, M. A., Mailman, J., & Galo, J. S. (2014). Economics of non-adherence to biologic therapies in rheumatoid arthritis. *Current Rheumatology Reports*, *16*(11), 460.

De Vincenzi, I. (1994). A longitudinal study of human immunodeficiency virus transmission by heterosexual partners. *New England Journal of Medicine*, *331*(6), 341–346.

de Vries, B., Utz, R., Caserta, M., & Lund, D. (2014). Friend and family contact and support in early widowhood. *The Journals of Gerontology Series B*, *69B*(1), 75–84.

De Vries, S., Verheij, R. A., Groenewegen, P. P., & Spreeuwenberg, P. (2003). Natural environments—healthy environments? An exploratory analysis of the relationship between greenspace and health. *Environment and Planning*, *35*(10), 1717–1731.

de Wit, J. B., Das, E., & Vet, R. (2008). What works best: Objective statistics or a personal testimonial? An assessment of the persuasive effects of different types of message evidence on risk perception. *Health Psychology*, *27*(1), 110–115.

Den Oudsten, B. L., Van Heck, G. L., Van der Steeg, A. F., Roukema, J. A., & De Vries, J. (2009). Predictors of depressive symptoms 12 months after surgical treatment of early-stage breast cancer. *Psycho-Oncology*, *18*(11), 1230–1237.

Degenholtz, H. B., Resnick, A., Tang, Y., Razdan, M., & Enos, M. (2015). Effect of web-based training for department of motor vehicle staff on donor designation rates: Results of a statewide randomized trial. *American Journal of Transplantation*, *15*(5), 1376–1383.

DeGood, D. E. (2000). Relationship of pain-coping strategies to adjustment and functioning. In R. J. Gatchel & J. N. Weisberg (Eds.), *Personality characteristics of patients with pain* (pp. 129–164). Washington, DC: American Psychological Association.

Degortes, D., Santonastaso, P., Zanetti, T., Tenconi, E., Veronese, A., & Favaro,

A. (2014). Stressful life events and binge eating disorder. *European Eating Disorders Review, 22*(5), 378–382.

Deimling, G. T., Wagner, L. J., Bowman, K. F., Sterns, S., Kercher, K., & Kahana, B. (2006). Coping among older-adult, long-term cancer survivors. *Psycho-Oncology, 15*(2), 143–159. **https://doi.org/10.1002/pon.931**

Delahanty, D. L., & Baum, A. (2001). Stress and breast cancer. In A. Baum, T. A. Revenson, & J. E. Singer (Eds.), *Handbook of health psychology* (pp. 747–756). Mahwah, NJ: Erlbaum.

Delbanco, T. L. (1992). Enriching the doctor–patient relationship by inviting the patient's perspective. *Annals of Internal Medicine, 116,* 414–418.

DeLeon, P. H. (2002). Presidential reflections: Past and future. *American Psychologist, 57,* 425–430.

Delin, C. R., & Lee, T. H. (1992). Drinking and the brain: Current evidence. *Alcohol and Alcoholism, 27*(2), 117–126.

Denissenko, M. E., Pao, A., Tang, M., & Pfeifer, G. P. (1996). Preferential formation of benzoapyrene adducts at lung cancer mutational hotspots in P53. *Science, 274,* 430–432.

Dennis, P., Watkins, L., Calhoun, P., Oddone, A., Sherwood, A., Dennis, M., . . . Beckham, J. (2014). Posttraumatic stress, heart-rate variability, and the mediating role of behavioral health risks. *Psychosomatic Medicine, 78*(8), 629–637.

Denollet, J., Schiffer, A. A., & Spek, V. (2010). A general propensity to psychological distress affects cardiovascular outcomes. *Circulation: Cardiovascular Quality and Outcomes, 3*(5), 546–557.

Department of Transportation (US). (2015). *Traffic safety facts 2014 data: Alcohol-impaired driving.* Washington, DC: National Highway Traffic Safety Administration (NHTSA).

DeSantana, J. M., Walsh, D. M., Vance, C., Rakel, B. A., & Sluka, K. A. (2008). Effectiveness of transcutaneous electrical nerve stimulation for treatment of hyperalgesia and pain. *Current Rheumatology Reports, 10*(6), 492–499.

Desmond, S. M., Price, J. H., Hallinan, C., & Smith, D. (1989). Black and White adolescents' perceptions of their weight. *Journal of School Health, 59*(8), 353–358.

Detweiler, J. B., Bedell, B. T., Salovey, P., Pronin, E., & Rothman, A. J. (1999). Message framing and sunscreen use: Gain-framed messages motivate beachgoers. *Health Psychology, 18*(2), 189–196.

Devins, G. M., & Binik, Y. M. (1996). Facilitating coping with chronic physical illness. In M. Zeidner, N. S. Endler, M. Zeidner, & N. S. Endler (Eds.), *Handbook of coping: Theory, research, applications* (pp. 640–696). Oxford, UK: Wiley.

Devins, G. M., Mandin, H., Hons, R. B., Burgess, E. D., Klassen, J., Taub, K., . . . Buckle, S. (1990). Illness intrusiveness and quality of life in end-stage renal disease: Comparison and stability across treatment modalities. *Health Psychology, 9*(2), 117–142.

Deyo, R. A., Walsh, N. E., & Martin, D. (1990). A controlled trial of transcutaneous electrical nerve stimulation (TENS) and exercise for chronic low back pain. *New England Journal of Medicine, 322,* 1627–1634.

Diamond, E. G., Kittle, C. F., & Crockett, J. F. (1960). Comparision of internal mammary artery ligation and sham operation for angina pectoris. *American Journal of Cardiology, 5,* 483–486.

Dich, N., Lange, T., Head, J., & Rod, N. (2015). Work stress, caregiving, and allostatic load: Prospective results from the Whitehall II cohort study. *Psychosomatic Medicine, 77*(5), 539–547.

DiClemente, C. C., Prochaska, J. O., Fairhurst, S. K., Velicer, W. F., Velasquez, M. M., & Rossi, J. S. (1991). The process of smoking cessation: An analysis of precontemplation, contemplation, and preparation stages of change. *Journal of Consulting and Clinical Psychology, 59*(2), 295–304.

DiClemente, R. J., Wingood, G. M., Sales, J. M., Brown, J. L., Rose, E. S., Davis, T. L., . . . Hardin, J. W. (2014). Efficacy of a telephone-delivered sexually transmitted infection/human immunodeficiency virus prevention maintenance intervention for adolescents: A randomized clinical trial. *JAMA Pediatrics, 168*(10), 938–946.

Diefenbach, M. A., Miller, S. M., & Daly, M. B. (1999). Specific worry about breast cancer predicts mammography use in women at risk for breast and ovarian cancer. *Health Psychology, 8*(5), 532–536.

Dieleman, J. L., Baral, R., Birger, M., Bui, A. L., Bulchis, A., Chapin, A., . . . Lavado, R. (2016). US spending on personal health care and public health, 1996-2013. *Journal of the American Medical Association, 316*(24), 2627–2646.

Diggins, A., Woods-Giscombe, C., & Waters, S. (2015). The association of perceived stress, contextualized stress, and emotional eating with body mass index in college-aged Black women. *Eating Behaviors, 19,* 188–192. **doi:10.1016/j.eatbeh.2015.09.006**

Dillard, A. J., Midboe, A. M., & Klein, W. M. (2009). The dark side of optimism: Unrealistic optimism about problems with alcohol predicts subsequent negative event experiences. *Personality and Social Psychology Bulletin, 35*(11), 1540–1550.

DiMatteo, M. R. (1994). Enhancing patient adherence to medical recommendations. *Journal of the American Medical Association, 271,* 79–83.

DiMatteo, M. R. (2004). Social support and patient adherence to medical treatment: A meta-analysis. *Health Psychology, 23*(2), 207–218.

DiMatteo, M. R., Hays, R. D., Gritz, E. R., Bar-toni, R., Crane, L., Elashoff, R., . . . Marcus, A. (1993). Patient adherence to cancer control regimens: Scale development and initial validation. *Psychological Assessment, 5,* 102–112.

Dimond, M. (1979). Social support and adaptation to chronic illness: The case of maintenance hemodialysis. *Research in Nursing & Health, 2*(3), 101–108.

Dinh, K. T., Sarason, I. G., Peterson, A. V., & Onstad, L. E. (1995). Children's perceptions of smokers and nonsmokers: A longitudinal study. *Health Psychology, 14*(1), 32–40.

DiNicola, D. D., & DeMatteo, M. R. (1984). Practitioners, patients, and compliance with medical regimens: A social psychological perspective. In A. Baum, S. E. Taylor, & J. E. Singer (Eds.), *Handbook of psychology and health: Vol. 4. Social psychological aspects of health* (pp. 55–84). Hillsdale, NJ: Erlbaum.

Ditto, P. H., Druley, J. A., Moore, K. A., Danks, H. J., & Smucker, W. D. (1996). Fates worse than death: The role of valued life activities in health-state evaluations. *Health Psychology, 15*, 332–343.

Ditto, P. H., & Hawkins, N. A. (2005). Advance directives and cancer decision making near the end of life. *Health Psychology, 24*(4S), S63–S70.

Dlin, B. (1985). Psychobiology and treatment of anniversary reactions. *Psychosomatics, 26*, 505–520.

Dodge, T., Williams, K. J., Marzell, M., & Turrisi, R. (2012). Judging cheaters: Is substance misuse viewed similarly in the athletic and academic domains? *Psychology of Addictive Behaviors, 26*(3), 678–682.

Doering, S., Katzlberger, F., Rumpold, G., Roessler, S., Hofstoetter, B., Schatz, D. S., . . . Schuessler, G. (2000). Videotape preparation of patients before hip replacement surgery reduces stress. *Psychosomatic Medicine, 62*(3), 365–373.

Doka, K. J. (1993). *Living with life-threatening illness.* Lexington, MA: Lexington Books.

Donaldson, E. A., Cohen, J. E., Villanti, A. C., Kanarek, N. F., Barry, C. L., & Rutkow, L. (2015). Patterns and predictors of state adult obesity prevention legislation enactment in US states: 2010–2013. *Preventive Medicine, 74*, 117–122.

Dowell, D., Haegerich, T. M., & Chou, R. (2016). CDC guideline for prescribing opioids for chronic pain— United States, 2016. *Journal of the American Medical Association, 315*(15), 1624–1645. **https://doi.org/10.1001/jama.2016.1464**

Downey, G., Silver, R. C., & Wortman, C. B. (1990). Reconsidering the attribution-adjustment relationship following a major negative event: Coping with the loss of a child. *Journal of Personality and Social Psychology, 59*, 925–940.

Dowson, D. I., Lewith, G. T., & Machin, C. (1985). The effects of acupuncture versus placebo in the treatment of headache. *Pain, 21*, 35–42.

Drach-Zahavy, A., & Somech, A. (2002). Coping with health problems: The distinctive relationships of hope sub-scales with constructive thinking and resource allocation. *Personality and Individual Differences, 33*(1), 103–117.

Drewnowski, A. (1996). The behavioral phenotype in human obesity. In E. D. Capaldi (Ed.), *Why we eat what we eat: The psychology of eating* (pp. 291–308). Washington, DC: American Psychological Association.

Druley, J. A., Stephens, M. A., & Coyne, J. C. (1997). Emotional and physical intimacy in coping with lupus. Women's dilemmas of disclosure and approach. *Health Psychology, 16*(6), 506 514. **doi:10.1037//0278-6133.16.6.506**

Du, A., Jiang, H., Xu, L., An, N., Liu, H., Li, Y., & Zhang, R. (2014). Damage of hippocampal neurons in rats with chronic alcoholism. *Neural Regeneration Research, 9*(17), 1610–1615.

Duarte, C., Ferreira, C., & Pinto-Gouveia, J. (2016). At the core of eating disorders: Overvaluation, social rank, self-criticism and shame in anorexia, bulimia and binge eating disorder. *Comprehensive Psychiatry, 66*, 123–131.

Dubus, R. (1959). *The mirage of health.* New York, NY: Harper.

Duchemin, A. M., Steinberg, B. A., Marks, D. R., Vanover, K., & Klatt, M. (2015). A small randomized pilot study of a workplace mindfulness-based intervention for surgical intensive care unit personnel: Effects on salivary α-amylase levels. *Journal of Occupational and Environmental Medicine, 57*(4), 393–399.

Dukes, J. W., Dewland, T. A., Vittinghoff, E., Olgin, J. E., Pletcher, M. J., Hahn, J. A., . . . Marcus, G. M. (2016). Access to alcohol and heart disease among patients in hospital: Observational cohort study using differences in alcohol sales laws. *British Medical Journal, 353*, i2714.

Dunbar-Jacob, J., Burke, L. E., & Puczynski, S. (1995). Clinical assessment and management of adherence to medical regimens. In P. M. Nicassio & T. M. Smith (Eds.), *Managing chronic illness: A biopsychosocial perspective* (pp. 313–349). Washington, DC: American Psychological Association.

Duncan, S. C., Duncan, T. E., & Strycker, L. A. (2005). Sources and types of social support in youth physical activity. *Health Psychology, 24*(1), 3–10.

Duncan, T. E., & McAuley, E. (1993). Social support and efficacy cognitions in exercise adherence: A latent growth curve analysis. *Journal of Behavioral Medicine, 16*(2), 199–218.

Dunkel Schetter, C. (1984). Social support and cancer: Findings based on patient interviews and their implications. *Journal of Social Issues, 40*, 77–98.

Dunkel Schetter, C., Feinstein, L. G., Taylor, S. E., & Falke, R. L. (1992). Patterns of coping with cancer. *Health Psychology, 11*(2), 79–87.

Dunkel Schetter, C., Schafer, P., Lanzi, R. G., Clark-Kauffman, E., Raju, T. N. K., Hillemeier, M. M., & the Community Child Health Network. (2013). Shedding light on the mechanisms underlying health disparities through community participatory methods: The stress pathway. *Perspectives on Psychological Science, 8*(6), 613–633. **http://doi .org/10.1177/1745691613506016**

Dunkel Schetter, C., & Wortman, C. B. (1982). The interpersonal dynamics of cancer: Problems in social relationships and their impact on the patient. In H. S. Friedman & M. R. DiMatteo (Eds.), *Interpersonal issues in health care* (pp. 69–100). New York, NY: Academic Press.

Dunlop, D. D., Song, J., Lee, J., Gilbert, A. L., Semanik, P. A., Ehrlich-Jones, L., . . . Chang, R. W. (2017). Physical activity minimum threshold predicting improved function in adults with lower-extremity symptoms. *Arthritis Care & Research, 69*(4), 475–483.

Dunn, A. L., Marcus, B. H., Kampert, J. B., Garcia, M. E., Kohl, H. W., III, & Blair, S. N. (1999). Comparison of lifestyle and structured interventions to increase physical activity and cardiorespiratory fitness: A randomized trial. *Journal of the American Medical Association, 281*(4), 327–334.

Dupre, M. E., & Lopes, R. D. (2016). Marital history and survival after stroke. *Journal of the American Heart Association, 5*, e004647. https://doi.org/10.1161/JAHA.116.004647

Durbin, D. R., Chen, I., Smith, R., Elliott, M. R., & Winston, F. K. (2005). Effects of seating position and appropriate restraint use on the risk of injury to children in motor vehicle crashes. *Pediatrics, 115*(3), 305–309.

Durkheim, É. (1951). *Suicide: A study in sociology.* London, UK: Routledge.

Dusseldorp, E., van Elderen, T., Maes, S., Meulman, J., & Kraaij, V. (1999). A meta-analysis of psychoeducational programs for coronary heart disease patients. *Health Psychology, 18*, 506–519.

Dvorak, R. D., Pearson, M. R., & Day, A. M. (2014). Ecological momentary assessment of acute alcohol use disorder symptoms: Associations with mood, motives, and use on planned drinking days. *Experimental and Clinical Psychopharmacology, 22*(4), 285–297.

Eakin, E., Reeves, M., Winkler, E., Lawler, S., & Owen, N. (2010). Maintenance of physical activity and dietary change following a telephone-delivered intervention. *Health Psychology, 29*(6), 566–573.

Earl, A., & Albarracín, D. (2007). Nature, decay, and spiraling of the effects of fear-inducing arguments and HIV counseling and testing: A meta-analysis of the short-and long-term outcomes of HIV-prevention interventions. *Health Psychology, 26*(4), 496–506.

Echeverría, S. E., Gundersen, D. A., Manderski, M. T. B., & Delnevo, C. D. (2015). Social norms and its correlates as a pathway to smoking among young Latino adults. *Social Science & Medicine (1982), 124*, 187–195. http://doi.org/10.1016/j.socscimed.2014.11.034

Eckardt, M. J., Harford, T. C., Kaelber, C. T., Parker, E. S., Rosenthal, L. S., Ryback, R. S., . . . Warren, K. R. (1981). Health hazards associated with alcohol consumption. *Journal of the American Medical Association, 246*(6), 648–666.

Eddy, K. T., Tabri, N., Thomas, J. J., Murray, H. B., Keshaviah, A., Hastings, E., . . . Franko, D. L. (2016). Recovery from anorexia nervosa and bulimia nervosa at 22-year follow-up. *The Journal of Clinical Psychiatry, 78*(2), 184–189.

Edelson, J., & Fitzpatrick, J. L. (1989). A comparison of cognitive-behavioral and hypnotic treatments of chronic pain. *Journal of Clinical Psychology, 45*, 316–323.

Edmondson, D., Park, C. L., Chaudoir, S. R., & Wortmann, J. H. (2008). Death without God. *Psychological Science, 19*(8), 754–758. https://doi.org/10.1111/j.1467-9280.2008.02152.x

Eggenberger Carroll, J., Smith, H., & Hillier, S. (2008). When will older patients follow doctors' recommendations? Interpersonal treatment, outcome favorability, and perceived age differences. *Journal of Applied Social Psychology, 38*, 1127–1146. doi:10.1111/j.1559-1816.2008.00342.x

Ehrensaft, M. K., Cohen, P., Brown, J., Smailes, E., Chen, H., & Johnson, J. G. (2003). Intergenerational transmission of partner violence: A 20-year prospective study. *Journal of Consulting and Clinical Psychology, 71*(4), 741–753.

Ehrenwald, J. (Ed.). (1976). *The history of psychotherapy: From healing magic to encounter.* New York, NY: Jason Aronson.

Ehsani, J. P., Li, K., Simons-Morton, B. G., Tree-McGrath, C. F., Perlus, J. G., O'Brien, F., & Klauer, S. G. (2015). Conscientious personality and young drivers' crash risk. *Journal of Safety Research, 54*, 83–87.

Eichstaedt, J. C., Schwartz, H. A., Kern, M. L., Park, G., Labarthe, D. R., Merchant, R. M., . . . Seligman, M. P. (2015). Psychological language on Twitter predicts county-level heart disease mortality. *Psychological Science, 26*(2), 159–169. doi:**10.1177/0956797614557867**

Eifert, G. H., Hodson, S. E., Tracey, D. R., Seville, L., & Gunawardane, K. (1996). Heart-focused anxiety, illness beliefs, and behavioral impairment: Comparing healthy heart-anxious patients with cardiac and surgical inpatients. *Journal of Behavioral Medicine, 19*(4), 385–399.

Eisenberg, D. M., Delbanco, T. L., Berkey, C. S., Kaptchuk, T. J., Kupelnick, B., Kuhl, J., & Chalmers, T. C. (1993). Cognitive behavioral techniques for hypertension: Are they effective? *Annals of Internal Medicine, 118*, 964–972. doi:**10.7326/0003-4819-118-12-199306150-00009**

Eisenberg, M. E., Olson, R. E., Neumark-Sztainer, D., Story, M., & Bearinger, L. H. (2004). Correlations between family meals and psychosocial well-being among adolescents. *Archives of Pediatrics and Adolescent Medicine, 158*, 792–796.

Eiser, C. (1982). The effects of chronic illness on children and their families. In J. R. Eiser (Ed.), *Social psychology and behavioral medicine* (pp. 459–481). New York, NY: Wiley.

Elfant, E., Burns, J. W., & Zeichner, A. (2008). Repressive coping style and suppression of pain-related thoughts: Effects on responses to acute pain induction. *Cognition and Emotion*, *22*(4), 671–696. https://doi.org/10.1080/02699930701483927

Ellington, L., & Wiebe, D. J. (1999). Neuroticism, symptom presentation, and medical decision making. *Health Psychology*, *18*(6), 634–643.

Elliott, A. M., Alexander, S. C., Mescher, C. A., Mohan, D., & Barnato, A. E. (2016). Differences in physicians' verbal and nonverbal communication with Black and White patients at the end of life. *Journal of Pain and Symptom Management*, *51*(1), 1–8.

Ellis, T. E., & Rufino, K. A. (2015). A psychometric study of the Suicide Cognitions Scale with psychiatric inpatients. *Psychological Assessment*, *27*(1), 82–89.

Elliston, K. G., Ferguson, S. G., Schüz, N., & Schüz, B. (2017). Situational cues and momentary food environment predict everyday eating behavior in adults with overweight and obesity. *Health Psychology*, *36*(4), 337–345. http://dx.doi.org/10.1037/hea0000439

Else-Quest, N. M., LoConte, N. K., Schiller, J. H., & Hyde, J. S. (2009). Perceived stigma, self-blame, and adjustment among lung, breast and prostate cancer patients. *Psychology & Health*, *24*(8), 949–964. https://doi.org/10.1080/08870440802074664

Elstein, A. S., Chapman, G. B., & Knight, S. J. (2005). Patients' values and clinical substituted judgments: The case of localized prostate cancer. *Health Psychology*, *24*(4S), S85–S92.

Elwert, F., & Christakis, N. A. (2008). The effect of widowhood on mortality by the causes of death of both spouses. *American Journal of Public Health*, *98*(11), 2092–2098. https://doi.org/10.2105/AJPH.2007.114348

Emanuel, E. J., Onwuteaka-Philipsen, B. D., Urwin, J. W., & Cohen, J. (2016). Attitudes and practices of euthanasia and physician-assisted suicide in the United States, Canada, and Europe. *Journal of the American Medical Association*, *316*(1), 79–90. https://doi.org/10.1001/jama.2016.8499

Emerson, E. (2009). Relative child poverty, income inequality, wealth, and health. *Journal of the American Medical Association*, *301*(4), 425–426.

Emlet, C. A. (2006). A comparison of HIV stigma and disclosure patterns between older and younger adults living with HIV/AIDS. *AIDS Patient Care and STDs*, *20*(5), 350–358. doi:10.1089/apc.2006.20.350

Emmett, C., & Ferguson, E. (1999). Oral contraceptive pill use, decisional balance, risk perception and knowledge: An exploratory study. *Journal of Reproductive and Infant Psychology*, *17*(4), 327–343.

Emmons, K. M., Wechsler, H., Dowdall, G., & Abraham, M. (1998). Predictors of smoking among US college students. *American Journal of Public Health*, *88*(1), 104–107.

Emmons, R. A. (2005). Striving for the sacred: Personal goals, life meaning, and religion. *Journal of Social Issues*, *61*(4), 731–745.

Endestad, T., Wortinger, L. A., Madsen, S. & Hortemo, S. (2016). Package design affects accuracy recognition for medications. *Human Factors: The Journal of the Human Factors and Ergonomics Society*, *58*(8), 1206–1216. doi:10.1177/0018720816664824

Eng, P. M., Rimm, E. B., Fitzmaurice, G., & Kawachi, I. (2002). Social ties and change in social ties in relation to subsequent total and cause-specific mortality and coronary heart disease incidence in men. *American Journal of Epidemiology*, *155*(8), 700–709.

Engel, G. (1977). The need for a new medical model: A challenge for biomedicine. *Science*, *196*(4286), 129–136. doi:10.1126/science.847460

Engel, G. L. (1980). The clinical application of the biopsychosocial model. *American Journal of Psychiatry*, *137*, 535–544.

Ennett, S. T., Tobler, N. S., Ringwalt, C. L., & Flewelling, R. L. (1994). How effective is drug abuse resistance education? A meta-analysis of Project DARE outcome evaluations. *American Journal of Public Health*, *84*(9), 1394–1401.

Enoch, M. A., Hodgkinson, C. A., Shen, P. H., Gorodetsky, E., Marietta, C. A., Roy, A., & Goldman, D. (2016). GABBR1 and SLC6A1, two genes involved in modulation of GABA synaptic transmission, influence risk for alcoholism: Results from three ethnically diverse populations. *Alcoholism: Clinical and Experimental Research*, *40*(1), 93–101.

Enright, M. F., Resnick, R., DeLeon, P. H., Sciara, A. D., & Tanney, F. (1990). The practice of psychology in hospital settings. *American Psychologist*, *45*(9), 1059–1065.

Epping-Jordan, J. E., Compas, B. E., Osowiecki, D. M., Oppedisano, G., Gerhardt, C., Primo, K., & Krag, D. N. (1999). Psychological adjustment in breast cancer: Processes of emotional distress. *Health Psychology*, *18*, 315–326.

Epstein, A. M., Taylor, W. C., & Seage, G. R. (1985). Effects of patients' socioeconomic status and physicians' training and practice on patient-doctor communication. *American Journal of Medicine*, *78*, 101–106.

Epstein, L. H., & Cluss, P. A. (1982). A behavioral medicine perspective on adherence to long-term medical regimens. *Journal of Consulting and Clinical Psychology*, *50*, 950–971.

Epstein, L. H., Paluch, R. A., Kilanowski, C. K., & Raynor, H. A. (2004). The effect of reinforcement or stimulus control to reduce sedentary behavior in the treatment of pediatric obesity. *Health Psychology*, *23*(4), 371–380.

Epton, T., & Harris, P. R. (2008). Self-affirmation promotes health behavior change. *Health Psychology*, *27*(6), 746–752.

Esterling, B. A., Kiecolt-Glaser, J. K., Bodnar, J. C., & Glaser, R. (1994). Chronic stress, social support, and persistent alterations in the natural kill cell response to cytokines in older adults. *Health Psychology, 13,* 291–298.

Esteve, R., Ramírez-Maestre, C., & López-Martínez, A. E. (2007). Adjustment to chronic pain: The role of pain acceptance, coping strategies, and pain-related cognitions. *Annals of Behavioral Medicine, 33*(2), 179–188. https://doi.org/10.1007/BF02879899

Evans, G. W., Bullinger, M., & Hygge, S. (1998). Chronic noise exposure and physiological response: A prospective study of children living under environmental stress. *Psychological Science, 9*(1), 75–77.

Evans, G. W., & Kim, P. (2007). Childhood poverty and health: Cumulative risk exposure and stress dysregulation. *Psychological Science, 18*(11), 953–957.

Evans, G. W., & Kutcher, R. (2011). Loosening the link between childhood poverty and adolescent smoking and obesity: The protective effects of social capital. *Psychological Science, 22*(1), 3–7.

Evans, R. I. (1988). Health promotion—science or ideology? *Health Psychology,* 7(3), 203–219.

Evans, R. I., Rozelle, R. M., Lasater, T. M., Dembroski, T. M., & Allen, B. P. (1970). Fear arousal, persuasion, and actual versus implied behavioral change: New perspective utilizing a real-life dental hygiene program. *Journal of Personality and Social Psychology, 16*(2), 220–227.

Evans, R. I., Rozelle, R. M., Maxwell, S. E., Raines, B. E., Dill, C. A., Guthrie, T. J., . . . Hill, P. C. (1981). Social modeling films to deter smoking in adolescents: Results of a three-year field investigation. *Journal of Applied Psychology, 66*(4), 399–414.

Evans, W. D., Powers, A., Hersey, J., & Renaud, J. (2006). The influence of social environment and social image on adolescent smoking. *Health Psychology,* 25(1), 26–33.

Evers, C., Stok, M. F., & de Ridder, D. T. (2010). Feeding your feelings: Emotion regulation strategies and emotional eating. *Personality and Social Psychology Bulletin, 36*(6), 792–804.

Everson, S. A., Goldberg, D. E., Kaplan, G. A., & Cohen, R. D. (1996). Hopelessness and risk of mortality and incidence of myocardial infarction and cancer. *Psychosomatic Medicine, 58,* 103–121.

Ewart, C. K., Harris, W. L., Iwata, M. M., Coates, T. J., Bullock, R., & Simon, B. (1987). Feasibility and effectiveness of school-based relaxation in lowering blood pressure. *Health Psychology, 6*(5), 399–416.

Eysenck, H. J. (1967). *The biological basis of personality.* Springfield, IL: Thomas.

Faasse, K., & Petrie, K. J. (2016). From me to you: The effect of social modeling on treatment outcomes. *Current Directions in Psychological Science, 25*(6), 438–443.

Fabio, A., Chen, C. Y., Dearwater, S., Jacobs, D. R., Jr., Erickson, D., Matthews, K. A., . . . Pereira, M. A. (2015). Television viewing and hostile personality trait increase the risk of injuries. *International Journal of Injury Control and Safety Promotion, 24*(1), 44–53.

Faden, R. R., Beauchamp, T. L., & King, N. P. (1986). *A history and theory of informed consent.* New York, NY: Oxford University Press.

Faden, R. R., & Kass, N. E. (1993). Genetic screening technology: Ethical issues in access to tests by employers and health insurance companies. *Journal of Social Issues, 49*(2), 75–88.

Falk, E. B., O'Donnell, M. B., Cascio, C. N., Tinney, F., Kang, Y., Lieberman, M. D., . . . Strecher, V. J. (2015). Self-affirmation alters the brain's response to health messages and subsequent behavior change. *Proceedings of the National Academy of Sciences of the United States of America, 112*(7), 1977–1982.

Falk, E. B., O'Donnell, M. B., Tompson, S., Gonzalez, R., Dal Cin, S., Strecher, V., . . . An, L. (2015). Functional brain imaging predicts public health campaign success. *Social Cognitive and Affective Neuroscience, 11*(2), 204–214.

Fallon, A. E., & Rozin, P. (1985). Sex differences in perception of desirable body shape. *Journal of Abnormal Psychology, 94,* 102–105.

Fang, C. Y., Ross, E. A., Pathak, H. B., Godwin, A. K., & Tseng, M. (2014). Acculturative stress and inflammation among Chinese immigrant women. *Psychosomatic Medicine, 76*(5), 320–326. http://doi.org/10.1097/PSY.0000000000000065

Farquhar, J. W., Fortmann, S. P., Flora, J. A., Taylor, C. B., Haskell, W. L., Williams, P. T., . . . Wood, P. D. (1990). Effects of communitywide education on cardiovascular disease risk factors: The Stanford Five-City Project. *Journal of the American Medical Association, 264*(3), 359–365.

Farrell, C. A., Fleegler, E. W., Monuteaux, M. C., Wilson, C. R., Christian, C. W., & Lee, L. K. (2017). Community poverty and child abuse fatalities in the United States. *Pediatrics, 139*(5), e20161616; doi:10.1542/peds.2016-1616

Farrelly, M. C., Davis, K. C., Haviland, M. L., Messeri, P., & Healton, C. G. (2005). Evidence of a dose—response relationship between "truth" antismoking ads and youth smoking prevalence. *American Journal of Public Health, 95*(3), 425–431.

Farrelly, M. C., Duke, J. C., Nonnemaker, J., MacMonegle, A. J., Alexander, T. N., Zhao, X., . . . Allen, J. A. (2017). Association between The Real Cost media campaign and smoking initiation among youths-United States, 2014-2016. *Morbidity and Mortality Weekly Report, 66*(2), 47–50.

Fawzy, F. I., Cousins, N., Fawzy, N. W., Kemeny, M. E., Elashoff, R., & Morton, D. (1990). A structured psychiatric intervention for cancer patients: I. Changes over time in methods of coping and affective disturbance. *Archives of General Psychiatry, 47,* 720–725.

Federal Bureau of Investigation. (2016). 2015 crime in the United States. Retrieved from https://ucr.fbi.gov/crime-in-the-u.s/2015/crime-in-the-u.s.-2015/offenses-known-to-law-enforcement/expanded-homicide

Fedewa, S. A., Sauer, A. G., Siegel, R. L., & Jemal, A. (2015). Prevalence of major risk factors and use of screening tests for cancer in the United States. *Cancer Epidemiology and Prevention Biomarkers, 24*(4), 637–652.

Fedirko, V., Tramacere, I., Bagnardi, V., Rota, M., Scotti, L., Islami, F., . . . Jenab, M. (2011). Alcohol drinking and colorectal cancer risk: An overall and dose–response meta-analysis of published studies. *Annals of Oncology, 22*(9), 1958–1972. https://doi.org/10.1093/annonc/mdq653

Feeg, V. D., & Elebiary, H. (2005). Exploratory study on end-of-life issues: Barriers to palliative care and advance directives. *American Journal of Hospice and Palliative Medicine®, 22*(2), 119–124. https://doi.org/10.1177/10499091050 2200207

Feifel, H. (1990). Psychology and death: Meaningful rediscovery. *American Psychologist, 45,* 537–543.

Feldman, S. I., Downey, G., & Schaffer-Neitz, R. (1999). Pain, negative mood, and perceived support in chronic pain patients: A daily diary study of people with reflex sympathetic dystrophy syndrome. *Journal of Consulting and Clinical Psychology, 67,* 776–785.

Feletti, G., Firman, D., & Sanson-Fisher, R. (1986). Patient satisfaction with primary-care consultations. *Journal of Behavioral Medicine, 9,* 389–399.

Fell, J. C., Fisher, D. A., Voas, R. B., Blackman, K., & Tippetts, A. S. (2008). The relationship of underage drinking laws to reductions in drinking drivers in fatal crashes in the United States.

Accident Analysis & Prevention, 40(4), 1430–1440.

Felson, D. T., Zhang, Y., Hannan, M. T., Kannel, W. B., & Kiel, D. P. (1995). Alcohol intake and bone mineral density in elderly men and women: The Framingham study. *American Journal of Epidemiology, 142*(5), 485–492.

Felton, B. J., & Revenson, T. A. (1984). Coping with chronic illness: A study of illness controllability and the influence of coping strategies on psychological adjustment. *Journal of Consulting and Clinical Psychology, 52*(3), 343–353.

Feng, R., Wang, D. B., Chai, J., Cheng, J., & Li, H. P. (2014). Total delay for treatment among cancer patients: A theory-guided survey in China. *Asian Pacific Journal of Cancer Prevention, 15*(10), 4339–4347.

Ferdinand, A. O., Menachemi, N., Sen, B., Blackburn, J. L., Morrisey, M., & Nelson, L. (2014). Impact of texting laws on motor vehicular fatalities in the United States. *American Journal of Public Health, 104*(8), 1370–1377.

Fernandez, E. (1986). A classification system of cognitive coping strategies for pain. *Pain, 26,* 141–151.

Feuille, M., & Pargament, K. (2015). Pain, mindfulness, and spirituality: A randomized controlled trial comparing effects of mindfulness and relaxation on pain-related outcomes in migraineurs. *Journal of Health Psychology, 20*(8), 1090–1106.

Feunekes, G. I., de Graaf, C., & Van Staveren, W. A. (1995). Social facilitation of food intake is mediated by meal duration. *Physiology & Behavior, 58*(3), 551–558.

Field, A. E., Camargo, C. A., Taylor, C. B., Berkey, C. S., Roberts, S. B., & Colditz, G. A. (2001). Peer, parent, and media influences on the development of weight concerns and frequent dieting among preadolescent and adolescent girls and boys. *Pediatrics, 107*(1), 54–60.

Field, N. P., Nichols, C., Holen, A., & Horowitz, M. J. (1999). The relation of continuing attachment to adjustment in conjugal bereavement. *Journal of Consulting and Clinical Psychology, 67,* 212–218.

Field, T. M. (1998). Massage therapy effects. *American Psychologist, 53,* 1270–1281.

Fielding, J. E., & Phenow, K. J. (1988). Health effects of involuntary smoking. *New England Journal of Medicine, 319,* 1452–1460.

Figaro, M. K., Russo, P. W., & Allegrante, J. P. (2004). Preferences for arthritis care among urban African Americans: "I don't want to be cut." *Health Psychology, 23*(3), 324–329.

Figaro, M. K., Williams-Russo, P., & Allegrante, J. P. (2005). Expectation and outlook: The impact of patient preference on arthritis care among African Americans. *The Journal of Ambulatory Care Management, 28*(1), 41–48.

Finch, E. A., Linde, J. A., Jeffery, R. W., Rothman, A. J., King, C. M., & Levy, R. L. (2005). The effects of outcome expectations and satisfaction on weight loss and maintenance: Correlational and experimental analyses—a randomized trial. *Health Psychology, 24*(6), 608–616.

Fine, P. R., Rousculp, M. D., Tomasek, A. D., & Horn, W. S. (1999). Intentional injury. In J. M. Raczynski & R. J. DiClemente (Eds.), *Handbook of health promotion and disease prevention* (pp. 287–308). New York, NY: Plenum.

Fiore, M. C., Jaen, C. R., Baker, T., Bailey, W. C., Benowitz, N. L., Curry, S. E. E. A., . . . Henderson, P. N. (2008). *Treating tobacco use and dependence: 2008 update.* Rockville, MD: US Department of Health and Human Services.

Fiscella, K., Franks, P., Gold, M. R., & Clancy, C. M. (2000). Inequality in quality: Addressing socioeconomic, racial, and ethnic disparities in health care. *Journal of the American Medical Association, 283*(19), 2579–2584.

Fishbein, M., & Ajzen, I. (1975). *Belief, attitude, intention, and behavior*. Reading, MA: Addison-Wesley.

Fitzgerald, T. E., Tennen, H., Affleck, G., & Pransky, G. S. (1993). The relative importance of dispositional optimism and control appraisals in quality of life after coronary artery bypass surgery. *Journal of Behavioral Medicine, 16*, 25–43.

Flack, J. M., Amaro, H., Jenkins, W., Kunitz, S., Levy, J., Mixon, M., & Yu, E. (1995). Panel I: Epidemiology of minority health. *Health Psychology, 14*(7), 592–600.

Flay, B. R., Hansen, W. B., Johnson, C. A., Collins, L. M., Dent, C. W., Dwyer, K. M., . . . Sobol, D. F. (1987). Implementation effectiveness trial of a social influences smoking prevention program using schools and television. *Health Education Research, 2*(4), 385–400.

Fleishman, J. A., & Fogel, B. (1994). Coping and depressive symptoms among young people with AIDS. *Health Psychology, 13*(2), 156–169.

Fleming, R., Baum, A., Gisriel, M. M., & Gatchel, R. J. (1982). Mediating influences of social support on stress at Three Mile Island. *Journal of Human Stress, 8*(3), 14–23.

Fletcher, A. M. (2001). *Sober for good: New solutions for drinking problems: Advice from those who have succeeded*. Boston, MA: Houghton, Mifflin and Company.

Flett, G. L., Hewitt, P. L., & Heisel, M. J. (2014). The destructiveness of perfectionism revisited: Implications for the assessment of suicide risk and the prevention of suicide. *Review of General Psychology, 18*(3), 156–172.

Flor, H., & Birbaumer, N. (1993). Comparison of the efficacy of electromyographic biofeedback, cognitive-behavioral therapy, and conservative medical interventions in the treatment of chronic musculoskeletal pain. *Journal of Consulting and Clinical Psychology, 61*, 653–658.

Flor, H., Elbert, T., Knecht, S., Wienbruch, C., Pantev, C., Birbaumer, N., . . . Taub, E. (1995). Phantom-limb pain as a perceptual correlate of cortical reorganization following arm amputation. *Nature, 375*, 482–484.

Flor, H., Fydrich, T., & Turk, D. C. (1992). Efficacy of multidisciplinary pain treatment centers: A meta-analytic review. *Pain, 49*, 221–230.

Flor, H., & Turk, C. D. (1988). Chronic back pain and rheumatoid arthritis: Predicting pain and disability from cognitive variables. *Journal of Behavioral Medicine, 11*, 251–265.

Florian, V., Mikulincer, M., & Taubman, O. (1995). Does hardiness contribute to mental health during a stressful real-life situation? The roles of appraisal and coping. *Journal of Personality and Social Psychology, 68*(4), 687–695.

Flynn, B. S., Worden, J. K., Secker-Walker, R. H., Badger, G. J., Geller, B. M., & Costanza, M. C. (1992). Prevention of cigarette smoking through mass media intervention and school programs. *American Journal of Public Health, 82*(6), 827–834.

Foege, W. (1983). The national pattern of AIDS. In K. M. Cahill (Ed.), *The AIDS epidemic* (pp. 1–17). New York, NY: St. Martin's Press.

Foerde, K., Steinglass, J. E., Shohamy, D., & Walsh, B. T. (2015). Neural mechanisms supporting maladaptive food choices in anorexia nervosa. *Nature Neuroscience, 18*(11), 1571–1573.

Foley, K. M. (1995). Pain, physician assisted dying, and euthanasia. *Pain Forum, 4*(3), 163–178.

Folkman, S., Chesney, M., Collette, L., Boccellari, A., & Cooke, M. (1996). Post-bereavement depressive mood and its prebereavement predictors in HIV+ and HIV– gay men. *Journal of Personality and Social Psychology, 70*, 336–348.

Folkman, S., Chesney, M. A., Cooke, M., Boccellari, A., & Collette, L. (1994). Caregiver burden in HIV-positive and HIV-negative partners of men with AIDS. *Journal of Consulting and Clinical Psychology, 62*, 746–756.

Folkman, S., & Lazarus, R. S. (1980). An analysis of coping in a middle-aged community sample. *Journal of Health and Social Behavior*, 219–239.

Folkman, S., Lazarus, R. S., Dunkel Schetter, C., DeLongis, A., & Gruen, R. J. (1986). Dynamics of a stressful encounter: Cognitive appraisal, coping, and encounter outcomes. *Journal of Personality and Social Psychology, 50*(5), 992–1003.

Folsom, A. R., Hughes, J. R., Buehler, J. F., Mittelmark, M. B., Jacobs, D. R., Jr., Grimm, R. H., Jr., & Multiple Risk Factor Intervention Trial Group. (1985). Do Type A men drink more frequently than Type B men? Findings in the multiple risk factor intervention trial (MRFIT). *Journal of Behavioral Medicine, 8*(3), 227–235.

Folsom, A. R., Kaye, S. A., Sellers, T. A., Hong, C. P., Cerhan, J. D., Potter, J. D., & Prineas, R. J. (1993). Body fat distribution and 5-year risk of death in older women. *Journal of the American Medical Association, 269*, 483–487.

Food and Agriculture Organization. (2015). *The state of food insecurity in the world 2015: Strengthening the enabling enviroment for food security and nutrition*. Rome, IT: FAO.

Forcier, K., Stroud, L. R., Papandonatos, G. D., Hitsman, B., Reiches, M., Krishnamoorthy, J., & Niaura, R. (2006). Links between physical fitness and cardiovascular reactivity and recovery to psychological stressors: A meta-analysis. *Health Psychology, 25*(6), 723–739.

Fordyce, W. E. (1988). Pain and suffering: A reappraisal. *American Psychologist, 43*, 276–283.

Fordyce, W. E., Brockway, J. A., Bergman, J. A., & Spengler, D. (1986). Acute back pain: A control-group comparison of behavioral vs.

traditional management methods. *Journal of Behavioral Medicine, 9,* 127–140.

Forsythe, C. J., & Compas, B. E. (1987). Interaction of cognitive appraisals of stressful events and coping: Testing the goodness of fit hypothesis. *Cognitive Therapy and Research, 11*(4), 473–485.

Fothergill, E., Guo, J., Howard, L., Kerns, J. C., Knuth, N. D., Brychta, R., . . . Hall, K. D. (2016). Persistent metabolic adaptation 6 years after "The Biggest Loser" competition. *Obesity, 24*(8), 1612–1619.

França-Pinto, A., Mendes, F. A., de Carvalho-Pinto, R. M., Agondi, R. C., Cukier, A., Stelmach, R., . . . Carvalho, C. R. (2015). Aerobic training decreases bronchial hyperresponsiveness and systemic inflammation in patients with moderate or severe asthma: A randomised controlled trial. *Thorax, 70*(8), 732–739. **doi:10.1136/thoraxjnl-2014-206070**

Francis, L. A., & Birch, L. L. (2005). Maternal influences on daughters' restrained eating behavior. *Health Psychology, 24*(6), 548–554.

Francis, L. E., Kypriotakis, G., O'Toole, E. E., & Rose, J. H. (2016). Cancer patient age and family caregiver bereavement outcomes. *Supportive Care in Cancer, 24*(9), 3987–3996. **https://doi.org/10.1007/s00520-016-3219-x**

Frank, R. G., Gluck, J. P., & Buckelew, S. P. (1990). Rehabilitation: Psychology's greatest opportunity? *American Psychologist, 45*(6), 757–761.

Frankenhaeuser, M. (1975). Sympathetic-adrenomedullary activity behavior and the psychosocial environment. In P. H. Venables & M. J. Christie (Eds.), *Research in psychophysiology* (pp. 71–94). New York, NY: Wiley.

Frankenhaeuser, M. (1978). Psycho-neuroendocrine approaches to the study of emotion as related to stress and coping. *Nebraska Symposium on Motivation, 26,* 123–162.

Franklin, G. M., & Nelson, L. M. (1993). Chronic neurologic disorders. In R. C. Brownson, P. L., Remington, & J. R. Davis (Eds.), *Chronic disease epidemiology and control* (pp. 307–335). Washington, DC: American Public Health Association.

Franko, D. L., Mintz, L. B., Villapiano, M., Green, T. C., Mainelli, D., Folensbee, L., . . . Kearns, M. (2005). Food, mood, and attitude: Reducing risk for eating disorders in college women. *Health Psychology, 24*(6), 567–578.

Frasure-Smith, N., & Prince, R. (1989). Long-term follow-up of the Ischemic Heart Disease Life Stress Monitoring Program. *Psychosomatic Medicine, 51,* 485–513.

Fredrickson, B. L. (2001). The role of positive emotions in positive psychology: The broaden-and-build theory of positive emotions. *American Psychologist, 56,* 218–226.

Fredrickson, B. L., & Joiner, T. (2002). Positive emotions trigger upward spirals toward emotional well-being. *Psychological Science, 13*(2), 172–175.

Freedman, N. S., Gazendam, J., Levan, L., Pack, A. I., & Schwab, R. J. (2001). Abnormal sleep/wake cycles and the effect of environmental noise on sleep disruption in the intensive care unit. *American Journal of Respiratory and Critical Care Medicine, 163*(2), 451–457.

Freeman, M. A., Hennessy, E. V., & Marzullo, D. M. (2001). Defensive evaluation of antismoking messages among college-age smokers: The role of possible selves. *Health Psychology, 20*(6), 424–433.

Freidson, E. (1961). *Patients' views of medical practice.* New York, NY: Russell Sage.

Freimuth, V. S., Hammond, S. L., Edgar, T., & Monahan, J. L. (1990). Reaching those at risk: A content-analytic study of AIDS PSAs. *Communication Research, 17*(6), 775–791.

Freisling, H., Arnold, M., Soerjomataram, I., O'Doherty, M. G., Ordóñez-Mena, J. M., Bamia, C., . . . Kee, F. (2017). Comparison of general obesity and measures of body fat distribution in older adults in relation to cancer risk: Meta-analysis of individual participant data of seven prospective cohorts in Europe. *British Journal of Cancer, 116*(11), 1486–1497.

French, S. A., Perry, C. L., Leon, G. R., & Fulkerson, J. A. (1994). Weight concerns, dieting behavior, and smoking initiation among adolescents: A prospective study. *American Journal of Public Health, 84*(11), 1818–1820.

Freud, S. (1963). *Dora: An analysis of a case of hysteria.* New York, NY: Macmillan.

Freudenberg, C., Jones, R. A., Livingston, G., Goetsch, V., Schaffner, A., & Buchanan, L. (2015). Effectiveness of individualized, integrative outpatient treatment for females with anorexia nervosa and bulimia nervosa. *Eating Disorders, 24*(3), 240–254.

Fried, L. P., Kronmal, R. A., Newman, A. B., Bild, D. E., Mittelmark, M. B., Polak, J. F., . . . Gardin, J. M. (1998). Risk factors for 5-year mortality in older adults: The Cardiovascular Health Study. *Journal of the American Medical Association, 279,* 585–592.

Fried, T. R., Bradley, E. H., Towle, V. R., & Allore, H. (2002). Treatment preferences of seriously ill patients. *New England Journal of Medicine, 2002*(347), 533–535.

Friedman, H. S., & Booth-Kewley, S. (1987a). The "disease-prone personality": A meta-analytic view of the construct. *The American Psychologist, 42*(6), 539–555.

Friedman, H. S., & Booth-Kewley, S. (1987b). Personality, type A behavior, and coronary heart disease: The role of emotional expression. *Journal of Personality and Social Psychology, 53*(4), 783–792.

Friedman, H. S., Hall, J. A., & Harris, M. J. (1985). Type A behavior, nonverbal expressive style, and health. *Journal of Personality and Social Psychology, 48*(5), 1299–1315.

Friedman, H. S., Tucker, J. S., Tomlinson-Keasey, C., Schwartz, J. E., Wingard, D. L., & Criqui, M. H. (1993). Does childhood personality predict longevity? *Journal of Personality and Social Psychology, 65*(1), 176–185. **doi:10.1037/0022-3514.65.1.176**

Friedman, M. A., & Brownell, K. D. (1995). Psychological correlates of obesity: Moving to the next research generation. *Psychological Bulletin, 117*(1), 3–20.

Friedman, M. J. (2015). The human stress response. In N. C. Bernardy & M. J. Friedman (Eds.), *A practical guide to PTSD treatment: Pharmacological and psychotherapeutic approaches* (pp. 9–19). Washington, DC: American Psychological Association. **http://dx.doi .org/10.1037/14522-002**

Friedman, M., & Rosenman, R. H. (1959). Association of specific overt pattern with blood and cardiovascular findings. *Journal of the American Medical Association, 169,* 1286–1296.

Friedman, M., & Rosenman, R. H. (1974). *Type A behavior and your heart.* New York, NY: Knopf.

Friedman, M., Thoresen, C., Gill, J., Ulmer, D., Powell, L. H., Price, V. A., . . . Dixon, T. (1986). Alteration of Type A behavior and its effects on cardiac recurrences in post myocardial infarction patients: Summary results of the recurrent coronary prevention project. *American Heart Journal, 112,* 653–665.

Friedman, R., Sobel, D., Myers, P., Caudill, M., & Benson, H. (1995). Behavioral medicine, clinical health psychology, and cost offset. *Health Psychology, 14*(6), 509–518.

Friedmann, E., & Thomas, S. A. (1995). Pet ownership, social support, and one-year survival after acute myocardial infarction in the Cardiac Arrhythmia Suppression Trial (CAST). *The American Journal of Cardiology, 76*(17), 1213–1217.

Friedrich, M. J. (2000). More healthy people in the 21st century? *Journal of the American Medical Association, 283,* 37–38.

Fries, J. F. (1998). Reducing the need and demand for medical services. *Psychosomatic Medicine, 60,* 140–142.

Fries, J. F., Koop, C. E., Beadle, C. E., Cooper, P. P., England, M. J., Greaves, R. F., . . . Wright, D. (1993). Reducing health care costs by reducing the need and demand for medical services. *New England Journal of Medicine, 329*(5), 321–325.

Fritz, H. L., Russek, L. N., & Dillon, M. M. (2017). Humor use moderates the relation of stressful life events with psychological distress. *Personality and Social Psychology Bulletin, 43*(6), 845–859. **doi:10.1177/0146167217699583**

Fröhlich, C., Jacobi, F., & Wittchen, H.-U. (2006). DSM–IV pain disorder in the general population. *European Archives of Psychiatry and Clinical Neuroscience, 256*(3), 187–196. **https:// doi.org/10.1007/s00406-005- 0625-3**

Frye, M. A., Hinton, D. J., Karpyak, V. M., Biernacka, J. M., Gunderson, L. J., Geske, J., . . . Port, J. D. (2016). Elevated glutamate levels in the left dorsolateral prefrontal cortex are associated with higher cravings for alcohol. *Alcoholism: Clinical and Experimental Research, 40*(8), 1609–1616.

Fuchs, C. S., Stampfer, M. J., Colditz, G. A., Giovannucci, E. L., Manson, J. E., Kawachi, I., . . . Speizer, F. E. (1995). Alcohol consumption and mortality among women. *New England Journal of Medicine, 332*(19), 1245–1250.

Fuemmeler, B. F., Mâsse, L. C., Yaroch, A. L., Resnicow, K., Campbell, M. K., Carr, C., . . . Williams, A. (2006). Psychosocial mediation of fruit and vegetable consumption in the body and soul effectiveness trial. *Health Psychology, 25*(4), 474–483.

Fuentes, J., Armijo-Olivo, S., Funabashi, M., Miciak, M., Dick, B., Warren, S., . . . Gross, D. P. (2014). Enhanced therapeutic alliance modulates pain intensity and muscle pain sensitivity in patients with chronic low back pain: An experimental controlled study. *Physical Therapy, 94*(4), 477–489.

Fujimoto, K., & Valente, T. W. (2013). Alcohol peer influence of participating in organized school activities: A network approach. *Health Psychology, 32*(10), 1084–1092.

Fuller-Thomson, E., Baird, S. L., Dhrodia, R., & Brennenstuhl, S. (2016). The association between adverse childhood experiences (ACEs) and suicide attempts in a population-based study. *Child: Care, Health and Development, 42*(5), 725–734.

Gable, P. A., Mechin, N. C., & Neal, L. B. (2016). Booze cues and attentional narrowing: Neural correlates of virtual alcohol myopia. *Psychology of Addictive Behaviors, 30*(3), 377–382.

Galanter, M., Josipovic, Z., Dermatis, H., Weber, J., & Millard, M. A. (2016). An initial fMRI study on neural correlates of prayer in members of Alcoholics Anonymous. *The American Journal of Drug and Alcohol Abuse, 43*(1), 44–54.

Galea, S., Brewin, C. R., Gruber, M., Jones, R. T., King, D. W., King, L. A., . . . Kessler, R. C. (2007). Exposure to hurricane-related stressors and mental illness after hurricane Katrina. *Archives of General Psychiatry, 64*(12), 1427–1435.

Gall, T. L., Guirguis-Younger, M., Charbonneau, C., & Florack, P. (2009). The trajectory of religious coping across time in response to the diagnosis of breast cancer. *Psycho-Oncology, 18,* 1165–1178.

Gall, T. L., Kristjansson, E., Charbonneau, C., & Florack, P. (2009). A longitudinal study on the role of spirituality in response to the diagnosis and treatment of breast cancer. *Journal of Behavioral Medicine, 32*(2), 174–186.

Gallagher, E. J., & LeRoith, D. (2015). Obesity and diabetes: The increased risk of cancer and cancer-related mortality. *Physiological Reviews, 95*(3), 727–748.

Gallagher, E. J., Viscoli, C. M., & Horwitz, R. I. (1993). The relationship of treatment adherence to the risk of death after myocardial infarction in women. *Journal of the American Medical Association, 270*, 742–743.

Gallagher, K. M., Updegraff, J. A., Rothman, A. J., & Sims, L. (2011). Perceived susceptibility to breast cancer moderates the effect of gain-and loss-framed messages on use of screening mammography. *Health Psychology, 30*(2), 145–152. **doi:10.1037/a0022264**

Gallart-Palau, X., Lee, B. S., Adav, S. S., Qian, J., Serra, A., Park, J. E., . . . Sze, S. K. (2016). Gender differences in white matter pathology and mitochondrial dysfunction in Alzheimer's disease with cerebrovascular disease. *Molecular Brain, 9*, 27. **doi:10.1186/s13041-016-0205-7**

Gallo, L. C., de los Monteros, K. E., & Shivpuri, S. (2009). Socioeconomic status and health: What is the role of reserve capacity? *Current Directions in Psychological Science, 18*(5), 269–274.

Gallo, L. C., & Matthews, K. A. (2003). Understanding the association between socioeconomic status and physical health: Do negative emotions play a role? *Psychological Bulletin, 129*(1), 10–51.

Gallup. (2016). Euthanasia still acceptable to solid majority in U.S. Retrieved from **http://www.gallup.com/poll/193082/euthanasia-acceptable-solid-majority.aspx**

Gallup, G. G., & Suarez, S. D. (1985). Alternatives to the use of animals in psychological research. *American Psychologist, 40*, 1104–1111.

Gandubert, C., Carrière, I., Escot, C., Soulier, M., Hermès, A., Boulet, P., . . . Chaudieu, I. (2009). Onset and relapse of psychiatric disorders following early breast cancer: A case–control study. *Psycho-Oncology, 18*(10), 1029–1037. **https://doi.org/10.1002/pon.1469**

Ganguli, A., Clewell, J., & Shillington, A. C. (2016). The impact of patient support programs on adherence, clinical, humanistic, and economic patient outcomes: A targeted systematic review. *Patient Preference and Adherence, 10*, 711–725.

Ganzini, L., Goy, E. R., & Dobscha, S. K. (2009). Oregonians' reasons for requesting physician aid in dying. *Archives of Internal Medicine, 169*(5), 489–492. **https://doi.org/10.1001/archinternmed.2008.579**

Ganzini, L., Harvath, T. A., Jackson, A., Goy, E. R., Miller, L. L., & Delorit, M. (2002). Experiences of Oregon nurses and social workers with hospice patients who requested assistance with suicide. *New England Journal of Medicine, 347*, 582–588.

García, M. C., Bastian, B., Rossen, L. M., Anderson, R., Miniño, A., Yoon, P. W., . . . Iademarco, M. F. (2016). Potentially preventable deaths among the five leading causes of death — United States, 2010 and 2014. *Morbidity and Mortality Weekly Report, 65*(45), 1245–1255. **doi:10.15585/mmwr.mm6545a1**

Gardner, M., & Steinberg, L. (2005). Peer influence on risk taking, risk preference, and risky decision making in adolescence and adulthood: An experimental study. *Developmental Psychology, 41*(4), 625–635.

Garfinkel, P. E., & Garner, D. M. (1984). Bulimia in anorexia nervosa. In R. C. Hawkins, W. J. Fremouw, & P. F. Clement (Eds.), *The binge–purge syndrome: Diagnosis, treatment and research* (pp. 27–46). New York, NY: Springer.

Garg, N., Wansink, B., & Inman, J. J. (2007). The influence of incidental affect on consumers' food intake. *Journal of Marketing, 71*(1), 194–206.

Garland, S. N., Carlson, L. E., Stephens, A. J., Antle, M. C., Samuels, C., & Campbell, T. S. (2014). Mindfulness-based stress reduction compared with cognitive behavioral therapy for the treatment of insomnia comorbid with cancer: A randomized, partially blinded, noninferiority trial. *Journal of Clinical Oncology, 32*(5), 449–457. **https://doi.org/10.1200/JCO.2012.47.7265**

Garner, D. M., & Garfinkel, P. E. (1980). Socio-cultural factors in the development of anorexia nervosa. *Psychological Medicine, 10*(4), 647–656.

Garner, D. M., Garfinkel, P. E., & Bemis, K. M. (1982). A multidimensional psychotherapy for anorexia nervosa. *International Journal of Eating Disorders, 1*(2), 3–46.

Garner, D. M., Garfinkel, P. E., Schwartz, D., & Thompson, M. (1980). Cultural expectations of thinness in women. *Psychological Reports, 47*(2), 483–491.

Garner, D. M., Rockert, W., & Davis, R. (1993). Comparison of cognitive-behavioral and supportive-expressive therapy for bulimia nervosa. *American Journal of Psychiatry, 150*, 37–46.

Garnier-Dykstra, L. M., Caldeira, K. M., Vincent, K. B., O'Grady, K. E., & Arria, A. M. (2012). Nonmedical use of prescription stimulants during college: Four-year trends in exposure opportunity, use, motives, and sources. *Journal of American College Health, 60*(3), 226–234.

Garrido, M. M., & Prigerson, H. G. (2014). The end-of-life experience: Modifiable predictors of caregivers' bereavement adjustment. *Cancer, 120*(6), 918–925. **https://doi.org/10.1002/cncr.28495**

Garvin, E. C., Cannuscio, C. C., & Branas, C. C. (2013). Greening vacant lots to reduce violent crime: a randomised controlled trial. *Injury Prevention: Journal of the International Society for Child and Adolescent Injury Prevention, 19*(3), 198–203. **http://doi.org/10.1136/injuryprev-2012-040439**

Gaskin, D. J., & Richard, P. (2012). The economic costs of pain in the United States. *The Journal of Pain, 13*(8), 715–724. **https://doi.org/10.1016/j.jpain.2012.03.009**

Gaziano, J. M., Buring, J. E., Breslow, J. L., Goldhaber, S. Z., Rosner, B., VanDenburgh, M., . . . Hennekens, C. H. (1993). Moderate alcohol intake, increased levels of high-density lipoprotein and its subfractions, and decreased risk of myocardial infarction. *New England Journal of Medicine, 329*(25), 1829–1834.

Geers, A. L., Wellman, J. A., Helfer, S. G., Fowler, S. L., & France, C. R. (2008). Dispositional optimism and thoughts of well-being determine sensitivity to an experimental pain task. *Annals of Behavioral Medicine, 36*(3), 304–313. https://doi.org/10.1007/s12160-008-9073-4

Geier, A., Wansink, B., & Rozin, P. (2012). Red potato chips: Segmentation cues can substantially decrease food intake. *Health Psychology, 31*(3), 398–401.

Gentry, W. D. (1984). Behavioral medicine: A new research paradigm. In W. D. Gentry (Ed.), *Handbook of behavioral medicine* (pp. 1–13). New York, NY: Guilford.

George, L. K., Ellison, C. G., & Larson, D. B. (2002). Explaining the relationships between religious involvement and health. *Psychological Inquiry, 13*(3), 190–200.

Gerteis, J., Izrael, D., Deitz, D., LeRoy, L., Ricciardi, R., Miller, T., & Basu, J. (2014). *Multiple chronic conditions chartbook*. AHRQ Publications No. Q14-0038. Rockville, MD: Agency for Healthcare Research and Quality.

Ghanbari, H., Dalloul, G., Hasan, R., Daccarett, M., Saba, S., David, S., & Machado, C. (2009). Effectiveness of implantable cardioverter-defibrillators for the primary prevention of sudden cardiac death in women with advanced heart failure: A meta-analysis of randomized controlled trials. *Archives of Internal Medicine, 169*(16), 1500–1506.

Gibbons, F. X., Gerrard, M., Lane, D. J., Mahler, H. I., & Kulik, J. A. (2005). Using UV photography to reduce use of tanning booths: A test of cognitive mediation. *Health Psychology, 24*(4), 358–363.

Gibbons, F. X., Pomery, E. A., Gerrard, M., Sargent, J. D., Weng, C. Y., Wills, T. A., . . . Tanski, S. E. (2010). Media as social influence: Racial differences in the effects of peers and media on adolescent alcohol cognitions and consumption. *Psychology of Addictive Behaviors, 24*(4), 649–659.

Gidron, Y., Davidson, K., & Bata, I. (1999). The short-term effects of a hostility-reduction intervention on male coronary heart disease patients. *Health Psychology, 18*, 416–420.

Gielen, A. C., Shields, W., McDonald, E., Frattaroli, S., Bishai, D., & Ma, X. (2012). Home safety and low-income urban housing quality. *Pediatrics, 130*(6), 1053–1059.

Gil, K. M., Carson, J. W., Porter, L. S., Scipio, C., Bediako, S. M., & Orringer, E. (2004). Daily mood and stress predict pain, health care use, and work activity in African American adults with sickle-cell disease. *Health Psychology, 23*(3), 267–274. https://doi.org/10.1037/0278-6133.23.3.267

Gil, K. M., Carson, J. W., Sedway, J. A., Porter, L. S., Schaeffer, J. J. W., & Orringer, E. (2000). Follow-up of coping skills training in adults with sickle cell disease: Analysis of daily pain and coping practice diaries. *Health Psychology, 19*(1), 85–90.

Gil, K. M., Williams, D. A., Keefe, F. J., & Beckham, J. C. (1990). The relationship of negative thoughts to pain and psychological distress. *Behavior Therapy, 21*, 349–362.

Gil, K. M., Wilson, J. J., Edens, J. L., Webster, D. A., Abrams, M. A., Orringer, E., . . . Janal, M. N. (1996). Effects of cognitive coping skills training on coping strategies and experimental pain sensitivity in African American adults with sickle cell disease. *Health Psychology, 15*(1), 3–10.

Gilchrist, J., & Parker, E. M. (2014). Racial/ethnic disparities in fatal unintentional drowning among persons aged ≤ 29 years—United States, 1999–2010. *Morbidity and Mortality Weekly Report, 63*, 421–426.

Giles, L. C., Glonek, G. F. V., Luszcz, M. A., & Andrews, G. R. (2005). Effect of social networks on 10 year survival in very old Australians: The Australian longitudinal study of aging. *Journal of Epidemiology and Community Health, 59*, 574–579.

Gilsanz, P., Walter, S., Tchetgen Tchetgen, E. J., Patton, K. K., Moon, J. R., Capistrant, B. D., . . . Glymour, M. M. (2015). Changes in depressive symptoms and incidence of first stroke among middle-aged and older US adults. *Journal of the American Heart Association: Cardiovascular and Cerebrovascular Disease, 4*(5), e001923. http://doi.org/10.1161/JAHA.115.001923

Ginis, K. A., Heisz, J., Spence, J. C., Clark, I. B., Antflick, J., Ardern, C. I., . . . Rotondi, M. A. (2017). Formulation of evidence-based messages to promote the use of physical activity to prevent and manage Alzheimer's disease. *BMC Public Health, 17*(1), 209. doi:10.1186/s12889-017-4090-5

Gintner, G. G., Rectanus, E. F., Achord, K., & Parker, B. (1987). Parental history of hypertension and screening attendance: Effects of wellness appeal versus threat appeal. *Health Psychology, 6*(5), 431–444.

Glaser, R., & Kiecolt-Glaser, J. K. (1994). *Handbook of human stress and immunity*. San Diego, CA: Academic Press.

Glaser, R., Thorn, B. E., Tarr, K. L., Kiecolt-Glaser, J. K., & D'Ambrosio, S. M. (1985). Effects of stress on methyltransferase synthesis: An important DNA repair enzyme. *Health Psychology, 4*, 403–412.

Glinder, J. G., & Compas, B. E. (1999). Self-blame attributions in women with newly diagnosed breast cancer: A prospective study of psychological adjustment. *Health Psychology, 18*, 475–481.

Gloria, C. T., & Steinhardt, M. A. (2014). Relationships among positive emotions, coping, resilience and mental health. *Stress and Health*, *2*(32), 145–156.

Glymour, M. M., & Manly, J. J. (2008). Lifecourse social conditions and racial and ethnic patterns of cognitive aging. *Neuropsychology Review*, *18*(3), 223–254. doi:10.1007/s11065-008-9064-z

Godin, G., & Kok, G. (1996). The theory of planned behavior: A review of its applications to health-related behaviors. *American Journal of Health Promotion*, *11*(2), 87–98.

Goel, M. S., McCarthy, E. P., Phillips, R. S., & Wee, C. C. (2004). Obesity among US immigrant subgroups by duration of residence. *Journal of the American Medical Association*, *292*(23), 2860–2867.

Gold, K. J., Leon, I., Boggs, M. E., & Sen, A. (2016). Depression and posttraumatic stress symptoms after perinatal loss in a population-based sample. *Journal of Women's Health*, *25*(3), 263–269.

Golden, N. H., Schneider, M., Wood, C., Committee on Nutrition, Committee on Adolescence, & Section on Obesity. (2016). Preventing obesity and eating disorders in adolescents. *Pediatrics*, *138*(3), e20161649. doi:10.1542/peds.2016-1649

Goldman, M. S., Del Boca, F. K., & Darkes, J. (1999). Alcohol expectancy theory: The application of cognitive neuroscience. *Psychological Theories of Drinking and Alcoholism*, *2*, 203–246.

Goldner, E. M., & Birmingham, C. L. (1994). Anorexia nervosa: Methods of treatment. In L. Alexander-Mott & D. B. Lumsden (Eds.), *Understanding eating disorders: Anorexia nervosa, bulimia nervosa, and obesity* (pp. 135–157). Philadelphia, PA: Taylor & Francis.

Goldring, A. B., Taylor, S. E., Kemeny, M. E., & Anton, P. A. (2002). Impact of health beliefs, quality of life, and the physician–patient relationship on the treatment intentions of inflammatory bowel disease patients. *Health Psychology*, *21*, 219–228.

Goldschmidt, A. B., Wonderlich, S. A., Crosby, R. D., Engel, S. G., Lavender, J. M., Peterson, C. B., . . . Mitchell, J. E. (2014). Ecological momentary assessment of stressful events and negative affect in bulimia nervosa. *Journal of Consulting and Clinical Psychology*, *82*(1), 30–39.

Goldstein, A. O., Sobel, R. A., & Newman, G. R. (1999). Tobacco and alcohol use in G-rated children's animated films. *Journal of the American Medical Association*, *281*(12), 1131–1136.

Goldstein, M., Murray, S. B., Griffiths, S., Rayner, K., Podkowka, J., Bateman, J. E., . . . Thornton, C. E. (2016). The effectiveness of family-based treatment for full and partial adolescent anorexia nervosa in an independent private practice setting: Clinical outcomes. *International Journal of Eating Disorders*, *49*(11), 1023–1026.

Goldzweig, G., Andritsch, E., Hubert, A., Walach, N., Perry, S., Brenner, B., & Baider, L. (2009). How relevant is marital status and gender variables in coping with colorectal cancer? A sample of middle-aged and older cancer survivors. *Psycho-Oncology*, *18*(8), 866–874. https://doi.org/10.1002/pon.1499

Gollwitzer, P. M. (1993). Goal achievement: The role of intentions. *European Review of Social Psychology*, *4*(1), 141–185.

Gomel, M., Oldenburg, B., Lemon, J., Owen, N., & Westbrook, F. (1993). Pilot study of the effects of a workplace smoking ban on indices of smoking, cigarette craving, stress and other health behaviours. *Psychology and Health*, *8*(4), 223–229.

Gonçalves, S., Machado, B. C., Martins, C., Hoek, H. W., & Machado, P. P. (2016). Retrospective correlates for bulimia nervosa: A matched case–control study. *European Eating Disorders Review*, *24*(3), 197–205.

Gonzalez, J. S., Penedo, F. J., Antoni, M. H., Durán, R. E., McPherson-Baker, S., Ironson, G., . . . Schneiderman, N. (2004). Social support, positive states of mind, and HIV treatment adherence in men and women living with HIV/AIDS. *Health Psychology*, *23*(4), 413–418.

Goodkin, K., Blaney, N. T., Feaster, D., Fletcher, M. A., Baum, M. K., Mantero-Atienza, E., . . . Eisdorfer, C. (1992). Active coping style is associated with natural killer cell cytotoxicity in asymptomatic HIV-1 seropositive homosexual men. *Journal of Psychosomatic Research*, *36*(7), 635–650.

Goodwin, J. S., Hunt, W. C., Key, C. R., & Samet, J. M. (1987). The effect of marital status on stage, treatment, and survival of cancer patients. *Journal of the American Medical Association*, *258*, 3125–3130.

Goodwin, P. J., Leszez, M., Ennis, M., Koopmans, J., Vincent, L., Guther, H., . . . Hunter, J. (2001). The effect of group psychosocial support on survival in metastatic breast cancer. *New England Journal of Medicine*, *345*(24), 1719–1726.

Goodwin, R. D., & Eaton, W. W. (2005). Asthma, suicidal ideation, and suicide attempts: Findings from the Baltimore epidemiologic catchment area follow-up. *American Journal of Public Health*, *95*(4), 717–722.

Goranson, A., Ritter, R. S., Waytz, A., Norton, M. I., & Gray, K. (2017). Dying is unexpectedly positive. *Psychological Science*, *28*(7), 988–999. https://doi.org/10.1177/0956797617701186

Gordon, C. M., Carey, M. P., & Carey, K. B. (1997). Effects of a drinking event on behavioral skills and condom attitudes in men: Implications for HIV risk from a controlled experiment. *Health Psychology*, *16*(5), 490–495.

Gornick, M. E., Eggers, P. W., Reilly, T. W., Mentnech, R. M., Fitterman, L. K., Kucken, L. E., & Vladeck, B. C. (1996). Effects of race and income on mortality and use of services among Medicare beneficiaries. *New England Journal of Medicine*, *335*(11), 791–799.

Gorsuch, R. L. (1995). Religious aspects of substance abuse and recovery. *Journal of Social Issues*, *51*(2), 65–83.

Gould, J. B., Davey, B., & Stafford, R. (1989). Socioeconomic differences in rates of cesearean section. *New England Journal of Medicine, 321,* 233–239.

Gould, M. S., & Lake, A. M. (2013). The contagion of suicidal behavior. *Contagion of violence: Workshop summary.* Washington, DC: National Academies Press.

Gould, M. S., & Shaffer, D. (1986). The impact of suicide in television movies. *New England Journal of Medicine, 315*(11), 690–694.

Goyal, M., Mehta, R. L., Schneiderman, L. J., & Sehgal, A. R. (2002). Economic and health consequences of selling a kidney in India. *Journal of the American Medical Association, 288*(13), 1589–1593.

Gracely, R. H., Dubner, R., Deeter, W. R., & Wolskee, P. J. (1985). Clinicians' expectations influence placebo analgesia. *Lancet, 1*(8419), 43.

Grady, K. E., Lemkau, J. P., McVay, J. M., & Reisine, S. T. (1992). The importance of physician encouragement in breast cancer screening of older women. *Preventive Medicine, 21*(6), 766–780.

Graham, J. E., Lobel, M., Glass, P., & Lokshina, I. (2008). Effects of written anger expression in chronic pain patients: Making meaning from pain. *Journal of Behavioral Medicine, 31*(3), 201–212. **https://doi.org/10.1007/s10865-008-9149-4**

Graham, J. W., Marks, G., & Hansen, W. B. (1991). Social influence processes affecting adolescent substance use. *Journal of Applied Psychology, 76*(2), 291–298.

Grahn, P., & Stigsdotter, U. A. (2003). Landscape planning and stress. *Urban Forestry & Urban Greening, 2*(1), 1–18.

Gram, I. T., Lund, E., & Slenker, S. E. (1990). Quality of life following a false positive mammogram. *British Journal of Cancer, 62*(6), 1018–1022.

Gramling, S. E., Clawson, E. P., & McDonald, M. K. (1996). Perceptual and cognitive abnormality model of hypochondriasis: Amplification and physiological reactivity in women. *Psychosomatic Medicine, 58*(5), 423–431.

Greeley, J., & Oei, T. (1999). Alcohol and tension reduction. In K. E. Leonard & H. T. Blane (Eds.), *Psychological theories of drinking and alcoholism* (2nd ed., pp. 14–53). New York, NY: Guilford Press.

Green, A. E., Mays, D., Falk, E. B., Vallone, D., Gallagher, N., Richardson, A., . . . Niaura, R. S. (2016). Young adult smokers' neural response to graphic cigarette warning labels. *Addictive Behaviors Reports, 3,* 28–32.

Green, B., Horel, T., & Papachristos, A. V. (2017). Modeling contagion through social networks to explain and predict gunshot violence in Chicago, 2006 to 2014. *JAMA Internal Medicine, 177*(3), 326–333. **doi:10.1001/jamainternmed.2016.8245**

Greenberg, M., & Schneider, D. (1994). Violence in American cities: Young Black males in the answer, but what was the question? *Social Science & Medicine, 39*(2), 179–187.

Greendale, G. A., Barrett-Connor, E., Edelstein, S., Ingles, S., & Haile, R. (1995). Lifetime leisure exercise and osteoporosis the Rancho Bemardo Study. *American Journal of Epidemiology, 141*(10), 951–959.

Greenfield, S., & Kaplan, S. (1985). Expanding patient involvment in care: Effects on patient outcomes. *Annals of Internal Medicine, 102,* 520–528.

Greenfield, S., Kaplan, S. H., Ware, J. E., Jr., Yano, E. M., & Frank, H. J. (1988). Patients' participation in medical care: Effects on blood sugar control and quality of life in diabetes. *Journal of General Internal Medicine, 3,* 448–457.

Greenspan, A. M., Kay, H. R., Berger, B. C., Greenberg, R. M., Greenspon, A. J., & Gaughan, M. J. S. (1988). Incidence of unwarranted implantation of permanent cardiac pacemakers in a large medical population. *New England Journal of Medicine, 318*(3), 158–163.

Greer, S. (1991). Psychological response to cancer and survival. *Psychological Medicine, 21,* 43–49.

Gregg, E. W., Chen, H., Wagenknecht, L. E., Clark, J. M., Delahanty, L. M., Bantle, J., . . . Pi-Sunyer, F. X. (2012). Association of an intensive lifestyle intervention with remission of type 2 diabetes. *Journal of the American Medical Association, 308*(23), 2489–2496.

Gremore, T. M., Baucom, D. H., Porter, L. S., Kirby, J. S., Atkins, D. C., & Keefe, F. J. (2011). Stress buffering effects of daily spousal support on women's daily emotional and physical experiences in the context of breast cancer concerns. *Health Psychology, 30*(1), 20–30.

Greville-Harris, M., & Dieppe, P. (2015). Bad is more powerful than good: The nocebo response in medical consultations. *American Journal of Medicine, 128*(2), 126–129.

Grewal, P., & Viswanathen, V. A. (2012). Liver cancer and alcohol. *Clinics in Liver Disease, 16*(4), 839–850. **https://doi.org/10.1016/j.cld.2012.08.011**

Griffith, R., Davies, K., & Lavender, V. (2015). The characteristics and experiences of anticipatory mourning in caregivers of teenagers and young adults. *International Journal of Palliative Nursing, 21*(11), 527–533. **doi:10.12968/ijpn.2015.21.11.527**

Grilo, C. M., & Pogue-Geile, M. F. (1991). The nature of environmental influences on weight and obesity: A behavior genetic analysis. *Psychological Bulletin, 110*(3), 520–537.

Grilo, C. M., Reas, D. L., & Mitchell, J. E. (2016). Combining pharmacological and psychological treatments for binge eating disorder: Current status, limitations, and future directions. *Current Psychiatry Reports, 18*(6), 55–55. **doi:10.1007/s11920-016-0696-z**

Grilo, C. M., Shiffman, S., & Wing, R. R. (1989). Relapse crises and coping among dieters. *Journal of Consulting and Clinical Psychology, 57*(4), 488–495.

Grimby, A. (1993). Bereavement among elderly people: Grief reactions, post-bereavement hallucinations and quality of life. *Acta Psychiatrica Scandinavica, 87,* 72–80.

Grisset, N. I., & Norvell, N. K. (1992). Perceived social support, social skills, and quality of relationships in bulimic women. *Journal of Consulting and Clinical Psychology, 60*(2), 293–299.

Grob, G. N. (1983). Disease and environment in American history. In D. Mechanic (Ed.), *Handbook of health, health care, and the health professions* (pp. 3–22). New York, NY: Free Press.

Grodstein, F., Stampfer, M. J., Manson, J. E., Colditz, G. A., Willett, W. C., Rosner, B., . . . Hennekens, C. H. (1996). Postmenopausal estrogen and progestin use and the risk of cardiovascular disease. *New England Journal of Medicine, 335,* 453–461.

Grol-Prokopczyk, H. (2017). Sociodemographic disparities in chronic pain, based on 12-year longitudinal data. *Pain, 158*(2), 313–322.

Gross, A. M., Stern, R. M., Levin, R. B., Dale, J., & Wojnilower, D. A. (1983). The effect of mother–child separation on the behavior of children experiencing a diagnostic procedure. *Journal of Consulting and Clinical Psychology, 51,* 783–785.

Grossi, G., Thomtén, J., Fandino-Losada, A., Soares, J. J. F., & Sundin, Ö. (2009). Does burnout predict changes in pain experiences among women living in Sweden? A longitudinal study. *Stress and Health, 25*(4), 297–311. https://doi.org/10.1002/smi.1281

Grow, J. C., Collins, S. E., Harrop, E. N., & Marlatt, G. A. (2015). Enactment of home practice following mindfulness-based relapse prevention and its association with substance-use outcomes. *Addictive Behaviors, 40,* 16–20.

Grube, J. W., & Wallack, L. (1994). Television beer advertising and drinking knowledge, beliefs, and intentions among schoolchildren. *American Journal of Public Health, 84*(2), 254–259.

Grunberg, N. E., Brown, K. J., & Klein, L. C. (1997). Tobacco smoking. In A. Baum, S. Newman, J. Weinman, R. West, & C. McManus (Eds.), *Cambridge handbook of psychology, health and medicine* (pp. 606–610). Cambridge, MA: Cambridge University Press.

Grunberg, N. E., Winders, S. E., & Wewers, M. E. (1991). Gender differences in tobacco use. *Health Psychology, 10*(2), 143–153.

Gu, J., Strauss, C., Bond, R., & Cavanagh, K. (2015). How do mindfulness-based cognitive therapy and mindfulness-based stress reduction improve mental health and wellbeing? A systematic review and meta-analysis of mediation studies. *Clinical Psychology Review, 37,* 1–12.

Guardino, C. M., Dunkel Schetter, C., Bower, J. E., Lu, M. C., & Smalley, S. L. (2014). Randomised controlled pilot trial of mindfulness training for stress reduction during pregnancy. *Psychology & Health, 29*(3), 334–349.

Gudenkauf, L. M., Antoni, M. H., Stagl, J. M., Lechner, S. C., Jutagir, D. R., Bouchard, L. C., . . . Carver, C. S. (2015). Brief cognitive-behavioral and relaxation training interventions for breast cancer: A randomized controlled trial. *Journal of Consulting and Clinical Psychology, 83*(4), 677–688.

Guerdjikova, A. I., Mori, N., Casuto, L. S., & McElroy, S. L. (2016). Novel pharmacologic treatment in acute binge eating disorder-role of lisdexamfetamine. *Neuropsychiatric Disease and Treatment, 12,* 833–841.

Guillory, J. E., Hancock, J. T., Woodruff, C., & Keilman, J. (2015). Text messaging reduces analgesic requirements during surgery. *Pain Medicine, 16*(4), 667–672. https://doi.org/10.1111/pme.12610

Guldin, M., Li, J., Pedersen, H., Obel, C., Agerbo, E., Gissler, M., . . . Vestergaard, M. (2015). Incidence of suicide among persons who had a parent who died during their childhood: A population-based cohort study. *JAMA Psychiatry, 72*(12),

1227–1234. https://doi.org/10.1001/jamapsychiatry.2015.2094

Gureje, O., Von Korff, M., Simon, G. E., & Gater, R. (1998). Persistent pain and well-being: A World Health Organization study in primary care. *Journal of the American Medical Association, 280,* 147–151.

Gustafson, D. H., McTavish, F. M., Chih, M. Y., Atwood, A. K., Johnson, R. A., Boyle, M. G., . . . Shah, D. (2014). A smartphone application to support recovery from alcoholism: A randomized clinical trial. *JAMA Psychiatry, 71*(5), 566–572.

Haase, C. M., Holley, S. R., Bloch, L., Verstaen, A., & Levenson, R. W. (2016). Interpersonal emotional behaviors and physical health: A 20-year longitudinal study of long-term married couples. *Emotion, 16*(7), 965–977. doi:10.1037/a0040239

Hacker, K., Collins, J., Gross-Young, L., Almeida, S., & Burke, N. (2008). Coping with youth suicide and overdose: One community's efforts to investigate, intervene, and prevent suicide contagion. *Crisis, 29*(2), 86–95.

Hadlow, J., & Pitts, M. (1991). The understanding of common health terms by doctors, nurses, and patients. *Social Science and Medicine, 32,* 193–196.

Haffner, S. M. (1998). Epidemiology of type 2 diabetes. Risk factors. *Diabetes Care, 21*(Suppl 3), C3–C6.

Hagman, J., Gardner, R. M., Brown, D. L., Gralla, J., Fier, J. M., & Frank, G. K. (2015). Body size overestimation and its association with body mass index, body dissatisfaction, and drive for thinness in anorexia nervosa. *Eating and Weight Disorders-Studies on Anorexia, Bulimia and Obesity, 4*(20), 449–455.

Hahn, R., Fuqua-Whitley, D., Wethington, H., Lowy, J., Crosby, A., Fullilove, M., . . . Snyder, S. (2007). Effectiveness of universal school-based programs to prevent violent and aggressive behavior: A systematic review. *American Journal of Preventive Medicine, 33*(2), 114–129.

Halkitis, P., Kapadia, F., & Ompad, D. (2015). Incidence of HIV infection in young gay, bisexual, and other YMSM. *Journal of Acquired Immune Deficiency Syndromes, 69*(4), 466–473. **doi:10.1097/qai.0000000000000616**

Hall, J. A., & Dornan, M. C. (1988a). Meta-analysis of satisfaction with medical care: Description of research done in and analysis of overall satisafction levels. *Social Science and Medicine, 26,* 637–644.

Hall, J. A., & Dornan, M. C. (1988b). What patients like about their medical care and how often they are asked: A meta-analysis of the satisfaction literature. *Social Science and Medicine, 27,* 935–939.

Hall, J. A., Epstein, A. M., DeCiantis, M. L., & McNeil, B. J. (1993). Physicians' liking for their patients: More evidence for the role of affect in medical care. *Health Psychology, 12,* 140–146.

Hall, J. A., Irish, J. T., Roter, D. L., Ehrlich, C. M., & Miller, L. H. (1994). Gender in medical encounters: An analysis of physician and patient communication in a primary care setting. *Health Psychology, 13*(5), 384–392.

Hall, J. A., Roter, D. L., & Katz, N. R. (1988). Meta-analysis of correlates of provider behavior in medical encounters. *Medical Care, 26,* 657–675.

Halpern, C. T., Udry, J. R., Campbell, B., & Suchindran, C. (1999). Effects of body fat on weight concerns, dating, and sexual activity: A longitudinal analysis of Black and White adolescent girls. *Developmental Psychology, 35*(3), 721–736.

Halpern, M. (1994). Effect of smoking characteristics on cognitive dissonance in current and former smokers. *Addictive Behaviors, 19,* 209–217.

Halpern, S. D., French, B., Small, D. S., Saulsgiver, K., Harhay, M. O., Audrain-McGovern, J., . . . Volpp, K. G. (2015). Randomized trial of four financial-incentive programs for smoking cessation. *New England Journal of Medicine, 372*(22), 2108–2117.

Hamano, J., Yamaguchi, T., Maeda, I., Suga, A., Hisanaga, T., Ishihara, T., . . . Morita, T. (2016). Multicenter cohort study on the survival time of cancer patients dying at home or in a hospital: Does place matter? *Cancer, 122*(9), 1453–1460. **https://doi.org/10.1002/cncr.29844**

Hamer, J., & Warner, E. (2017). Lifestyle modifications for patients with breast cancer to improve prognosis and optimize overall health. *Canadian Medical Association Journal, 189*(7), E268–E274.

Hamilton, T. K., & Schweitzer, R. D. (2000). The cost of being perfect: Perfectionism and suicide ideation in university students. *Australian and New Zealand Journal of Psychiatry, 34*(5), 829–835.

Hampel, P., Rudolph, H., Stachow, R., Laß-Lentzsch, A., & Petermann, F. (2005). Coping among children and adolescents with chronic illness. *Anxiety, Stress & Coping, 18*(2), 145–155.

Hampson, S. E., Edmonds, G. W., Goldberg, L. R., Dubanoski, J. P., & Hillier, T. A. (2013). Childhood conscientiousness relates to objectively measured adult physical health four decades later. *Health Psychology, 32*(8), 925–928.

Hampson, S. E., Goldberg, L. R., Vogt, T. M., & Dubanoski, J. P. (2006). Forty years on: Teachers' assessments of children's personality traits predict self-reported health behaviors and outcomes at midlife. *Health Psychology, 25,* 57–64.

Hampson, S. E., Tildesley, E., Andrews, J. A., Luyckx, K., & Mroczek, D. K. (2010). The relation of change in hostility and sociability during childhood to substance use in mid adolescence. *Journal of Research in Personality, 44*(1), 103–114.

Hanks, A. S., Just, D. R., & Brumberg, A. (2016). Marketing vegetables in elementary school cafeterias to increase uptake. *Pediatrics, 138*(2), e20151720. **doi:10.1542/peds.2015-1720**

Hannerz, H., Albertsen, K., Nielsen, M. L., Tüchsen, F., & Burr, H. (2004).

Occupational factors and 5-year weight change among men in a Danish national cohort. *Health Psychology, 23*(3), 283–288.

Hansen, W. B., Raynor, A. E., & Wolkenstein, B. H. (1991). Perceived personal immunity to the consequences of drinking alcohol: The relationship between behavior and perception. *Journal of Behavioral Medicine, 14*(3), 205–224.

Harding, D. J. (2010). *Living the drama: Community, conflict, and culture among inner-city boys.* Chicago, IL: University of Chicago Press.

Harper, M., O'Connor, R. C., & O'Carroll, R. E. (2014). Factors associated with grief and depression following the loss of a child: A multivariate analysis. *Psychology, Health & Medicine, 19*(3), 247–252. **https://doi.org/10.1080/13548506.2013.811274**

Harrell, E., Kelly, K. S., & Stutts, W. (1996). Situational determinants of correlations between serum cortisol and self-reported stress measures. *Psychology, 33,* 22–25.

Harrell, E., Langton, L., Berzofsky, M., Couzens, L., & Smiley-McDonald, H. (2014). *Household poverty and nonfatal violent victimization, 2008–2012.* Washington, DC: Bureau of Justice Statistics.

Harriger, J. A., Calogero, R. M., Witherington, D. C., & Smith, J. E. (2010). Body size stereotyping and internalization of the thin ideal in preschool girls. *Sex Roles, 63*(9), 609–620.

Harris, P. L. (1992). Reducing the mortality from abdominal aortic aneurysms: Need for a national screening programme. *BMJ: British Medical Journal, 305*(6855), 697–699.

Harris, P. R., Mayle, K., Mabbott, L., & Napper, L. (2007). Self-affirmation reduces smokers' defensiveness to graphic on-pack cigarette warning labels. *Health Psychology, 26*(4), 437–446.

Harris, P. R., & Napper, L. (2005). Self-affirmation and the biased processing of threatening health-risk information. *Personality and Social Psychology Bulletin, 31*(9), 1250–1263.

Hartmann, A. S., Thomas, J. J., Greenberg, J. L., Elliott, C. M., Matheny, N. L., & Wilhelm, S. (2015). Anorexia nervosa and body dysmorphic disorder: A comparison of body image concerns and explicit and implicit attractiveness beliefs. *Body Image, 14,* 77–84.

Hartmann, L. C., Schaid, D. J., Woods, J. E., Crotty, T. P., Myers, J. L., Arnold, P. G., . . . Jenkins, R. B. (1999). Efficacy of bilateral prophylactic mastectomy in women with a family history of breast cancer. *New England Journal of Medicine, 340*(2), 77–84.

Harvey, J. H., & Hansen, A. M. (2000). Loss and bereavement in close romantic relationships. In J. H. Harvey & A. M. Hansen (Eds.), *Close relationships* (pp. 359–370). Thousand Oaks, CA: Sage.

Hashim, S. A., & Van Itallie, T. B. (1965). Studies in normal and obese subjects with a monitored food dispensing device. *Annals of the New York Academy of Sciences, 131*(1), 654–661.

Hashish, I., Hai, H. K., Harvey, W., Feinmann, C., & Harris, M. (1988). Reduction of postoperative pain and swelling by ultrasound treatment: A placebo effect. *Pain, 33*(3), 303–311. **https://doi.org/10.1016/0304-3959(88)90289-8**

Haskard, K. B., Williams, S. L., DiMatteo, M. R., Rosenthal, R., White, M. K., & Goldstein, M. G. (2008). Physician and patient communication training in primary care: Effects on participation and satisfaction. *Health Psychology, 27*(5), 513–522. **doi:10.1037/0278-6133.27.5.513**

Hassler, M., Pulverer, W., Lakshminarasimhan, R., Redl, E., Hacker, J., Garland, G., . . . Egger, G. (2016). Insights into the pathogenesis of anaplastic large-cell lymphoma through genome-wide DNA methylation profiling. *Cell Reports, 17*(2), 596–608. **doi:10.1016/j.celrep.2016.09.018**

Hatchett, L., Friend, R., Symister, P., & Wadhwa, N. (1997). Interpersonal expectations, social support, and adjustment to chronic illness. *Journal of Personality and Social Psychology, 73*(3), 560–573.

Hatzenbuehler, M. L. (2011). The social environment and suicide attempts in lesbian, gay, and bisexual youth. *Pediatrics, 127*(5), 896–903. **doi:10.1037//0022-3514.73.3.560**

Hawkley, L. C., & Cacioppo, J. T. (2010). Loneliness matters: A theoretical and empirical review of consequences and mechanisms. *Annals of Behavioral Medicine, 40*(2), 218–227. **https://doi.org/10.1007/s12160-010-9210-8**

Hawthorne, D. M., Youngblut, J. M., & Brooten, D. (2016). Parent spirituality, grief, and mental health at 1 and 3 months after their infant's/child's death in an intensive care unit. *SI: Achievements, Challenges, and Implications for Pediatric Nursing in the Post-Genomic Era, 31*(1), 73–80. **https://doi.org/10.1016/j.pedn.2015.07.008**

Hayman, L., Lucas, T., & Porcerelli, J. (2014). Cognitive appraisal vs. exposure-based stress measures links to perceived mental and physical health in low-income Black women. *Journal of Nervous and Mental Disease, 202*(11), 807–812.

Hays, R. B., Turner, H., & Coates, T. J. (1992). Social support, AIDS-related symptoms, and depression among gay men. *Journal of Consulting and Clinical Psychology, 60*(3), 463–469.

Hays, R. D., Kravitz, R. L., Mazel, R. M., Sherbourne, C. D., DiMatteo, M. R., Rogers, W. H., & Greenfield, S. (1994). The impact of patient adherence on health outcomes for patients with chronic disease in the Medical Outcomes Study. *Journal of Behavioral Medicine, 17,* 347–360.

He, L. F. (1987). Involvement of endogenous opiod peptides in acupuncture analgesia. *Pain, 31,* 99–121.

Heath, A. C., & Madden, P. A. (1995). Genetic influences on smoking. In J. R. Turner, L. R. Cardon, & J. K. Hewitt (Eds.), *Behavior genetic approaches in behavioral medicine* (pp. 45–66). New York, NY: Plenum.

Heath, A. C., & Martin, N. G. (1993). Genetic models for the natural history of smoking: Evidence for a genetic influence on smoking persistence. *Addictive Behaviors, 18*(1), 19–34.

Heatherton, T. F., & Sargent, J. D. (2009). Does watching smoking in movies promote teenage smoking? *Current Directions in Psychological Science, 18*(2), 63–67.

Heatherton, T. F., Striepe, M., & Wittenberg, L. (1998). Emotional distress and disinhibited eating: The role of self. *Personality and Social Psychology Bulletin, 24*(3), 301–313.

Hebert, L. E., Weuve, J., Scherr, P. A., & Evans, D. A. (2013). Alzheimer disease in the United States (2010-2050) estimated using the 2010 census. *Neurology, 80*(19), 1778–1783. **doi:10.1212/wnl.0b013e31828726f5**

Heckman, B. D., Fisher, E. B., Monsees, B., Merbaum, M., Ristvedt, S., & Bishop, C. (2004). Coping and anxiety in women recalled for additional diagnostic procedures following an abnormal screening mammogram. *Health Psychology, 23*(1), 42–48.

Heckman, T. G., Barcikowski, R., Ogles, B., Suhr, J., Carlson, B., Holroyd, K., & Garske, J. (2006). A telephone-delivered coping improvement group intervention for middle-aged and older adults living with HIV/AIDS. *Annals of Behavioral Medicine, 32*(1), 27–38.

Heckman, T. G., Kelly, J. A., & Somlai, A. M. (1998). Predictors of continued high-risk sexual behavior in a community sample of persons living with HIV/AIDS. *AIDS and Behavior, 2*(2), 127–135.

Hedegaard, U., Kjeldsen, L. J., Pottegård, A., Henriksen, J. E., Lambrechtsen, J., Hangaard, J., &

Hallas, J. (2015). Improving medication adherence in patients with hypertension: A randomized trial. *American Journal of Medicine, 128*(12), 1351–1361. doi:10.1016/j.amjmed.2015.08.011

Hegel, M. T., Ayllon, T., Thiel, G., & Oulton, B. (1992). Improving adherence to fluid restrictions in male hemodialysis patients: A comparision of cognitive and behavioral approaches. *Health Psychology, 11,* 324–330.

Heinberg, L. J., & Thompson, J. K. (1995). Body image and televised images of thinness and attractiveness: A controlled laboratory investigation. *Journal of Social and Clinical Psychology, 14*(4), 325–338.

Heishman, S. J., Kozlowski, L. T., & Henningfield, J. E. (1997). Nicotine addiction: Implications for public health policy. *Journal of Social Issues, 53*(1), 13–33.

Helgeson, V. S. (1991). The effects of masculinity and social support on recovery from myocardial infarction. *Psychosomatic Medicine, 53*(6), 621–633.

Helgeson, V. S. (1992). Moderators of the relation between perceived control and adjustment to chronic illness. *Journal of Personality and Social Psychology, 63*(4), 656–666. doi:10.1037/0022-3514.63.4.656

Helgeson, V. S., & Cohen, S. (1996). Social support and adjustment to cancer: Reconciling descriptive, correlational, and intervention research. *Health Psychology, 15*(2), 135–148.

Helgeson, V. S., Cohen, S., & Fritz, H. L. (1998). Social ties and cancer. In J. C. Holland (Ed.), *Psycho-Oncology* (pp. 99–109). New York, NY: Oxford University Press.

Helgeson, V. S., Cohen, S., Schulz, R., & Yasko, J. (1999). Education and peer discussion group interventions and adjustment to breast cancer. *Archives of General Psychiatry, 56,* 340–347.

Helgeson, V. S., Cohen, S., Schulz, R., & Yasko, J. (2000). Group support interventions for women with breast cancer: Who benefits from what? *Health Psychology, 19,* 107–114.

Helgeson, V. S., Cohen, S., Schulz, R., & Yasko, J. (2001). Long-term effects of educational and peer discussion group interventions on adjustment to breast cancer. *Health Psychology, 20,* 387–392.

Helgeson, V. S., Lepore, S. J., & Eton, D. T. (2006). Moderators of the benefits of psychoeducational interventions for men with prostate cancer. *Health Psychology, 25*(3), 348–354.

Helgeson, V. S., Snyder, P., & Seltman, H. (2004). Psychological and physical adjustment to breast cancer over 4 years: Identifying distinct trajectories of change. *Health Psychology, 23*(1), 3–15.

Helgeson, V. S., & Tomich, P. L. (2005). Surviving cancer: A comparison of 5-year disease-free breast cancer survivors with healthy women. *Psycho-Oncology, 14*(4), 307–317. https://doi.org/10.1002/pon.848

Helmrich, S. P., Ragland, D. R., Leung, R. W., & Paffenbarger R. S., Jr. (1991). Physical activity and reduced occurrence of non-insulin-dependent diabetes mellitus. *New England Journal of Medicine, 325*(3), 147–152.

Helms, J. M. (1987). Acupuncture for the management of primary dysmenorrhea. *Obstetrics and Gynecology, 69,* 51–56.

Helsing, K., & Szklo, M. (1981). Mortality after bereavement. *American Journal of Epidemiology, 114,* 41–52.

Hemenover, S. H. (2001). Self-reported processing bias and naturally occurring mood: Mediators between personality and stress appraisals. *Personality and Social Psychology Bulletin, 27*(4), 387–394.

Hemenover, S. H., & Dienstbier, R. A. (1996). Prediction of stress appraisals from mastery, extraversion, neuroticism, and general appraisal tendencies. *Motivation and Emotion, 20*(4), 299–317.

Hendrickson, K. L., & Rasmussen, E. B. (2017). Mindful eating reduces impulsive food choice in adolescents and adults. *Health Psychology, 36*(3), 226–235.

Henifin, M. S. (1993). New reproductive technologies: Equity and access to reproductive health care. *Journal of Social Issues, 49*(2), 61–74.

Henley, S. J., Richards, T. B., Underwood, J. M., Eheman, C. R., Plescia, M., & McAfee, T. A. (2014). Lung cancer incidence trends among men and women—United States, 2005-2009. *Morbidity and Mortality Weekly Report, 63*(1), 1–5.

Henoch, I., Berg, C., & Benkel, I. (2015). The shared experience help the bereavement to flow. *American Journal of Hospice and Palliative Medicine®, 33*(10), 959–965. https://doi.org/10.1177/1049909115607204

Herbert, T. B., & Cohen, S. (1993). Depression and immunity: A meta-analytic review. *Psychological Bulletin, 113*(3), 472–486.

Herman, C. P., & Polivy, J. (1984). A boundary model for the regulation of eating. *Research Publications-Association for Research in Nervous and Mental Disease, 62,* 141–156.

Hernandez, D. C., & Pressler, E. (2015). Gender disparities among the association between cumulative family-level stress & adolescent weight status. *Preventive Medicine, 73,* 60–66.

Hernandez-Reif, M., Field, T., Krasnegor, J., & Theakston, H. (2001). Lower back pain is reduced and range of motion increased after massage therapy. *International Journal of Neuroscience, 106*(3–4), 131–145. https://doi.org/10.3109/00207450109149744

Heron, M. (2016). Deaths: Leading causes for 2014. *National Vital Statistics Reports, 65*(5), 1–96.

Hershey, J. C., Niederdeppe, J., Evans, W. D., Nonnemaker, J., Blahut, S.,

Holden, D., . . . Haviland, M. L. (2005). The theory of "truth": How counterindustry campaigns affect smoking behavior among teens. *Health Psychology, 24*(1), 22–31.

Hertel, A. W., Finch, E. A., Kelly, K. M., King, C., Lando, H., Linde, J. A., . . . Rothman, A. J. (2008). The impact of expectations and satisfaction on the initiation and maintenance of smoking cessation: An experimental test. *Health Psychology, 27*(3), 197–206.

Herzog, T. A. (2008). Analyzing the transtheoretical model using the framework of Weinstein, Rothman, and Sutton (1998): The example of smoking cessation. *Health Psychology, 27*(5), 548–556.

Herzog, T. A., Abrams, D. B., Emmons, K. M., Linnan, L. A., & Shadel, W. G. (1999). Do processes of change predict smoking stage movements? A prospective analysis of the transtheoretical model. *Health Psychology, 18*(4), 369–375.

Herzog, T. A., & Blagg, C. O. (2007). Are most precontemplators contemplating smoking cessation? Assessing the validity of the stages of change. *Health Psychology, 26*(2), 222–231.

Heuch, I., Kvale, G., Jacobsen, B. K., & Bjelke, E. (1983). Use of alcohol, tobacco and coffee, and risk of pancreatic cancer. *British Journal of Cancer, 48,* 637–643.

Hewitt, J. K. (1997). Behavior genetics and eating disorders. *Psychopharmacology Bulletin, 33*(3), 355–358.

Hewitt, P. L., & Flett, G. L. (1996). Personality traits and the coping process. In M. Zeidner & N. S. Endler (Eds.), *Handbook of coping* (pp. 410–433). New York, NY: Wiley.

Hewitt, P. L., Flett, G. L., & Mosher, S. W. (1992). The Perceived Stress Scale: Factor structure and relation to depression symptoms in a psychiatric sample. *Journal of Psychopathology and Behavioral Assessment, 14*(3), 247–257.

Hewitt, P. L., Flett, G. L., Sherry, S. B., & Caelian, C. (2006). Trait perfectionism dimensions and suicidal behavior.

In T. E. Ellis (Ed.), *Cognition and suicide: Theory, research, and therapy* (pp. 215–235). Washington, DC: American Psychological Association.

Higbee, K. L. (1969). Fifteen years of fear arousal: Research on threat appeals: 1953-1968. *Psychological Bulletin, 72*(6), 426–444.

Hilgard, E. R. (1975). The alleviation of pain by hypnosis. *Pain, 1,* 213–231.

Hilgard, E. R., & Hilgard, J. R. (1983). *Hypnosis in the relief of pain.* Los Altos, CA: Kaufman.

Hill-Briggs, F., Gary, T. L., Bone, L. R., Hill, M. N., Levine, D. M., & Brancati, F. L. (2005). Medication adherence and diabetes control in urban African Americans with type 2 diabetes. *Health Psychology, 24,* 349–357.

Hill, J. O., & Peters, J. C. (1998). Environmental contributions to the obesity epidemic. *Science, 280*(5368), 1371–1374.

Himmelstein, M. S., & Sanchez, D. T. (2016). Masculinity impediments: Internalized masculinity contributes to healthcare avoidance in men and women. *Journal of Health Psychology, 21*(7), 1283–1292. doi:10.1177/1359105314551623

Hinshaw, S. P., Owens, E. B., Zalecki, C., Huggins, S. P., Montenegro-Nevado, A. J., Schrodek, E., & Swanson, E. N. (2012). Prospective follow-up of girls with attention-deficit/hyperactivity disorder into early adulthood: Continuing impairment includes elevated risk for suicide attempts and self-injury. *Journal of Consulting and Clinical Psychology, 80*(6), 1041–1051. doi:10.1037/a0029451

Hinton, J. (1979). Comparison of places and policies for terminal care. *Lancet, 1,* 29–32.

Ho, R., & Chantagul, N. (2015). Support for voluntary and nonvoluntary euthanasia. *OMEGA – Journal of Death and Dying, 70*(3), 251–277. https://doi.org/10.1177/0030222815568958

Hodeib, M., Chang, J., Liu, F., Ziogas, A., Dilley, S., Randall, L. M., . . . Bristow,

R. E. (2015). Socioeconomic status as a predictor of adherence to treatment guidelines for early-stage ovarian cancer. *Gynecologic Oncology, 138*(1), 121–127. http://doi.org/10.1016/j.ygyno.2015.04.011

Hodge, A. M., & Zimmet, P. Z. (1994). The epidemiology of obesity. *Bailliere's Clinical Endocrinology and Metabolism, 8*(3), 577–599.

Hodgins, D. C., el-Guebaly, N., & Armstrong, S. (1995). Prospective and retrospective reports of mood states before relapse to substance use. *Journal of Consulting and Clinical Psychology, 63,* 400–407.

Hoerger, M., Perry, L. M., Gramling, R., Epstein, R. M., & Duberstein, P. R. (2017). Does educating patients about the Early Palliative Care Study increase preferences for outpatient palliative cancer care? Findings from Project EMPOWER. *Health Psychology, 36*(6), 538–548. https://doi.org/10.1037/hea0000489

Hoffman, C., Rice, D., & Sung, H. (1996). Persons with chronic conditions: Their prevalence and costs. *Journal of the American Medical Association, 276*(18), 1473–1479. doi:10.1001/jama.1996.03540180029029

Hoffman, K. M., Trawalter, S., Axt, J. R., & Oliver, M. N. (2016). Racial bias in pain assessment and treatment recommendations, and false beliefs about biological differences between Blacks and Whites. *Proceedings of the National Academy of Sciences of the United States of America, 113*(16), 4296–4301. https://doi.org/10.1073/pnas.1516047113

Hoffmann, T. C., Maher, C. G., Briffa, T., Sherrington, C., Bennell, K., Alison, J., . . . Glasziou, P. P. (2016). Prescribing exercise interventions for patients with chronic conditions. *Canadian Medical Association Journal, 188*(7), 510–518.

Hohwü, L., Li, J., Olsen, J., Sørensen, T. I., & Obel, C. (2014). Severe maternal stress exposure due to bereavement before, during and after pregnancy and risk of overweight and obesity in young adult men: A Danish national cohort study. *PLOS ONE*, *9*(5), e97490.

Holderness, C. C., Brooks-Gunn, J., & Warren, M. P. (1994). Co-morbidity of eating disorders and substance abuse review of the literature. *International Journal of Eating Disorders*, *16*(1), 1–34.

Hole, J., Hirsch, M., Ball, E., & Meads, C. (2015). Music as an aid for postoperative recovery in adults: A systematic review and meta-analysis. *The Lancet*, *386*(10004), 1659–1671. https://doi.org/10.1016/S0140-6736(15)60169-6

Holford, T. R., Levy, D. T., & Meza, R. (2016). Comparison of smoking history patterns among African American and White cohorts in the United States born 1890 to 1990. *Nicotine & Tobacco Research*, *18*(Suppl 1), S16–S29.

Hollands, G. J., Prestwich, A., & Marteau, T. M. (2011). Using aversive images to enhance healthy food choices and implicit attitudes: An experimental test of evaluative conditioning. *Health Psychology*, *30*(2), 195–203. doi:10.1037/a0022261

Hollis, J. F., Gullion, C. M., Stevens, V. J., Brantley, P. J., Appel, L. J., Ard, J. D., . . . Laferriere, D. (2008). Weight loss during the intensive intervention phase of the weight-loss maintenance trial. *American Journal of Preventive Medicine*, *35*(2), 118–126.

Holm, J., Holroyd, K., Hursey, K., & Penzien, D. (1986). The role of stress in recurrent tension headache. *Headache*, *26*, 160–167.

Holman, E. A., Garfin, D. R., & Silver, R. C. (2014). Media's role in broadcasting acute stress following the Boston Marathon bombings. *Proceedings of the National Academy of Sciences of the United States of America*, *111*(1), 93–98.

Holmes, T. H., & Rahe, R. H. (1967). The social readjustment rating scale. *Journal of Psychosomatic Research*, *11*(2), 213–218.

Holroyd, K. A., & Lipchik, G. L. (1999). Psychological management of recurrent headache disorders: Progress and prospects. In R. J. Gatchel & D. C. Turk (Eds.), *Psychological factors in pain: Critical perspectives* (pp. 193–212). New York, NY: Guilford.

Holroyd, K. A., O'Donnell, F. J., Stensland, M., Lipchik, G. L., Cordingley, G. E., & Carlson, B. W. (2001). Management of chronic tension-type headache with tricyclic antidepressant medication, stress management therapy, and their combination: A randomized controlled trial. *Journal of the American Medical Association*, *285*, 2208–2215.

Holt, C. L., Clark, E. M., Kreuter, M. W., & Scharff, D. P. (2000). Does locus of control moderate the effects of tailored health education materials? *Health Education Research*, *15*(4), 393–403.

Holtgrave, D. R., & Kelly, J. A. (1996). Preventing HIV/AIDS among high-risk urban women: The cost-effectiveness of a behavioral group intervention. *American Journal of Public Health*, *86*(10), 1442–1445.

Holt-Lunstad, J., & Smith, T. B. (2016). Loneliness and social isolation as risk factors for CVD: Implications for evidence-based patient care and scientific inquiry. *Heart*, *102*(13), 987–989. https://doi.org/10.1136/heartjnl-2015-309242

Holtzman, S., Newth, S., & Delongis, A. (2004). The role of social support in coping with daily pain among patients with rheumatoid arthritis. *Journal of Health Psychology*, *9*(5), 677–695. https://doi.org/10.1177/1359105304045381

Horgen, K. B., Choate, M., & Brownell, K. D. (2001). Television food advertising. In D. G. Singer & J. L. Singer (Eds.), *Handbook of children and media* (pp. 447–461). Thousand Oaks, CA: Sage.

Horndasch, S., Heinrich, H., Kratz, O., Mai, S., Graap, H., & Moll, G. H. (2015). Perception and evaluation of women's bodies in adolescents and adults with anorexia nervosa. *European Archives of Psychiatry and Clinical Neuroscience*, *265*(8), 677–687.

Horne, Z., Powell, D., Hummel, J. E., & Holyoak, K. J. (2015). Countering antivaccination attitudes. *Proceedings of the National Academy of Sciences of the United States of America*, *112*(33), 10321–10324. http://doi.org/10.1073/pnas.1504019112

Horwitz, R. I., Viscoli, C. M., Berkman, L., Donaldson, R. M., Horwitz, S. M., Murray, C. J., . . . Sindelar, J. (1990). Treatment adherence and risk of death after myocardial infarction. *Lancet*, *336*, 542–545.

House, J. S. (1981). *Work stress and social support*. Reading, MA: Addison-Wesley.

House, J. S., & Kahn, R. L. (1985). Measures and concepts of social support. In C. Sheldon & S. Leonard (Eds.), *Social support and health* (pp. 83–108). New York, NY: Academic Press.

House, J. S., Robbins, C., & Metzner, H. L. (1982). The association of social relationships and activities with mortality: Prospective evidence from the Tecumseh Community Health Study. *American Journal of Epidemiology*, *116*(1), 123–140.

Houston, B. K., & Vavak, C. R. (1991). Cynical hostility: Developmental factors, psychosocial correlates, and health behaviors. *Health Psychology*, *10*(1), 9–17.

Howell, D., Osternig, L., Van Donkelaar, P., Mayr, U., & Chou, L. S. (2013). Effects of concussion on attention and executive function in adolescents. *Medicine and Science in Sports and Exercise*, *45*(6), 1030–1037.

Howlader, N., Noone, A. M., Krapcho, M., Miller, D., Bishop, K., Kosary, C. L., . . . Cronin, K. A. (Eds.). (2017). *SEER Cancer Statistics Review, 1975-2014, National Cancer Institute*. Bethesda, MD: National Cancer Institutde.

Howsepian, B. A., & Merluzzi, T. V. (2009). Religious beliefs, social support, self-efficacy and adjustment to cancer. *Psycho-Oncology*, *18*(10), 1069 1079.

Hoyt, L. T., Chase-Lansdale, P. L., McDade, T. W., & Adam, E. K. (2012). Positive youth, healthy adults: Does positive well-being in adolescence predict better perceived health and fewer risky health behaviors in young adulthood? *Journal of Adolescent Health, 50*(1), 66–73.

Hu, G., Wilcox, H. C., Wissow, L., & Baker, S. P. (2008). Mid-life suicide: An increasing problem in U.S. Whites, 1999-2005. *American Journal of Preventive Medicine, 35*(6), 589–593. doi:10.1016/j.amepre.2008.07.005

Huang, G. C., Unger, J. B., Soto, D., Fujimoto, K., Pentz, M. A., Jordan-Marsh, M., & Valente, T. W. (2014). Peer influences: The impact of online and offline friendship networks on adolescent smoking and alcohol use. *Journal of Adolescent Health, 54*(5), 508–514.

Huang, H. P., He, M., Wang, H. Y., & Zhou, M. (2016). A meta-analysis of the benefits of mindfulness-based stress reduction (MBSR) on psychological function among breast cancer (BC) survivors. *Breast Cancer, 23*(4), 568–576.

Huang, K., Marcora, E., Pimenova, A., Narzo, A. D., Kapoor, M., Jin, S. C., . . . Goate, A. (2017). A common haplotype lowers PU.1 expression in myeloid cells and delays onset of Alzheimers disease. *Nature Neuroscience, 20*(8), 1052–1061. doi:10.1101/110957

Hudson, J. I., Hiripi, E., Pope, H. G., & Kessler, R. C. (2007). The prevalence and correlates of eating disorders in the National Comorbidity Survey Replication. *Biological Psychiatry, 61*(3), 348–358.

Huebner, D. M., Neilands, T. B., Rebchook, G. M., & Kegeles, S. M. (2011). Sorting through chickens and eggs: A longitudinal examination of the associations between attitudes, norms, and sexual risk behavior. *Health Psychology, 30*(1), 110–118. doi:10.1037/a0021973

Huggins, M., Bloch, M., Wiggins, S., Adam, S., Suchowersky, O., Trew, M., . . . Knight, J. (1992). Predictive testing for Huntington disease in Canada: Adverse effects and unexpected results in those receiving a decreased risk. *American Journal of Medical Genetics Part A, 42*(4), 508–515.

Hughes, A., McMunn, A., Bartley, M., & Kumari, M. (2015). Elevated inflammatory biomarkers during unemployment: Modification by age and country in the UK. *Journal of Epidemiology & Community Health, 69*(7), 673–680.

Hughes, J. R., & Hatsukami, D. (1986). Signs and symptoms of tobacco withdrawal. *Archives of General Psychiatry, 43*(3), 289–294.

Hughes, M., Brymer, M., Chiu, W. T., Fairbank, J. A., Jones, R. T., Pynoos, R. S., . . . Kessler, R. C. (2011). Posttraumatic stress among students after the shootings at Virginia Tech. *Psychological Trauma: Theory, Research, Practice, and Policy, 3*(4), 403–411.

Humphrey, L. L. (1986). Family dynamics in bulimia. *Adolescent Psychiatry, 13*, 315–332.

Humphrey, L. L. (1988). Relationships within subtypes of anorexic, bulimic, and normal families. *Journal of the American Academy of Child & Adolescent Psychiatry, 27*(5), 544–551.

Humphreys, K., Blodgett, J. C., & Wagner, T. H. (2014). Estimating the efficacy of Alcoholics Anonymous without self-selection bias: An instrumental variables re-analysis of randomized clinical trials. *Alcoholism: Clinical and Experimental Research, 38*(11), 2688–2694.

Hunt, K. A., Gaba, A., & Lavizzo-Mourey, R. (2005). Racial and ethnic disparities and perceptions of health care: Does health plan type matter? *Health Services Research, 40*(2), 551–576. http://doi.org/10.1111/j.1475-6773.2005.00372

Hunt, W. A., Barnett, L. W., & Branch, L. G. (1971). Relapse rates in addiction programs. *Journal of Clinical Psychology, 27*(4), 455–456.

Hunter, D. J., Manson, J. E., Colditz, G. A., Stampfer, M. J., Rosner, B., Hennekens, C. H., . . . Willett, W. C. (1993). A prospective study of the intake of vitamins C, E, and A and the risk of breast cancer. *New England Journal of Medicine, 329*(4), 234–240.

Hurwitz, E. L., Morgenstern, H., & Chiao, C. (2005). Effects of recreational physical activity and back exercises on low back pain and psychological distress: Findings from the UCLA low back pain study. *American Journal of Public Health, 95*(10), 1817–1824. https://doi.org/10.2105/AJPH.2004.052993

Hygge, S., Evans, G. W., & Bullinger, M. (2002). A prospective study of some effects of aircraft noise on cognitive performance in schoolchildren. *Psychological Science, 13*(5), 469–474.

IARC Working Group on the Evaluation of Carcinogenic Risks to Humans. (2012). Pharmaceuticals. A review of human carcinogens. *IARC Monographs on the Evaluation of Carcinogenic Risks to Humans, 100*(PT A), 1–401.

Iida, M., Gleason, M., Green-Rapaport, A. S., Bolger, N., & Shrout, P. E. (2017). The influence of daily coping on anxiety under examination stress: A model of interindividual differences in intraindividual change. *Personality and Social Psychology Bulletin, 43*(7), 907–923. doi:10.1177/0146167217700605

Iida, M., Stephens, M. A. P., Franks, M. M., & Rook, K. S. (2013). Daily symptoms, distress and interaction quality among couples coping with type 2 diabetes. *Journal of Social and Personal Relationships, 30*(3), 293–300.

Iihara, N., Nishio, T., Okura, M., Anzai, H., Kagawa, M., Houchi, H., & Kirino, Y. (2013). Comparing patient dissatisfaction and rational judgment in intentional medication non-adherence versus unintentional non-adherence. *Journal of Clinical Pharmacy and Therapeutics, 39*(1), 45–52. doi:10.1111/jcpt.12100

Ilacqua, G. E. (1994). Migraine headaches: Coping efficacy of guided imagery training. *Headache: The Journal of Head and Face Pain, 34*(2), 99–102. https://doi.org/10.1111/j.1526-4610.1994.hed3402099.x

Inagaki, T. K., Bryne, H. K., Suzuki, S., Jevtic, I., Hornstein, E., Bower, J. E., & Eisenberger, N. I. (2016). The neurobiology of giving versus receiving support: The role of stress-related and social reward-related neural activity. *Psychosomatic Medicine*, 78(4), 443–453.

Infurna, F. J., & Luthar, S. S. (2017). Parents' adjustment following the death of their child: Resilience is multidimensional and differs across outcomes examined. *Journal of Research in Personality*, 68, 38–53. https://doi.org/10.1016/j .jrp.2017.04.004

Inoue-Choi, M., Liao, L. M., Reyes-Guzman, C., Hartge, P., Caporaso, N., & Freedman, N. D. (2017). Association of long-term, low-intensity smoking with all-cause and cause-specific mortality in the National Institutes of Health–AARP Diet and Health Study. *JAMA Internal Medicine*, 177(1), 87–95.

International Association for the Study of Pain. (1979). Pain terms: A list with definitions and a note on usage. *Pain*, 6, 249–252.

Ironson, G., Stuetzle, R., & Fletcher, M. A. (2006). An increase in religiousness/spirituality occurs after HIV diagnosis and predicts slower disease progression over 4 years in people with HIV. *Journal of General Internal Medicine*, 21(5), 62–68.

Ironson, G., Wynings, C., Schneiderman, N., Baum, A., Rodriguez, M., Greenwood, D., . . . Klimas, N. (1997). Posttraumatic stress symptoms, intrusive thoughts, loss, and immune function after Hurricane Andrew. *Psychosomatic Medicine*, 59(2), 128–141.

Irvin, J. E., Bowers, C. A., Dunn, M. E., & Wang, M. C. (1999). Efficacy of relapse prevention: A meta-analytic review. *Journal of Consulting and Clinical Psychology*, 67, 563–570.

Irwin, M., Mascovich, A., Gillin, J. C., Willoughby, R., Pike, J., & Smith, T. L. (1994). Partial sleep deprivation reduced natural killer cell activity in humans. *Psychosomatic Medicine*, 56(6), 493–498. doi:10.1097/00006842-199411 000-00004

Isaacs, S. L., & Knickman, J. R. (1997). *To improve health and health care*. San Francisco, CA: Jossey Bass.

Iturralde, E., Weissberg-Benchell, J., & Hood, K. K. (2017). Avoidant coping and diabetes-related distress: Pathways to adolescents' Type 1 diabetes outcomes. *Health Psychology*, 36(3), 236–244. doi:10.1037/hea000044

Ivanova, I. V., Tasca, G. A., Hammond, N., Balfour, L., Ritchie, K., Koszycki, D., & Bissada, H. (2015). Negative affect mediates the relationship between interpersonal problems and binge-eating disorder symptoms and psychopathology in a clinical sample: A test of the interpersonal model. *European Eating Disorders Review*, 23(2), 133–138.

Izard, C. E., Libero, D. Z., Putnam, P., & Haynes, O. M. (1993). Stability of emotion experiences and their relations to traits of personality. *Journal of Personality and Social Psychology*, 64(5), 847–860.

Jackson, E. R., Shanafelt, T. D., Hasan, O., Satele, D. V., & Dyrbye, L. N. (2016). Burnout and alcohol abuse/dependence among U.S. medical students. *Academic Medicine*, 91(9), 1251–1256. doi:10.1097/ACM.0000000000001138

Jackson, J. S., & Inglehart, M. R. (1995). Reverberation theory: Stress and racism in hierarchically structured communities. In S. E. Hobfoff & M. W. De Vries (Eds.), *Extreme stress and communities: Impact and intervention* (pp. 353–373). Dordrecht, NL: Kluwer Academic Publishers.

Jackson, J. S., Knight, K. M., & Rafferty, J. A. (2010). Race and unhealthy behaviors: Chronic stress, the HPA axis, and physical and mental health disparities over the life course. *American Journal of Public Health*, 100(5), 933–939.

Jackson, K. M., & Aiken, L. S. (2000). A psychosocial model of sun protection and sunbathing in young women: The impact of health beliefs, attitudes, norms, and self-efficacy for sun protection. *Health Psychology*, 19(5), 469–478.

Jackson, T., Pope, L., Nagasaka, T., Fritch, A., Iezzi, T., & Chen, H. (2005). The impact of threatening information about pain on coping and pain tolerance. *British Journal of Health Psychology*, 10(3), 441–451. https://doi .org/10.1348/135910705X27587

Jackson, V. P., Lex, A. M., & Smith, D. J. (1988). Patient discomfort during screen-film mammography. *Radiology*, 168(2), 421–423.

Jacob, J. A. (2016). As opioid prescribing guidelines tighten, mindfulness meditation holds promise for pain relief. *Journal of the American Medical Association*, 315(22), 2385–2387. https:// doi.org/10.1001/jama.2016.4875

Jacobi, C., Morris, L., Beckers, C., Bronisch-Holtze, J., Winter, J., Winzelberg, A. J., & Taylor, C. B. (2007). Maintenance of internet-based prevention: A randomized controlled trial. *International Journal of Eating Disorders*, 40(2), 114–119.

Jacobs, I. J., Menon, U., Ryan, A., Gentry-Maharaj, A., Burnell, M., Kalsi, J. K., . . . Crump, D. N. (2015). Ovarian cancer screening and mortality in the UK Collaborative Trial of Ovarian Cancer Screening (UKCTOCS): A randomized controlled trial. *The Lancet*, 387(10022), 945–956.

Jacobs, L. M., Burns, K., & Bennett Jacobs, B. (2008). Trauma death: Views of the public and trauma professionals on death and dying from injuries. *Archives of Surgery*, 143(8), 730–735. doi:10.1001/archsurg.143.8.730

Jacobs, T. J., & Charles, E. (1980). Life events and the occurrence of cancer in children. *Psychosomatic Medicine*, 42(1), 11–24.

Jacobson, E. (1938). *Progressive relaxation: A physiological and clinical investigation of muscle states and their significance in psychology and medical practice* (2nd ed.). Chicago, IL: University of Chicago Press.

Jacobson, P. D., Wasserman, J., & Anderson, J. R. (1997). Historical overview of tobacco legislation and regulation. *Journal of Social Issues, 53*(1), 75–95.

Jaffe, A. J., Rounsaville, B., Chang, G., Schottenfeld, R. S., Meyer, R. E., & O'Malley, S. S. (1996). Naltrexone, relapse prevention, and supportive therapy with alcoholics: An analysis of patient treatment matching. *Journal of Consulting and Clinical Psychology, 64*(5), 1044–1053.

Jakicic, J. M., Winters, C., Lang, W., & Wing, R. R. (1999). Effects of intermittent exercise and use of home exercise equipment on adherence, weight loss, and fitness in overweight women: A randomized trial. *Journal of the American Medical Association, 282*(16), 1554–1560.

Jamal, A., Gentzke, A., Hu, S. S., Cullen, K. A., Apelberg, B. J., Homa, D. M., & King, B. A. (2017). Tobacco use among middle and high school students — United States, 2011–2016. *Morbidity and Mortality Weekly Report, 66,* 597–603. **http://dx.doi.org/10.15585/mmwr .mm6623a1**

Jamal, A., King, B. A., Neff, L. J., Whitmill, J., Babb, S. D., & Graffunder, C. M. (2016). Current cigarette smoking among adults — United States, 2005–2015. *Morbidity and Mortality Weekly Report, 65*(44), 1205–1211. **http://dx.doi.org/10.15585/mmwr .mm6544a2**

Janis, I. L. (1967). Effects of fear arousal on attitude change: Recent developments in theory and experimental research. In L. Berkowitz (Ed.), *Advances in experimental social psychology* (Vol. 3, pp. 166–224). San Diego, CA: Academic Press.

Janis, I. L., & Feshbach, S. (1953). Effects of fear-arousing communications. *The Journal of Abnormal and Social Psychology, 48*(1), 78–92.

Janis, I. L., & Mann, L. (1965). Effectiveness of emotional role-playing in modifying smoking habits and attitudes. *Journal of Experimental Research in Personality, 1,* 84–90.

Janis, I. L., & Terwilliger, R. F. (1962). An experimental study of psychological resistances to fear arousing communications. *The Journal of Abnormal and Social Psychology, 65*(6), 403–410.

Janoff-Bulman R. (1992). *Shattered assumptions: Towards a new psychology of trauma.* New York, NY: Free Press.

Jansen, L., Hoffmeister, M., Chang-Claude, J., Brenner, H., & Arndt, V. (2011). Benefit finding and post-traumatic growth in long-term colorectal cancer survivors: Prevalence, determinants, and associations with quality of life. *British Journal of Cancer, 105*(8), 1158–1165. **https://doi.org/10.1038/ bjc.2011.335**

Janssen, C., Ommen, O., Ruppert, G., & Pfaff, H. (2008). Patient- and hospital-related determinants on subjective evaluation of medical treatment outcome of severely injured patients. *International Journal of Public Health, 16*(1), 53–60.

Janz, N. K., & Becker, M. H. (1984). The health belief model: A decade later. *Health Education Quarterly, 11*(1), 1–47.

Jaremka, L. M., Fagundes, C. P., Glaser, R., Bennett, J. M., Malarkey, W. B., & Kiecolt-Glaser, J. K. (2013). Loneliness predicts pain, depression, and fatigue: Understanding the role of immune dysregulation. *Psychoneuroendocrinology, 38*(8), 1310–1317. **http://doi.org/ 10.1016/j.psyneuen.2012.11.016**

Jarlais, D. C. D., Friedman, S. R., Casriel, C., & Kott, A. (1987). AIDS and preventing initiation into intravenous (V) drug use. *Psychology and Health, 1*(2), 179–194.

Jarpe-Ratner, E., Folkens, S., Sharma, S., Daro, D., & Edens, N. K. (2016). An experiential cooking and nutrition education program increases cooking self-efficacy and vegetable consumption in children in grades 3–8. *Journal of Nutrition Education and Behavior, 48*(10), 697–705.

Jay, S. M., Elliott, C. H., Katz, E., & Siegel, S. E. (1987). Cognitive-behavioral and pharmacologic interventions for childrens' distress during painful medical procedures. *Journal of Consulting and Clinical Psychology, 55*(6), 860–865.

Jeffery, R. W., Bjornson-Benson, W. M., Rosenthal, B. S., Lindquist, R. A., Kurth, C. L., & Johnson, S. L. (1984). Correlates of weight loss and its maintenance over two years of follow-up among middle-aged men. *Preventive Medicine, 13*(2), 155–168.

Jeffery, R. W., Hennrikus, D. J., Lando, H. A., Murray, D. M., & Liu, J. W. (2000). Reconciling conflicting findings regarding postcessation weight concerns and success in smoking cessation. *Health Psychology, 19*(3), 242–246.

Jeffery, R. W., Wing, R. R., Thorson, C., & Burton, L. R. (1998). Use of personal trainers and financial incentives to increase exercise in a behavioral weight-loss program. *Journal of Consulting and Clinical Psychology, 66*(5), 777–783.

Jeitler, M., Brunnhuber, S., Meier, L., Lüdtke, R., Büssing, A., Kessler, C., & Michalsen, A. (2015). Effectiveness of jyoti meditation for patients with chronic neck pain and psychological distress—a randomized controlled clinical trial. *The Journal of Pain, 16*(1), 77–86.

Jemmott, J. B., Jemmott, L. S., O'Leary, A., Ngwane, Z., Icard, L. D., Bellamy, S. L., . . . Makiwane, M. B. (2010). School-based randomized controlled trial of an HIV/STD risk-reduction intervention for South African adolescents. *Archives of Pediatrics & Adolescent Medicine, 164*(10), 923–929.

Jemmott, J. B., III, Jemmott, L. S., O'Leary, A., Ngwane, Z., Icard, L. D., Heeren, G. A., . . . Carty, C. (2014). Cluster-randomized controlled trial of an HIV/sexually transmitted infection risk-reduction intervention for South African men. *American Journal of Public Health, 104*(3), 467–473.

Jemmott, J. B., III, & Jones, J. M. (1993). Social psychology and AIDS among ethnic minority individuals: Risk behaviors and strategies for changing them. In J. B. Pryor & G. D. Reeder (Eds.), *The social psychology of HIV infection* (pp. 183–224). Hillsdale, NJ: Erlbaum.

Jemmott, J. B., & Locke, S. E. (1984). Psychosocial factors, immunologic mediation, and human susceptibility to infectious diseases: How much do we know? *Psychological Bulletin*, *95*(1), 78–108.

Jemmott, J. B., & Magloire, K. (1988). Academic stress, social support, and secretory immunoglobulin A. *Journal of Personality and Social Psychology*, *55*(5), 803–810.

Jemmott, J. I., Sanderson, C. A., & Miller, S. M. (1995). Changes in psychological distress and HIV risk-associated behavior: Consequences of HIV antibody testing? In R. T. Croyle (Ed.), *Psychosocial effects of screening for disease prevention and detection* (pp. 82–125). New York, NY: Oxford University Press.

Jena, A. B., Mann, N. C., Wedlund, L. N., & Olenski, A. (2017). Delays in emergency care and mortality during major U.S. marathons. *New England Journal of Medicine*, *376*(15), 1441–1450. https://doi.org/10.1056/NEJMsa1614073

Jennings, B. (1993). Health policy in a new key: Setting democratic priorities. *Journal of Social Issues*, *49*, 169–184.

Jennings-Bey, T., Lane, S. D., Rubinstein, R. A., Bergen-Cico, D., Haygood-El, A., Hudson, H., . . . Fowler, F. L. (2015). The trauma response team: A community intervention for gang violence. *Journal of Urban Health*, *92*(5), 947–954.

Jensen, M. P., Day, M. A., & Miró, J. (2014). Neuromodulatory treatments for chronic pain: Efficacy and mechanisms. *Nature Reviews Neurology*, *10*(3), 167–178.

Jensen, M. P., Karoly, P., & Harris, P. (1991). Assessing the affective component of chronic pain: Development of the Pain Discomfort Scale. *Journal of Psychosomatic Research*, *35*, 149–154.

Jensen, M. P., & Patterson, D. R. (2014). Hypnotic approaches for chronic pain management: Clinical implications of recent research findings. *American Psychologist*, *69*(2), 167–177. doi:10.1037/a0035644

Jensen, M. P., Turner, J. A., & Romano, J. M. (2001). Change in beliefs, catastrophizing, and coping are associated with improvement in multidisciplinary pain treatment. *Journal of Consulting and Clinical Psychology*, *69*, 655–662.

Jensen, M. P., Turner, J. A., Romano, J. M., & Karoly, P. (1991). Coping with chronic pain: A critical review of the literature. *Pain*, *47*, 249–283.

Jepson, C., & Rimer, B. K. (1993). Determinants of mammography intentions among prior screenees and non-screenees. *Journal of Applied Social Psychology*, *23*(1), 40–51.

Jewell, S. L., Luecken, L. J., Gress-Smith, J., Crnic, K. A., & Gonzales, N. A. (2015). Economic stress and cortisol among postpartum low-income Mexican American women: Buffering influence of family support. *Behavioral Medicine*, *41*(3), 138–144.

Jilcott Pitts, S. B., Keyserling, T. C., Johnston, L., Smith, T. W., McGuirt, J. T., Evenson, K. R., . . . Ammerman, A. S. (2015). Associations between neighborhood-level factors related to a healthful lifestyle and dietary intake, physical activity, and support for obesity prevention polices among rural adults. *Journal of Community Health*, *40*(2), 276–284. http://doi.org/10.1007/s10900-014-9927-6

Johns, S. A., Brown, L. F., Beck-Coon, K., Monahan, P. O., Tong, Y., & Kroenke, K. (2015). Randomized controlled pilot study of mindfulness-based stress reduction for persistently fatigued cancer survivors. *Psycho-Oncology*, *24*(8), 885–893.

Johnson, A., Kent, P., Swanson, B., Rosdil, A., Owen, E., Fogg, L., & Keithley, J. (2015). The use of acupuncture for pain management in pediatric patients: A single-arm feasibility study. *Alternative and Complementary Therapies*, *21*(6), 255–260.

Johnson, C. J., Heckman, T. G., Hansen, N. B., Kochman, A., & Sikkema, K. J. (2009). Adherence to antiretroviral medication in older adults living with HIV/AIDS: A comparison of alternative models. *AIDS Care*, *21*(5), 541–551. http://doi.org/10.1080/09540120802385611

Johnson, E. J., & Goldstein, D. G. (2003). Do defaults save lives? *Science*, *302*, 1338–1339.

Johnson, J. R., Crespin, D. J., Griffin, K. H., Finch, M. D., & Dusek, J. A. (2014). Effects of integrative medicine on pain and anxiety among oncology inpatients. *JNCI Monographs*, *2014*(50), 330–337. https://doi.org/10.1093/jncimonographs/lgu030

Johnson, K. W., Anderson, N. B., Bastida, E., Kramer, B., Williams, D., & Wong, M. (1995). Panel II: Macrosocial and environmental influences on minority health. *Health Psychology*, *14*(7), 601–612.

Johnson, L. M., Zautra, A. J., & Davis, M. C. (2006). The role of illness uncertainty on coping with fibromyalgia symptoms. *Health Psychology*, *25*(6), 696–703. https://doi.org/10.1037/0278-6133.25.6.696

Johnson, M. O., Elliott, T. R., Neilands, T. B., Morin, S. F., & Chesney, M. A. (2006). A social problem-solving model of adherence to HIV medications. *Health Psychology*, *25*(3), 355–363. http://doi.org/10.1037/0278-6133.25.3.355

Johnson, S. B., & Millstein, S. G. (2003). Prevention opportunities in health care settings. *American Psychologist*, *58*(6–7), 475–481.

Johnston, M., & Vögele, C. (1993). Benefits of psychological preparation for surgery: A meta-analysis. *Annals of Behavioral Medicine*, *15*, 245–245.

Jones, A., Cremin, I., Abdullah, F., Idoko, J., Cherutich, P., Kilonzo, N., . . . Schwartlander, B. (2014). Transformation of HIV from pandemic to low-endemic levels: A public health approach to combination prevention. *Lancet*, *384*(9939), 272–279.

Jones, C. M., Logan, J., Gladden, R. M., & Bohm, M. K. (2015). Vital signs: Demographic and substance use trends among heroin users-United States, 2002-2013. *Morbidity and Mortality Weekly Report, 64*(26), 719–725.

Jones, J. L., & Leary, M. R. (1994). Effects of appearance-based admonitions against sun exposure on tanning intentions in young adults. *Health Psychology, 13*(1), 86–90.

Jorgensen, R. S., Johnson, B. T., Kolodziej, M. E., & Schreer, G. E. (1996). Elevated blood pressure and personality: A meta-analytic review. *Psychological Bulletin, 120*(2), 293–320.

Joshi, P., Islam, S., Pais, P., Reddy, S., Dorairaj, P., Kazmi, K., . . . Yusuf, S. (2007). Risk factors for early myocardial infarction in South Asians compared with individuals in other countries. *Journal of the American Medical Association, 297*(3), 286–294. doi:10.1001/jama.297.3.286

Judge, T. A., Ilies, R., & Zhang, Z. (2012). Genetic influences on core self-evaluations, job satisfaction, and work stress: A behavioral genetics mediated model. *Organizational Behavior and Human Decision Processes, 117*(1), 208–220. doi:10.1016/j.obhdp.2011.08.005

Julliard, K., Vivar, J., Delgado, C., Cruz, E., Kabak, J., & Sabers, H. (2008). What Latina patients don't tell their doctors: A qualitative study. *The Annals of Family Medicine, 6*(6), 543–549.

Juster, R., Smith, N., Ouellet, E., Sindi, S., & Lupien, S. (2013). Sexual orientation and disclosure in relation to psychiatric symptoms, diurnal cortisol, and allostatic load. *Psychosomatic Medicine, 75*(2), 103–116.

Juth, V., Smyth, J. M., Carey, M. P., & Lepore, S. J. (2015). Social constraints are associated with negative psychological and physical adjustment in bereavement. *Applied Psychology: Health and Well-Being, 7*(2), 129–148. https://doi.org/10.1111/aphw.12041

Kabat-Zinn, J. (2003). Mindfulness-based interventions in context: Past, present, and future. *Clinical Psychology: Science and Practice, 10*(2), 144–156. https://doi.org/10.1093/clipsy.bpg016

Kabat-Zinn, J., Lipworth, L., & Burney, R. (1985). The clinical use of mindfulness meditation for the self-regulation of chronic pain. *Journal of Behavioral Medicine, 8,* 163–190.

Kadden, R. M., Cooney, N. L., Getter, H., & Litt, M. D. (1989). Matching alcoholics to coping skills or interactional therapies: Posttreatment results. *Journal of Consulting and Clinical Psychology, 57*(6), 698–704.

Kakkar, A. K., & Dahiya, N. (2015). Drug treatment of obesity: Current status and future prospects. *European Journal of Internal Medicine, 26*(2), 89–94.

Kalesan, B., Mobily, M. E., Keiser, O., Fagan, J. A., & Galea, S. (2016). Firearm legislation and firearm mortality in the USA: A cross-sectional, state-level study. *Lancet, 387*(10030), 1847–1855.

Kalichman, S. C., Carey, M. P., & Johnson, B. T. (1996). Prevention of sexually transmitted HIV infection: A meta-analytic review of the behavioral outcome literature. *Annals of Behavioral Medicine, 18*(1), 6–15.

Kalichman, S. C., & Coley, B. (1995). Context framing to enhance HIV-antibody-testing messages targeted to African American women. *Health Psychology, 14*(3), 247–254.

Kalichman, S. C., Heckman, T., Kochman, A., Sikkema, K., & Bergholte, J. (2000). Depression and thoughts of suicide among middle-aged and older persons living with HIV-AIDS. *Psychiatric Services, 51*(7), 903–907.

Kalichman, S. C., Kelly, J. A., Hunter, T. L., Murphy, D. A., & Tyler, R. (1993). Culturally tailored HIV-AIDS risk-reduction messages targeted to African-American urban women: Impact on risk sensitization and risk reduction. *Journal of Consulting and Clinical Psychology, 61,* 291–295.

Kalichman, S. C., & Nachimson, D. (1999). Self-efficacy and disclosure of HIV-positive serostatus to sex partners. *Health Psychology, 18*(3), 281–287. doi:10.1037/0278-6133.18.3.281

Kallmes, D. F., Comstock, B. A., Heagerty, P. J., Turner, J. A., Wilson, D. J., Diamond, T. H., . . . Jarvik, J. G. (2009). A randomized trial of vertebroplasty for osteoporotic spinal fractures. *New England Journal of Medicine, 361*(6), 569–579. https://doi.org/10.1056/NEJMoa0900563

Kamarck, T. W., & Lichtenstein, E. (1985). Current trends in clinic-based smoking control. *Annals of Behavioral Medicine, 7*(2), 19–23. doi:10.1207/s15324796abm0702_4

Kamarck, T. W., Manuck, S. B., & Jennings, J. R. (1990). Social support reduces cardiovascular reactivity to psychological challenge: A laboratory model. *Psychosomatic Medicine, 52*(1), 42–58.

Kamarck, T. W., Muldoon, M. F., Shiffman, S. S., & Sutton-Tyrrell, K. (2007). Experiences of demand and control during daily life are predictors of carotid atherosclerotic progression among healthy men. *Health Psychology, 26*(3), 324–332.

Kamarck, T. W., Muldoon, M. F., Shiffman, S., Sutton-Tyrrell, K., Gwaltney, C., & Janicki, D. L. (2004). Experiences of demand and control in daily life as correlates of subclinical carotid atherosclerosis in a healthy older sample. *Health Psychology, 23*(1), 24–32.

Kane, R. L., Wales, J., Bernstein, L., Leibowitz, A., & Kaplan, S. (1984). A randomised controlled trial of hospice care. *Lancet, 1*(8382), 890–894.

Kang, C. D., Tsang, P. P., Li, W. T., Wang, H. H., Liu, K. Q., Griffiths, S. M., & Wong, M. C. (2015). Determinants of medication adherence and blood pressure control among hypertensive patients in Hong Kong:

A cross-sectional study. *International Journal of Cardiology, 182,* 250–257. doi:10.1016/j.ijcard.2014.12.064

Kangas, M., Henry, J. L., & Bryant, R. A. (2005). The course of psychological disorders in the 1st year after cancer diagnosis. *Journal of Consulting and Clinical Psychology, 73*(4), 763–768.

Kaniasty, K., & Norris, F. H. (1993). A test of the social support deterioration model in the context of natural disaster. *Journal of Personality and Social Psychology, 64*(3), 395–408.

Kaniasty, K., & Norris, F. H. (1995). Mobilization and deterioration of social support following natural disasters. *Current Directions in Psychological Science, 4*(3), 94–98.

Kann, L., McManus, T., Harris, W. A., Shanklin, S. L., Flint, K. H., Hawkins, W. A., . . . Zaza, S. (2016). Youth risk behavior surveillance — United States, 2015. *Morbidity and Mortality Weekly Report: Surveillance Summaries, 65*(No. SS-6), 1–174.

Kanner, A. D., Coyne, J. C., Schaefer, C., & Lazarus, R. S. (1981). Comparison of two modes of stress measurement: Daily hassles and uplifts versus major life events. *Journal of Behavioral Medicine, 4*(1), 1–39.

Kaplan, G. A., & Keil, J. E. (1993). Socioeconomic factors and cardiovascular disease: A review of the literature. *Circulation, 88*(4), 1973–1998.

Kaplan, G. A., Salonen, J. T., Cohen, R. D., Brand, R. J., Syme, S. L., & Puska, P. (1988). Social connections and mortality from all causes and from cardiovascular disease: Prospective evidence from eastern Finland. *American Journal of Epidemiology, 128*(2), 370–380.

Kaplan, R. M. (1989). Health outcome models for policy analysis. *Health Psychology, 8*(6), 723–735.

Kaplan, R. M. (1991). Health-related quality of life in patient decision making. *Journal of Social Issues, 47*(4), 69–90.

Kaplan, R. M. (2000). Two pathways to prevention. *American Psychologist, 55*(4), 382–396.

Kaplan, R. M., & Bush, J. W. (1982). Health-related quality of life measurement for evaluation research and policy analysis. *Health Psychology, 1*(1), 61–80.

Kaplan, R. M., & Groessl, E. J. (2002). Applications of cost-effectiveness methodologies in behavioral medicine. *Journal of Consulting and Clinical Psychology, 70*(3), 482–493.

Kaplan, R. M., Orleans, C. T., Perkins, K. A., & Pierce, J. P. (1995). Marshaling the evidence for greater regulation and control of tobacco products: A call for action. *Annals of Behavioral Medicine, 17*(1), 3–14.

Kaplan, S. H., Greenfield, S., Gandek, B., Rogers, W. H., & Ware, J. E., Jr. (1996). Characteristics of physicans with participatory decision-making styles. *Annals of Internal Medicine, 124,* 497–504.

Karoly, P., & Ruehlman, L. S. (1996). Motivational implications of pain: Chronicity, psychological distress, and work goal construal in a national sample of adults. *Health Psychology, 15,* 383–390.

Kasat, V., Gupta, A., Ladda, R., Kathariya, M., Saluja, H., & Farooqui, A.-A. (2014). Transcutaneous electric nerve stimulation (TENS) in dentistry-A review. *Journal of Clinical and Experimental Dentistry, 6*(5), e562–e568. https://doi.org/10.4317/jced.51586

Kask, J., Ekselius, L., Brandt, L., Kollia, N., Ekbom, A., & Papadopoulos, F. C. (2016). Mortality in women with anorexia nervosa: The role of comorbid psychiatric disorders. *Psychosomatic Medicine, 78*(8), 910–919.

Kasl, S. V., & Cobb, S. (1966a). Health behavior, illness behavior and sick role behavior: I. Health and illness behavior. *Archives of Environmental Health: An International Journal, 12*(2), 246–266.

Kasl, S. V., & Cobb, S. (1966b). Health behavior, illness behavior, and sick-role behavior: II. Sick-role behavior. *Archives of Environmental Health: An International Journal, 12*(4), 531–541.

Kastenbaum, R. (1999). Dying and bereavement. In J. C. Cavanaugh & S. K. Whitbourne (Eds.), *Gerontology: An interdisciplinary perspective* (pp. 155–185). New York, NY: Oxford University Press.

Kastenbaum, R. (2000). *The psychology of death* (3rd ed.). New York, NY: Springer.

Katan, M. B., Grundy, S. M., & Willett, W. C. (1997). Should a low-fat, high-carbohydrate diet be recommended for everyone? Beyond low-fat diets. *New England Journal of Medicine, 337*(8), 563–566, discussion 566–567.

Kato, K., Sullivan, P. F., Evengård, B., & Pedersen, N. L. (2006). Chronic widespread pain and its comorbidities: A population-based study. *Archives of Internal Medicine, 166*(15), 1649–1654. https://doi.org/10.1001/archinte.166.15.1649

Katon, W. J., Lin, E. H., Von Korff, M., Ciechanowski, P., Ludman, E. J., Young, B., . . . McCulloch, D. (2010). Collaborative care for patients with depression and chronic illnesses. *New England Journal of Medicine, 363*(27), 2611–2620.

Katritsis, D. G., & Ioannidis, J. P. (2005). Percutaneous coronary intervention versus conservative therapy in nonacute coronary artery disease. *Circulation, 111*(22), 2906–2912.

Kauffman, N. A., Herman, C. P., & Polivy, J. (1995). Hunger-induced finickiness in humans. *Appetite, 24*(3), 203–218.

Kaye, W. H. (1997). Anorexia nervosa, obessional behavior, and serotonin. *Psychopharmacology Bulletin, 33*(3), 335–344.

Kearney, D. J., Simpson, T. L., Malte, C. A., Felleman, B., Martinez, M. E., & Hunt, S. C. (2016). Mindfulness-based stress reduction in addition to usual care is associated with improvements in pain, fatigue, and cognitive failures among veterans with gulf war illness. *American Journal of Medicine, 129*(2), 204–214.

Kearney, M. S., & Levine, P. B. (2015). Media influences on social outcomes: The impact of MTV's 16 and pregnant on teen childbearing. *American Economic Review, 105*(12), 3597–3632.

Keefe, F. J., & Block, A. R. (1982). Development of an observation method for assessing pain behavior in chronic low back pain patients. *Behavior Therapy, 13*, 363–375.

Keefe, F. J., Brown, G. K., Wallston, K. A., & Caldwell, D. S. (1989). Coping with rheumatoid arthritis pain: Catastrophizing as a maladaptive strategy. *Pain, 37*, 51–56.

Keefe, F. J., Caldwell, D. S., Queen, K. T., Gil, K. M., Martinez, S., Crissor, J. E., . . . Nunley, J. (1987). Pain coping strategies in osteoarthritis patients. *Journal of Consulting and Clinical Psychology, 55*, 208–212.

Keefe, F. J., Hauck, E. R., Egert, J., Rimer, B., & Kornguth, P. (1994). Mammography pain and discomfort: A cognitive-behavioral perspective. *Pain, 56*, 247–260.

Keesee, N. J., Currier, J. M., & Neimeyer, R. A. (2008). Predictors of grief following the death of one's child: The contribution of finding meaning. *Journal of Clinical Psychology, 64*(10), 1145–1163. https://doi.org/10.1002/jclp.20502

Keesey, R. E. (1995). A set-point model of body weight regulation. In K. D. Brownell & C. G. Fairburn (Eds.), *Eating disorders and obesity: A comprehensive handbook* (pp. 46–51). New York, NY: Guilford.

Keesey, R. E., & Powley, T. L. (1975). Hypothalamic regulation of body weight: Experiments suggest that the lateral and ventromedial hypothalamus jointly determine the regulation level or "set point" for body fat. *American Scientist, 63*(5), 558–565.

Kellerman, A. L., Rivara, F. P., & Rushford, N. B. (1992). Suicide in the home in relationship to gun ownership. *New England Journal of Medicine, 327*, 467–472.

Kellerman, Q. D., Christensen, A. J., Baldwin, A. S., & Lawton, W. J. (2010). Association between depressive symptoms and mortality risk in chronic kidney disease. *Health Psychology, 29*(6), 594–600. **doi:10.1037/a0021235**

Kellermann, A. L., Rivara, F. P., Rushforth, N. B., Banton, J. G., Reay, D. T., Francisco, J. T., . . . Somes, G. (1993). Gun ownership as a risk factor for homicide in the home. *New England Journal of Medicine, 329*(15), 1084–1091.

Kelly, K. E., & Houston, B. K. (1985). Type A behavior in employed women: Relation to work, marital, and leisure variables, social support, stress, tension, and health. *Journal of Personality and Social Psychology, 48*(4), 1067–1079.

Kelly, P. J., Leung, J., Deane, F. P., & Lyons, G. C. B. (2016). Predicting client attendance at further treatment following drug and alcohol detoxification: Theory of Planned Behaviour and implementation intentions. *Drug and Alcohol Review, 35*, 678–685.

Kelly, S. J., & Ismail, M. (2015). Stress and type 2 diabetes: A review of how stress contributes to the development of type 2 diabetes. *Annual Review of Public Health, 36*, 441–462.

Kelsey, M. M., Zaepfel, A., Bjornstad, P., & Nadeau, K. J. (2014). Age related consequences of childhood obesity. *Gerontology, 60*(3), 222–228.

Kemeny, M. E. (1994). Stressful events, psychological responses, and progression of HIV infection. In R. Glaser & J. Kiecolt-Glaser (Eds.), *Handbook of human stress and immunity* (pp. 245–266). New York, NY: Academic Press.

Kemeny, M. E., Weiner, H., Duran, R., Taylor, S. E., Visscher, B., & Fahey, J. L. (1995). Immune system changes following the death of a partner in HIV positive gay men. *Psychosomatic Medicine, 57*, 549–554.

Kemeny, M. E., Weiner, H., Taylor, S. E., Schneider, S., Visscher, B., & Fahey, J. L. (1994). Repeated bereavement, depressed mood, and immune parameters in HIV seropositive and seronegative gay men. *Health Psychology, 13*(1), 14–24.

Kendler, K. S., MacLean, C., Neale, M., Kessler, R., Heath, A., & Eaves, L. (1991). The genetic epidemiology of bulimia nervosa. *The American Journal of Psychiatry, 148*(12), 1627–1637.

Kendzor, D. E., Businelle, M. S., Poonawalla, I. B., Cuate, E. L., Kesh, A., Rios, D. M., . . . Balis, D. S. (2015). Financial incentives for abstinence among socioeconomically disadvantaged individuals in smoking cessation treatment. *American Journal of Public Health, 105*(6), 1198–1205.

Kennedy, S., Kiecolt-Glaser, J. K., & Glaser, R. G. (1990). Social support, stress and the immune system. In I. G. Sarason, B. Sarason, & G. Pierce (Eds.), *Social support: An interactional view* (pp. 253–266). New York, NY: Wiley.

Kennell, J., Klaus, M., McGrath, S., Robertson, S., & Hinkley, C. (1991). Continuous emotional support during labor in a US hospital. A randomized controlled trial. *Journal of the American Medical Association, 265*(17), 2197–2201. **doi:10.1001/jama.265.17.2197**

Kent, G. (1985). Memory of dental pain. *Pain, 21*, 187–194.

Kern, M. L., & Friedman, H. S. (2008). Do conscientious individuals live longer? A quantitative review. *Health Psychology, 27*(5), 505–512.

Kerns, R. D., Turk, D. C., & Rudy, T. E. (1985). The West Haven-Yale Multidimensional Pain Inventory. *Pain, 23*, 345–356.

Kerrison, R. S., Shukla, H., Cunningham, D., Oyebode, O., & Friedman, E. (2015). Text-message reminders increase uptake of routine breast screening appointments: A randomised controlled trial in a hard-to-reach population. *British Journal of Cancer, 112*(6), 1005–1010.

Kershaw, K. N., Mezuk, B., Abdou, C. M., Rafferty, J. A., & Jackson, J. S. (2010).

Socioeconomic position, health behaviors, and C-reactive protein: A moderated-mediation analysis. *Health Psychology*, *29*(3), 307–316. **doi:10.1037/a0019286**

Kessels, L. T., Ruiter, R. A., & Jansma, B. M. (2010). Increased attention but more efficient disengagement: Neuroscientific evidence for defensive processing of threatening health information. *Health Psychology*, *29*(4), 346–354. **doi:10.1037/a0019372**

Kessler, R. C., Crum, R. M., Warner, L. A., Nelson, C. B., Schulenberg, J., & Anthony, J. C. (1997). Lifetime co-occurrence of DSM-III-R alcohol abuse and dependence with other psychiatric disorders in the National Comorbidity Survey. *Archives of General Psychiatry*, *54*(4), 313–321.

Kharsany, A. B., & Karim, Q. A. (2016). HIV infection and AIDS in Sub-Saharan Africa: Current status, challenges and opportunities. *Open AIDS Journal*, *10*, 34–48. **doi:10.2174/1874613601610010034**

Khoury, B., Sharma, M., Rush, S. E., & Fournier, C. (2015). Mindfulness-based stress reduction for healthy individuals: A meta-analysis. *Journal of Psychosomatic Research*, *78*(6), 519–528.

Kiecolt-Glaser, J. K., Dura, J. R., Speicher, C. E., Trask, O. J., & Glaser, R. (1991). Spousal caregivers of dementia victims: Longitudinal changes in immunity and health. *Psychosomatic Medicine*, *53*(4), 345–362.

Kiecolt-Glaser, J. K., Fisher, L., Ogrocki, P., Stout, J. C., Speicher, C. E., & Glaser, R. (1987). Marital quality, marital disruption, and immune function. *Psychosomatic Medicine*, *49*, 31–34.

Kiecolt-Glaser, J. K., & Glaser, R. (1986). Psychological influences on immunity. *Psychosomatics*, *27*, 621–624.

Kiecolt-Glaser, J. K., & Glaser, R. (1989). Psychoneuroimmunology: Past, present, and future. *Health Psychology*, *8*, 677–682.

Kiecolt-Glaser, J. K., & Glaser, R. (2002). Depression and immune function: Central pathways to morbidity and mortality. *Journal of Psychosomatic Research*, *53*(4), 873–876.

Kiecolt-Glaser, J. K., Glaser, R., Shuttleworth, E. C., Dyer, C. S., Ogrocki, P., & Speicher, C. E. (1987). Chronic stress and immunity in family caregivers of Alzheimer's disease victims. *Psychosomatic Medicine*, *49*(5), 523–535.

Kiecolt-Glaser, J. K., Kennedy, S., Malkoff, S., Fisher, L., Speicher, C. E., & Glaser, R. (1988). Marital discord and immunity in males. *Psychosomatic Medicine*, *50*(3), 213–229.

Kiecolt-Glaser, J. K., McGuire, L., Robles, T. F., & Glaser, R. (2002). Psychoneuroimmunology: Psychological influences on immune function and health. *Journal of Consulting and Clinical Psychology*, *70*(3), 537–547.

Kiecolt-Glaser, J. K., & Williams, D. A. (1987). Self-blame, compliance, and distress among burn patients. *Journal of Personality and Social Psychology*, *53*(1), 187–193.

Kiefe, C. I., McKay, S. V., Halevy, A., & Brody, B. A. (1994). Is cost a barrier to screening mammography for low-income women receiving Medicare benefits? A randomized trial. *Archives of Internal Medicine*, *154*(11), 1217–1224.

Kiene, S. M., Barta, W. D., Zelenski, J. M., & Cothran, D. L. (2005). Why are you bringing up condoms now? The effect of message content on framing effects of condom use messages. *Health Psychology*, *24*(3), 321–326.

Kilbey, M. M., Downey, K., & Breslau, N. (1998). Predicting the emergence and persistence of alcohol dependence in young adults: The role of expectancy and other risk factors. *Experimental and Clinical Psychopharmacology*, *6*(2), 149–156.

Killen, J. D., Taylor, C. B., Hammer, L. D., Litt, I., Wilson, D. M., Rich, T., . . . Varady, A. (1993). An attempt to modify unhealthful eating attitudes and weight regulation practices of young adolescent girls. *International Journal of Eating Disorders*, *13*(4), 369–384.

Kilmer, B., Nicosia, N., Heaton, P., & Midgette, G. (2013). Efficacy of frequent monitoring with swift, certain, and modest sanctions for violations: Insights from South Dakota's 24/7 Sobriety Project. *American Journal of Public Health*, *103*(1), e37–e43.

Kim, E. S., Hagan, K. A., Grodstein, F., DeMeo, D. L., De Vivo, I., & Kubzansky, L. D. (2017). Optimism and cause-specific mortality: A prospective cohort study. *American Journal of Epidemiology*, *185*(1), 21–29. **https://doi.org/10.1093/aje/kww182**

Kim, E. S., Hawes, A. M., & Smith, J. (2014). Perceived neighborhood social cohesion and myocardial infarction. *Journal of Epidemiology and Community Health*, *68*(11), 1020–1026.

Kim, E. S., Park, N., & Peterson, C. (2011). Dispositional optimism protects older adults from stroke. *Stroke*, *42*(10), 2855–2859.

Kim, S. H. (2009). The influence of finding meaning and worldview of accepting death on anger among bereaved older spouses. *Aging & Mental Health*, *13*(1), 38–45. **https://doi.org/10.1080/13607860802154457**

Kim, S. H., De Vries, R. G., & Peteet, J. R. (2016). Euthanasia and assisted suicide of patients with psychiatric disorders in the Netherlands 2011 to 2014. *JAMA Psychiatry*, *73*(4), 362–368. **https://doi.org/10.1001/jamapsychiatry.2015.2887**

Kimzey, S. L. (1975). The effects of extended spaceflight on hematologic and immunologic systems. *Journal of the American Medical Women's Association*, *30*(5), 218–232.

King, K. A., Strunk, C. M., & Sorter, M. T. (2011). Preliminary effectiveness of surviving the Teens® suicide prevention and depression awareness program on adolescents' suicidality and self-efficacy in performing help-seeking behaviors. *Journal of School Health*, *81*(9), 581–590.

King, K. B., & Reis, H. T. (2012). Marriage and long-term survival after coronary artery bypass grafting. *Health Psychology, 31*(1), 55–62. **doi:10.1037/a0025061**

King, K. B., Reis, H. T., Porter, L. A., & Norsen, L. H. (1993). Social support and long-term recovery from coronary artery surgery: Effects on patients and spouses. *Health Psychology, 12*(1), 56–63.

Kirkman, M. S., Rowan-Martin, M. T., Levin, R., Fonseca, V. A., Schmittdiel, J. A., Herman, W. H., & Aubert, R. E. (2015). Determinants of adherence to diabetes medications: Findings from a large pharmacy claims database. *Diabetes Care, 38*(4), 604–609.

Kirsch, I., & Sapirstein, G. (1999). Listening to Prozac but hearing placebo: A meta-analysis of antidepressant medications. In I. Kirsch (Ed.), *How expectancies shape experience* (pp. 303–320). Washington, DC: American Psychological Asssociation.

Kirscht, J. P. (1988). The health belief model and predictions of health actions. In D. S. Gochman (Ed.), *Health behavior: Emerging research perspectives* (pp. 27–42). New York, NY: Plenum.

Kirscht, J. P., Kirscht, J. L., & Rosenstock, I. M. (1981). A test of interventions to increase adherence to hypertensive medical regimens. *Health Education Quarterly, 8*(3), 261–272.

Kirscht, J. P., & Rosenstock, I. M. (1979). Patients' problems in following recommendations of health experts. In G. C. Stone, F. Cohen, & N. E. Adler (Eds.), *Health psychology: A handbook* (pp. 198–215). San Francisco, CA: Jossey-Bass.

Kitayama, S., Park, J., Boylan, J. M., Miyamoto, Y., Levine, C. S., Markus, H. R., . . . Ryff, C. D. (2015). Expression of anger and ill health in two cultures: An examination of inflammation and cardiovascular risk. *Psychological Science, 26*(2), 211–220.

Kitzmann, K. M., Dalton, W. T., Stanley, C. M., Beech, B. M., Reeves, T. P., Buscemi, J., . . . Midgett, E. L. (2010). Lifestyle interventions for youth who are overweight: A meta-analytic review. *Health Psychology, 29*(1), 91–101.

Kitzman-Ulrich, H., Wilson, D. K., Van Horn, M. L., & Lawman, H. G. (2010). Relationship of body mass index and psychosocial factors on physical activity in underserved adolescent boys and girls. *Health Psychology, 29*(5), 506–513.

Kivimaki, M., Leino-Arjas, P., Luukkonen, R., Riihimaki, H., Vahtera, J., & Kirjonen, J. (2002). Work stress and risk of cardiovascular mortality: Prospective cohort study of industrial employees. *British Medical Journal, 325*(7369), 857–861.

Kivlahan, D. R., Marlatt, G. A., Fromme, K., Coppel, D. B., & Williams, E. (1990). Secondary prevention with college drinkers: Evaluation of an alcohol skills training program. *Journal of Consulting and Clinical Psychology, 58*(6), 805–810.

Klag, M. J., Ford, D. E., Mead, L. A., He, J., Whelton, P. K., Liang, K. Y., & Levine, D. M. (1993). Serum cholesterol in young men and subsequent cardiovascular disease. *New England Journal of Medicine, 328*(5), 313–318.

Klapow, J., Slater, M., Patterson, T., & Atkinson, J. (1995). Psychological factors discriminate multidimensional clinical groups of chronic low back-pain patients. *Pain, 62*(3), 349–355.

Klass, P. (1987). *A not entirely benign procedure: Four years as a medical student.* New York, NY: Putnam.

Klassen, T. P., MacKay, J. M., Moher, D., Walker, A., & Jones, A. L. (2000). Community-based injury prevention interventions. *The Future of Children, 10*(1), 83–110.

Klatsky, A. L., Friedman, G. D., & Siegelaub, A. B. (1981). Alcohol and mortality: A ten-year Kaiser-Permanente experience. *Annals of Internal Medicine, 95*(2), 139–145.

Klevens, J., Luo, F., Xu, L., Peterson, C., & Latzman, N. E. (2016). Paid family leave's effect on hospital admissions for pediatric abusive head trauma. *Injury Prevention, 22*(6), 442–445.

Klingspon, K. L., Holland, J. M., Neimeyer, R. A., & Lichtenthal, W. G. (2015). Unfinished business in bereavement. *Death Studies, 39*(7), 387–398. **https://doi.org/10.1080/07481187.2015.1029143**

Klohn, L. S., & Rogers, R. W. (1991). Dimensions of the severity of a health threat: The persuasive effects of visibility, time of onset, and rate of onset on young women's intentions to prevent osteoporosis. *Health Psychology, 10*(5), 323–329.

Klonoff, E. A., & Landrine, H. (1993). Cognitive representations of bodily parts and products: Implications for health behavior. *Journal of Behavioral Medicine, 16*(5), 497–508.

Knott, S., Woodward, D., Hoefkens, A., & Limbert, C. (2015). Cognitive behaviour therapy for bulimia nervosa and eating disorders not otherwise specified: Translation from randomized controlled trial to a clinical setting. *Behavioural and Cognitive Psychotherapy, 43*(6), 641–654.

Knowler, W. C., Barrett-Conner, E., Fowler, S. E., Hammon, R. F., Lachin, J. M., Walker, E. A., & Nathan, D. M. (2002). Reduction in the incidence of type 2 diabetes with lifestyle intervention or metformin. *New England Journal of Medicine, 346*(6), 393–403.

Knowles, E. D., Wearing, J. R., & Campos, B. (2011). Culture and the health benefits of expressive writing. *Social Psychological and Personality Science, 2*(4), 408–415.

Knowles, J. H. (1977). The responsibility of the individual. In J. H. Knowles (Ed.), *Doing better and feeling worse: Health in the United States* (pp. 57–80). New York, NY: Norton.

Knutson, K. L. (2012). Does inadequate sleep play a role in vulnerability to obesity? *American Journal of Human Biology, 24*(3), 361–371.

Kobasa, S. C., Maddi, S. R., & Kahn, S. (1982). Hardiness and health: A prospective study. *Journal of Personality and Social Psychology*, *42*(1), 168–177.

Koçak, N. D., Eren, A., Boğa, S., Aktürk, Ü. A., Öztürk, Ü. A., Arınç, S., & Şengül, A. (2015). Relapse rate and factors related to relapse in a 1-year follow-up of subjects participating in a smoking cessation program. *Respiratory Care*, *60*(12), 1796–1803.

Kochanek, K. D., Murphy, S. L., Xu, J., & Tejada-Vera, B. (2016). Deaths: Final data for 2014. *National Vital Statistics Reports*, *65*(4), 1–122.

Koenig, H. G., McCullough, M. E., & Larson, D. B. (2001). *Religion and health*. New York, NY: Oxford University Press.

Koenig, L. B., & Vaillant, G. E. (2009). A prospective study of church attendance and health over the lifespan. *Health Psychology*, *28*(1), 117–124.

Koetting O'Byrne, K., Peterson, L., & Saldana, L. (1997). Survey of pediatric hospitals' preparation programs: Evidence of the impact of health psychology research. *Health Psychology*, *16*(2), 147–154.

Kog, E., & Vandereycken, W. (1985). Family characteristics of anorexia nervosa and bulimia: A review of the research literature. *Clinical Psychology Review*, *5*(2), 159–180.

Koh, H. K., Bak, S. M., Geller, A. C., Mangione, T. W., Hingson, R. W., Levenson, S. M., . . . Howland, J. (1997). Sunbathing habits and sunscreen use among White adults: Results of a national survey. *American Journal of Public Health*, *87*(7), 1214–1217.

Kohen, J. A. (1983). Old but not alone: Informal social supports among the elderly by marital status and sex. *Gerontologist*, *23*(1), 57–63.

Kohn, P. M., Lafreniere, K., & Gurevich, M. (1991). Hassles, health and personality. *Journal of Personality and Social Psychology*, *61*(3), 478–483.

Kokkinos, P. F., Narayan, P., Colleran, J. A., Pittaras, A., Notargiacomo, A., Reda, D., & Papademetriou, V. (1995). Effects of regular exercise on blood pressure and left ventricular hypertrophy in African-American men with severe hypertension. *New England Journal of Medicine*, *333*(22), 1462–1467.

Kole-Snijders, A. M. J., Vlaeyen, J. W., Goossens, M. E., Rutten-van Molken, M. P., Heuts, P. H., van Breukelen, G., & van Eek, H. (1999). Chronic low-back pain: What does cognitive coping skills training add to operant behavioral treatment? Results of a randomized clinical trial. *Journal of Consulting and Clinical Psychology*, *67*(6), 931–944.

Kondo, M. C., Keene, D., Hohl, B. C., MacDonald, J. M., & Branas, C. C. (2015). A difference-in-differences study of the effects of a new abandoned building remediation strategy on safety. *PLOS ONE*, *10*(7), e0129582.

Kop, W. J., Gottdiener, J. S., & Krantz, D. S. (2001). Stress and silent ischemia. In A. Baum, T. A. Revenson, & J. E. Singer (Eds.), *Handbook of health psychology* (pp. 669–682). Mahwah, NJ: Erlbaum.

Korotkov, D. (2008). Does personality moderate the relationship between stress and health behavior? Expanding the nomological network of the five-factor model. *Journal of Research in Personality*, *42*(6), 1418–1426.

Korsch, B. M., Gozzi, E. K., & Francis, V. (1968). Gaps in doctor–patient communications: 1. Doctor–patient interaction and patient satisfaction. *Paediatrics*, *42*, 855–871.

Kosenko, K. A., Binder, A. R., & Hurley, R. (2016). Celebrity influence and identification: A test of the Angelina effect. *Journal of Health Communication*, *21*(3), 318–326.

Kosinski, M., Stillwell, D., & Graepel, T. (2013). Private traits and attributes are predictable from digital records of human behavior. *Proceedings of the National Academy of Sciences of the United States of America*, *110*(15), 5802–5805. **doi:10.1073/pnas.1218772110**

Kotov, R., Bromet, E., Schechter, C., Broihier, J., Feder, A., Friedman-Jimenez, G., . . . Luft, B. (2015). Posttraumatic stress disorder and the risk of respiratory problems in World Trade Center responders: Longitudinal test of a pathway. *Psychosomatic Medicine*, *77*(4), 438–448.

Kozhimannil, K. B., Pereira, M. A., & Harlow, B. L. (2009). Association between diabetes and perinatal depression among low-income mothers. *Journal of the American Medical Association*, *301*(8), 842–847.

Kozuki, N., Lee, A. C., Silveira, M. F., Victora, C. G., Adair, L., Humphrey, J., . . . Katz, J. (2013). The associations of birth intervals with small-for-gestational-age, preterm, and neonatal and infant mortality: A meta-analysis. *BMC Public Health*, *13*(3), S3.

Krahn, M. D., Mahoney, J. E., Eckman, M. H., Trachtenberg, J., Pauker, S. G., & Detsky, A. S. (1994). Screening for prostate cancer: A decision analytic view. *Journal of the American Medical Association*, *272*(10), 773–780.

Kral, J. G. (1992). Overview of surgical techniques for treating obesity. *The American Journal of Clinical Nutrition*, *55*(2), 552–555.

Kranjac, A. W., Kimbro, R. T., Denney, J. T., Osiecki, K. M., Moffett, B. S., & Lopez, K. N. (2017). Comprehensive neighborhood portraits and child asthma disparities. *Maternal and Child Health Journal*, *21*(7), 1552–1562. **doi:10.1007/s10995-017-2286-z**

Krantz, D. S., Baum, A., & Wideman, M. V. (1980). Assessment of Preferences for self-treatment and information in health care. *Journal of Personality and Social Psychology*, *39*(5), 977–990.

Krauss, M. J., Cavazos-Rehg, P. A., Plunk, A. D., Bierut, L. J., & Grucza, R. A. (2014). Effects of state cigarette excise taxes and smoke-free air policies on state per capita alcohol consumption in the United States, 1980 to 2009. *Alcoholism: Clinical and Experimental Research*, *38*(10), 2630–2638.

Krawczyk, A., Knäuper, B., Gilca, V., Dubé, E., Perez, S., Joyal-Desmarais, K., & Rosberger, Z. (2015). Parents' decision-making about the human papillomavirus vaccine for their daughters: I. Quantitative results. *Human Vaccines & Immunotherapeutics, 11*(2), 322–329.

Krawczyk, A. L., Perez, S., Lau, E., Holcroft, C. A., Amsel, R., Knäuper, B., & Rosberger, Z. (2012). Human papillomavirus vaccination intentions and uptake in college women. *Health Psychology, 31*(5), 685–693. **doi:10.1037/a0027012**

Krebs, C., Lindquist, C., Berzofsky, M., Shook-Sa, B., Peterson, K., Planty, M., . . . Stroop, J. (2016). *Campus climate survey validation study final technical report.* Washington, DC: Bureau of Justice Statistics, U.S. Department of Justice.

Krebs, C. P., Lindquist, C. H., Warner, T. D., Fisher, B. S., & Martin, S. L. (2007). *The Campus Sexual Assault (CSA) Study.* Washington, DC: National Institute of Justice, U.S. Department of Justice.

Kreicbergs, U., Valdimarsdóttir, U., Onelöv, E., Henter, J.-I., & Steineck, G. (2004). Talking about death with children who have severe malignant disease. *New England Journal of Medicine, 351,* 1175–1186. **doi:10.1056/NEJMoa040366**

Kremer, E. F., Block, A., & Gaylor, M. S. (1981). Behavioral approaches to treatment of chronic pain: The inaccuracy of patient self-report measures. *Archives of Physical Medicine and Rehabilitation, 62,* 188–191.

Kreuter, M. W., Bull, F. C., Clark, E. M., & Oswald, D. L. (1999). Understanding how people process health information: A comparison of tailored and non-tailored weight-loss materials. *Health Psychology, 18*(5), 487–494.

Kreuter, M. W., & Holt, C. L. (2001). How do people process health information? Applications in an age of individualized communication. *Current Directions in Psychological Science, 10*(6), 206–209.

Kreuter, M. W., & Skinner, C. S. (2000). Tailoring: What's in a name? *Health Education Research, 15,* 1–3.

Kreuter, M. W., & Strecher, V. J. (1996). Do tailored behavior change messages enhance the effectiveness of health risk appraisal? Results from a randomized trial. *Health Education Research, 11*(1), 97–105.

Kreuter, M. W., Strecher, V. J., & Glassman, B. (1999). One size does not fit all: The case for tailoring print materials. *Annals of Behavioral Medicine, 21*(4), 276–283.

Krieger, N., & Sidney, S. (1996). Racial discrimination and blood pressure: The CARDIA Study of young Black and White adults. *American Journal of Public Health, 86*(10), 1370–1378.

Krieger, N., Sidney, S., & Coakley, E. (1998). Racial discrimination and skin color in the CARDIA study: Implications for public health research. *American Journal of Public Health, 88,* 1308–1313.

Kroenke, C. H., Kwan, M. L., Neugut, A. I., Ergas, I. J., Wright, J. D., Caan, B. J., . . . Kushi, L. H. (2013). Social networks, social support mechanisms, and quality of life after breast cancer diagnosis. *Breast Cancer Research and Treatment, 139*(2), 515–527. **https://doi.org/10.1007/s10549-013-2477-2**

Kroenke, C. H., Michael, Y. L., Poole, E. M., Kwan, M. L., Nechuta, S., Leas, E., . . . Chen, W. Y. (2017). Postdiagnosis social networks and breast cancer mortality in the After Breast Cancer Pooling Project. *Cancer, 123*(7), 1228–1237. **https://doi.org/10.1002/cncr.30440**

Kroenke, C. H., Michael, Y. L., Shu, X.-O., Poole, E. M., Kwan, M. L., Nechuta, S., . . . Chen, W. Y. (2017). Postdiagnosis social networks, and lifestyle and treatment factors in the After Breast Cancer Pooling Project. *Psycho-Oncology, 26*(4), 544–552. **https://doi.org/10.1002/pon.4059**

Kroenke, K., Bair, M. J., Damush, T. M., Wu, J., Hoke, S., Sutherland, J., &

Tu, W. (2009). Optimized antidepressant therapy and pain self-management in primary care patients with depression and musculoskeletal pain: A randomized controlled trial. *Journal of the American Medical Association, 301*(20), 2099–2110. **https://doi.org/10.1001/jama.2009.723**

Krohne, H. W., & Slangen, K. E. (2005). Influence of social support on adaptation to surgery. *Health Psychology, 24*(1), 101–105.

Kroshus, E., Garnett, B., Hawrilenko, M., Baugh, C. M., & Calzo, J. P. (2015). Concussion under-reporting and pressure from coaches, teammates, fans, and parents. *Social Science & Medicine, 134,* 66–75.

Krueger, P. M., Bond, H., Rogers, R. G., & Hummer, R. A. (2004). Neighbourhoods and homicide mortality: An analysis of race/ethnic differences. *Journal of Epidemiology and Community Health, 58*(3), 223–230.

Kruger, D. J., Greenberg, E., Murphy, J. B., DiFazio, L. A., & Youra, K. R. (2014). Local concentration of fast-food outlets is associated with poor nutrition and obesity. *American Journal of Health Promotion, 28*(5), 340–343.

Krupat, E., Rosenkranz, S. L., Yeager, C. M., Barnard, K., Putnam, S. M., & Inui, T. S. (2000). The practice orientations of physicians and patients: The effect of doctor-patient congruence on satisfaction. *Patient Education and Counseling, 39,* 49–59.

Kübler-Ross, E. (1969). *On death and dying.* London, UK: Macmillan.

Kubzansky, L. D., Cole, S. R., Kawachi, I., Vokonas, P., & Sparrow, D. (2006). Shared and unique contributions of anger, anxiety, and depression to coronary heart disease: A prospective study in the normative aging study. *Annals of Behavioral Medicine, 31*(1), 21–29.

Kubzansky, L. D., & Thurston, R. C. (2007). Emotional vitality and incident coronary heart disease: Benefits of healthy psychological functioning.

Archives of General Psychiatry, 64(12), 1393–1401. https://doi.org/10.1001/archpsyc.64.12.1393

Kuhlman, S. T., Walch, S. E., Bauer, K. N., & Glenn, A. D. (2017). Intention to enact and enactment of gatekeeper behaviors for suicide prevention: An application of the theory of planned behavior. *Prevention Science, 18*(6), 704–715. doi:10.1007/s11121-017-0786-0

Kujala, U. M., Kaprio, J., Sarna, S., & Koskenvuo, M. (1998). Relationship of leisure-time physical activity and mortality: The Finnish twin cohort. *Journal of the American Medical Association, 279*(6), 440–444.

Kukihara, H., Yamawaki, N., Uchiyama, K., Arai, S., & Horikawa, E. (2014). Trauma, depression, and resilience of earthquake/tsunami/nuclear disaster survivors of Hirono, Fukushima, Japan. *Psychiatry and Clinical Neurosciences, 68*(7), 524–534. doi:10.1111/pcn.12159

Kulik, J. A., & Mahler, H. I. (1989). Social support and recovery from surgery. *Health Psychology, 8*(2), 221–238.

Kulik, J. A., Mahler, H. I., & Moore, P. J. (1996). Social comparison and affiliation under threat: Effects on recovery from major surgery. *Journal of Personality and Social Psychology, 71*(5), 967–979.

Kumsar, A. N., & Dilbaz, N. (2015). Relationship between craving and ghrelin, adiponectin, and resistin levels in patients with alcoholism. *Alcoholism: Clinical and Experimental Research, 39*(4), 702–709.

Kunda, Z. (1990). The case for motivated reasoning. *Psychological Bulletin, 108*(3), 480–498.

Kung, H.-C., Hoyert, D. L., Xu, J., & Murphy, S. L. (2008). Deaths: Final data for 2005. *National Vital Statistics Report, 56*(10), 1–120.

Kung, W. W. (2016). Culture- and immigration-related stress faced by Chinese American families with a patient having schizophrenia. *Journal of Marital and Family Therapy, 42*(3), 409–422.

Kuntsche, E., van der Vorst, H., & Engels, R. (2009). The earlier the more? Differences in the links between age at first drink and adolescent alcohol use and related problems according to quality of parent–child relationships. *Journal of Studies on Alcohol and Drugs, 70*(3), 346–354.

Kuo, M. (2015). How might contact with nature promote human health? Promising mechanisms and a possible central pathway. *Frontiers in Psychology, 6*, 1093.

Kushlev, K., & Dunn, E. W. (2015). Checking email less frequently reduces stress. *Computers in Human Behavior, 43*, 220–228. http://dx.doi.org/10.1016/j.chb.2014.11.005

Kushner, M. G. (1996). Relationship between alcohol problems and anxiety disorders. *The American Journal of Psychiatry, 153*(1), 139–140.

Lac, A., & Crano, W. D. (2009). Monitoring matters meta-analytic review reveals the reliable linkage of parental monitoring with adolescent marijuana use. *Perspectives on Psychological Science, 4*(6), 578–586.

LaCrosse, M. B. (1975). Nonverbal behaviour and perceived counsellor attractiveness and persuasiveness. *Journal of Counseling Psychology, 22*, 563–566.

Ladwig, K. H., Baumert, J., Marten-Mittag, B., Lukachek, K., Johar, H., Fang, X., . . . KORA Investigators. (2017). Room for depressed and exhausted mood as a risk predictor for all-cause and cardiovascular mortality beyond the contribution of the classical somatic risk factors in men. *Atherosclerosis, 257*, 224–231. doi:10.1016/j.atherosclerosis.2016

Lahey, B. B. (2009). Public health significance of neuroticism. *American Psychologist, 64*(4), 241 256. doi:10.1037/a0015309

Laine, C., & Davidoff, F. (1996). Patient-centered medicine: A professional evolution. *Journal of the American Medical Association, 275*, 152–156.

Lalonde, M. (1974). *A new perspective on the health of Canadians*. Ottawa, ON: Government of Canada.

Lamaze, F. (1970). *Painless childbirth: Psychoprophylactic method*. Chicago, IL: Regnery.

Lamme, S., Dykstra, P. A., & Brose Van Groenou, M. I. (1996). Rebuilding the network: New relationships in widowhood. *Personal Relationships, 3*, 337–349.

Lamont, E. B., & Christakis, N. A. (2001). Prognostic disclosure to patients with cancer near the end of life. *Annals of Internal Medicine, 134*(12), 1096–1105. https://doi.org/10.7326/0003-4819-134-12-200106190-00009

Landrine, H., & Klonoff, E. A. (1994). Cultural diversity in causal attributions for illness: The role of the supernatural. *Journal of Behavioral Medicine, 17*(2), 181–193.

Lang, A. R., & Marlatt, G. A. (1982). Problem drinking: A social learning perspective. In R. J. Gatchel, A. Baum, J. E. Singer, R. J. Gatchel, A. Baum, & J. E. Singer (Eds.), *Handbook of psychology and health, Vol. 1: Clinical psychology and behavioral medicine: Overlapping disciplines* (pp. 121–169). Hillsdale, NJ: Lawrence Erlbaum Associates, Inc.

Langens, T. A., & Schuler, J. (2007). Effects of written emotional expression: The role of positive expectancies. *Health Psychology, 26*, 174–182.

Lannin, D. R., Mathews, H. F., Mitchell, J., Swanson, M. S., Swanson, F. H., & Edwards, M. S. (1998). Influence of socioeconomic and cultural factors on racial differences in late-stage presentation of breast cancer. *Journal of the American Medical Association, 279*(22), 1801–1807.

LaPerriere, A. R., Antoni, M. H., Schneiderman, N., Ironson, G., Klimas, N., Caralis, P., & Fletcher, M. A. (1990). Exercise intervention attenuates emotional distress and natural killer cell decrements following notification of positive serologic status for HIV-1. *Biofeedback and Self-regulation, 15*(3), 229–242.

Larroque, B., Kaminski, M., Dehaene, P., Subtil, D., Delfosse, M. J., & Querleu, D. (1995). Moderate prenatal alcohol exposure and psychomotor development at preschool age. *American Journal of Public Health*, *85*(12), 1654–1661.

Larson, P. C. (1992). Neuropsychological counseling in hospital settings. *The Counseling Psychologist*, *20*(4), 556–570. doi:10.1177/0011000092204002

Larson, R. J., Woloshin, S., Schwartz, L. M., & Welch, H. G. (2005). Celebrity endorsements of cancer screening. *Journal of the National Cancer Institute*, *97*(9), 693–695.

Laslett, A. M., Room, R., Dietze, P., & Ferris, J. (2012). Alcohol's involvement in recurrent child abuse and neglect cases. *Addiction*, *107*(10), 1786–1793.

Latimer, E. A., & Lave, L. B. (1987). Initial effects of the New York State auto safety belt law. *American Journal of Public Health*, *77*(2), 183–186.

Lauby-Secretan, B., Scoccianti, C., Loomis, D., Grosse, Y., Bianchini, F., & Straif, K. (2016). Body fatness and cancer—viewpoint of the IARC Working Group. *New England Journal of Medicine*, *375*(8), 794–798.

Lautrette, A., Darmon, M., Megarbane, B., Joly, L. M., Chevret, S., Adrie, C., . . . Azoulay, E. (2007). A communication strategy and brochure for relatives of patients dying in the ICU. *New England Journal of Medicine*, *356*(5), 469–478. https://doi.org/10.1056/NEJMoa063446

Lavender, J. M., Wonderlich, S. A., Engel, S. G., Gordon, K. H., Kaye, W. H., & Mitchell, J. E. (2015). Dimensions of emotion dysregulation in anorexia nervosa and bulimia nervosa: A conceptual review of the empirical literature. *Clinical Psychology Review*, *40*, 111–122.

Lavoie, K. L., Bouchard, A., Joseph, M., Campbell, T. S., Favreau, H., & Bacon, S. L. (2008). Association of asthma self-efficacy to asthma control and quality of life. *Annals of Behavioral Medicine*, *36*(1), 100–106.

Law, A., Logan, H., & Baron, R. S. (1994). Desire for control, felt control, and stress inoculation training during dental treatment. *Journal of Personality and Social Psychology*, *67*(5), 926–936.

Law, C. K., Sveticic, J., & De Leo, D. (2014). Restricting access to a suicide hotspot does not shift the problem to another location. An experiment of two river bridges in Brisbane, Australia. *Australian and New Zealand Journal of Public Health*, *38*(2), 134–138.

Lawes, C. M., Vander Hoorn, S., & Rodgers, A. (2008). Global burden of blood-pressure-related disease, 2001. *Lancet*, *371*(9623), 1513–1518. https://doi.org/10.1016/S0140-6736(08)60655-8

Lawton, R., Conner, M., & McEachan, R. (2009). Desire or reason: Predicting health behaviors from affective and cognitive attitudes. *Health Psychology*, *28*(1), 56–65. doi:10.1037/a0013424

Laye-Gindhu, A., & Schonert-Reichl, K. A. (2005). Nonsuicidal self harm among community adolescents: Understanding the "whats" and "whys" of self-harm. *Journal of Youth and Adolescence*, *34*(5), 447–457.

Lazarus, R. S., & Folkman, S. (1984). *Stress, appraisal, and coping*. New York, NY: Guilford.

Lazarus, R. S., Kanner, A., & Folkman, S. (1980). Emotions: A cognitive-phenomenological analysis. In R. Plutchik & H. Hellerman (Eds.), *Theories of emotion* (pp. 189–217). New York, NY: Academic Press.

le Grange, D., Crosby, R. D., Rathouz, P. J., & Leventhal, B. L. (2007). A randomized controlled comparison of family-based treatment and supportive psychotherapy for adolescent bulimia nervosa. *Archives of General Psychiatry*, *64*(9), 1049–1056.

le Grange, D., Lock, J., Agras, W. S., Bryson, S. W., & Jo, B. (2015). Randomized clinical trial of family-based treatment and cognitive-behavioral therapy for adolescent bulimia nervosa. *Journal of the American Academy of Child & Adolescent Psychiatry*, *54*(11), 886–894.

Leahey, T. M., LaRose, J. G., Fava, J. L., & Wing, R. R. (2011). Social influences are associated with BMI and weight loss intentions in young adults. *Obesity (Silver Spring)*, *19*(6), 1157–1162.

Leake, R., Friend, R., & Wadhwa, N. (1999). Improving adjustment to chronic illness through strategic self-presentation: An experimental study on a renal dialysis unit. *Health Psychology*, *18*(1), 54–62.

Leary, M. R., & Jones, J. L. (1993). The Social psychology of tanning and sunscreen use: Self-presentational motives as a predictor of health risk. *Journal of Applied Social Psychology*, *23*(17), 1390–1406.

Lecci, L., & Cohen, D. J. (2002). Perceptual consequences of an illness-concern induction and its relation to hypochondriacal tendencies. *Health Psychology*, *21*(2), 147–156.

Lecci, L., Karoly, P., Ruehlman, L. S., & Lanyon, R. I. (1996). Goal-relevant dimensions of hypochondriacal tendencies and their relation to symptom manifestation and psychological distress. *Journal of Abnormal Psychology*, *105*(1), 42–45.

Lee, C., Sui, X., & Blair, S. N. (2009). Combined effects of cardiorespiratory fitness, not smoking, and normal waist girth on morbidity and mortality in men. *Archives of Internal Medicine*, *169*(22), 2096–2101.

Lee, D. B., Kim, E. S., & Neblett, E. W., Jr. (2017). The link between discrimination and telomere length in African American adults. *Health Psychology*, *36*(5), 458–467.

Lee, D. J., Mendes de Leon, C. F., Jenkins, C. D., Croog, S. H., Levine, S., & Sudilovsky, A. (1992). Relation of hostility to medication adherence, symptom complaints, and blood pressure reduction in a clinical field trial of antihypertensive medication. *Journal of Psychosomatic Research*, *36*(2), 181–190.

Lee, I.-M., Paffenbarger, R. S., Jr., & Hsieh, C.-C. (1992). Physical activity and risk of prostatic cancer among college alumni. *American Journal of Epidemiology, 135*, 169–179.

Lee, J., Hardesty, L. A., Kunzler, N. M., & Rosenkrantz, A. B. (2016). Direct interactive public education by breast radiologists about screening mammography: Impact on anxiety and empowerment. *Journal of the American College of Radiology, 13*(11), 89–97.

Lee, K. H., Seow, A., Luo, N., & Koh, D. (2008). Attitudes towards the doctor-patient relationship: A prospective study in an Asian medical school. *Medical Education, 42*(11), 1092–1099.

Lee, K. K., Raja, E. A., Lee, A. J., Bhattacharya, S., Bhattacharya, S., Norman, J. E., & Reynolds, R. M. (2015). Maternal obesity during pregnancy associates with premature mortality and major cardiovascular events in later life. *Hypertension, 66*(5), 938–944.

Lee, S., Chen, L., Jung, M. Y., Baezconde-Garbanati, L., & Juon, H. S. (2014). Acculturation and cancer screening among Asian Americans: Role of health insurance and having a regular physician. *Journal of Community Health, 39*(2), 201–212.

Lee, S., & Tsang, A. (2009). A population-based study of depression and three kinds of frequent pain conditions and depression in Hong Kong. *Pain Medicine, 10*(1), 155–163.

Lefcourt, H. M., Davidson, K., Prkachin, K. M., & Mills, D. E. (1997). Humor as a stress moderator in the prediction of blood pressure obtained during five stressful tasks. *Journal of Research in Personality, 31*(4), 523–542.

Lefcourt, H. M., Davidson-Katz, K., & Kueneman, K. (1990). Humor and immune-system functioning. *Humor: International Journal of Humor Research, 3*(3), 305–321.

Legate, N., Ryan, R. M., & Rogge, R. D. (2017). Daily autonomy support and sexual identity disclosure predicts daily mental and physical health outcomes. *Personality and Social Psychology Bulletin, 43*(6), 860–873.

Lehrer, P., Feldman, J., Giardino, N., Song, H.-S., & Schmaling, K. (2002). Psychological aspects of asthma. *Journal of Consulting and Clinical Psychology, 70*, 691–711.

Leibel, R. L., Berry, E. M., & Hirsch, J. (1983). Biochemistry and development of adipose tissue in man. *Health and Obesity*, pp. 21–48.

Leiker, M., & Hailey, B. J. (1988). A link between hostility and disease: Poor health habits? *Behavioral Medicine, 14*(3), 129–133.

Leitner, J. B., Hehman, E., Ayduk, O., & Mendoza-Denton, R. (2016). Racial bias is associated with ingroup death rate for Blacks and Whites: Insights from Project Implicit. *Social Science & Medicine, 170*, 220–228. **doi:10.1016/j.socscimed.2016.10.007**

Leitzell, J. D. (1977). Patient and physician: Is either objective? *New England Journal of Medicine, 296*(18), 1070.

Lengacher, C. A., Johnson-Mallard, V., Post-White, J., Moscoso, M. S., Jacobsen, P. B., Klein, T. W., . . . Kip, K. E. (2009). Randomized controlled trial of mindfulness-based stress reduction (MBSR) for survivors of breast cancer. *Psycho-Oncology, 18*(12), 1261–1272. **https://doi.org/10.1002/pon.1529**

Lengacher, C. A., Shelton, M. M., Reich, R. R., Barta, M. K., Johnson-Mallard, V., Moscoso, M. S., . . . Lucas, J. (2014). Mindfulness based stress reduction (MBSR (BC)) in breast cancer: Evaluating fear of recurrence (FOR) as a mediator of psychological and physical symptoms in a randomized control trial (RCT). *Journal of Behavioral Medicine, 37*(2), 185–195.

Lepore, S. J. (1995). Cynicism, social support, and cardiovascular reactivity. *Health Psychology, 14*(3), 210–216.

Lepore, S. J., Silver, R. C., Wortman, C. B., & Wayment, H. A. (1996). Social constraints, intrusive thoughts, and depressive symptoms among bereaved mothers. *Journal of Personality and Social Psychology, 70*, 271–282.

Lerman, C. (1997). Psychological aspects of genetic testing: Introduction to the special issue. *Health Psychology, 16*(1), 3–7.

Lerman, C., Daly, M., Sands, C., Balshem, A., Lustbader, E., Heggan, T., . . . Engstrom, P. (1993). Mammography adherence and psychological distress among women at risk for breast cancer. *JNCI: Journal of the National Cancer Institute, 85*(13), 1074–1080.

Lerman, C., Hughes, C., Croyle, R. T., Main, D., Durham, C., Snyder, C., . . . Lynch, H. T. (2000). Prophylactic surgery decisions and surveillance practices one year following BRCA1/2 testing. *Preventive Medicine, 31*(1), 75–80.

Lerman, C., & Rimer, B. K. (1995). Psychosocial impact of cancer screening. In R. T. Croyle (Ed.), *Psychosocial effects of screening for disease prevention and detection* (pp. 65–81). New York, NY: Oxford University Press.

Lerman, C., Rimer, B., Trock, B., Balshem, A., & Engstrom, P. F. (1990). Factors associated with repeat adherence to breast cancer screening. *Preventive Medicine, 19*(3), 279–290.

Leserman, J., Jackson, E. D., Petitto, J. M., Golden, R. N., Silva, S. G., Perkins, D. O., . . . Evans, D. L. (1999). Progression to AIDS: The effects of stress, depressive symptoms, and social support. *Psychosomatic Medicine, 61*(3), 397–406.

Leserman, J., Perkins, D. O., & Evans, D. L. (1992). Coping with the threat of AIDS: The role of social support. *American Journal of Psychiatry, 149*, 1514–1520.

Leung, S., Croft, R. J., Jackson, M. L., Howard, M. E., & McKenzie, R. J. (2012). A comparison of the effect of mobile phone use and alcohol consumption on driving simulation performance. *Traffic Injury Prevention, 13*(6), 566–574.

Leventhal, E. A., Hansell, S., Diefenbach, M., Leventhal, H., & Glass, D. C. (1996). Negative affect and self-report of physical symptoms: Two longitudinal studies of older adults. *Health Psychology, 15*(3), 193–199.

Leventhal, E. A., Leventhal, H., Shacham, S., & Easterling, D. V. (1989). Active coping reduces reports of pain from childbirth. *Journal of Consulting and Clinical Psychology, 57,* 365–371.

Leventhal, H. (1970). Findings and theory in the study of fear communications. In L. Berkowitz (Ed.), *Advances in experimental social psychology* (Vol. 5, pp. 119–185). San Diego, CA: Academic Press.

Leventhal, H., & Cleary, P. D. (1980). The smoking problem: A review of the research and theory in behavioral risk modification. *Psychological Bulletin, 88*(2), 370–405.

Leventhal, H., Meyer, D., & Nerenz, D. (1980). The common sense model of illness danger. In S. Rachman (Ed.), *Medical psychology* (Vol. 2, pp. 7–30). New York, NY: Pergamon.

Leventhal, H., Singer, R., & Jones, S. (1965). Effects of fear and specificity of recommendation upon attitudes and behavior. *Journal of Personality and Social Psychology, 2*(1), 20–29.

Leventhal, H., & Watts, J. C. (1966). Sources of resistance to fear-arousing communications on smoking and lung cancer. *Journal of Personality, 34*(2), 155–175.

Levin, I. P., Schnittjer, S. K., & Thee, S. L. (1988). Information framing effects in social and personal decisions. *Journal of Experimental Social Psychology, 24*(6), 520–529.

Levin, J. (2015). Religious differences in self-rated health among US Jews: Findings from five urban population surveys. *Journal of Religion and Health, 54*(2), 765–778.

Levin, J. S. (1994). Religion and health: Is there an association, is it valid, and is it causal? *Social Science & Medicine, 38*(11), 1475–1482.

Levine, A. J., Hinkin, C. H., Marion, S., Keuning, A., Castellon, S. A., Lam, M. M., . . . Durvasula, R. S. (2006). Adherence to antiretroviral medications in HIV: Differences in data collected via self-report and electronic monitoring. *Health Psychology, 25*(3), 329–335.

Levine, F. M., & DeSimone, L. L. (1991). The effects of experimenter gender on pain report in male and female subjects. *Pain, 44*(1), 69–72.

Levine, J. A., Eberhardt, N. L., & Jensen, M. D. (1999). Role of nonexercise activity thermogenesis in resistance to fat gain in humans. *Science, 283*(5399), 212–214.

Levine, J. D., Gordon, N. C., & Fields, H. L. (1978). The mechanism of placebo analgesia. *Lancet, 2,* 654–657.

Levine, R. V. (1990). The pace of life. *American Scientist, 79,* 450–459.

Levy, D. J., Heissel, J. A., Richeson, J. A., & Adam, E. K. (2016). Psychological and biological responses to race-based social stress as pathways to disparities in educational outcomes. *American Psychologist, 71*(6), 455–473. doi:10.1037/a0040322

Levy, R. K. (1997). The transtheoretical model of change: An application to bulimia nervosa. *Psychotherapy: Theory, Research, Practice, Training, 34*(3), 278–285.

Levy, S. M. (1983). The process of death and dying: Behavioral and social factors. In T. G. Burish & L. A. Bradley (Eds.), *Coping with chronic disease: Research and applications* (pp. 425–446). New York, NY: Academic Press.

Levy, S. M. (1985). *Behavior and cancer: Life-style and psychosocial factors in the initiation and progression of cancer.* San Francisco, CA: Jossey-Bass.

Levy, S. M., Lee, J., Bagley, C., & Lippman, M. (1988). Survival hazards analysis in first recurrent breast cancer patients: Seven-year follow-up. *Psychosomatic Medicine, 50*(5), 520–528.

Lew, E. A. (1985). Mortality and weight: Insured lives and the American Cancer Society studies. *Annals of Internal Medicine, 103*(6), 1024–1029.

Lewin, K. (1935). *A dynamic theory of personality.* New York, NY: McGraw-Hill.

Ley, P. (1982). Satisfaction, compliance and communication. *British Journal of Clinical Psychology, 21*(4), 241–254.

Li, J., Laursen, T. M., Precht, D. H., Olsen, J., & Mortensen, P. B. (2005). Hospitalization for mental illness among parents after the death of a child. *New England Journal of Medicine, 352*(12), 1190–1196. https://doi.org/10.1056/NEJMoa033160

Li, J., Stroebe, M., Chan, C. L. W., & Chow, A. Y. M. (2014). Guilt in bereavement: A review and conceptual framework. *Death Studies, 38*(3), 165–171. https://doi.org/10.1080/07481187.2012.738770

Li, Q. (2010). Effect of forest bathing trips on human immune function. *Environmental Health and Preventive Medicine, 15*(1), 9–17.

Li, S., Stampfer, M. J., Williams, D. R., & VanderWeele, T. J. (2016). Association of religious service attendance with mortality among women. *JAMA Internal Medicine, 176*(6), 777–785.

Liberman, A., & Chaiken, S. (1992). Defensive processing of personally relevant health messages. *Personality and Social Psychology Bulletin, 18*(6), 669–679.

Liberman, R. (1962). An analysis of the placebo phenomenon. *Journal of Chronic Diseases, 15,* 761–783.

Lichtenstein, E., & Mermelstein, R. (1984). Review of approaches to smoking treatment strategies. In J. D. Matarazzo, N. E. Miller, S. M. Weiss, & J. A. Herd (Eds.), *Behavioral health: A handbook of health enhancement and disease prevention* (pp. 695–712). New York, NY: Wiley.

Lichtenstein, P., Gatz, M., Pedersen, N. L., Berg, S., & McClearn, G. E. (1996).

A co-twin-control study of response to widowhood. *Journal of Gerontology: Psychological Sciences, 51*, 279–289.

Lichtenstein, P., Holm, N. V., Verkasalo, P. K., Iliadou, A., Kaprio, J., Koskenvuo, M., . . . Hemminki, K. (2000). Environmental and heritable factors in the causation of cancer — Analyses of cohorts of twins from Sweden, Denmark, and Finland. *New England Journal of Medicine, 343*(2), 78–85. https://doi.org/10.1056/NEJM200007133430201

Lilienfeld, A. M., & Lilienfeld, D. E. (1980). *Foundations of epidemiology* (2nd ed.). New York, NY: Oxford University Press.

Lillberg, K., Verkasalo, P. K., Kaprio, J., Teppo, L., Helenius, H., & Koskenvuo, M. (2003). Stressful life events and risk of breast cancer in 10,808 women: A cohort study. *American Journal of Epidemiology, 157*(5), 415–423.

Lima, J., Nazarian, L., Charney, E., & Lahti, B. A. (1976). Compliance with short-term antimicrobial therapy: Some techniques that help. *Pediatrics, 57*, 383–386.

Lin, M.-Y., & Kressin, N. R. (2015). Race/ethnicity and Americans' experiences with treatment decision making. *Patient Education and Counseling, 98*(12), 1636–1642.

Linde, K., Streng, A., Jürgens, S., Hoppe, A., Brinkhaus, B., Witt, C., . . . Melchart, D. (2005). Acupuncture for patients with migraine: A randomized controlled trial. *Journal of the American Medical Association, 293*(17), 2118–2125. https://doi.org/10.1001/jama.293.17.2118

Linden, W., Chambers, L., Maurice, J., & Lenz, J. W. (1993). Sex differences in social support, self-deception, hostility, and ambulatory cardiovascular activity. *Health Psychology, 12*(5), 376–380.

Lindstrom, T. C. (1995). Experiencing the presence of the dead: Discrepancies in "the sensing experience" and their psychological concomitants. *Omega-Journal of Death and Dying, 31*, 11–21.

Linn, S., Carroll, M., Johnson, C., Fulwood, R., Kalsbeek, W., & Briefel, R. (1993). High-density lipoprotein cholesterol and alcohol consumption in US White and Black adults: Data from NHANES II. *American Journal of Public Health, 83*(6), 811–816.

Linville, P. W., Fischer, G. W., & Fischhoff, B. (1993). AIDS risk perceptions and decision biases. In J. B. Pryor & G. D. Reeder (Eds.), *The social psychology of HIV infection* (pp. 5–38). Hillsdale, NJ: Erlbaum.

Liossi, C., White, P., & Hatira, P. (2006). Randomized clinical trial of local anesthetic versus a combination of local anesthetic with self-hypnosis in the management of pediatric procedure-related pain. *Health Psychology, 25*(3), 307–315.

Lipkus, I. M., McBride, C. M., Pollak, K. I., Lyna, P., & Bepler, G. (2004). Interpretation of genetic risk feedback among African American smokers with low socioeconomic status. *Health Psychology, 23*(2), 178–188.

Lipowski, Z. J. (1986). What does the word "psychosomatic" really mean? A historical and semantic inquiry. In M. J. Christie & P. G. Mellett (Eds.), *The psychosomatic approach: Contemporary practice and wholeperson care* (pp. 17–38). New York, NY: Wiley.

Lippke, S., & Plotnikoff, R. C. (2014). Testing two principles of the Health Action Process Approach in individuals with type 2 diabetes. *Health Psychology, 33*(1), 77–84.

Lippold, M., Davis, K. D., McHale, S. M., Buxton, O., & Almeida, D. M. (2016). Daily stressor reactivity during adolescence: The buffering role of parental warmth. *Health Psychology, 35*(9), 1027–1035.

Lipton, R. I. (1994). The effect of moderate alcohol use on the relationship between stress and depression. *American Journal of Public Health, 84*(12), 1913–1917.

Lisspers, J., Sundin, O., Ohman, A., Hofman-Bang, C., Rydén, L., & Nygren, A. (2005). Long-term effects of lifestyle behavior change in coronary artery disease: Effects on recurrent coronary events after percutaneous coronary intervention. *Health Psychology, 24*(1), 41–48.

Listing, M., Reißhauer, A., Krohn, M., Voigt, B., Tjahono, G., Becker, J., . . . Rauchfuß, M. (2009). Massage therapy reduces physical discomfort and improves mood disturbances in women with breast cancer. *Psycho-Oncology, 18*(12), 1290–1299. https://doi.org/10.1002/pon.1508

Litt, M. D., Kalinowski, L., & Shafer, D. (1999). A dental fears typology of oral surgery patients: Matching patients to anxiety interventions. *Health Psychology, 18*(6), 614–624.

Litt, M. D., Nye, C., & Shafer, D. (1995). Preparation for oral surgery: Evaluating elements of coping. *Journal of Behavioral Medicine, 18*(5), 435–459.

Litt, M. D., Shafer, D., & Napolitano, C. (2004). Momentary mood and coping processes in TMD pain. *Health Psychology, 23*(4), 354–362. https://doi.org/10.1037/0278-6133.23.4.354

Litt, M. D., Tennen, H., Affleck, G., & Klock, S. (1992). Coping and cognitive factors in adaptation to in vitro fertilization failure. *Journal of Behavioral Medicine, 15*(2), 171–187.

Liu, H. (2009). Till death do us part: Marital status and US mortality trends, 1986–2000. *Journal of Marriage and Family, 71*(5), 1158–1173.

Liu, H., Waite, L., & Shen, S. (2016). Diabetes risk and disease management in later life: A national longitudinal study of the role of marital quality. *Journals of Gerontology Series B: Psychological Sciences and Social Sciences, 71*(6), 1070–1080.

Lloyd-Jones, D. M., Nam, B. H., D'Agostino, R. B., Sr., Levy, D., Murabito, J. M., Wang, T. J., . . . O'Donnell, C. J. (2004). Parental cardiovascular disease as a risk factor for cardiovascular disease in middle-aged adults: A prospective study of parents and offspring. *Journal of the American Medical Association, 291*(18), 2204–2211. **https://doi.org/10.1001/jama.291.18.2204**

LoConto, D. G. (1998). Death and dreams: A sociological approach to grieving and identity. *Omega-Journal of Death and Dying, 37,* 171–185.

Loeber, R., & Farrington, D. P. (1998). Never too early, never too late: Risk factors and successful interventions for serious and violent juvenile offenders. *Studies on Crime and Crime Prevention, 7*(1), 7–30.

Loeber, R., Pardini, D., Homish, D. L., Wei, E. H., Crawford, A. M., Farrington, D. P., . . . Rosenfeld, R. (2005). The prediction of violence and homicide in young men. *Journal of Consulting and Clinical Psychology, 73*(6), 1074–1088.

Logan, D. E., & Marlatt, G. A. (2010). Harm reduction therapy: A practice-friendly review of research. *Journal of Clinical Psychology, 66*(2), 201–214. **http://doi.org/10.1002/jclp.20669**

Lombard, D. N., Lombard, T. N., & Winett, R. A. (1995). Walking to meet health guidelines: The effect of prompting frequency and prompt structure. *Health Psychology, 14*(2), 164–170.

Lopez, E. N., Drobes, D. J., Thompson, J. K., & Brandon, T. H. (2008). Effects of a body image challenge on smoking motivation among college females. *Health Psychology, 27*(3), 243–251.

López-Martínez, A. E., Esteve-Zarazaga, R., & Ramírez-Maestre, C. (2008). Perceived social support and coping responses are independent variables explaining pain adjustment among chronic pain patients. *The Journal of Pain, 9*(4), 373–379. **https://doi.org/10.1016/j.jpain.2007.12.002**

Lorber, J. (1975). Good patients and problem patients: Conformity and deviance in a general hospital. *Journal of Health and Social Behavior, 16*(2), 213–225.

Lovallo, W. R. (2015). Can exaggerated stress reactivity and prolonged recovery predict negative health outcomes? The case of cardiovascular disease. *Psychosomatic Medicine, 77*(3), 212–214. **doi:10.1097/PSY.0000000000000173**

Low, C. A., Stanton, A. L., & Danoff-Burg, S. (2006). Expressive disclosure and benefit finding among breast cancer patients: Mechanisms for positive health effects. *Health Psychology, 25,* 181–189.

Lowe, M. R. (1993). The effects of dieting on eating behavior: A three-factor model. *Psychological Bulletin, 114*(1), 100–121.

Lowe, M. R., Whitlow, J. W., & Bellwoar, V. (1991). Eating regulation: The role of restraint, dieting, and weight. *International Journal of Eating Disorders, 10*(4), 461–471.

Lox, C. L., Mcauley, E., & Tucker, R. S. (1996). Physical training effects on acute exercise-induced feeling states in HIV-1-positive individuals. *Journal of Health Psychology, 1*(2), 235–240. **doi:10.1177/135910539600100207**

Ludwick-Rosenthal, R., & Neufeld, R. W. (1993). Preparation for undergoing an invasive medical procedure: Interacting effects of information and coping style. *Journal of Consulting and Clinical Psychology, 61*(1), 156–164.

Lumeng, J. C., & Hillman, K. H. (2007). Eating in larger groups increases food consumption. *Archives of Disease in Childhood, 92*(5), 384–387.

Lund, A. K., & Kegeles, S. S. (1984). Rewards and adolescent health behavior. *Health Psychology, 3*(4), 351–369.

Luo, F., Florence, C. S., Quispe-Agnoli, M., Ouyang, L., & Crosby, A. E. (2011). Impact of business cycles on US suicide rates, 1928–2007. *American Journal of Public Health, 101*(6), 1139–1146.

Lu, Q., Wong, C. C. Y., Gallagher, M. W., Tou, R. Y., Young, L., & Loh, A. (2017). Expressive writing among Chinese American breast cancer survivors: A randomized controlled trial. *Health Psychology, 36*(4), 370–379. **doi:10.1037/hea000044**

Lustria, M. L. A., Cortese, J., Gerend, M. A., Schmitt, K., Kung, Y. M., & McLaughlin, C. (2016). A model of tailoring effects: A randomized controlled trial examining the mechanisms of tailoring in a web-based STD screening intervention. *Health Psychology, 35*(11), 1214–1224.

Luszczynska, A., Sobczyk, A., & Abraham, C. (2007). Planning to lose weight: Randomized controlled trial of an implementation intention prompt to enhance weight reduction among overweight and obese women. *Health Psychology, 26*(4), 507–512.

Lutgendorf, S. K., Russell, D., Ullrich, P., Harris, T. B., & Wallace, R. (2004). Religious participation, interleukin-6, and mortality in older adults. *Health Psychology, 23*(5), 465–475.

Ly, J., McGrath, J. J., & Gouin, J. (2015). Poor sleep as a pathophysiological pathway underlying the association between stressful experiences and the diurnal cortisol profile among children and adolescents. *Psychoneuroendocrinology, 57,* 51–60.

Lyles, J. N., Burish, T. G., Krozely, M. G., & Oldham, R. K. (1982). Efficacy of relaxation training and guided imagery in reducing the aversiveness of cancer chemotherapy. *Journal of Consulting and Clinical Psychology, 50,* 509–524.

Lynch, D. J., Birk, T. J., Weaver, M. T., Gohara, A. F., Leighton, R. F., Repka, F. J., & Walsh, M. E. (1992). Adherence to exercise interventions in the treatment of hypercholesterolemia. *Journal of Behavioral Medicine, 15,* 365–377.

Lynch, H., & Watson, P. (1992). Genetic counselling and hereditary breast/ovarian cancer. *The Lancet, 339*(8802), 1181.

Lyness, S. A. (1993). Predictors of differences between Type A and B individuals in heart rate and blood pressure reactivity. *Psychological Bulletin, 114*(2), 266–295.

Lynn, J. (2001). Serving patients who may die soon and their families: The role of hospice and other services. *Journal of the American Medical Association, 285,* 925–932.

Lyubomirsky, S., King, L., & Diener, E. (2005). The benefits of frequent positive affect: Does happiness lead to success? *Psychological Bulletin, 131*(6), 803–855.

Lyubomirsky, S., & Nolen-Hoeksema, S. (1995). Effects of self-focused rumination on negative thinking and interpersonal problem solving. *Journal of Personality and Social Psychology, 69*(1), 176–190. **doi:10.1037//0022-3514.69.1.176**

Mabe, A. G., Forney, K. J., & Keel, P. K. (2014). Do you "like" my photo? Facebook use maintains eating disorder risk. *International Journal of Eating Disorders, 47*(5), 516–523.

MacDonald, T. K., Zanna, M. P., & Fong, G. T. (1995). Decision making in altered states: Effects of alcohol on attitudes toward drinking and driving. *Journal of Personality and Social Psychology, 68*(6), 973–985.

MacDougall, E. E., & Farreras, I. G. (2016). The multidimensional orientation toward dying and death inventory (MODDI-F): Factorial validity and reliability in a U.S. sample. *Journal of Pain and Symptom Management, 51*(6), 1062–1069. **doi:10.1016/j.jpainsymman.2015.12.322**

Machado, B. C., Gonçalves, S. F., Martins, C., Brandão, I., Roma-Torres, A., Hoek, H. W., & Machado, P. P. (2015). Anorexia nervosa versus bulimia nervosa: Differences based on retrospective correlates in a case-control study. *Eating and Weight Disorders: EWD, 21*(2), 185–197.

Macharia, W. M., Leon, G., Rowe, B. H., Stephenson, B. J., & Haynes, R. B. (1992). An overview of interventions to improve compliance with appointment keeping for medical services. *Journal of the American Medical Association, 267,* 1813–1817.

Mackenzie, T., Gifford, A. H., Sabadosa, K. A., Quinton, H. B., Knapp, E. A., Goss, C. H., & Marshall, B. C. (2014). Longevity of patients with cystic fibrosis in 2000 to 2010 and beyond: Survival analysis of the Cystic Fibrosis Foundation Patient Registry. *Annals of Internal Medicine, 161*(4), 233–241. **doi:10.7326/m13-0636**

MacKinnon, D. P., Johnson, C. A., Pentz, M. A., Dwyer, J. H., Hansen, W. B., Flay, B. R., & Wang, E. Y. I. (1991). Mediating mechanisms in a school-based drug prevention program: first-year effects of the Midwestern Prevention Project. *Health Psychology, 10*(3), 164–172.

MacLeod, R. D. (2001). On reflection: Doctor's learning to care for people who are dying. *Social Science and Medicine, 52,* 1719–1727.

Maclure, M. (1993). Demonstration of deductive meta-analysis: Ethanol intake and risk of myocardial infarction. *Epidemiologic Reviews, 15*(2), 328–351.

MacNell, L., Elliott, S., Hardison-Moody, A., & Bowen, S. (2017). Black and Latino urban food desert residents' perceptions of their food environment and factors that influence food shopping decisions. *Journal of Hunger & Environmental Nutrition, 12*(3), 375–393. **doi:10.1080/19320248.2017.1284025**

Macrodimitris, S. D., & Endler, N. S. (2001). Coping, control, and adjustment in Type 2 diabetes. *Health Psychology, 20*(3), 208–216.

Madden, S., Hay, P., & Touyz, S. W. (2015). Systematic review of evidence for different treatment settings in anorexia nervosa. *World Journal of Psychiatry, 5*(1), 147–153.

Maes, M., Hendriks, D., Van Gastel, A., Demedts, P., Wauters, A., Neels, H., . . . Scharpé, S. (1997). Effects of psychological stress on serum immunoglobulin, complement and acute phase protein concentrations in normal volunteers. *Psychoneuroendocrinology, 22*(6), 397–409.

Magni, G., Moreschi, C., Rigatti-Luchini, S., & Merskey, H. (1994). Prospective study on the relationship between depressive symptoms and chronic musculoskeletal pain. *Pain, 56,* 289–297.

Magni, G., Silvestro, A., Tamiello, M., Zanesco, L., & Carl, M. (1988). An integrated approach to the assessment of family adjustment to acute lymphocytic leukemia in children. *Acta Psychiatrica Scandinavia, 78,* 639–642.

Maguire, P. (1985). Barriers to psychological care of the dying. *British Medical Journal, 291*(6510), 1711–1713.

Maher, V. M., Brown, B. G., Marcovina, S. M., Hillger, L. A., & Zhao, X. (1995). Effects of lowering elevated LDL cholesterol on the cardiovascular risk of lipoprotein. *Journal of the American Medical Association, 22,* 1771–1774.

Mahler, H. I., Kulik, J. A., Gerrard, M., & Gibbons, F. X. (2007). Long-term effects of appearance-based interventions on sun protection behaviors. *Health Psychology, 26*(3), 350–360.

Maisto, S. A., Carey, K. B., & Bradizza, C. M. (1999). Social learning theory. In K. E. Leonard & H. T. Blane (Eds.), *Psychological theories of drinking and alcoholism* (2nd ed., pp. 106–163). New York, NY: Guilford Press.

Ma-Kellams, C., Or, F., Baek, J. H., & Kawachi, I. (2015). Rethinking suicide surveillance: Google search data and self-reported suicidality differentially estimate completed suicide risk. *Clinical Psychological Science, 4*(3), 480–484.

Malek, L., Umberger, W. J., Makrides, M., & Zhou, S. (2017). Predicting healthy eating intention and adherence to dietary recommendations during pregnancy in Australia using the Theory of Planned Behaviour. *Appetite, 116,* 431–441. **doi:10.1016/j.appet.2017.05.028**

Males, M. (2015). Age, poverty, homicide, and gun homicide: Is young age or poverty level the key issue? *Sage Open, 5*(1).

Manasse, S. M., Forman, E. M., Ruocco, A. C., Butryn, M. L., Juarascio, A. S., & Fitzpatrick, K. K. (2015). Do executive functioning deficits underpin binge eating disorder? A comparison of overweight women with and without binge eating pathology. *International Journal of Eating Disorders, 48*(6), 677–683.

Manfredi, M., Bini, G., Cruccu, G., Accornero, N., Berardelli, A., & Medolago, L. (1981). Congenital absence of pain. *Archives of Neurology, 38*, 507–511.

Mann, J. J., Apter, A., Bertolote, J., Beautrais, A., Currier, D., Haas, A., . . . Mehlum, L. (2005). Suicide prevention strategies: A systematic review. *Journal of the American Medical Association, 294*(16), 2064–2074.

Mann, T., Nolen-Hoeksema, S., Huang, K., Burgard, D., Wright, A., & Hanson, K. (1997). Are two interventions worse than none? Joint primary and secondary prevention of eating disorders in college females. *Health Psychology, 16*(3), 215–225.

Manne, S. L., Bakeman, R., Jacobsen, P. B., Gorfinkle, K., Bernstein, D., & Redd, W. H. (1992). Adult-child interaction during invasive medical procedures. *Health Psychology, 11*(4), 241–249.

Manne, S., Jacobsen, P. B., Ming, M. E., Winkel, G., Dessureault, S., & Lessin, S. R. (2010). Tailored versus generic interventions for skin cancer risk reduction for family members of melanoma patients. *Health Psychology, 29*(6), 583–593.

Manne, S., Markowitz, A., Winawer, S., Meropol, N. J., Haller, D., Rakowski, W., . . . Jandorf, L. (2002). Correlates of colorectal cancer screening compliance and stage of adoption among siblings of individuals with early onset colorectal cancer. *Health Psychology, 21*(1), 3–15.

Manne, S. L., Norton, T. R., Ostroff, J. S., Winkel, G., Fox, K., & Grana, G. (2007). Protective buffering and psychological distress among couples coping with breast cancer: The moderating role of relationship satisfaction. *Journal of Family Psychology, 21*(3), 380–388.

Manne, S., Ostroff, J. S., & Winkel, G. (2007). Social-cognitive processes as moderators of a couple-focused group intervention for women with early stage breast cancer. *Health Psychology, 26*(6), 735–744.

Manne, S. L., Ostroff, J., Winkel, G., Grana, G., & Fox, K. (2005). Partner unsupportive responses, avoidant coping, and distress among women with early stage breast cancer: Patient and partner perspectives. *Health Psychology, 24*(6), 635–641.

Manne, S. L., & Zautra, A. J. (1989). Spouse criticism and support: Their association with coping and psychological adjustment among women with rheumatoid arthritis. *Journal of Personality and Social Psychology, 56*(4), 608–617.

Manners, M. T., Ertel, A., Yuzhen, T., & Ajit, S. K. (2016). Genome-wide redistribution of MeCP2 in dorsal root ganglia after peripheral nerve injury. *Epigenetics & Chromatin, 9*, 1–15. doi:10.1186/s13072-016-0073-5

Manning, M. M., & Wright, T. L. (1983). Self-efficacy expectancies, outcome expectancies, and the persistence of pain control in childbirth. *Journal of Personality and Social Psychology, 45*(2), 421–431.

Manson, J. E., Colditz, G. A., Stampfer, M. J., Willett, W. C., Rosner, B., Monson, R. R., . . . Hennekens, C. H. (1990). A prospective study of obesity and risk of coronary heart disease in women. *New England Journal of Medicine, 322*(13), 882–889.

Manson, J. E., Nathan, D. M., Krolewski, A. S., Stampfer, M. J., Willett, W. C., & Hennekens, C. H. (1992). A prospective study of exercise and incidence of diabetes among US male physicians. *Journal of the American Medical Association, 268*(1), 63–67.

Manstead, A. S., Proffitt, C., & Smart, J. L. (1983). Predicting and understanding mothers' infant-feeding intentions and behavior: Testing the theory of reasoned action. *Journal of Personality and Social Psychology, 44*(4), 657–671.

Manyande, A., Berg, S., Gettins, D., Stanford, S. C., Mazhero, S., Marks, D. F., & Salmon, P. (1995). Preoperative rehearsal of active coping imagery influences subjective and hormonal responses to abdominal surgery. *Psychosomatic Medicine, 57*(2), 177–182.

Manzardo, A. M., McGuire, A., & Butler, M. G. (2015). Clinically relevant genetic biomarkers from the brain in alcoholism with representation on high resolution chromosome ideograms. *Gene, 560*(2), 184–194.

Maranda, L., & Gupta, O. T. (2016). Association between responsible pet ownership and glycemic control in youths with type 1 diabetes. *PLOS ONE, 11*(4), e0152332.

Marcus, B. H., Dubbert, P. M., Forsyth, L. H., McKenzie, T. L., Stone, E. J., Dunn, A. L., & Blair, S. N. (2000). Physical activity behavior change: issues in adoption and maintenance. *Health Psychology, 19*(1), 32–41.

Marcus, B. H., Lewis, B. A., Williams, D. M., Dunsiger, S., Jakicic, J. M., Whiteley, J. A., . . . Sciamanna, C. N. (2007). A comparison of Internet and print-based physical activity interventions. *Archives of Internal Medicine, 167*(9), 944–949.

Mares, S. H., van der Vorst, H., Engels, R. C., & Lichtwarck-Aschoff, A. (2011). Parental alcohol use, alcohol-related problems, and alcohol-specific attitudes, alcohol-specific communication, and adolescent excessive alcohol use and alcohol-related problems: An indirect path model. *Addictive Behaviors, 36*(3), 209–216.

Marin, B. V., & Marin, G. (1992). Predictors of condom accessibility among Hispanics in San Francisco. *American Journal of Public Health, 82*(4), 592–595.

Marin, G., & Marin, B. V. (1991). *Research with Hispanic populations.* Newbury Park, CA: Sage.

Marin, M., Zhang, J. X., & Seward, J. F. (2011). Near elimination of varicella deaths in the US after implementation of the vaccination program. *Pediatrics, 128*(2), 214–220.

Marin, T. J., Martin, T. M., Blackwell, E., Stetler, C., & Miller, G. E. (2007). Differentiating the impact of episodic and chronic stressors on hypothalamic-pituitary-adrenocortical axis regulation in young women. *Health Psychology, 26*(4), 447–455.

Markowitz, J. H., Matthews, K. A., Kannel, W. B., Cobb, J. L., & D'Agostino, R. B. (1993). Psychological predictors of hypertension in the Framingham Study: Is there tension in hypertension? *Journal of the American Medical Association, 270*, 2439–2443.

Marks, G., Graham, J. W., & Hansen, W. B. (1992). Social projection and social conformity in adolescent alcohol use: A longitudinal analysis. *Personality and Social Psychology Bulletin, 18*(1), 96–101.

Marks, G., Richardson, J. L., Graham, J. W., & Levine, A. (1986). Role of health locus of control beliefs and expectations of treatment efficacy in adjustment to cancer. *Journal of Personality and Social Psychology, 51*(2), 443–450.

Marks, G., Richardson, J. L., Ruiz, M. S., & Maldonado, N. (1992). HIV-infected men's practices in notifying past sexual partners of infection risk. *Public Health Reports, 107*(1), 100–105.

Marlatt, G. A. (1985a). Relapse prevention: Theoretical rationale and overview of the model. In G. A. Marlatt & J. R. Gordon (Eds.), *Relapse prevention* (pp. 3–70). New York, NY: Guilford Press.

Marlatt, G. A. (1985b). Situational determinants of relapse and skill-training interventions. In G. A. Marlatt & J. R. Gordon (Eds.), *Relapse prevention* (pp. 71–127). New York, NY: Guilford Press.

Marlatt, G. A., Baer, J. S., Kivlahan, D. R., Dimeff, L. A., Larimer, M. E., Quigley, L. A., . . . Williams, E. (1998). Screening and brief intervention for high-risk college student drinkers: Results from a 2-year follow-up assessment. *Journal of Consulting and Clinical Psychology, 66*(4), 604–615.

Marlatt, G. A., & George, W. H. (1984). Relapse prevention: Introduction and overview of the model.

Addiction, (4), 261–273. **doi:10.1111/ j.1360-0443.1984.tb00274.x**

Marlatt, G. A., & Gordon, J. R. (1980). Determinants of relapse: Implication for the maintenance of behavior change. In P. O. Davidson & S. M. Davidson (Eds.), *Behavioral medicine: Changing health lifestyles* (pp. 410–452). New York, NY: Brunner/Mazel.

Marsland, A. L., Cohen, S., Rabin, B. S., & Manuck, S. B. (2001). Associations between stress, trait negative affect, acute immune reactivity, and antibody response to hepatitis B vaccination. *Health Psychology, 20*, 4–11.

Marteau, T. M. (1989). Framing of information: Its influence upon decisions of doctors and patients. *British Journal of Social Psychology, 28*(1), 89–94.

Marteau, T. M., Dundas, R., & Axworthy, D. (1997). Long-term cognitive and emotional impact of genetic testing for carriers of cystic fibrosis: The effects of test result and gender. *Health Psychology, 16*(1), 51–62.

Martelli, M. F., Auerbach, S. M., Alexander, J., & Mercuri, L. G. (1987). Stress management in the health care setting: Matching interventions with patient coping styles. *Journal of Consulting and Clinical Psychology, 55*(2), 201–207.

Martikainen, P., & Valkonen, T. (1996). Mortality after the death of a spouse: Rates and causes of death in a large Finnish cohort. *American Journal of Public Health, 86*, 1087–1093.

Martin, J. L., & Dean, L. (1993). Effects of AIDS-related bereavement and HIV-related illness on psychological distress among gay men: A 7-year longitudinal study, 1985–1991. *Journal of Consulting and Clinical Psychology, 61*, 94–103.

Martin, L. R., Friedman, H. S., & Schwartz, J. E. (2007). Personality and mortality risk across the lifespan: The importance of conscientiousness as a biopsychosocial attribute. *Health Psychology, 26*, 428–436.

Martin, L. R., Friedman, H. S., Tucker, J. S., Tomlinson-Keasey, C., Criqui, M. H., & Schwartz, J. E. (2002). A life course perspective on childhood cheerfulness and its relation to mortality risk. *Personality and Social Psychology Bulletin, 28*(9), 1155–1165. **doi:10.1177/01461672022812001**

Martinez, M. E., & Ward, B. W. (2016). Health care access and utilization among adults aged 18-64, by poverty level: United States, 2013-2015. *National Center for Health Statistics Data Brief, 262*, 1–8.

Martinez, M. E., Ward, B. W., & Adams, P. F. (2015). Health care access and utilization among adults aged 18–64, by race and Hispanic origin: United States, 2013 and 2014. *National Center for Health Statistics Data Brief, 208*, 1–8.

Marván, M. L., & Cortés-Iniestra, S. (2001). Women's beliefs about the prevalence of premenstrual syndrome and biases in recall of premenstrual changes. *Health Psychology, 20*(4), 276–280.

Marvel, M. K., Epstein, R. M., Flowers, K., & Beckman, H. B. (1999). Soliciting the patient's agenda: Have we improved? *Journal of the American Medical Association, 281*, 283–287.

Maslach, C. (1982). Understanding burnout: Definitional issues in analyzing a complex phenomenon. In W. S. Paine (Ed.), *Job stress and burnout* (pp. 29–40). Beverly Hills, CA: Sage.

Maslach, C., & Jackson, S. E. (1982). Burnout in health professions: A social psychological analysis. In G. S. Sanders & J. Suls (Eds.), *Social psychology of health and illness* (pp. 227–251). Hillsdale, NJ: Erlbaum.

Mason, J. W. (1975). A historical view of the stress field. *Journal of Human Stress, 1*(2), 22–36.

Master, S. L., Eisenberger, N. I., Taylor, S. E., Naliboff, B. D., Shirinyan, D., & Lieberman, M. D. (2009). A picture's worth. *Psychological Science, 20*(11), 1316–1318. **https://doi.org/10.1111/j.1467-9280.2009.02444.x**

Masters, R. K., Hummer, R. A., Powers, D. A., Beck, A., Lin, S. F., & Finch, B. K. (2014). Long-term trends in adult mortality for US Blacks and Whites: An examination of period-and cohort-based changes. *Demography, 51*(6), 2047–2073.

Matarazzo, J. D. (1980). Behavioral health and behavioral medicine: Frontiers for a new health psychology. *American Psychologist, 35*(9), 807–817.

Matarazzo, J. D. (1984). Behavioral health: A 1990 challenge for the health sciences professions. In J. D. Matarazzo, S. M. Weiss, J. A. Herd, N. E. Miller, & S. M. Weiss (Eds.), *Behavioral health: A handbook of health enhancement and disease prevention* (pp. 3–40). New York, NY: Wiley.

Mather, M., Jacobsen, L. A., & Pollard, K. M. (2015). Aging in the United States. *Population Reference Bureau, 70*, 1–23.

Mathews, T. J., & Driscoll, A. K. (2017). Trends in infant mortality in the United States, 2005-2014. *National Center for Health Statistics Data Brief, 279*, 1–8.

Mathias, R. A. (2014). Introduction to genetics and genomics in asthma: Genetics of asthma. *Advances in Experimental Medicine and Biology, 795*, 125–155. **doi:10.1007/978-1-4614-8603-9_9**

Matthews, K. A. (1988). Coronary heart disease and type A behaviors: Update on and alternative to the Booth-Kewley and Friedman (1987) quantitative review. *Psychological Bulletin, 104*(3), 373–380.

Matthews, K. A., & Gump, B. B. (2002). Chronic work stress and marital dissolution increase risk of post-trial mortality in men from the Multiple Risk Factor Intervention Trial. *Archives of Internal Medicine, 162*, 309–315.

Matthews, K. A., Gump, B. B., & Owens, J. F. (2001). Chronic stress influences cardiovascular and neuroendocrine responses during acute stress and recovery, especially in men. *Health Psychology, 20*(6), 403–411.

Matthews, K. A., Kuller, L. H., Siegel, J. M., Thompson, M., & Varat, M. (1983). Determinants of decisions to seek medical treatment by patients with acute myocardial infarction symptoms. *Journal of Personality and Social Psychology, 44*(6), 1144–1156.

Matthews, K. A., Owens, J. F., Allen, M. T., & Stoney, C. M. (1992). Do cardiovascular responses to laboratory stress relate to ambulatory blood pressure levels?: Yes, in some of the people, some of the time. *Psychosomatic Medicine, 54*(6), 686–698.

Matthews, K. A., Owens, J. F., Kuller, L. H., Sutton-Tyrrell, K., & Jansen-McWilliams, L. (1998). Are hostility and anxiety associated with carotid atherosclerosis in healthy postmenopausal women? *Psychosomatic Medicine, 60*(5), 633–638.

Matthews, K. A., Räikkönen, K., Gallo, L., & Kuller, L. H. (2008). Association between socioeconomic status and metabolic syndrome in women: Testing the reserve capacity model. *Health Psychology, 27*(5), 576–583.

Matthews, K. A., Shumaker, S. A., Bowen, D. J., Langer, R. D., Hunt, J. R., Kaplan, R. M., . . . Ritenbaugh, C. (1997). Women's Health Initiative: Why now? What is it? What's new? *American Psychologist, 52*(2), 101–116.

Mayer, J. (1980). The best diet is exercise. In P. J. Collipp (Ed.), *Childhood obesity* (2nd ed., pp. 207–222). Littleton, MA: PSG.

Mayer-Davis, E. J., Lawrence, J. M., Dabelea, D., Divers, J., Isom, S., Dolan, L., . . . Wagenknecht, L. (2017). Incidence trends of type 1 and type 2 diabetes among youths, 2002–2012. *New England Journal of Medicine, 376*(15), 1419–1429.

Mayne, S. L., Auchincloss, A. H., Stehr, M. F., Kern, D. M., Navas-Acien, A., Kaufman, J. D., . . . Roux, A. V. D. (2017). Longitudinal associations of local cigarette prices and smoking bans with smoking behavior in the Multi-ethnic Study of Atherosclerosis (MESA). *Epidemiology, 28*(6), 863–871. **doi:10.1097/EDE .0000000000000736**

Mays, V. M., & Cochran, S. D. (1988). Issues in the perception of AIDS risk and risk reduction activities by Black and Hispanic/Latina women. *American Psychologist, 43*(11), 949–957.

Mazzullo, J. M., Lasagna, L., & Griner, P. F. (1974). Variations in interpretation of prescription instructions. *Journal of the American Medical Association, 227*(8), 929–931.

McAllister, T. W., Ford, J. C., Ji, S., Beckwith, J. G., Flashman, L. A., Paulsen, K., & Greenwald, R. M. (2012). Maximum principal strain and strain rate associated with concussion diagnosis correlates with changes in corpus callosum white matter indices. *Annals of Biomedical Engineering, 40*(1), 127–140.

McBride, C. M., Curry, S. J., Grothaus, L. C., Nelson, J. C., Lando, H., & Pirie, P. L. (1998). Partner smoking status and pregnant smoker's perceptions of support for and likelihood of smoking cessation. *Health Psychology, 17*(1), 63–69.

McCaffery, J. M., Papandonatos, G. D., Stanton, C., Lloyd-Richardson, E. E., & Niaura, R. (2008). Depressive symptoms and cigarette smoking in twins from the National Longitudinal Study of Adolescent Health. *Health Psychology, 27*(3), 207–215.

McCanlies, E. C., Mnatsakanova, A., Andrew, M. E., Burchfiel, C. M., & Violanti, J. M. (2014). Positive psychological factors are associated with lower PTSD symptoms among police officers: Post Hurricane Katrina. *Stress and Health, 30*(5), 405–415.

McCann, I. L., & Holmes, D. S. (1984). Influence of aerobic exercise on depression. *Journal of Personality and Social Psychology, 46*(5), 1142–1147.

McCaul, K. D., Branstetter, A. D., Schroeder, D. M., & Glasgow, R. E. (1996). What is the relationship between breast cancer risk and mammography screening? A meta-analytic review. *Health Psychology, 15*(6), 423–449.

McCaul, K. D., & Marlatt, J. M. (1984). Distraction and coping with pain. *Psychological Bulletin, 95*, 516–533.

McCaul, K. D., Schroeder, D. M., & Reid, P. A. (1996). Breast cancer worry and screening: Some prospective data. *Health Psychology, 15*(6), 430–433.

McCaul, M. E., Hutton, H. E., Stephens, M. A. C., Xu, X., & Wand, G. S. (2017). Anxiety, anxiety sensitivity, and perceived stress as predictors of recent drinking, alcohol craving, and social stress response in heavy drinkers. *Alcoholism: Clinical and Experimental Research, 41*(4), 836–845.

McConnell, A. R., Brown, C. M., Shoda, T. M., Stayton, L. E., & Martin, C. E. (2011). Friends with benefits: On the positive consequences of pet ownership. *Journal of Personality and Social Psychology, 101*(6), 1239–1252.

Mccormick, J. (1989). Cervical smears: A questionable practice? *The Lancet, 334*(8656), 207–209.

McCoy, S. B., Gibbons, F. X., Reis, T. J., Gerrard, M., Luus, C. E., & Sufka, A. V. W. (1992). Perceptions of smoking risk as a function of smoking status. *Journal of Behavioral Medicine, 15*(5), 469–488.

McCrady, B. S., Epstein, E. E., & Kahler, C. W. (2004). Alcoholics anonymous and relapse prevention as maintenance strategies after conjoint behavioral alcohol treatment for men: 18-month outcomes. *Journal of Consulting and Clinical Psychology, 72*(5), 870–878.

McCrae, R. R., & Costa, P. T. (1986). Personality, coping, and coping effectiveness in an adult sample. *Journal of Personality, 54*(2), 385–404.

McCrae, R. R., & Costa, P. T. (1987). Validation of the five-factor model of personality across instruments and observers. *Journal of Personality and Social Psychology, 52*(1), 81–90.

McCullough, M., Hoyt, W. T., Larson, D. B., Koenig, H. G., & Thoresen, C. (2000). Religious involvement and mortality. *Health Psychology, 19*(3), 211–222.

Mccutchan, J. A. (1990). Virology, immunology, and clinical course of HIV infection. *Journal of Consulting and Clinical Psychology, 58*(1), 5–12. doi:10.1037/0022-006x.58.1.5

McDonough, M. H., Sabiston, C. M., & Wrosch, C. (2014). Predicting changes in posttraumatic growth and subjective well-being among breast cancer survivors: The role of social support and stress. *Psycho-Oncology, 23*(1), 114–120.

McElroy, S. L., Mitchell, J. E., Wilfley, D., Gasior, M., Ferreira-Cornwell, M. C., McKay, M., . . . Hudson, J. I. (2016). Lisdexamfetamine dimesylate effects on binge eating behaviour and obsessive-compulsive and impulsive features in adults with binge eating disorder. *European Eating Disorders Review, 24*(3), 223–231.

McEwen, B. S. (1998). Seminars in medicine of the Beth Israel Deaconess Medical Center: Protective and damaging effects of stress mediators. *New England Journal of Medicine, 338*(3), 171–179. doi:10.1056/NEJM199801153380307

McEwen, B. S. (2000). The neurobiology of stress: From serendipity to clinical relevance. *Brain Research, 886*(1–2), 172–189. doi:10.1016/S0006-8993(00)02950-4

McEwen, B. S., & Stellar, E. (1993). Stress and the individual: Mechanisms leading to disease. *Archives of Internal Medicine, 153*(18), 2093–2101.

McFadden, S. H. (1995). Religion and well-being in aging persons in an aging society. *Journal of Social Issues, 51*(2), 161–175.

McGregor, M. (1989). Technology and the allocation of the resource. *New England Journal of Medicine, 320*, 118–120.

McGue, M. (1999). The behavioral genetics of alcoholism. *Current Directions in Psychological Science, 8*(4), 109–115.

McIntosh, D. N., Silver, R. C., & Wortman, C. B. (1993). Religion's role in adjustment to a negative life event: Coping with the loss of a child. *Journal of Personality and Social Psychology, 65*(4), 812–821.

McKenna, M. C., Zevon, M. A., Corn, B., & Rounds, J. (1999). Psychosocial factors and the development of breast cancer: A meta-analysis. *Health Psychology, 18*(5), 520–531.

McKinlay, J. B. (1975). A case for re-focusing upstream: The political economy of illness. In A. J. Enelow & J. B. Henderson (Eds.), *Applying behavioral science to cardiovascular risk* (pp. 7–18). Seattle, WA: American Heart Association. doi:10.1037/0278-6133.18.5.520

McKinlay, J. B. (1996). More appropriate evaluation methods for community-level health interventions: Introduction to the special issue. *Evaluation Review, 20*(3), 237–243.

McKinney, C. M., Caetano, R., Harris, T. R., & Ebama, M. S. (2009). Alcohol availability and intimate partner violence among US couples. *Alcoholism: Clinical and Experimental Research, 33*(1), 169–176.

McKinney, C. M., Caetano, R., Rodriguez, L. A., & Okoro, N. (2010). Does alcohol involvement increase the severity of intimate partner violence? *Alcoholism: Clinical and Experimental Research, 34*(4), 655–658.

McLaughlin, K. A., Busso, D. S., Duys, A., Green, J. G., Alves, S., Way, M., & Sheridan, M. A. (2014). Amygdala response to negative stimuli predicts PTSD symptom onset following a terrorist attack. *Depression and Anxiety, 31*(10), 834–842.

McLaughlin, T. J., Aupont, O., Bambauer, K. Z., Stone, P., Mullan, M. G., Colagiovanni, J., . . . Locke, S. E. (2005). Improving psychologic adjustment to chronic illness in cardiac patients. *Journal of General Internal Medicine, 20*(12), 1084–1090.

McLean, H. Q., Fiebelkorn, A. P., Temte, J. L., & Wallace, G. S. (2013). Prevention of measles, rubella, congenital rubella syndrome, and mumps, 2013: Summary recommendations of the Advisory Committee on Immunization Practices (ACIP). *Morbidity and Mortality Weekly Report: Recommendations and Reports, 62*(4), 1–34.

McLean, S., Gomes, B., & Higginson, I. J. (2017). The intensity of caregiving is a more important predictor of adverse bereavement outcomes for adult–child than spousal caregivers of patients who die of cancer. *Psycho-Oncology, 26*(3), 316–322. **https://doi.org/10.1002/pon.4132**

McNeil, B. J., Pauker, S. G., Sox, H. C., Jr., & Tversky, A. (1982). On the elicitation of preferences for alternative therapies. *New England Journal of Medicine, 306*(21), 1259–1262.

McVey, E., Duchesne, J. C., Sarlati, S., O'Neal, M., Johnson, K., & Avegno, J. (2014). Operation CeaseFire–New Orleans: An infectious disease model for addressing community recidivism from penetrating trauma. *Journal of Trauma and Acute Care Surgery, 77*(1), 123–128.

Meadows, J., Jenkinson, S., Catalan, J., & Gazzard, B. (1990). Voluntary HIV testing in the antenatal clinic: Differing uptake rates for individual counselling midwives. *AIDS Care, 2*(3), 229–233.

Mechanic, D. (1972). Social psychologic factors affecting the presentation of bodily complaints. *New England Journal of Medicine, 286*(21), 1132–1139.

Meert, K. L., Donaldson, A. E., Newth, C. L., Harrison, R., Berger, J., Zimmerman, J., . . . Eunice Kennedy Shriver National Institute of Child Health and Human Development Collaborative Pediatric Critical Care Research Network. (2010). Complicated grief and associated risk factors among parents following a child's death in the pediatric intensive care unit. *Archives of Pediatrics & Adolescent Medicine, 164*(11), 1045–1051. **https://doi.org/10.1001/archpediatrics.2010.187**

Meghani, S. H., Byun, E., & Gallagher, R. M. (2012). Time to take stock: A meta-analysis and systematic review of analgesic treatment disparities for pain in the United States. *Pain Medicine, 13*(2), 150–174.

Mehler, P. S. (2010). Medical complications of bulimia nervosa and their treatments. *International Journal of Eating Disorders, 44*(2), 95–104.

Mehler, P. S., & Rylander, M. (2015). Bulimia nervosa – medical complications. *Journal of Eating Disorders, 3*, 12. **http://doi.org/10.1186/s40337-015-0044-4**

Meijer, S. A., Sinnema, G., Bijstra, J. O., Mellenbergh, G. J., & Wolters, W. H. (2000). Social functioning in children with a chronic illness. *The Journal of Child Psychology and Psychiatry and Allied Disciplines, 41*(3), 309–317.

Meijers-Heijboer, H., van Geel, B., van Putten, W. L., Henzen-Logmans, S. C., Seynaeve, C., Menke-Pluymers, M. B., . . . Brekelmans, C. T. (2001). Breast cancer after prophylactic bilateral mastectomy in women with a BRCA1 or BRCA2 mutation. *New England Journal of Medicine, 345*(3), 159–164.

Meissen, G. J., Myers, R. H., Mastromauro, C. A., Koroshetz, W. J., Klinger, K. W., Farrer, L. A., . . . Martin, J. B. (1988). Predictive testing for Huntingtons disease with use of a linked DNA marker. *New England Journal of Medicine, 318*(9), 535–542.

Melamed, S. (2009). Burnout and risk of regional musculoskeletal pain—a prospective study of apparently healthy employed adults. *Stress and Health, 25*(4), 313–321. **https://doi.org/10.1002/smi.1265**

Mellon, S., Janisse, J., Gold, R., Cichon, M., Berry-Bobovski, L., Tainsky, M. A., & Simon, M. S. (2009). Predictors of decision making in families at risk for inherited breast/ovarian cancer. *Health Psychology, 28*(1), 38–47.

Melzack, R. (1993). Labour pain as a model of acute pain. *Pain, 53*, 117–120.

Melzack, R., Taenzer, P., Feldman, P., & Kinch, R. A. (1981). Labour is still painful after prepared childbirth training. *Candian Medical Association Journal, 125*, 357–363.

Melzack, R., & Torgerson, W. S. (1971). On the language of pain. *Anesthesiology, 34*, 50–59.

Melzack, R., & Wall, P. D. (1965). Pain mechanisms: A new theory. *Science, 150*, 971–979.

Melzack, R., & Wall, P. D. (1982). *The challenge of pain.* New York, NY: Basic Books.

Melzack, R., & Wall, P. D. (1988). *The challenge of pain* (2nd ed.). New York, NY: Basic Books.

Mentzer, S. J., & Snyder, M. L. (1982). The doctor and the patient: A psychological perspective. In G. S. Sanders & J. Suls (Eds.), *Social psychology of health and illness* (pp. 161–181). Hillsdale, NJ: Erlbaum.

Menzies, V., & Jallo, N. (2011). Guided imagery as a treatment option for fatigue. *Journal of Holistic Nursing, 29*(4), 279–286. **https://doi.org/10.1177/0898010111412187**

Menzies, V., & Taylor, A. G. (2004). The idea of imagination: An analysis of "imagery." *Advances in Mind-Body Medicine, 20*(2), 4–10.

Mercado, A. C., Carroll, L. J., Cassidy, J. D., & Cote, P. (2000). Coping with neck and low back pain in the general population. *Health Psychology, 19*, 333–338.

Mercken, L., Candel, M., Willems, P., & de Vries, H. (2009). Social influence and selection effects in the context of smoking behavior: Changes during early and mid adolescence. *Health Psychology, 28*(1), 73–82.

Mermelstein, R., Cohen, S., Lichtenstein, E., Baer, J. S., & Kamarck,

T. (1986). Social support and smoking cessation and maintenance. *Journal of Consulting and Clinical Psychology*, *54*(4), 447–453.

Merritt, M. M., Bennett, G. G., Jr., Williams, R. B., Edwards, C. L., & Sollers, J. J., III. (2006). Perceived racism and cardiovascular reactivity and recovery to personally relevant stress. *Health Psychology*, *25*(3), 364–370.

Mertz, K. J., & Weiss, H. B. (2008). Changes in motorcycle-related head injury deaths, hospitalizations, and hospital charges following repeal of Pennsylvania's mandatory motorcycle helmet law. *American Journal of Public Health*, *98*(8), 1464–1467.

Merz, E. L., Fox, R. S., & Malcarne, V. L. (2014). Expressive writing interventions in cancer patients: A systematic review. *Health Psychology Review*, *8*(3), 339–361. **https://doi.org/10.1080/17437199.2 014.882007**

Messina, C. R., Lane, D. S., Glanz, K., West, D. S., Taylor, V., Frishman, W., & Powell, L. (2004). Relationship of social support and social burden to repeated breast cancer screening in the women's health initiative. *Health Psychology*, *23*(6), 582–594.

Meyer, D., Leventhal, H., & Gutmann, M. (1985). Common-sense models of illness: The example of hypertension. *Health Psychology*, *4*(2), 115–135.

Meyerhardt, J. A., Giovannucci, E. L., Ogino, S., Kirkner, G. J., Chan, A. T., Willett, W., & Fuchs, C. S. (2009). Physical activity and male colorectal cancer survival. *Archives of Internal Medicine*, *169*(22), 2102–2108.

Meyerhardt, J. A., Niedzwiecki, D., Hollis, D., Saltz, L. B., Hu, F. B., Mayer, R. J., ... Fuchs, C. S. (2007). Association of dietary patterns with cancer recurrence and survival in patients with stage III colon cancer. *Journal of the American Medical Association*, *298*(7), 754–764. **https://doi.org/10.1001/ jama.298.7.754**

Meyerowitz, B. E., Richardson, J., Hudson, S., & Leedham, B. (1998). Ethnicity and cancer outcomes: Behavioral and psychosocial considerations. *Psychological Bulletin*, *123*, 47–70.

Mez, J., Daneshvar, D. H., Kiernan, P. T., Abdolmohammadi, B., Alvarez, V. E., Huber, B. R., . . . McKee, A. C. (2017). Clinicopathological evaluation of chronic traumatic encephalopathy in players of American football. *Journal of the American Medical Association*, *318*(4), 360–370. **doi:10.1001/jama.2017.8334**

Micali, N., Field, A. E., Treasure, J. L., & Evans, D. M. (2015). Are obesity risk genes associated with binge eating in adolescence? *Obesity*, *23*(8), 1729–1736.

Michael, R. T., Gagnon, J. H., Laumann, E. O., & Kolata, G. (1994). *Sex in America: A definitive survey*. New York, NY: Little, Brown.

Michels, N., Sioen, I., Boone, L., Clays, E., Vanaelst, B., Huybrechts, I., & De Henauw, S. (2015). Cross-lagged associations between children's stress and adiposity: The Children's Body Composition and Stress Study. *Psychosomatic Medicine*, *77*(1), 50–58.

Mickey, R. M., Durski, J., Worden, J. K., & Danigelis, N. L. (1995). Breast cancer screening and associated factors for low-income African-American women. *Preventive Medicine*, *24*(5), 467–476.

Milbury, K., Spelman, A., Wood, C., Matin, S. F., Tannir, N., Jonasch, E., . . . Cohen, L. (2014). Randomized controlled trial of expressive writing for patients with renal cell carcinoma. *Journal of Clinical Oncology*, *32*(7), 663–670. **https://doi.org/10.1200/ JCO.2013.50.3532**

Miller, D. K., Chibnall, J. T., Videen, S. D., & Duckro, P. N. (2005). Supportive-affective group experience for persons with life-threatening illness: Reducing spiritual, psychological, and death-related distress in dying patients. *Journal of Palliative Medicine*, *8*(2), 333–343.

Miller, G. E., & Chen, E. (2010). Harsh family climate in early life presages the emergence of a proinflammatory phenotype in adolescence. *Psychological Science*, *21*(6), 848–856.

Miller, L., Bansal, R., Wickramaratne, P., Hao, X., Tenke, C. E., Weissman, M. M., & Peterson, B. S. (2013). Neuroanatomical correlates of religiosity and spirituality: A study in adults at high and low familial risk for depression. *JAMA Psychiatry*, *71*, 128–135.

Miller, M. F., Barabasz, A. F., & Barabasz, M. (1991). Effects of active alert and relaxation hypnotic inductions on cold pressor pain. *Journal of Abnormal Psychology*, *100*, 223–226.

Miller, M., Lippmann, S. J., Azrael, D., & Hemenway, D. (2007). Household firearm ownership and rates of suicide across the 50 United States. *Journal of Trauma and Acute Care Surgery*, *62*(4), 1029–1034.

Miller, N. E. (1985). The value of behavioral research on animals. *American Psychologist*, *40*(4), 423–440.

Miller, S. M., Brody, D. S., & Summerton, J. (1988). Styles of coping with threat: Implications for health. *Journal of Personality and Social Psychology*, *54*(1), 142–148.

Miller, S. M., & Mangan, C. E. (1983). Interacting effects of information and coping style in adapting to gynecologic stress: Should the doctor tell all? *Journal of Personality and Social Psychology*, *45*(1), 223–236.

Miller, T. Q., Smith, T. W., Turner, C. W., Guijarro, M. L., & Hallet, A. J. (1996). A meta-analytic review of research on hostility and physical health. *Psychological Bulletin*, *119*(2), 322–348.

Miller, T. R., & Spicer, R. S. (2012). Hospital-admitted injury attributable to alcohol. *Alcoholism, Clinical and Experimental Research*, *36*(1), 104–112.

Miller, W. R., & Hester, R. R. (1980). Treating the problem drinker: Modern approaches. In W. R. Miller (Ed.), *The addictive behaviors: Treatment of alcoholism, drug abuse, smoking and obesity* (pp. 11–141). Oxford, UK: Pergamon Press.

Miloh, T., Annunziato, R., Arnon, R., Warshaw, J., Parkar, S., Suchy, F. J., . . . Kerkar, N. (2009). Improved adherence and outcomes for pediatric liver transplant recipients by using text messaging. *Pediatrics, 124*(5), e844–e850. doi:10.1542/peds.2009-0415

Miranda, J., Perez-Stable, E. J., Muñoz, R. F., Hargreaves, W., & Henke, C. J. (1991). Somatization, psychiatric disorder, and stress in utilization of ambulatory medical services. *Health Psychology, 10*(1), 46–51.

Mitchell, J. E. (2015). Medical comorbidity and medical complications associated with binge-eating disorder. *International Journal of Eating Disorders, 49*(3), 319–323.

Mitchell, K. S., Porter, B., Boyko, E. J., & Field, A. E. (2016). Longitudinal associations among posttraumatic stress disorder, disordered eating, and weight gain in military men and women. *American Journal of Epidemiology, 184*(1), 33–48.

Mittelmark, M. B., Murray, D. M., Luepker, R. V., Pechacek, T. F., Pirie, P. L., & Pallonen, U. E. (1987). Predicting experimentation with cigarettes: The childhood antecedents of smoking study (CASS). *American Journal of Public Health, 77*(2), 206–208.

Miyajima, K., Fujisawa, D., Yoshimura, K., Ito, M., Nakajima, S., Shirahase, J., . . . Miyashita, M. (2014). Association between quality of end-of-life care and possible complicated grief among bereaved family members. *Journal of Palliative Medicine, 17*(9), 1025–1031.

Miyashita, M., Morita, T., Sato, K., Hirai, K., Shima, Y., & Uchitomi, Y. (2008). Good Death Inventory: A measure for evaluating good death from the bereaved family member's perspective. *Journal of Pain and Symptom Management, 35*(5), 486–498. https://doi.org/10.1016/j.jpainsymman.2007.07.009

Mo, P. K., & Mak, W. W. (2009). Intentionality of medication non-adherence among individuals living with HIV/AIDS in Hong Kong. *AIDS Care, 21*(6), 785–795. doi:10.1080/09540120802511968

Modica, M., Ferratini, M., Spezzaferri, R., De Maria, R., Previtali, E., & Castiglioni, P. (2014). Gender differences in illness behavior after cardiac surgery. *Journal of Cardiopulmonary Rehabilitation and Prevention, 34*(2), 123–129.

Mohr, C. D., Armeli, S., Tennen, H., Carney, M. A., Affleck, G., & Hromi, A. (2001). Daily interpersonal experiences, context, and alcohol consumption. *Journal of Personality and Social Psychology, 80*(3), 489–500.

Mohr, D. C., Dick, L. P., Russo, D., Pinn, J., Boudewyn, A. C., Likosky, W., & Goodkin, D. E. (1999). The psychosocial impact of multiple sclerosis: Exploring the patient's perspective. *Health Psychology, 18*(4), 376–382.

Mok, L. C., & Lee, I. F.-K. (2008). Anxiety, depression and pain intensity in patients with low back pain who are admitted to acute care hospitals. *Journal of Clinical Nursing, 17*(11), 1471–1480. https://doi.org/10.1111/j.13652702.2007.02037.x

Molloy, G. J., Messerli-Bürgy, N., Hutton, G., Wikman, A., Perkins-Porras, L., & Steptoe, A. (2014). Intentional and unintentional non-adherence to medications following an acute coronary syndrome: A longitudinal study. *Journal of Psychosomatic Research, 76*(5), 430–432. http://doi.org/10.1016/j.jpsychores.2014.02.007

Mols, F., Vingerhoets, A. J. J. M., Coebergh, J. W. W., & van de Poll-Franse, L. V. (2009). Well-being, posttraumatic growth and benefit finding in long-term breast cancer survivors. *Psychology & Health, 24*(5), 583–595. https://doi.org/10.1080/08870440701671362

Monane, M., Bohn, R. L., Gurwitz, J. H., Glynn, R. J., Levin, R., & Avorn, J. (1996). Compliance with anti-hypertensive therapy among elderly Medicaid employees: The rates of age, gender, and race. *American Journal of Public Health, 86*(12), 1805–1808.

Mondanaro, J., Homel, P., Lonner, B., Shepp, J., Lichtenszetin, M., & Loewy, J. (2017). Music therapy increases comfort and reduces pain in patients recovering from spine surgery. *American Journal of Orthopedics (Belle Mead, NJ), 46*(1), E13–E22.

Montgomery, G. H., Bovbjerg, D. H., Schnur, J. B., David, D., Goldfarb, A., Weltz, C. R., . . . Silverstein, J. H. (2007). A randomized clinical trial of a brief hypnosis Intervention to control side effects in breast surgery patients. *Journal of the National Cancer Institute, 99*(17), 1304–1312. https://doi.org/10.1093/jnci/djm106

Montgomery, G. H., Kangas, M., David, D., Hallquist, M. N., Green, S., Bovbjerg, D. H., & Schnur, J. B. (2009). Fatigue during breast cancer radiotherapy: An initial randomized study of cognitive–behavioral therapy plus hypnosis. *Health Psychology, 28*(3), 317–322.

Monti, P. M., Rohsenow, D. J., Rubonis, A. V., Niaura, R. S., Sirota, A. D., Colby, S. M., & Abrams, D. B. (1993). Alcohol cue reactivity: Effects of detoxification and extended exposure. *Journal of Studies on Alcohol, 54*(2), 235–245.

Moody, D. L. B., Waldstein, S. R., Tobin, J., Cassels, A., Schwartz, J. C., & Brondolo, E. (2016). Lifetime racial/ethnic discrimination and ambulatory blood pressure: The moderating effect of age. *Health Psychology, 35*(4), 333–342.

Moonaz, S. H., Bingham, C. O., Wissow, L., & Bartlett, S. J. (2015). Yoga in sedentary adults with arthritis: Effects of a randomized controlled pragmatic trial. *The Journal of Rheumatology, 42*(7), 1194–1202. http://doi.org/10.3899/jrheum.141129

Moos, R. H. (1977). *Coping with physical illness*. New York, NY: Plenum.

Moreno, M. A., & Whitehill, J. M. (2014). Influence of social media on alcohol use in adolescents and young adults. *Alcohol Research: Current Reviews, 36*(1), 91–100.

Moriarty, J., Maguire, A., O'Reilly, D., & McCann, M. (2015). Bereavement after informal caregiving: Assessing mental health burden using linked population data. *American Journal of Public Health*, *105*(8), 1630–1637.

Mori, D., Chaiken, S., & Pliner, P. (1987). "Eating lightly" and the self-presentation of femininity. *Journal of Personality and Social Psychology*, *53*(4), 693–702.

Morin-Major, J. K., Marin, M., Durand, N., Wan, N., Juster, R., & Lupien, S. J. (2016). Facebook behaviors associated with diurnal cortisol in adolescents: Is befriending stressful? *Psychoneuroendocrinology*, *63*, 238–247. **doi:10.1016/j.psyneuen.2015.10.005**

Morisky, D. E., Levine, D. M., Green, L. W., Shapiro, S., Russell, R. P., & Smith, C. R. (1983). Five-year blood pressure control and mortality following health education for hypertensive patients. *American Journal of Public Health*, *73*, 153–162.

Morisky, D. E., Stein, J. A., Chiao, C., Ksobiech, K., & Malow, R. (2006). Impact of a social influence intervention on condom use and sexually transmitted infections among establishment-based female sex workers in the Philippines: A multilevel analysis. *Health Psychology*, *25*(5), 595–603. **http://doi.org/10.1037/0278-6133.25.5.595**

Morozink, J. A., Friedman, E. M., Coe, C. L., & Ryff, C. D. (2010). Socioeconomic and psychosocial predictors of interleukin-6 in the MIDUS national sample. *Health Psychology*, *29*(6), 626–635. **doi:10.1037/a0021360**

Morrell, H. E., Song, A. V., & Halpern-Felsher, B. L. (2010). Predicting adolescent perceptions of the risks and benefits of cigarette smoking: A longitudinal investigation. *Health Psychology*, *29*(6), 610–617.

Morris, A. T., Gabert-Quillen, C., Friebert, S., Carst, N., & Delahanty, D. L. (2016). The indirect effect of positive parenting on the relationship between parent and sibling bereavement outcomes after the death of a child. *Journal of Pain and Symptom Management*, *51*(1), 60–70. **https://doi.org/10.1016/j.jpainsymman.2015.08.011**

Morrongiello, B. A., & Kiriakou, S. (2004). Mothers' home-safety practices for preventing six types of childhood injuries: What do they do, and why? *Journal of Pediatric Psychology*, *29*(4), 285–297.

Morrow, G. R., Asbury, R., Hammon, S., & Dobkin, P. (1992). Comparing the effectiveness of behavioral treatment for chemotherapy-induced nausea and vomiting when administered by oncologists, oncology nurses, and clinical psychologists. *Health Psychology*, *11*(4), 250–256.

Morse, D. S., Edwardsen, E. A., & Gordon, H. S. (2008). Missed opportunities for interval empathy in lung cancer communication. *Archives of Internal Medicine*, *168*(17), 1853–1858. **http://doi.org/10.1001/archinte.168.17.1853**

Morton, P. M., Schafer, M. H., & Ferraro, K. F. (2012). Does childhood misfortune increase cancer risk in adulthood? *Journal of Aging and Health*, *24*(6), 948–984. **https://doi.org/10.1177/0898264312449184**

Moseley, J. B., O'Malley, K., Peterson, N. J., Menke, T. J., Brady, B. A., Kuykendall, D. H., . . . Wray, N. P. (2002). A controlled trial of arthroscopic surgery for osteoarthritis of the knee. *New England Journal of Medicine*, *347*, 81–88.

Moskowitz, J. T. (2003). Positive affect predicts lower risk of AIDS mortality. *Psychosomatic Medicine*, *65*(4), 620–626.

Moskowitz, J. T., Carrico, A. W., Duncan, L. G., Cohn, M. A., Cheung, E. O., Batchelder, A., . . . Folkman, S. (2017). Randomized controlled trial of a positive affect intervention for people newly diagnosed with HIV. *Journal of Consulting and Clinical Psychology*, *85*(5), 409–423. **doi:10.1037/ccp0000188**

Mostofsky, E., Penner, E. A., & Mittleman, M. A. (2014). Outbursts of anger as a trigger of acute cardiovascular events: A systematic review and meta-analysis†. *European Heart Journal*, *35*(21), 1404–1410. **https://doi.org/10.1093/eurheartj/ehu033**

Moum, T. (1995). Screening for disease detection and prevention: Some comments and future perspectives. In R. T. Croyle (Ed.), *Psychosocial effects of screening for disease prevention and detection* (pp. 200–213). New York, NY: Oxford University Press.

Moyer, A. (1997). Psychosocial outcomes of breast-conserving surgery versus mastectomy: A meta-analytic review. *Health Psychology*, *16*, 284–298.

Moyer, A., & Salovey, P. (1996). Psychosocial sequelae of breast cancer and its treatment. *Annals of Behavioral Medicine*, *18*, 110–125.

Moynihan, J. A., & Ader, R. (1996). Psychoneuroimmunology: Animal models of disease. *Psychosomatic Medicine*, *58*(6), 546–558.

Mozaffarian, D., Benjamin, E. J., Go, A. S., Arnett, D. K., Blaha, M. J., Cushman, M., . . . Turner, M. B. (2016). Heart disease and stroke statistics—2016 update. *Circulation*, *133*, e38–e360.

Mueller, A. S., & Abrutyn, S. (2016). Adolescents under pressure: A new Durkheimian framework for understanding adolescent suicide in a cohesive community. *American Sociological Review*, *81*(5), 877–899.

Muennig, P. A., Epstein, M., Li, G., & DiMaggio, C. (2014). The cost-effectiveness of New York City's Safe Routes to School Program. *American Journal of Public Health*, *104*(7), 1294–1299.

Multhaup, M., Seldin, M., Jaffe, A., Lei, X., Kirchner, H., Mondal, P., . . . Feinberg, A. (2015). Mouse-human experimental epigenetic analysis unmasks dietary targets and genetic liability for diabetic phenotypes. *Cell Metabolism*, *21*(1), 138–149. **doi:10.1016/j.cmct.2014.12.014**

Murabito, J. M., Pencina, M. J., Nam, B., D'Agostino, R. B., Sr., Wang, T. J., Lloyd-Jones, D., . . . O'Donnell, C. J. (2005). Sibling cardiovascular disease as a risk factor for cardiovascular disease in middle-aged adults. *Journal of the American Medical Association, 294*(24), 3117–3123. **https://doi.org/10.1001/jama.294.24.3117**

Murdock, K. W., Fagundes, C. P., Peek, M. K., Vohra, V., & Stowe, R. P. (2016). The effect of self-reported health on latent herpesvirus reactivation and inflammation in an ethnically diverse sample. *Psychoneuroendocrinology, 72*, 113–118.

Murphy, S. T., Monahan, J. L., & Miller, L. C. (1998). Inference under the influence: The impact of alcohol and inhibition conflict on women's sexual decision making. *Personality and Social Psychology Bulletin, 24*(5), 517–528.

Murray, D. M., Johnson, C. A., Luepker, R. V., & Mittelmark, M. B. (1984). The prevention of cigarette smoking in children: A comparison of four strategies. *Journal of Applied Social Psychology, 14*(3), 274–288.

Murray, S. B., Anderson, L. K., Cusack, A., Nakamura, T., Rockwell, R., Griffiths, S., & Kaye, W. H. (2015). Integrating family-based treatment and dialectical behavior therapy for adolescent bulimia nervosa: Preliminary outcomes of an open pilot trial. *Eating Disorders, 23*(4), 336–344.

Musick, K., Meier, A., & Flood, S. (2016). How parents fare: Mothers' and fathers' subjective well-being in time with children. *American Sociological Review, 81*(5), 1069–1095. **doi:10.1177/0003122416663917**

Mutterperl, J. A., & Sanderson, C. A. (2002). Mind over matter: Internalization of the thinness norm as a moderator of responsiveness to norm misperception education in college women. *Health Psychology, 21*(5), 519–523.

Myers, H. F., Kagawa-Singer, M., Kumanyika, S. K., Lex, B. W., & Markides, K. S. (1995). Panel III: Behavioral risk factors related to chronic diseases in ethnic minorities. *Health Psychology, 14*(7), 613–621. **doi:10.1037/0278-6133.14.7.613**

Myers, J. (2003). Exercise and cardiovascular health. *Circulation, 107*(1), e2. **https://doi.org/10.1161/01.CIR.0000048890.59383.8D**

Nadkarni, A., Endsley, P., Bhatia, U., Fuhr, D. C., Noorani, A., Naik, A., . . . Velleman, R. (2016). Community detoxification for alcohol dependence: A systematic review. *Drug and Alcohol Review, 36*(3), 389–399.

Nagl, M., Jacobi, C., Paul, M., Beesdo-Baum, K., Höfler, M., Lieb, R., & Wittchen, H. U. (2016). Prevalence, incidence, and natural course of anorexia and bulimia nervosa among adolescents and young adults. *European Child & Adolescent Psychiatry, 25*(8), 903–918.

Nahin, R. L. (2015). Estimates of pain prevalence and severity in adults: United States, 2012. *The Journal of Pain, 16*(8), 769–780. **https://doi.org/10.1016/j.jpain.2015.05.002**

Naimi, T. S., Xuan, Z., Cooper, S. E., Coleman, S. M., Hadland, S. E., Swahn, M. H., & Heeren, T. C. (2016). Alcohol involvement in homicide victimization in the United States. *Alcoholism: Clinical and Experimental Research, 40*(12), 2614–2621.

Nakaya, N., Hansen, P. E., Schapiro, I. R., Eplov, L. F., Saito-Nakaya, K., Uchitomi, Y., & Johansen, C. (2006). Personality traits and cancer survival: A Danish cohort study. *British Journal of Cancer, 95*(2), 146–152.

Namir, S., Alumbaugh, M. J., Fawzy, F. I., & Wolcott, D. L. (1989). The relationship of social support to physical and psychological aspects of AIDS. *Psychology and Health, 3*(2), 77–86.

Nation, M., Crusto, C., Wandersman, A., Kumpfer, K. L., Seybolt, D., Morrissey-Kane, E., & Davino, K. (2003). What works in prevention: Principles of effective prevention programs. *American Psychologist, 58*(6–7), 449–456.

National Center for Health Statistics. (2016). *Wide-ranging online data for epidemiologic research (WONDER)*. Atlanta, GA: CDC.

National Center for Health Statistics. (2017). *Health, United States, 2016: With chartbook on long-term trends in health*. Hyattsville, MD: National Center for Health Statistics.

National Center for Health Statistics. (2006). *Health, United States, 2006, with chartbook on trends in the health of Americans*. Hyattsville, MD: US Government Printing Office.

National Center for Statistics and Analysis. (2017). *Distracted driving: 2015. Traffic Safety Facts: Research Notes, DOT HS 812 381*. Washington, DC: National Highway Traffic Safety Administration.

National Human Genome Research Institute. (2013, December 27). Learning about cystic fibrosis. Retrieved from **https://www.genome.gov/10001213/learning-about-cystic-fibrosis/**

Nayyar, D., & Hwang, S. W. (2015). Cardiovascular health issues in inner city populations. *Canadian Journal of Cardiology, 31*(9), 1130–1138. **https://doi.org/10.1016/j.cjca.2015.04.011**

Ndumele, C. E., Matsushita, K., Lazo, M., Bello, N., Blumenthal, R. S., Gerstenblith, G., . . . Coresh, J. (2016). Obesity and subtypes of incident cardiovascular disease. *Journal of the American Heart Association, 5*(8), pii: e003921. **https://doi.org/10.1161/JAHA.116.003921**

Nederkoorn, C., Houben, K., Hofmann, W., Roefs, A., & Jansen, A. (2010). Control yourself or just eat what you like? Weight gain over a year is predicted by an interactive effect of response inhibition and implicit preference for snack foods. *Health Psychology, 29*(4), 389–393.

Neighbors, C., Lee, C. M., Lewis, M. A., Fossos, N., & Walter, T. (2009). Internet-based personalized feedback to reduce 21st-birthday drinking: a randomized controlled trial of an event-specific prevention intervention. *Journal of Consulting and Clinical Psychology, 77*(1), 51–63. **doi:10.1037/a0014386**

Neighbors, C., Lewis, M. A., Atkins, D. C., Jensen, M. M., Walter, T., Fossos, N., . . . Larimer, M. E. (2010). Efficacy of web-based personalized normative feedback: A two-year randomized controlled trial. *Journal of Consulting and Clinical Psychology*, *78*(6), 898–911. **doi:10.1037/a0020766**

Neighbors, C., Lewis, M. A., Bergstrom, R. L., & Larimer, M. E. (2006). Being controlled by normative influences: Self-determination as a moderator of a normative feedback alcohol intervention. *Health Psychology*, *25*(5), 571–579. **doi:10.1037/0278-6133.25.5.571**

Neilson, K., Ftanou, M., Monshat, K., Salzberg, M., Bell, S., Kamm, M. A., . . . Castle, D. (2016). A controlled study of a group mindfulness intervention for individuals living with inflammatory bowel disease. *Inflammatory Bowel Diseases*, *22*(3), 694–701.

Neimeyer, R. A. (2000). Searching for the meaning of meaning: Grief therapy and the process of reconstruction. *Death Studies*, *24*(6), 541–558. **https://doi.org/10.1080/07481180050121480**

Neufeld, H. N., & Goldbourt, U. (1983). Coronary heart disease: Genetic aspects. *Circulation*, *67*(5), 943–954. **https://doi.org/10.1161/01.CIR.67.5.943**

Neumark-Sztainer, D., Wall, M., Story, M., & Fulkerson, J. A. (2004). Are family meal patterns associated with disordered eating behaviors among adolescents? *Journal of Adolescent Health*, *35*(5), 350–359.

Newlin, D. B., & Thomson, J. B. (1990). Alcohol challenge with sons of alcoholics: A critical review and analysis. *Psychological Bulletin*, *108*(3), 383–402.

Newsom, J. T., & Schulz, R. (1998). Caregiving from the recipient's perspective: Negative reactions to being helped. *Health Psychology*, *17*(2), 172–181.

Ng, B., Dimsdale, J. E., Shragg, G. P., & Deutsch, R. (1996). Ethnic differences in analgesic consumption for postoperative pain. *Psychosomatic Medicine*, *58*, 125–129.

Ng, D. M., & Jeffery, R. W. (2003). Relationships between perceived stress and health behaviors in a sample of working adults. *Health Psychology*, *22*(6), 638–642.

Nicholson, A., Rose, R., & Bobak, M. (2010). Associations between different dimensions of religious involvement and self-rated health in diverse European populations. *Health Psychology*, *29*(2), 227–235.

Nichter, M., & Nichter, M. (1991). Hype and weight. *Medical Anthropology*, *13*(3), 249–284.

Nielsen, K. M., Faergeman, O., Larsen, M. L., & Foldspang, A. (2006). Danish singles have a twofold risk of acute coronary syndrome: Data from a cohort of 138,290 persons. *Journal of Epidemiology and Community Health*, *60*(8), 721–728. **https://doi.org/10.1136/jech.2005.041541**

Nielsen, M. K., Neergaard, M. A., Jensen, A. B., Bro, F., & Guldin, M.-B. (2016). Do we need to change our understanding of anticipatory grief in caregivers? A systematic review of caregiver studies during end-of-life caregiving and bereavement. *Clinical Psychology Review*, *44*, 75–93. **https://doi.org/10.1016/j.cpr.2016.01.002**

Nieto, A., Mazon, A., Pamies, R., Linana, J. J., Lanuza, A., Jiménez, F. O., . . . Nieto F. J. (2007). Adverse effects of inhaled corticosteroids in funded and nonfunded studies. *Archives of Internal Medicine*, *167*(19), 2047–2053. **doi:10.1001/archinte.167.19.2047**

Nigl, A. J. (1984). *Biofeedback and behavioral strategies in pain treatment*. New York, NY: Medical and Scientific Books.

Nihtilä, E., & Martikainen, P. (2008). Institutionalization of older adults after the death of a spouse. *American Journal of Public Health*, *98*(7), 1228–1234. **https://doi.org/10.2105/AJPH.2007.119271**

Nijs, J., Van de Putte, K., Louckx, F., Truijen, S., & De Meirleir, K. (2008). Exercise performance and chronic pain in chronic fatigue syndrome: The role of pain catastrophizing. *Pain Medicine*, *9*(8), 1164–1172. **https://doi.org/10.1111/j.1526-4637.2007.00368.x**

Nikiforov, S. V., & Mamaev, V. B. (1998). The development of sex differences in cardiovascular disease mortality: A historical perspective. *American Journal of Public Health*, *88*, 1348–1353.

Noar, S. M., Hall, M. G., Francis, D. B., Ribisl, K. M., Pepper, J. K., & Brewer, N. T. (2016). Pictorial cigarette pack warnings: A meta-analysis of experimental studies. *Tobacco Control*, *25*(3), 341–354. **http://doi.org/10.1136/tobaccocontrol-2014-051978**

Noble, R. E. (1997). The incidence of parental obesity in overweight individuals. *International Journal of Eating Disorders*, *22*(3), 265–271.

Noland, M. P. (1989). The effects of self-monitoring and reinforcement on exercise adherence. *Research Quarterly for Exercise and Sport*, *60*(3), 216–224.

Nolen-Hoeksema, S., Parker, L. E., & Larson, J. (1994). Ruminative coping with depressed mood following loss. *Journal of Personality and Social Psychology*, *67*, 92–104.

Nordentoft, M., Mortensen, P. B., & Pedersen, C. B. (2011). Absolute risk of suicide after first hospital contact in mental disorder. *Archives of General Psychiatry*, *68*(10), 1058–1064.

Norris, F. H., & Kaniasty, K. (1996). Received and perceived social support in times of stress: A test of the social support deterioration deterrence model. *Journal of Personality and Social Psychology*, *71*(3), 498–511.

Nsamenang, S., & Hirsch, J. (2015). Positive psychological determinants of treatment adherence among primary care patients. *Primary Health Care Research & Development*, *16*(4), 398–406.

Ober, C., & Yao, T. (2011). The genetics of asthma and allergic disease: A 21st century perspective. *Immunological Reviews*, *242*(1), 10–30.

O'Carroll, R. E., Foster, C., McGeechan, G., Sandford, K., & Ferguson, E. (2011). The "ick" factor, anticipated regret, and willingness to become an organ donor. *Health Psychology, 30*(2), 236–245.

Ockene, J. K., Mermelstein, R. J., Bonollo, D. S., Emmons, K. M., Perkins, K. A., Voorhees, C. C., & Hollis, J. F. (2000). Relapse and maintenance issues for smoking cessation. *Health Psychology, 19*(1S), 17–31.

O'Cleirigh, C., Ironson, G., Fletcher, M. A., & Schneiderman, N. (2008). Written emotional disclosure and processing of trauma are associated with protected health status and immunity in people living with HIV/AIDS. *British Journal of Health Psychology, 13*(1), 81–84.

O'Cleirigh, C., Ironson, G., Weiss, A., & Costa, P. T., Jr. (2007). Conscientiousness predicts disease progression (CD4 number and viral load) in people living with HIV. *Health Psychology, 26*(4), 473–480.

O'Connor, D. B., Jones, F., Conner, M., McMillan, B., & Ferguson, E. (2008). Effects of daily hassles and eating style on eating behavior. *Health Psychology, 27*(1), 20–31.

O'Connor, P. (2002). Incidence and patterns of spinal cord injury in Australia. *Accident Analysis & Prevention, 34*(4), 405–415.

O'Connor, R. C., & Nock, M. K. (2014). The psychology of suicidal behaviour. *The Lancet Psychiatry, 1*(1), 73–85.

Odongo, J., Makumbi, T., Kalungi, S., & Galukande, M. (2015). Patient delay factors in women presenting with breast cancer in a low income country. *BMC Research Notes, 8*(467). **doi:10.1186/s13104-015-1438-8.**

O'Donnell, C. R. (1995). Firearm deaths among children and youth. *American Psychologist, 50*(9), 771–776.

O'Donnell, M. P., Schultz, A. B., & Yen, L. (2015). The portion of health care costs associated with lifestyle-related modifiable health risks based on a sample of 223,461 employees in seven industries: The UM-HMRC Study. *Journal of Occupational and Environmental Medicine, 57*(12), 1284–1290.

Ogden, C. L., Carroll, M. D., Fryar, C. D., & Flegal, K. M. (2015). Prevalence of obesity among adults and youth: United States, 2011-2014. *National Center for Health Statistics Data Brief, No. 219.* Hyattsville, MD: National Center for Health Statistics.

Ogden, C. L., Carroll, M. D., Kit, B. K., & Flegal, K. M. (2014). Prevalence of childhood and adult obesity in the United States, 2011-2012. *Journal of the American Medical Association, 311*(8), 806–814.

Ogden, J., Oikonomou, E., & Alemany, G. (2015). Distraction, restrained eating and disinhibition: An experimental study of food intake and the impact of "eating on the go." *Journal of Health Psychology, 22*(1), 39–50.

Ogedegbe, G. O., Boutin-Foster, C., Wells, M. T., Allegrante, J. P., Isen, A. M., Jobe, J. B., & Charlson, M. E. (2012). A randomized controlled trial of positive-affect intervention and medication adherence in hypertensive African Americans. *Archives of Internal Medicine, 172*(4), 322–326. **http://doi.org/10.1001/archinternmed.2011.1307**

O'Hara, R. E., Gibbons, F. X., Gerrard, M., Li, Z., & Sargent, J. D. (2012). Greater exposure to sexual content in popular movies predicts earlier sexual debut and increased sexual risk taking. *Psychological Science, 23*(9), 984–993.

Oken, B. S., Chamine, I., & Wakeland, W. (2015). A systems approach to stress, stressors and resilience in humans. *Behavioural Brain Research, 282*, 144–155. **doi:10.1016/j.bbr.2014.12.047**

Okuyama, T., Endo, C., Seto, T., Kato, M., Seki, N., Akechi, T., . . . Hosaka, T. (2008). Cancer patients' reluctance to disclose their emotional distress to their physicians: A study of Japanese patients with lung cancer. *Psycho-Oncology, 17*(5), 460–465. **doi:10.1002/pon.1255**

Olbrisch, M. E. (1996). Ethical issues in psychological evaluation of patients for organ transplant surgery. *Rehabilitation Psychology, 41*(1), 53–71.

Olbrisch, M. E., Benedict, S. M., Ashe, K., & Levenson, J. L. (2002). Psychological assessment and care of organ transplant patients. *Journal of Consulting and Clinical Psychology, 70*(3), 771–783.

O'Leary, A. (1992). Self-efficacy and health: Behavioral and stress-physiological mediation. *Cognitive Therapy and Research, 16*(2), 229–245.

Olenski, A. R., Abola, M. V., & Jena, A. B. (2015). Do heads of government age more quickly? *British Medical Journal, 351*(8038), 8–10.

Oles, K. S., & Penry, J. K. (1987). Epilepsy. In C. S. Rogers, J. D. McCue, & P. Gal (Eds.), *Managing chronic disease* (pp. 43–57). Oradell, NJ: Medical Economics Books.

Oliveira, A. J., Rostila, M., Saarela, J., & Lopes, C. S. (2014). The influence of bereavement on body mass index: Results from a national Swedish survey. *PLOS ONE, 9*(4), e95201. **https://doi.org/10.1371/journal.pone.0095201**

Olmsted, M. P., Kaplan, A. S., & Rockert, W. (1994). Rate and prediction of relapse in bulimia nervosa. *American Journal of Psychiatry, 151*(5), 738–743.

Olson, D. P., & Windish, D. M. (2010). Communication discrepancies between physicians and hospitalized patients. *Archives of Internal Medicine, 170*(15), 1302–1307. **doi:10.1001/archinternmed.2010.239**

Omalu, B. I., DeKosky, S. T., Hamilton, R. L., Minster, R. L., Kamboh, M. I., Shakir, A. M., & Wecht, C. H. (2006). Chronic encephalopathy in a National Football League player: Part II. *Neurosurgery, 59*(5), 1086–1093. **doi:10.1227/01.NEU.0000245601.69451.2**

Omalu, B. I., Hamilton, R. L., Kamboh, M. I., DeKosky, S. T., & Bailes, J. (2010). Chronic traumatic encephalopathy (CTE) in a National Football League player: Case report and emerging medicolegal practice questions. *Journal of Forensic Nursing, 6*(1), 40–46. doi:10.1111/j.1939-3938.2009.01064.x

Onengut-Gumuscu, S., Chen, W.-M., Burren, O., Cooper, N. J., Quinlan, A. R., Mychaleckyj, J. C., . . . Rich, S. S. (2015). Fine mapping of type 1 diabetes susceptibility loci and evidence for colocalization of causal variants with lymphoid gene enhancers. *Nature Genetics, 47*(4), 381–386. http://doi.org/10.1038/ng.3245

Ormel, J., & Wohlfarth, T. (1991). How neuroticism, long-term difficulties, and life situation change influence psychological distress: A longitudinal model. *Journal of Personality and Social Psychology, 60*(5), 744–755.

Ornish, D., Brown, S. E., Billings, J. H., Scherwitz, L. W., Armstrong, W. T., Ports, T. A., . . . Brand, R. J. (1990). Can lifestyle changes reverse coronary heart disease? The lifestyle heart trial. *The Lancet, 336*(8708), 129–133.

Ornish, D., Scherwitz, L. W., Billings, J. H., Gould, K. L., Merritt, T. A., Sparler, S., . . . Brand, R. J. (1998). Intensive lifestyle changes for reversal of coronary heart disease. *Journal of the American Medical Association, 280*(23), 2001–2007.

Ornstein, K. A., Aldridge, M. D., Garrido, M. M., Gorges, R., Meier, D. E., & Kelley, A. S. (2015). Association between hospice use and depressive symptoms in surviving spouses. *JAMA Internal Medicine, 175*(7), 1138–1146. https://doi.org/10.1001/jamainternmed.2015.1722

Ortega, D. F., & Pipal, J. E. (1984). Challenge seeking and the type A coronary-prone behavior pattern. *Journal of Personality and Social Psychology, 46*(6), 1328–1334.

Ortega, F. B., Lee, D., Katzmarzyk, P. T., Ruiz, J. R., Sui, X., Church, T. S., & Blair, S. N. (2013). The intriguing metabolically healthy but obese phenotype:

Cardiovascular prognosis and role of fitness. *European Heart Journal, 34*(5), 389–397. http://doi.org/10.1093/eurheartj/ehs174

Orth-Gomér, K., Wamala, S. P., Horsten, M., Schenck-Gustafsson, K., Schneiderman, N., & Mittleman, M. A. (2000). Marital stress worsens prognosis in women with coronary heart disease: The stockholm female coronary risk study. *Journal of the American Medical Association, 284*(23), 3008–3014.

Otten, M. W., Jr., Zaidi, A. A., Wroten, J. E., Witte, J. J., & Peterman, T. A. (1993). Changes in sexually transmitted disease rates after HIV testing and posttest counseling, Miami, 1988 to 1989. *American Journal of Public Health, 83*(4), 529–533.

Otten, R., Bricker, J. B., Liu, J., Comstock, B. A., & Peterson, A. V. (2011). Adolescent psychological and social predictors of young adult smoking acquisition and cessation: A 10-year longitudinal study. *Health Psychology, 30*(2), 163–170.

Otten, R., van Lier, P. A., & Engels, R. C. (2011). Disentangling two underlying processes in the initial phase of substance use: Onset and frequency of use in adolescent smoking. *Addictive Behaviors, 36*(3), 237–240.

Outcalt, S. D., Kroenke, K., Krebs, E. E., Chumbler, N. R., Wu, J., Yu, Z., & Bair, M. J. (2015). Chronic pain and comorbid mental health conditions: Independent associations of posttraumatic stress disorder and depression with pain, disability, and quality of life. *Journal of Behavioral Medicine, 38*(3), 535–543.

Oxman, T. E., Freeman, D. H., & Manheimer, E. D. (1995). Lack of social participation or religious strength and comfort as risk factors for death after cardiac surgery in the elderly. *Psychosomatic Medicine, 57*(1), 5–15.

Pacak, K., Palkovits, M., Yadid, G., Kvetnansky, R., Kopin, I. J., & Goldstein, D. S. (1998). Heterogeneous neurochemical responses to different stressors:

A test of Selye's doctrine of nonspecificity. *The American Journal of Physiology, 275*(4), 1247–1256.

Pacelli, B., Carretta, E., Spadea, T., Caranci, N., Di Felice, E., Stivanello, E., . . . Fantini, M. P. (2014). Does breast cancer screening level health inequalities out? A population-based study in an Italian region. *The European Journal of Public Health, 24*(2), 280–285.

Page, N., Sivarajasingam, V., Matthews, K., Heravi, S., Morgan, P., & Shepherd, J. (2016). Preventing violence-related injuries in England and Wales: A panel study examining the impact of on-trade and off-trade alcohol prices. *Injury Prevention, 23*(1), 33–39.

Pakenham, K. I. (1999). Adjustment to multiple sclerosis: Application of a stress and coping model. *Health Psychology, 18*(4), 383–392.

Pakenham, K. I. (2005). Benefit finding in multiple sclerosis and associations with positive and negative outcomes. *Health Psychology, 24*(2), 123–132.

Pakenham, K. I., Dadds, M. R., & Terry, D. J. (1994). Relationship between adjustment to HIV and both social support and coping. *Journal of Consulting and Clinical Psychology, 62*(6), 1194–1203.

Pakpour, A., Gellert, P., Asefzadeh, S., Updegraff, J. A., Molloy, G. J., & Sniehotta, F. F. (2014). Motivation and planning predict medication adherence following coronary artery bypass graft surgery. *Journal of Psychosomatic Research, 77*, 287–295.

Palermo, T. M., & Drotar, D. (1996). Prediction of children's postoperative pain: The role of presurgical expectations and anticipatory emotions. *Journal of Pediatric Psychology, 21*(5), 683–698.

Pan, A., Sun, Q., Okereke, O. I., Rexrode, K. M., & Hu, F. B. (2011). Depression and risk of stroke morbidity and mortality: A meta-analysis and systematic review. *Journal of the American Medical Association, 306*(11), 1241–1249.

Papadatou, D. (1997). Training health proessionals in caring for dying children and grieving families. *Death Studies, 21*(6), 575–600. https://doi.org/10.1080/074811897201787

Papaioannou, M., Skapinakis, P., Damigos, D., Mavreas, V., Broumas, G., & Palgimesi, A. (2009). The role of catastrophizing in the prediction of postoperative pain. *Pain Medicine, 10*(8), 1452–1459.

Pargament, K. I. (1997). *The psychology of religion and coping: Theory, research, practice.* New York, NY: Guilford Press. https://doi.org/10.1111/j.1526-4637.2009.00730.x

Park, A., Zid, D., Russell, J., Malone, A., Rendon, A., Wehr, A., & Li, X. (2013). Effects of a formal exercise program on Parkinson's disease: A pilot study using a delayed start design. *Parkinsonism and Related Disorders, 30*, 1–6.

Park, S. H., & Mattson, R. H. (2009). Therapeutic influences of plants in hospital rooms on surgical recovery. *HortScience, 44*(1), 102–105.

Parker, J. C. (1995). Stress management. In P. M. Nicassio & T. W. Smith (Eds.), *Managing chronic illness: A biopsychosocial perspective* (pp. 285–312). Washington, DC: American Psychological Association.

Parker, P. A., & Kulik, J. A. (1995). Burnout, self-and supervisor-rated job performance, and absenteeism among nurses. *Journal of Behavioral Medicine, 18*(6), 581–599.

Parks, K. A., Frone, M. R., Muraven, M., & Boyd, C. (2017). Nonmedical use of prescription drugs and related negative sexual events: Prevalence estimates and correlates in college students. *Addictive Behaviors, 65*, 258–263.

Parr, M. N., Ross, L. A., McManus, B., Bishop, H. J., Wittig, S. M., & Stavrinos, D. (2016). Differential impact of personality traits on distracted driving behaviors in teens and older adults. *Accident Analysis & Prevention, 92*, 107–112.

Parschau, L., Barz, M., Richert, J., Knoll, N., Lippke, S., & Schwarzer, R. (2014). Physical activity among adults with obesity: Testing the health action process approach. *Rehabilitation Psychology, 59*(1), 42–49. doi:10.1037/a0035529

Parsons, J. T., Rosof, E., & Mustanski, B. (2008). The temporal relationship between alcohol consumption and HIV-medication adherence: A multilevel model of direct and moderating effects. *Health Psychology, 27*(5), 628–637. http://doi.org/10.1037/a0012664

Parsons, O. A. (1977). Neuropsychological deficits in alcoholics: Facts and fancies. *Alcoholism: Clinical and Experimental Research, 1*(1), 51–56.

Parsons, T. (1951). Illness and the role of the physician: A sociological perspective. *American Journal of Orthopsychiatry, 21*(3), 452–460.

Parsons, T. (1975). The sick role and the role of the physician reconsidered. *The Milbank Memorial Fund Quarterly. Health and Society, 53*(3), 257–278.

Pasulka, J., Jayanthi, N., McCann, A., Dugas, L. R., & LaBella, C. (2017). Specialization patterns across various youth sports and relationship to injury risk. *The Physician and Sportsmedicine, 45*(3), 344–352. doi:10.1080/00913847.2017.1313077

Patenaude, A. F., Guttmacher, A. E., & Collins, F. S. (2002). Genetic testing and psychology: New roles, new responsibilities. *American Psychologist, 57*(4), 271–282. doi:10.1037/0003-066X.57.4.271

Patlamazoglou, L., Simmonds, J. G., & Snell, T. L. (2017). Same-sex partner bereavement. *OMEGA – Journal of Death and Dying.* doi:10.1177/0030222817690160

Patterson, T. L., Shaw, W. S., Semple, S. J., Cherner, M., McCutchan, J. A., Atkinson, J. H., . . . HIV Neurobehavioral Research Center (HNRC) Group. (1996). Relationship of psychosocial factors to HIV disease progression. *Annals of Behavioral Medicine, 18*(1), 30–39.

Paul, L. A., Felton, J. W., Adams, Z. W., Welsh, K., Miller, S., & Ruggiero, K. J. (2015). Mental health among adolescents exposed to a tornado: The influence of social support and its interactions with sociodemographic characteristics and disaster exposure. *Journal of Traumatic Stress, 28*(3), 232–239.

Pavlov, I. (1927). *Conditioned reflexes.* Oxford, UK: Oxford University Press.

Paxton, S. J., Wertheim, E. H., Gibbons, K., Szmukler, G. I., Hillier, L., & Petrovich, J. L. (1991). Body image satisfaction, dieting beliefs, and weight loss behaviors in adolescent girls and boys. *Journal of Youth and Adolescence, 20*(3), 361–379.

Payne, A., & Blanchard, E. B. (1995). A controlled comparison of cognitive therapy and self-help support groups in the treatment of irritable bowel syndrome. *Journal of Consulting and Clinical Psychology, 63*(5), 779–786.

Pearl, R. L., & Lebowitz, M. S. (2014). Beyond personal responsibility: Effects of causal attributions for overweight and obesity on weight-related beliefs, stigma, and policy support. *Psychology & Health, 29*(10), 1176–1191.

Pearlman, R., Frankel, W. L., Swanson, B., Zhao, W., Yilmaz, A., Miller, K., . . . Hampel, H. (2017). Prevalence and spectrum of germline cancer susceptibility gene mutations among patients with early-onset colorectal cancer. *JAMA Oncology, 3*(4), 464–471.

Pearson, T. A. (1996). Alcohol and heart disease. *Circulation, 94*(11), 3023–3025. https://doi.org/10.1161/01.CIR.94.11.3023

Pechmann, C. (1997). Does antismoking advertising combat underage smoking: A review of past practices and research. In M. E. Goldberg, M. Fishbein, & S. E. Middlestadt (Eds.), *Social marketing: Theoretical and practical perspectives* (pp. 189–216). Mahwah, NJ: Lawrence Erlbaum Associates Publishers.

Pechmann, C., & Reibling, E. T. (2006). Antismoking advertisements for youths: An independent evaluation of health, counter-industry, and industry approaches. *American Journal of Public Health, 96*(5), 906–913.

Pechmann, C., & Shih, C. F. (1999). Smoking scenes in movies and anti-smoking advertisements before movies: Effects on youth. *The Journal of Marketing, 63*(3), 1–13.

Peña-Oliver, Y., Carvalho, F. M., Sanchez-Roige, S., Quinlan, E. B., Jia, T., Walker-Tilley, T., . . . Bokde, A. L. (2016). Mouse and human genetic analyses associate kalirin with ventral striatal activation during impulsivity and with alcohol misuse. *Frontiers in Genetics, 7*(52). **doi:10.3389/fgene.2016.00052.**

Pendleton, D., & Bochner, S. (1980). The communciation of medical information as a function of patients' social class. *Social Science and Medicine, 14A,* 669–673.

Penley, J. A., Tomaka, J., & Wiebe, J. S. (2002). The association of coping to physical and psychological health outcomes: A meta-analytic review. *Journal of Behavioral Medicine, 25*(6), 551–603.

Pennebaker, J. W. (1982). *The psychology of physical symptoms*. New York, NY: Springer-Verlag.

Pennebaker, J. W. (1989). Confession, inhibition and disease. *Advances in Experimental Social Psychology, 22,* 211–244.

Pennebaker, J. W., & Beall, S. K. (1986). Confronting a traumatic event: Toward an understanding of inhibition and disease. *Journal of Abnormal Psychology, 95*(3), 274–281.

Pennebaker, J. W., Hughes, C. F., & O'Heeron, R. C. (1987). The psychophysiology of confession: Linking inhibitory and psychosomatic processes. *Journal of Personality and Social Psychology, 52*(4), 781–791.

Pennebaker, J. W., & O'Heeron, R. C. (1984). Confiding in others and illness rate among spouses of suicide and accidental-death victims. *Journal of Abnormal Psychology, 93*(4), 473–476.

Pennebaker, J. W., & Skelton, J. (1981). Selective monitoring of bodily sensations. *Journal of Personality and Social Psychology, 41,* 213–223.

Pepper, J. K., Ribisl, K. M., & Brewer, N. T. (2016). Adolescents' interest in trying flavoured e-cigarettes. *Tobacco Control, 25,* ii62–ii66.

Péquignot, R., Dufouil, C., Prugger, C., Pérès, K., Artero, S., Tzourio, C., & Empana, J.-P. (2016). High level of depressive symptoms at repeated study visits and risk of coronary heart disease and stroke over 10 years in older adults: The three-city study. *Journal of the American Geriatrics Society, 64*(1), 118–125. **doi:10.1111/jgs.13872**

Pergament, K. I. (1997). *The psychology of religion and coping: Theory, research, practice*. London, UK: Guilford.

Periyakoil, V. S., Kraemer, H., & Neri, E. (2016). Multi-ethnic attitudes toward physician-assisted death in California and Hawaii. *Journal of Palliative Medicine, 19*(10), 1060–1065. **https://doi .org/10.1089/jpm.2016.0160**

Perkins, H. S., Cortez, J. D., & Hazuda, H. P. (2009). Cultural beliefs about a patient's right time to die: An exploratory study. *Journal of General Internal Medicine, 24*(11), 1240–1247. **https:// doi.org/10.1007/s11606-009-1115-5**

Perri, M. G., Martin, A. D., Leermakers, E. A., Sears, S. F., & Notelovitz, M. (1997). Effects of group-versus home-based exercise in the treatment of obesity. *Journal of Consulting and Clinical Psychology, 65*(2), 278–285.

Persky, V. W., Kempthorne-Rawson, J., & Shekelle, R. B. (1987). Personality and risk of cancer: 20-year follow-up of the Western Electric Study. *Psychosomatic Medicine, 49,* 435–439.

Pestinger, M., Stiel, S., Elsner, F., Widdershoven, G., Voltz, R., Nauck, F., & Radbruch, L. (2015). The desire to hasten death: Using grounded theory for a better understanding "When perception of time tends

to be a slippery slope." *Palliative Medicine, 29*(8), 711–719. **https://doi .org/10.1177/0269216315577748**

Peters, E., Baker, D. P., Dieckmann, N. F., Leon, J., & Collins, J. (2010). Explaining the effect of education on health: A field study in Ghana. *Psychological Science, 21*(10), 1369–1376.

Peters, M. N., Moscona, J. C., Katz, M. J., Deandrade, K. B., Quevedo, H. C., Tiwari, S., . . . Irimpen, A. M. (2014). Natural disasters and myocardial infarction: The six years after Hurricane Katrina. *Mayo Clinic Proceedings, 89*(4), 472–478. **doi:10.1016/j .mayocp.2013.12.013**

Peters, S., Rogers, A., Salmon, P., Gask, L., Dowrick, C., Towey, M., . . . Morriss, R. (2009). What do patients choose to tell their doctors? Qualitative analysis of potential barriers to reattributing medically unexplained symptoms. *Journal of General Internal Medicine, 24*(4), 443–449.

Peters, S. A., Huxley, R. R., & Woodward, M. (2014). Diabetes as a risk factor for stroke in women compared with men: A systematic review and meta-analysis of 64 cohorts, including 775,385 individuals and 12,539 strokes. *The Lancet, 383*(993), 1973–1980. **doi:10.1016/S0140-6736(14)60040-4**

Peterson, C. (2000). The future of optimism. *American Psychologist, 55*(1), 44–55. **doi:10.1037/0003-066X.55.1.44**

Peterson, C., & Seligman, M. E. (1987). Explanatory style and illness. *Journal of Personality, 55*(2), 237–265.

Peterson, C., Seligman, M. E., & Vaillant, G. E. (1988). Pessimistic explanatory style is a risk factor for physical illness: A thirty-five-year longitudinal study. *Journal of Personality and Social Psychology, 55*(1), 23–27.

Peterson, C., Seligman, M. E., Yurko, K. H., Martin, L. R., & Friedman, H. S. (1998). Catastrophizing and untimely death. *Psychological Science, 9*(2), 127–130.

Peterson, J. L., & Marin, G. (1988). Issues in the prevention of AIDS among Black and Hispanic men. *American Psychologist, 43*(11), 871–877.

Petrie, K. J., Booth, R. J., & Pennebaker, J. W. (1998). The immunological effects of thought suppression. *Journal of Personality and Social Psychology, 75*(5), 1264–1272.

Petrie, K. J., Fontanilla, I., Thomas, M. G., Booth, R. J., & Pennebaker, J. W. (2004). Effect of written emotional expression on immune function in patients with human immunodeficiency virus infection: A randomized trial. *Psychosomatic Medicine, 66*(2), 272–275.

Petry, N. M., Martin, B., Cooney, J. L., & Kranzler, H. R. (2000). Give them prizes and they will come: Contingency management for treatment of alcohol dependence. *Journal of Consulting and Clinical Psychology, 68*(2), 250–257.

Petterson, H., & Olson, B. L. (2016). Effects of mindfulness-based interventions in high school and college athletes for reducing stress and injury, and improving quality of life. *Journal of Sport Rehabilitation*, pp. 1–18.

Pettingale, K. W., Morris, T., Greer, S., & Haybittle, J. L. (1985). Mental attitudes to cancer: An additional prognostic factor. *Lancet, 1*(8431), 750.

Pew Research Center (2015, May 11). *Religious landscape study*. Retrieved from **http://www.pewforum.org/religious-landscape-study/belief-in-god/**

Phelan, C. M., Kuchenbaecker, K. B., Tyrer, J. P., Kar, S. P., Lawrenson, K., Winham, S. J., . . . Chornokur, G. (2017). Identification of 12 new susceptibility loci for different histotypes of epithelial ovarian cancer. *Nature Genetics, 49*(5), 680–691. **doi:10.1038/ng.3826**

Phelps, A. C., Maciejewski, P. K., Nilsson, M., Balboni, T. A., Wright, A. A., Paulk, M. E., . . . Prigerson, H. G. (2009). Association between religious coping and use of intensive life-prolonging care near death among patients with advanced cancer. *Journal of*

the *American Medical Association, 301*(11), 1140–1147. **http://doi.org/10.1001/jama.2009.341**

Phillips, D. P. (1982). The impact of fictional television stories on US adult fatalities: New evidence on the effect of the mass media on violence. *American Journal of Sociology, 87*(6), 1340–1359.

Phillips, D. P., & Carstensen, L. L. (1986). Clustering of teenage suicides after television news stories about suicide. *New England Journal of Medicine, 315*(11), 685–689.

Pike, K. M., & Dunne, P. E. (2015). The rise of eating disorders in Asia: A review. *Journal of Eating Disorders, 3*, 33. **https://doi.org/10.1186/s40337-015-0070-2**

Pike, K. M., & Striegel-Moore, R. H. (1997). Disordered eating and eating disorders. In S. J. Gallant, G. P. Keita, & R. Royak-Schaler (Eds.), *Health care for women* (pp. 97–114). Washington, DC: American Psychological Association.

Pilkington, S. (2013). Causes and consequences of sleep deprivation in hospitalised patients. *Nursing Standard, 27*(49) 35–42.

Pinto, R. P., & Hollandsworth, J. G. (1989). Using videotape modeling to prepare children psychologically for surgery: Influence of parents and costs versus benefits of providing preparation services. *Health Psychology, 8*(1), 79–95.

Pirkis, J., Too, S. L., Spittal, M. J., Krysinska, K., Robinson, J., & Cheung, Y. T. D. (2015). Interventions to reduce suicides at suicide hotspots: A systematic review and meta-analysis. *The Lancet Psychiatry, 2*(11), 994–1001.

Pischke, C. R., Scherwitz, L., Weidner, G., & Ornish, D. (2008). Long-term effects of lifestyle changes on well-being and cardiac variables among coronary heart disease patients. *Health Psychology, 27*(5), 584–592. **doi:10.1037/0278-6133.27.5.584**

Pitman, A. L., Osborn, D. P., Rantell, K., & King, M. B. (2016). Bereavement

by suicide as a risk factor for suicide attempt: A cross-sectional national UK-wide study of 3432 young bereaved adults. *BMJ Open, 6*(1). **doi:10.1136/bmjopen-2015-009948**

Pitts, S. B. J., Keyserling, T. C., Johnston, L. F., Smith, T. W., McGuirt, J. T., Evenson, K. R., . . . Ammerman, A. S. (2015). Associations between neighborhood-level factors related to a healthful lifestyle and dietary intake, physical activity, and support for obesity prevention polices among rural adults. *Journal of Community Health, 40*(2), 276–284.

Placek, P. J., Taffel, S. M., & Moien, M. (1988). 1986 C-sections rise; VBACs inch upward. *American Journal of Public Health, 78*(5), 562–563.

Plante, T. G., & Sherman, A. C. (Eds.). (2001). *Faith and health: Psychological perspectives*. New York, NY: Guilford.

Plesh, O., Adams, S., & Gansky, S. (2011). Racial/ethnic and gender prevalences in reported common pains in a national sample. *Journal of Orofacial Pain, 25*(1), 25–31.

Plous, S. (1996a). Attitudes toward the use of animals in psychological research and education: Results from a national survey of psychologists. *American Psychologist, 51*(11), 1167–1180.

Plous, S. (1996b). Attitudes toward the use of animals in psychological research and education: Results from a national survey of psychology majors. *Psychological Science, 7*(6), 352–358.

Poijula, S., Wahlberg, K. E., & Dyregrov, A. (2001). Adolescent suicide and suicide contagion in three secondary schools. *International Journal of Emergency Mental Health, 3*(3), 163–170.

Pollak, K. I., Alexander, S. C., Coffman, C. J., Tulsky, J. A., Lyna, P., Dolor, R. J., . . . Østbye, T. (2010). Physician communication techniques and weight loss in adults: Project CHAT. *American Journal of Preventive Medicine, 39*(4), 321–328. **http://doi.org/10.1016/j.amepre.2010.06.005**

Polnay, A., James, V. A. W., Hodges, L., Murray, G. D., Munro, C., & Lawrie, S. M. (2014). Group therapy for people with bulimia nervosa: Systematic review and meta-analysis. *Psychological Medicine*, 44(11), 2241–2254.

Polusny, M. A., & Follette, V. M. (1995). Long-term correlates of child sexual abuse: Theory and review of the empirical literature. *Applied and Preventive Psychology*, 4(3), 143–166.

Pomerleau, O. F., Collins, A. C., Shiffman, S., & Pomerleau, C. S. (1993). Why some people smoke and others do not: New perspectives. *Journal of Consulting and Clinical Psychology*, 61(5), 723–731.

Pomerleau, O. F., & Pomerleau, C. S. (1989). A biobehavioral perspective on smoking. In T. Ney & A. Gale (Eds.), *Smoking and human behavior* (pp. 69–90). Oxford, UK: John Wiley & Sons.

Pope, H. G., Olivardia, R., Gruber, A., & Borowiecki, J. (1999). Evolving ideals of male body image as seen through action toys. *International Journal of Eating Disorders*, 26(1), 65–72.

Portanova, J., Irvine, K., Yi, J. Y., & Enguidanos, S. (2015). It isn't like this on TV: Revisiting CPR survival rates depicted on popular TV shows. *Resuscitation*, 96, 148–150.

Poston, W. S., Ericsson, M., Linder, J., Nilsson, T., Goodrick, G. K., & Foreyt, J. P. (1999). Personality and the prediction of weight loss and relapse in the treatment of obesity. *International Journal of Eating Disorders*, 25(3), 301–309.

Powell, H., Krall, J. R., Wang, Y., Bell, M. L., & Peng, R. D. (2015). Ambient coarse particulate matter and hospital admissions in the Medicare Cohort Air Pollution Study, 1999–2010. *Environmental Health Perspectives*, 123(11), 1152–1158. https://doi.org/10.1289/ehp.1408720

Powell, L. M., Szczypka, G., Chaloupka, F. J., & Braunschweig, C. L. (2007). Nutritional content of television food advertisements seen by children and adolescents in the United States. *Pediatrics*, 120(3), 576–583.

Prat, J., Ribé, A., & Gallardo, A. (2005). Hereditary ovarian cancer. *Human Pathology*, 36(8), 861–870. https://doi.org/10.1016/j.humpath.2005.06.006

Prather, A. A., Janicki-Deverts, D., Hall, M. H., & Cohen, S. (2015). Behaviorally assessed sleep and susceptibility to the common cold. *Sleep*, 38(9), 1353–1359.

Préau, M., Bouhnik, A. D., Roussiau, N., Lert, F., & Spire, B. (2008). Disclosure and religion among people living with HIV/AIDS in France. *AIDS Care*, 20(5), 521–526. doi:10.1080/09540120701867230

Prentice, D. A., & Miller, D. T. (1993). Pluralistic ignorance and alcohol use on campus: Some consequences of misperceiving the social norm. *Journal of Personality and Social Psychology*, 64(2), 243–256.

Prescott, C. A., Neale, M. C., Corey, L. A., & Kendler, K. S. (1997). Predictors of problem drinking and alcohol dependence in a population-based sample of female twins. *Journal of Studies on Alcohol*, 58(2), 167–181.

Pressman, S. D., & Cohen, S. (2005). Does positive affect influence health? *Psychological Bulletin*, 131(6), 925–971.

Prestwich, A., Perugini, M., & Hurling, R. (2010). Can implementation intentions and text messages promote brisk walking? A randomized trial. *Health Psychology*, 29(1), 40–49.

Prochaska, J. J., & Benowitz, N. L. (2016). The past, present, and future of nicotine addiction therapy. *Annual Review of Medicine*, 67, 467–486.

Prochaska, J. O., DiClemente, C. C., & Norcross, J. C. (1992). In search of how people change: Applications to addictive behaviors. *American Psychologist*, 47(9), 1102–1114.

Prochaska, J. O., DiClemente, C. C., Velicer, W. F., & Rossi, J. S. (1993). Standardized, individualized, interactive, and personalized self-help programs for smoking cessation. *Health Psychology*, 12(5), 399–405.

Prochaska, J. O., & Velicer, W. F. (1997). The transtheoretical model of health behavior change. *American Journal of Health Promotion*, 12(1), 38–48.

Prochaska, J. O., Velicer, W. F., Rossi, J. S., Goldstein, M. G., Marcus, B. H., Rakowski, W., . . . Rossi, S. R. (1994). Stages of change and decisional balance for 12 problem behaviors. *Health Psychology*, 13(1), 39–46.

Procopio, M., & Marriott, P. (2007). Intrauterine hormonal environment and risk of developing anorexia nervosa. *Archives of General Psychiatry*, 64(12), 1402–1407.

Proctor, B. D., Semega, J. L., & Kollar, M. A. (2016). *US Census Bureau, current population reports, P60-256 (RV): Income and poverty in the United States: 2015.* Washington, DC: U.S. Government Printing Office.

Prohaska, T. R., Keller, M. L., Leventhal, E. A., & Leventhal, H. (1987). Impact of symptoms and aging attribution on emotions and coping. *Health Psychology*, 6(6), 495–514.

Provencal, N., & Binder, E. B. (2015). The neurobiological effects of stress as contributors to psychiatric disorders: Focus on epigenetics. *Current Opinion in Neurobiology*, 30(3), 1–37. doi:10.1016/j.conb.2014.08.007

Psaty, B. M., Koepsell, T. D., Wagner, E. H., LoGerfo, J. P., & Inui, T. S. (1990). The relative risk of incident coronary heart disease associated with recently stopping the use of β-blockers. *Journal of the Amercian Medical Association*, 263(12), 1653–1657. doi:10.1001/jama.1990.03440120075040

Ptacek, J. T., Smith, R. E., & Zanas, J. (1992). Gender, appraisal, and coping: A longitudinal analysis. *Journal of Personality*, 60(4), 747–770.

Pulkki-Råback, L., Elovainio, M., Kivimäki, M., Raitakari, O. T., & Keltikangas-Järvinen, L. (2005).

Temperament in childhood predicts body mass in adulthood: The cardiovascular risk in young Finns Study. *Health Psychology, 24*(3), 307–315.

Purohit, V., Khalsa, J., & Serrano, J. (2005). Mechanisms of alcohol-associated cancers: Introduction and summary of the symposium. *Alcohol, 35*(3), 155–160. https://doi.org/10.1016/j.alcohol.2005.05.001

Puzziferri, N., Zigman, J. M., Thomas, B. P., Mihalakos, P., Gallagher, R., Lutter, M., . . . Tamminga, C. A. (2016). Brain imaging demonstrates a reduced neural impact of eating in obesity. *Obesity, 24*(4), 829–836.

Quartana, P. J., Burns, J. W., & Lofland, K. R. (2007). Attentional strategy moderates effects of pain catastrophizing on symptom-specific physiological responses in chronic low back pain patients. *Journal of Behavioral Medicine, 30*(3), 221–231. https://doi.org/10.1007/s10865-007-9101-z

Quick, J. C. (1999). Occupational health psychology: Historical roots and future directions. *Health Psychology, 18*(1), 82–88.

Quittner, A. L., Espelage, D. L., Opipari, L. C., Carter, B., Eid, N., & Eigen, H. (1998). Role strain in couples with and without a child with a chronic illness: Associations with marital satisfaction, intimacy, and daily mood. *Health Psychology, 17*(2), 112–124.

Rabin, B. S. (1999). *Stress, immune function, and health: The connection.* New York, NY: Wiley.

Rabin, B. S. (2000). Changes in the immune system during aging. In S. B. Manuck (Ed.), *Behavior, health, and aging* (pp. 59–68). Mahwah, NJ: Erlbaum.

Rabins, P. V., Fitting, M. D., Eastham, J., & Zabora, J. (1990). Emotional adaptation over time in care-givers for chronically ill elderly people. *Age and Ageing, 19*(3), 185–190.

Rabkin, J. G., & Struening, E. L. (1976). Life events, stress, and illness. *Science, 194*(4269), 1013–1020.

Racine, N. M., Pillai Riddell, R. R., Flora, D. B., Taddio, A., Garfield, H., & Greenberg, S. (2016). Predicting preschool pain-related anticipatory distress: The relative contribution of longitudinal and concurrent factors. *Pain, 157*(9), 1918–1932.

Racine, S. E., Burt, S. A., Keel, P. K., Sisk, C. L., Neale, M. C., Boker, S., & Klump, K. L. (2015). Examining associations between negative urgency and key components of objective binge episodes. *International Journal of Eating Disorders, 48*(5), 527–531.

Rackow, P., Scholz, U., & Hornung, R. (2015). Received social support and exercising: An intervention study to test the enabling hypothesis. *British Journal of Health Psychology, 20*(4), 763–776.

Rafferty, M. R., Schmidt, P. N., Luo, S. T., Li, K., Marras, C., Davis, T. L., . . . Simuni, T. (2017). Regular exercise, quality of life, and mobility in Parkinson's disease: A longitudinal analysis of national parkinson foundation quality improvement initiative data. *Journal of Parkinson's disease, 7*(1), 193–202.

Rahe, R. H., & Arthur, R. J. (1978). Life change and illness studies: Past history and future directions. *Journal of Human Stress, 4*(1), 3–15.

Rahe, R. H., Biersner, R., Ryman, D., & Arthur, R. (1972). Psychosocial predictors of illness behavior and failure in stressful training. *Journal of Health and Social Behavior, 13*(4), 393–397.

Rahe, R. H., Mahan, J. L., & Arthur, R. J. (1970). Prediction of near-future health change from subjects' preceding life changes. *Journal of Psychosomatic Research, 14*(4), 401–406.

Räikkönen, K., Matthews, K. A., Flory, J. D., & Owens, J. F. (1999). Effects of hostility on ambulatory blood pressure and mood during daily living in healthy adults. *Health Psychology, 18*(1), 44–53.

Rainey, L. C. (1988). The experience of dying. In H. Wass, F. M. Berado, & R. A.

Neimeyer (Eds.), *Dying: Facing the facts* (2nd ed., pp. 137–157). New York, NY: Hemisphere.

Rajaee, S. S., Bae, H. W., Kanim, L. E. A., & Delamarter, R. B. (2012). Spinal fusion in the United States: Analysis of trends from 1998 to 2008. *Spine, 37*(1), 67–76. doi:10.1097/BRS.0b013e31820cccfb

Rajasagaram, U., Taylor, D. M., Braitberg, G., Pearsell, J. P., & Capp, B. A. (2009). Paediatric pain assessment: Differences between triage nurse, child and parent. *Journal of Paediatrics and Child Health, 45*(4), 199–203. https://doi.org/10.1111/j.1440-1754.2008.01454.x

Rakowski, W., Ehrich, B., Goldstein, M. G., Rimer, B. K., Pearlman, D. N., Clark, M. A., . . . Woolverton, H. (1998). Increasing mammography among women aged 40–74 by use of a stage-matched, tailored intervention. *Preventive Medicine, 27*(5), 748–756.

Ramchand, R., Roth, E., Acosta, J. D., & Eberhart, N. K. (2015). *Adults newly exposed to the "Know the Signs" campaign report greater gains in confidence to intervene with those who might be at risk for suicide than those unexposed to the campaign.* Santa Monica, CA: RAND Corporation.

Rapaport, M. H., Schettler, P., & Bresee, C. (2010). A preliminary study of the effects of a single session of Swedish massage on hypothalamic–pituitary–adrenal and immune function in normal individuals. *The Journal of Alternative and Complementary Medicine, 16*(10), 1079–1088.

Raphael, B., & Dobson, M. (2000). College student grief and loss. In J. H. Harvey & E. D. Miller (Eds.), *Loss and trauma* (pp. 45–61). Philadelphia, PA: Brunner-Rutledge.

Raposa, E. B., Laws, H. B., & Ansell, E. B. (2016). Prosocial behavior mitigates the negative effects of stress in everyday life. *Clinical Psychological Science, 4*(4), 691–698.

Rathore, S. S., Chen, J., Wang, Y., Radford, M. J., Vaccarino, V., &

Krumholz, H. M. (2001). Sex differences in cardiac catheterization: The role of physician gender. *Journal of the American Medical Association, 286*(22), 2849–2856.

Ravussin, E., Lillioja, S., Knowler, W. C., Christin, L., Freymond, D., Abbott, W. G., . . . Bogardus, C. (1988). Reduced rate of energy expenditure as a risk factor for body-weight gain. *New England Journal of Medicine, 318*(8), 467–472.

Ray, O. (2004). How the mind hurts and heals the body. *American Psychologist, 59*(1), 29–40.

Rebbeck, T. R., Mitra, N., Wan, F., Sinilnikova, O. M., Healey, S., McGuffog, L., . . . Andrulis, I. (2015). Association of type and location of BRCA1 and BRCA2 mutations with risk of breast and ovarian cancer. *Journal of the American Medical Association, 313*(13), 1347–1361. **https://doi.org/10.1001/jama.2014.5985**

Reed, G. M., Kemeny, M. E., Taylor, S. E., & Visscher, B. R. (1999). Negative HIV-specific expectancies and AIDS-related bereavement as predictors of symptom onset in asymptomatic HIV-positive gay men. *Health Psychology, 18*(4), 354–363.

Reed, G. M., Kemeny, M. E., Taylor, S. E., Wang, H. Y. J., & Visscher, B. R. (1994). Realistic acceptance as a predictor of decreased survival time in gay men with AIDS. *Health Psychology, 13*(4), 299–307.

Reed, M. B., Anderson, C. M., Vaughn, J. W., & Burns, D. M. (2008). The effect of cigarette price increases on smoking cessation in California. *Prevention Science, 9*(1), 47–54.

Reeves, B., Lang, A., Thorson, E., & Rothschild, M. (1989). Emotional television scenes and hemispheric specialization. *Human Communication Research, 15*(4), 493–508.

Regier, D. A., Farmer, M. E., Rae, D. S., Locke, B. Z., Keith, S. J., Judd, L. L., & Goodwin, F. K. (1990). Comorbidity of mental disorders with alcohol and other drug abuse: Results from the Epidemiologic Catchment Area (ECA) study. *Journal of the American Medical Association, 264*(19), 2511–2518.

Reiff, M., Zakut, H., & Weingarten, M. A. (1999). Illness and treatment perceptions of Ethiopian immigrants and their doctors in Israel. *American Journal of Public Health, 89*(12), 1814–1818.

Reininghaus, E., Reininghaus, B., Fitz, W., Hecht, K., & Bonelli, R. M. (2012). Sexual behavior, body image, and partnership in chronic illness. *The Journal of Nervous and Mental Disease, 200*(8), 716–720. **doi:10.1097/nmd.0b013e318261410f**

Reis, H. T., Wheeler, L., Kernis, M. H., Spiegel, N., & Nezlek, J. (1985). On specificity in the impact of social participation on physical and psychological health. *Journal of Personality and Social Psychology, 48*(2), 456–471.

Remor, E., Penedo, F. J., Shen, B. J., & Schneiderman, N. (2007). Perceived stress is associated with CD4+ cell decline in men and women living with HIV/AIDS in Spain. *AIDS Care, 19*(2), 215–219.

Resneck, J. S., Lipton, S., & Pletcher, M. J. (2007). Short wait times for patients seeking cosmetic botulinum toxin appointments with dermatologists. *Journal of the American Academy of Dermatology, 57*(6), 985–989.

Resnick, M. D., Bearman, P. S., Blum, R. W., Bauman, K. E., Harris, K. M., Jones, J., . . . Ireland, M. (1997). Protecting adolescents from harm: Findings from the National Longitudinal Study on Adolescent Health. *Journal of the American Medical Association, 278*(10), 823–832.

Rey, M., & Rey, H. A. (1966). *Curious George goes to the hospital.* Boston, MA: Houghton Mifflin Harcourt.

Reynolds, D. V. (1969). Surgery in the rat during electrical analgesia induced by focal brain stimulation. *Science, 164*(3878), 444–445.

Reynolds, K. D., Buller, D. B., Yaroch, A. L., Maloy, J. A., & Cutter, G. R. (2006). Mediation of a middle school skin cancer prevention program. *Health Psychology, 25*(5), 616–625.

Reynolds, P., & Kaplan, G. A. (1990). Social connections and risk for cancer: Prospective evidence from the Alameda Country Study. *Behavioral Medicine, 16*(3), 101–110.

Rhodes, N., Roskos-Ewoldsen, D. R., Edison, A., & Bradford, M. B. (2008). Attitude and norm accessibility affect processing of anti-smoking messages. *Health Psychology, 27*(3S), S224–S232.

Rhodewalt, E., & Smith, T. W. (1991). Current issues in Type A behavior, coronary proneness, and coronary heart disease. In C. R. Snyder & D. R. Forsyth (Eds.), *Handbook of social and clinical psychology: The health perspective* (pp. 197–220). Elmsford, NY: Pergamon Press.

Rhodewalt, F., Hays, R. B., Chemers, M. M., & Wysocki, J. (1984). Type A behavior, perceived stress, and illness: A person-situation analysis. *Personality and Social Psychology Bulletin, 10*(1), 149–159.

Richardson, P. H., & Vincent, C. A. (1986). Acupuncture for the treatment of pain: A review of evaluative research. *Pain, 24*(1), 15–40.

Rickard, K. (1988). The occurrence of maladaptive health-related behaviors and teacher-related conduct problems in children of chronic low back pain patients. *Journal of Behavioral Medicine, 11*(2), 107–116.

Ridker, P. M., Vaughan, D. E., Stampfer, M. J., Glynn, R. J., & Hennekens, C. H. (1994). Association of moderate alcohol consumption and plasma concentration of endogenous tissue-type plasminogen activator. *Journal of the American Medical Association, 272*(12), 929–933.

Rigby, K., Brown, M., Anagnostou, P., Ross, M. W., & Rosser, B. R. S. (1989). Shock tactics to counter AIDS: The Australian experience. *Psychology and Health, 3*(3), 145–159.

Rimal, R. N. (2000). Closing the knowledge-behavior gap in health promotion:

the mediating role of self-efficacy. *Health Communication, 12*(3), 219–237.

Rimer, B. K. (1994). Mammography use in the US: Trends and the impact of interventions. *Annals of Behavioral Medicine, 16*(4), 317–326.

Rimer, B. K., Meissner, H., Breen, N., Legler, J., & Coyne, C. A. (2001). Social and behavioral interventions to increase breast cancer screening. In N. Schneiderman, M. A. Speers, J. M. Silva, H. Tomes, & J. H. Gentry (Eds.), *Integrating behavioral and social sciences with public health* (pp. 177–201). Washington, DC: American Psychological Association.

Rimer, B. K., Resch, N., King, E., Ross, E., Lerman, C., Boyce, A., . . . Engstrom, P. F. (1992). Multistrategy health education program to increase mammography use among women ages 65 and older. *Public Health Reports, 107*(4), 369–380.

Rimm, E., Giovannucci, E., Willett, W., Colditz, G., Ascherio, A., Rosner, B., & Stampfer, M. (1991). Prospective study of alcohol consumption and risk of coronary disease in men. *Lancet, 338*(8765), 464–468. https://doi.org/10.1016/0140-6736(91)90542-W

Rinaldis, M., Pakenham, K. I., & Lynch, B. M. (2010). Relationships between quality of life and finding benefits in a diagnosis of colorectal cancer. *British Journal of Psychology, 101*(2), 259–275. https://doi.org/10.1348/000712609X448676

Rini, C., Jandorf, L., Valdimarsdottir, H., Brown, K., & Itzkowitz, S. H. (2008). Distress among inflammatory bowel disease patients at high risk for colorectal cancer: A preliminary investigation of the effects of family history of cancer, disease duration, and perceived social support. *Psycho-Oncology, 17*(4), 354–362.

Riskin, A., Erez, A., Foulk, T. A., Kugelman, A., Gover, A., Shoris, I., . . . Bamberger, P. A. (2015). The impact of rudeness on medical team performance: A randomized trial. *Pediatrics, 136*(3), 487–495.

Rivara, F. P., Thompson, D. C., Thompson, R. S., Rogers, L. W., Alexander, B., Felix, D., & Bergman, A. B. (1994). The Seattle children's bicycle helmet campaign: Changes in helmet use and head injury admissions. *Pediatrics, 93*(4), 567–569.

Roberts, A. H. (1987). Biofeedback and chronic pain: An update. *Journal of Pain and Symptom Management, 2,* 169–171.

Roberts, A. H., Kewman, D. C., Mercier, L., & Hovell, M. (1993). The power of nonspecific effects in healing: Implications for psychosocial and biological treatments. *Clinical Psychology Review, 13,* 375–391.

Roberts, A. H., & Reinhardt, L. (1980). The behavioral management of chronic pain: Long-term follow-up with comparison groups. *Pain, 8*(2), 151–162.

Roberts, F. D., Newcomb, P. A., Trentham-Dietz, A., & Storer, B. E. (1996). Self-reported stress and breast cancer. *Cancer, 77*(6), 1089–1093.

Robertson, E. K., & Suinn, R. M. (1968). The determination of rate of progress of stroke patients through empathy measures of patient and family. *Journal of Psychosomatic Research, 12*(3), 189–191.

Robie, P. W. (1987). Compliance. In C. S. Rogers, J. D. McCue, & P. Gal (Eds.), *Managing chronic disease* (pp. 13–17). Oradell, NJ: Medical Economics Books.

Robiner, W. N., Dixon, K. E., Miner, J. L., & Hong, B. A. (2014). Psychologists in medical schools and academic medical centers: Over 100 years of growth, influence, and partnership. *American Psychologist, 69*(3), 230–248.

Robinson, E., & Sutin, A. R. (2017). Parents' perceptions of their children as overweight and children's weight concerns and weight gain. *Psychological Science, 28*(3), 320–329.

Robinson, E., Sutin, A., & Daly, M. (2017). Perceived weight discrimination mediates the prospective relation between obesity and depressive symptoms in US

and UK adults. *Health Psychology, 36*(2), 112–121.

Robinson, T. N., Borzekowski, D. L., Matheson, D. M., & Kraemer, H. C. (2007). Effects of fast food branding on young children's taste preferences. *Archives of Pediatrics & Adolescent Medicine, 161*(8), 792–797.

Robinson, E., Thomas, J., Aveyard, P., & Higgs, S. (2014). What everyone else is eating: A systematic review and meta-analysis of the effect of informational eating norms on eating behavior. *Journal of the Academy of Nutrition and Dietetics, 114*(3), 414–429.

Rockhill, B., Willett, W. C., Hunter, D. J., Manson, J. E., Hankinson, S. E., & Colditz, G. A. (1999). A prospective study of recreational physical activity and breast cancer risk. *Archives of Internal Medicine, 159*(19), 2290–2296.

Rodger, A. J., Cambiano, V., Bruun, T., Vernazza, P., Collins, S., Lunzen, J. V., . . . Lundgren, J. (2016). Sexual activity without condoms and risk of HIV transmission in serodifferent couples when the HIV-positive partner is using suppressive antiretroviral therapy. *Journal of the American Medical Association, 316*(2), 171–181. doi:10.1001/jama.2016.5148

Rodin, J. (1981). Current status of the internal–external hypothesis for obesity: What went wrong? *American Psychologist, 36*(4), 361–372.

Rodin, J., & Ickovics, J. R. (1990). Women's health: Review and research agenda as we approach the 21st century. *American Psychologist, 45*(9), 1018–1034.

Rogers, E. M., Vaughan, P. W., Swalehe, R., Rao, N., Svenkerud, P., & Sood, S. (1999). Effects of an entertainment-education radio soap opera on family planning behavior in Tanzania. *Studies in Family Planning, 30*(3), 193–211.

Rogers, R. W. (1975). A protection motivation theory of fear appeals and attitude change. *The Journal of Psychology, 91*(1), 93–114.

Rohling, M. L., Binder, L. M., & Langhin-Rich-sen-Rohling, J. (1995). Money matters: A meta-analytic review of the association between financial compensation and the experience and treatment of chronic pain. *Health Psychology, 14*(6), 537–547.

Rollman, G. B., & Harris, G. (1987). The detectability, discriminability, and perceived magnitude of painful electrical shock. *Perception and Psychophysics, 42*(3), 257–268.

Rolls, B. J., Rowe, E. A., Rolls, E. T., Kingston, B., Megson, A., & Gunary, R. (1981). Variety in a meal enhances food intake in man. *Physiology & Behavior, 26*(2), 215–221.

Romano, J. M., Turner, J. A., Friedman, L. S., Bulcroft, R. A., Jensen, M. P., Hops, H., & Wright, S. F. (1992). Sequential analysis of chronic pain behaviors and spouse responses. *Journal of Consulting and Clinical Psychology, 60*, 777–782.

Ronaldson, A., Poole, L., Kidd, T., Leigh, E., Jahangiri, M., & Steptoe, A. (2014). Optimism measured pre-operatively is associated with reduced pain intensity and physical symptom reporting after coronary artery bypass graft surgery. *Journal of Psychosomatic Research, 77*(4), 278–282.

Rook, K. S. (1987). Social support versus companionship: Effects on life stress, loneliness, and evaluations by others. *Journal of Personality and Social Psychology, 52*(6), 1132–1147.

Rooks, D. S., Gautam, S., Romeling, M., Cross, M. L., Stratigakis, D., Evans, B., . . . Katz, J. N. (2007). Group exercise, education, and combination self-management in women with fibromyalgia: A randomized trial. *Archives of Internal Medicine, 167*(20), 2192–2200. https://doi.org/10.1001/archinte.167.20.2192

Rosemann, T., Laux, G., Szecsenyi, J., Wensing, M., & Grol, R. (2008). Pain and osteoarthritis in primary care: Factors associated with pain perception in a sample of 1,021 patients. *Pain Medicine, 9*(7), 903–910. https://doi.org/10.1111/j.1526-4637.2008.00498.x

Rosen, C. S. (2000). Is the sequencing of change processes by stage consistent across health problems? A meta-analysis. *Health Psychology, 19*(6), 593–604.

Rosenbaum, M., & Ben-Ari Smira, K. (1986). Cognitive and personality factors in the delay of gratification of hemodialysis patients. *Journal of Personality and Social Psychology, 51*(2), 357–364.

Rosenbaum, S., Vancampfort, D., Steel, Z., Newby, J., Ward, P. B., & Stubbs, B. (2015). Physical activity in the treatment of post-traumatic stress disorder: A systematic review and meta-analysis. *Psychiatry Research, 230*(2), 130–136.

Rosenberg, M. (1965). *Society and the adolescent self-image*. Princeton, NJ: Princeton University Press.

Rosenberger, P. H., Kerns, R., Jokl, P., & Ickovics, J. R. (2009). Mood and attitude predict pain outcomes following arthroscopic knee surgery. *Annals of Behavioral Medicine, 37*(1), 70–76. https://doi.org/10.1007/s12160-008-9078-z

Rosenbloom, J. I., Wilker, E. H., Mukamal, K. J., Schwartz, J., & Mittleman, M. A. (2012). Residential proximity to major roadway and 10-year all-cause mortality after myocardial infarction. *Circulation, 125*(18), 2197–2203. https://doi.org/10.1161/CIRCULATIONAHA.111.085811

Rosengren, A., Hawken, S., Ôunpuu, S., Sliwa, K., Zubaid, M., Almahmeed, W. A., . . . INTERHEART investigators. (2004). Association of psychosocial risk factors with risk of acute myocardial infarction in 11119 cases and 13648 controls from 52 countries (the INTERHEART study): Case-control study. *The Lancet, 364*(9438), 953–962. doi:10.1016/S0140-6736(04)17019-0

Rosengren, A., Orth-Gomér, K., Wedel, H., & Wilhelmsen, L. (1993). Stressful life events, social support, and mortality in men born in 1933. *British Medical Journal, 307*(6912), 1102–1105.

Rosengren, A., Teo, K., Rangarajan, S., Kabali, C., Khumalo, I., Kutty, V. R., . . . Altuntas, Y. (2015). Psychosocial factors and obesity in 17 high-, middle- and low-income countries: The Prospective Urban Rural Epidemiologic study. *International Journal of Obesity, 39*(8), 1217–1223.

Rosenman, R. H., & Friedman, M. (1961). Association of specific behavior pattern in women with blood and cardiovascular findings. *Circulation, 24*(5), 1173–1184.

Rosenstock, I. M. (1960). What research in motivation suggests for public health. *American Journal of Public Health, 50*, 295–301.

Rosenstock, I. M. (1990). The health belief model: Explaining health behavior through expectancies. In K. Glanz, F. M. Lewis, & B. K. Rimer (Eds.), *Health behavior and health education: Theory, research, and practice* (pp. 39–62). San Francisco, CA: Jossey-Bass.

Ross, H., Powell, L. M., Tauras, J. A., & Chaloupka, F. J. (2005). New evidence on youth smoking behavior based on experimental price increases. *Contemporary Economic Policy, 23*(2), 195–210. doi:10.1093/cep/byi015

Rossetto, K. R., Lannutti, P. J., & Strauman, E. C. (2015). Death on Facebook: Examining the roles of social media communication for the bereaved. *Journal of Social and Personal Relationships, 32*(7), 974–994.

Roter, D. L., Hall, J. A., & Aoki, Y. (2002). Physician gender effects in medical communication: A meta-analytic review. *Journal of the American Medical Association, 288*(6), 756–764. doi:10.1001/jama.288.6.756

Roter, D. L., Lipkin, M., Jr., & Korsgaard, A. (1991). Gender differences in patients' and physicians' communication during primary care medical visits. *Medical Care, 29*(11), 1083–1093.

Roth, D. L., Wiebe, D. J., Fillingim, R. B., & Shay, K. A. (1989). Life events, fitness, hardiness, and health: A simultaneous analysis of proposed stress-resistance effects. *Journal of Personality and Social Psychology*, *57*(1), 136–143.

Roth, S., & Cohen, L. J. (1986). Approach, avoidance, and coping with stress. *American Psychologist*, *41*(7), 813–819.

Rothenberg, K. H., & Paskey, S. J. (1995). The risk of domestic violence and women with HIV infection: Implications for partner notification, public policy, and the law. *American Journal of Public Health*, *85*(11), 1569–1576. **doi:10.2105/ajph.85.11.1569**

Rothman, A. J., & Salovey, P. (1997). Shaping perceptions to motivate healthy behavior: The role of message framing. *Psychological Bulletin*, *121*(1), 3–19.

Rothman, A. J., Salovey, P., Antone, C., Keough, K., & Martin, C. D. (1993). The influence of message framing on intentions to perform health behaviors. *Journal of Experimental Social Psychology*, *29*(5), 408–433.

Rotter, J. B. (1966). Generalized expectancies for internal versus external control of reinforcement. *Psychological Monographs: General and Applied*, *80*(1), 1–28. **doi:10.1037/h0092976**

Roulston, A., Campbell, A., Cairnduff, V., Fitzpatrick, D., Donnelly, C., & Gavin, A. (2016). Bereavement outcomes: A quantitative survey identifying risk factors in informal carers bereaved through cancer. *Palliative Medicine*, *31*(2), 162–170. **https://doi.org/10.1177/0269216316649127**

Rovario, S., Holmes, D. S., & Holmsten, R. D. (1984). Influence of a cardiac rehabilitation program on the cardiovascular, psychological, and social functioning of cardiac patients. *Journal of Behavioral Medicine*, *7*(1), 61–81.

Rowsell, M., MacDonald, D. E., & Carter, J. C. (2016). Emotion regulation difficulties in anorexia nervosa: Associations with improvements in eating psychopathology. *Journal of Eating Disorders*, *4*, 17.

Roy, S. S., Foraker, R. E., Girton, R. A., & Mansfield, A. J. (2015). Posttraumatic stress disorder and incident heart failure among a community-based sample of US veterans. *American Journal of Public Health*, *105*(4), 757–784.

Rozema, H., Völlink, T., & Lechner, L. (2009). The role of illness representations in coping and health of patients treated for breast cancer. *Psycho-Oncology*, *18*(8), 849–857. **https://doi.org/10.1002/pon.1488**

Ruberman, W., Weinblatt, E., Goldberg, J. D., & Chaudhary, B. S. (1984). Psychosocial influences on mortality after myocardial infarction. *New England Journal of Medicine*, *311*(9), 552–559.

Rubonis, A. V., & Bickman, L. (1991). A test of the consensus and distinctiveness attribution principles in victims of disaster. *Journal of Applied Social Psychology*, *21*(10), 791–810.

Ruiter, R. A., Kessels, L. T., Jansma, B. M., & Brug, J. (2006). Increased attention for computer-tailored health communications: An event-related potential study. *Health Psychology*, *25*(3), 300–306.

Rutjes, A. W., Nüesch, E., Sterchi, R., Kalichman, L., Hendriks, E., Osiri, M., . . . Jüni, P. (2009). Transcutaneous electrostimulation for osteoarthritis of the knee. *Cochrane Database of Systematic Reviews*, *4*. **doi:10.1002/14651858.CD002823.pub2**

Rutledge, T., Stucky, E., Dollarhide, A., Shively, M., Jain, S., Wolfson, T., . . . Dresselhaus, T. (2009). A real-time assessment of work stress in physicians and nurses. *Health Psychology*, *28*(2), 194–200.

Rutte, A., Van Splunter, M. M., Van Der Heijden, A. A., Welschen, L. M., Elders, P. J., Dekker, J. M., . . . Nijpels, G. (2015). Prevalence and correlates of sexual dysfunction in men and women with type 2 diabetes. *Journal of Sex & Marital Therapy*, *41*(6), 680–690.

Ryan, C., Huebner, D., Diaz, R. M., & Sanchez, J. (2009). Family rejection as a predictor of negative health outcomes in White and Latino lesbian, gay, and bisexual young adults. *Pediatrics*, *123*(1), 346–352. **doi:10.1080/0092623x.2014.966399**

Ryan, R. M., Weinstein, N., Bernstein, J., Brown, K. W., Mistretta, L., & Gagne, M. (2010). Vitalizing effects of being outdoors and in nature. *Journal of Environmental Psychology*, *30*(2), 159–168.

Ryckman, R. M., Robbins, M. A., Kaczor, L. M., & Gold, J. A. (1989). Male and female raters' stereotyping of male and female physiques. *Personality and Social Psychology Bulletin*, *15*(2), 244–251.

Saab, P. G., McCalla, J. R., Coons, H. L., Christensen, A. J., Kaplan, R., Johnson, S. B., . . . Melamed, B. (2004). Technological and medical advances: Implications for health psychology. *Health Psychology*, *23*(2), 142–146.

Sabel, M. S., & Dal Cin, S. (2016). Trends in media reports of celebrities' breast cancer treatment decisions. *Annals of Surgical Oncology*, *23*(9), 2795–2801.

Sackett, D. L. (1979). A compliance practicum for the busy practitioner. In R. B. Haynes, D. W. Taylor, & D. L. Sackett (Eds.), *Compliance in health care* (pp. 286–294). Baltimore, MD: Johns Hopkins Press.

Sacks, J. J., Holmgreen, P., Smith, S. M., & Sosin, D. M. (1991). Bicycle-associated head injuries and deaths in the United States from 1984 through 1988: How many are preventable? *Journal of the American Medical Association*, *266*(21), 3016–3018.

Safe Kids Worldwide. (2017). *Safe medicine storage: A look at the disconnect between parent knowledge and behavior.* Washington, DC: Safe Kids Worldwide.

Safer, M. A., Tharps, Q. J., Jackson, T. C., & Leventhal, H. (1979). Determinants of three stages of delay in seeking care at a medical clinic. *Medical Care*, *17*(1), 11–29.

Safren, S. A., O'Cleirigh, C., Tan, J., Raminani, S., Reilly, L. C., Otto, M. W., & Mayer, K. H. (2009). A randomized controlled trial of cognitive behavioral therapy for adherence and depression (CBT-AD) in HIV-infected individuals. *Health Psychology, 28*(1), 1–10. http://doi.org/10.1037/a0012715

Saito-Nakaya, K., Nakaya, N., Akechi, T., Inagaki, M., Asai, M., Goto, K., . . . Uchitomi, Y. (2008). Marital status and non-small cell lung cancer survival: The lung cancer database project in Japan. *Psycho-Oncology, 17*(9), 869–876. https://doi.org/10.1002/pon.1296

Saleh, F., Mumu, S. J., Ara, F., Hafez, M. A., & Ali, L. (2014). Non-adherence to self-care practices and medication and health related quality of life among patients with type 2 diabetes: A cross-sectional study. *BMC Public Health, 14*, 431. http://doi.org/10.1186/1471-2458-14-431

Salomon, K., & Jagusztyn, N. E. (2008). Cardiovascular reactivity to an interpersonal conflict is moderated by reports of ethnic discrimination. *Health Psychology, 27*, 473–481.

Salyers, M. P., Bonfils, K. A., Luther, L., Firmin, R. L., White, D. A., Adams, E. L., & Rollins, A. L. (2017). The relationship between professional burnout and quality and safety in healthcare: A meta-analysis. *Journal of General Internal Medicine, 32*(4), 475–483. doi:10.1007/s11606-016-3886-9

Sanda, M. G., Dunn, R. L., Michalski, J., Sandler, H. M., Northouse, L., Hembroff, L., . . . Wei, J. T. (2008). Quality of life and satisfaction with outcome among prostate-cancer survivors. *New England Journal of Medicine, 358*(12), 1250–1261. https://doi.org/10.1056/NEJMoa074311

Sanders, M. R., Shepherd, R. W., Cleghorn, G., & Woolford, H. (1994). The treatment of recurrent abdominal pain in children: A controlled comparison of cognitive-behavioral family intervention and standard pediatric care. *Journal of Consulting and Clinical Psychology, 62*, 306–314.

Sanders, S. H., Brena, S. F., Spier, C. J., Beltrutti, D., McConnell, H., & Quintero, O. (1992). Chronic low back pain patients around the world: Cross-cultural similarities and differences. *Clinical Journal of Pain, 8*(4), 317–323.

Sanderson, C. A., & Cantor, N. (1995). Social dating goals in late adolescence: Implications for safer sexual activity. *Journal of Personality and Social Psychology, 68*(6), 1121–1134.

Sanderson, C. A., Darley, J. M., & Messinger, C. S. (2002). "I'm not as thin as you think I am": The development and consequences of feeling discrepant from the thinness norm. *Personality and Social Psychology Bulletin, 28*(2), 172–183.

Sanderson, C. A., & Holloway, R. M. (2003). Who benefits from what? Drive for thinness as a moderator of responsiveness to different eating disorder prevention messages. *Journal of Applied Social Psychology, 33*(9), 1837–1861.

Sanftner, J. L., Crowther, J. H., Crawford, P. A., & Watts, D. D. (1996). Maternal influences (or lack thereof) on daughters' eating attitudes and behaviors. *Eating Disorders, 4*(2), 147–159.

Sangeda, R. Z., Mosha, F., Prosperi, M., Aboud, S., Vercauteren, J., Camacho, R. J., . . . Vandamme, A.-M. (2014). Pharmacy refill adherence outperforms self-reported methods in predicting HIV therapy outcome in resource-limited settings. *BMC Public Health, 14*, 1035. http://doi.org/10.1186/1471-2458-14-1035

Santaella-Tenorio, J., Cerdá, M., Villaveces, A., & Galea, S. (2016). What do we know about the association between firearm legislation and firearm-related injuries? *Epidemiologic Reviews, 38*(1), 140–57.

Sapolsky, R. M. (1992). *Stress, the aging brain, and the mechanisms of neuron death.* Cambridge, MA: MIT Press.

Sapolsky, R. M. (1994). *Why zebras don't get ulcers.* New York, NY: Freeman.

Sapolsky, R. M. (1998). *Why zebras don't get ulcers: An updated guide to stress, stress-related diseases, and coping.* New York, NY: Freeman

Saquib, N., Saquib, J., & Ioannidis, J. P. (2015). Does screening for disease save lives in asymptomatic adults? Systematic review of meta-analyses and randomized trials. *International Journal of Epidemiology, 44*(1), 264–277.

Sarason, I. G., Johnson, J. H., & Siegel, J. M. (1978). Assessing the impact of life changes: Development of the Life Experiences Survey. *Journal of Consulting and Clinical Psychology, 46*(5), 932–946.

Sarason, I. G., Sarason, B. R., Keefe, D. E., Hayes, B. E., & Shearin, E. N. (1986). Cognitive interference: Situational determinants and traitlike characteristics. *Journal of Personality and Social Psychology, 51*, 215–226.

Sarason, I. G., Sarason, B. R., & Shearin, E. N. (1986). Social support as an individual difference variable: Its stability, origins, and relational aspects. *Journal of Personality and Social psychology, 50*(4), 845–855.

Sargent, J. D., Beach, M. L., Adachi-Mejia, A. M., Gibson, J. J., Titus-Ernstoff, L. T., Carusi, C. P., . . . Dalton, M. A. (2005). Exposure to movie smoking: Its relation to smoking initiation among US adolescents. *Pediatrics, 116*(5), 1183–1191.

Sargent, J. D., Tanski, S. E., & Gibson, J. (2007). Exposure to movie smoking among US adolescents aged 10 to 14 years: A population estimate. *Pediatrics, 119*(5), 1167–1176.

Sassaroli, S., Fiore, F., Mezzaluna, C., & Ruggiero, G. M. (2015). Stressful task increases drive for thinness and bulimia: A laboratory study. *Frontiers in Psychology, 6*, 591.

Sasson, I., & Umberson, D. J. (2014). Widowhood and depression: New light on gender differences, selection, and psychological adjustment. *The Journals of Gerontology: Series B, 69B*(1), 135–145. https://doi.org/10.1093/geronb/gbt058

Sawyer, K. S., Oscar-Berman, M., Ruiz, M. S., Gálvez, D. A., Makris, N., Harris, G. J., & Valera, E. M. (2016). Associations between cerebellar subregional morphometry and alcoholism history in men and women. *Alcoholism: Clinical and Experimental Research, 40*(6), 1262–1272.

Sayette, M. A. (1999). Cognitive theory and research. In K. E. Leonard & H. T. Blane (Eds.), *Psychological theories of drinking and alcoholism* (2nd ed., pp. 247–291). New York, NY: Guilford Press.

Sbarra, D. A., & Nietert, P. J. (2009). Divorce and death: Forty years of the Charleston heart study. *Psychological Science, 20*(1), 107–113. http://doi.org/10.1111/j.1467-9280.2008.02252.x

Scarmeas, N., Luchsinger, J. A., Schupf, N., Brickman, A. M., Cosentino, S., Tang, M. X., & Stern, Y. (2009). Physical activity, diet, and risk of alzheimer disease. *Journal of the American Medical Association, 302*(6), 627–637. doi:10.1001/jama.2009.1144

Schachter, S. (1968). Obesity and eating. Internal and external cues differentially affect the eating behavior of obese and normal subjects. *Science, 161*(3843), 751–756.

Schachter, S. (1977). Studies of the interaction of psychological and pharmacological determinants of smoking: I. Nicotine regulation in heavy and light smokers. *Journal of Experimental Psychology: General, 106*(1), 5–12.

Schaefer, C., Quesenberry, C. P., Jr., & Wi, S. (1995). Mortality following conjugal bereavement and the effects of a shared environment. *American Journal of Epidemiology, 141*(12), 1142–1152.

Scheier, M. F., & Carver, C. S. (1985). Optimism, coping, and health: Assessment and implications of generalized outcome expectancies. *Health Psychology, 4*(3), 219–247.

Scheier, M. F., & Carver, C. S. (1987). Dispositional optimism and physical well-being: The influence of generalized outcome expectancies on health. *Journal of Personality, 55*(2), 169–210.

Scheier, M. F., & Carver, C. S. (1992). Effects of optimism on psychological and physical well-being: Theoretical overview and empirical update. *Cognitive Therapy and Research, 16*(2), 201–228.

Scheier, M. F., & Carver, C. S. (1993). On the power of positive thinking: The benefits of being optimistic. *Current Directions in Psychological Science, 2*(1), 26–30.

Scheier, M. F., Carver, C. S., & Bridges, M. W. (1994). Distinguishing optimism from neuroticism (and trait anxiety, self-mastery, and self-esteem): A reevaluation of the Life Orientation Test. *Journal of Personality and Social Psychology, 67*(6), 1063–1078.

Scheier, M. F., Matthews, K. A., Owens, J. F., Magovern, G. J., Lefebvre, R. C., Abbott, R. A., & Carver, C. S. (1989). Dispositional optimism and recovery from coronary artery bypass surgery: The beneficial effects on physical and psychological well-being. *Journal of Personality and Social Psychology, 57*(6), 1024–1040. doi:10.1037/0022-3514.57.6.1024

Scheier, M. F., Matthews, K. A., Owens, J. F., Schulz, R., Bridges, M. W., Magovern, G. J., & Carver, C. S. (1999). Optimism and rehospitalization after coronary artery bypass graft surgery. *Archives of Internal Medicine, 159*(8), 829–835.

Scherer, K. P. (1986). Voice, stress, and emotion. In M. H. Appley & R. Trumbull (Eds.), *Dynamics of stress: Physiological, psychological, and social perspectives* (pp. 157–179). New York, NY: Plenum.

Scherer, L. D., Caverly, T. J., Burke, J., Zikmund-Fisher, B. J., Kullgren, J. T., Steinley, D., . . . Fagerlin, A. (2016). Development of the Medical Maximizer-Minimizer Scale. *Health Psychology, 35*(11), 1276–1287.

Schiffer, A. A., Denollet, J., Widdershoven, J. W., Hendriks, E. H., & Smith, O. R. F. (2007). Failure to consult for symptoms of heart failure in patients with a type-D personality. *Heart, 93*(7), 814–818. https://doi.org/10.1136/hrt.2006.102822

Schlenger, W. E., Caddell, J. M., Ebert, L., Jordan, B. K., Rourke, K. M., Wilson, D., . . . Kulka, R. A. (2002). Psychological reactions to terrorist attacks: Findings from the national study of Americans' reactions to September 11. *Journal of the American Medical Association, 288*(5), 581–588. doi:10.1001/jama.288.5.581

Schmidt, J. E., & Andrykowski, M. A. (2004). The role of social and dispositional variables associated with emotional processing in adjustment to breast cancer: An internet-based study. *Health Psychology, 23*(3), 259–266.

Schneider, D., Harknett, K., & McLanahan, S. (2016). Intimate partner violence in the Great Recession. *Demography, 53*(2), 471–505.

Schneider, T. R., Salovey, P., Apanovitch, A. M., Pizarro, J., McCarthy, D., Zullo, J., & Rothman, A. J. (2001). The effects of message framing and ethnic targeting on mammography use among low-income women. *Health Psychology, 20*(4), 256–266.

Schofield, T. J., Conger, R. D., & Robins, R. W. (2015). Early adolescent substance use in Mexican origin families: Peer selection, peer influence, and parental monitoring. *Drug and Alcohol Dependence, 157*, 129–135.

Scholer, S. J., Hickson, G. B., & Ray, W. A. (1999). Sociodemographic factors identify US infants at high risk of injury mortality. *Pediatrics, 103*(6), 1183–1188.

Scholer, S. J., Mitchel, E. F., & Ray, W. A. (1997). Predictors of injury mortality in early childhood. *Pediatrics, 100*(3), 342–347.

Scholz, U., Stadler, G., Ochsner, S., Rackow, P., Hornung, R., & Knoll, N. (2016). Examining the relationship between daily changes in support and smoking around a self-set quit date. *Health Psychology, 35*(5), 514–517.

Schorr, L., Burger, A., Hochner, H., Calderon, R., Manor, O., Friedlander, Y., . . . Paltiel, O. (2016). Mortality, cancer incidence, and survival in parents after bereavement. *Annals of Epidemiology, 26*(2), 115–121. https://doi.org/10.1016/j.annepidem.2015.12.008

Schreiber, G. B., Robins, M., Striegel-Moore, R., Obarzanek, E., Morrison, J. A., & Wright, D. J. (1996). Weight modification efforts reported by Black and White preadolescent girls: National Heart, Lung, and Blood Institute Growth and Health Study. *Pediatrics, 98*(1), 63–70.

Schroeder, D. H., & Costa, P. T. (1984). Influence of life event stress on physical illness: Substantive effects or methodological flaws? *Journal of Personality and Social Psychology, 46*(4), 853–863.

Schroevers, M. J., Helgeson, V. S., Sanderman, R., & Ranchor, A. V. (2010). Type of social support matters for prediction of posttraumatic growth among cancer survivors. *Psycho-Oncology, 19*(1), 46–53. https://doi.org/10.1002/pon.1501

Schuckit, M. A. (1985). The clinical implications of primary diagnostic groups among alcoholics. *Archives of General Psychiatry, 42*(11), 1043–1049.

Schuckit, M. A., & Smith, T. L. (1996). An 8-year follow-up of 450 sons of alcoholic and control subjects. *Archives of General Psychiatry, 53*(3), 202–210.

Schulman, K. A., Berlin, J. A., Harless, W., Kerner, J. F., Sistrunk, S., Gersh, B. J., . . . Eisenberg, J. M. (1999). The effect of race and sex on physicians' recommendations for cardiac catheterization. *New England Journal of Medicine, 340*(8), 618–626.

Schulz, R., Beach, S. R., Lind, B., Martire, L. M., Zdaniuk, B., Hirsch, C., . . . Burton, L. (2001). Involvement in caregiving and adjustment to death of a spouse: Findings from the Caregiver Health Effects Study. *Journal of the American Medical Association, 285*, 3123–3129.

Schut, H. A. W., van den Bout, J., De Keijser, J., & Stroebe, M. S. (1996). Cross-modality grief therapy: Description and assessment of a new program. *Journal of Clinical Psychology, 52*(3), 357–365.

Schüz, B., Wurm, S., Ziegelmann, J. P., Warner, L. M., Tesch-Römer, C., & Schwarzer, R. (2011). Changes in functional health, changes in medication beliefs, and medication adherence. *Health Psychology, 30*(1), 31–39. doi:10.1037/a0021881

Schwartz, B. S., Stewart, W. F., Simon, D., & Lipton, R. B. (1998). Epidemiology of tension-type headache. *Journal of the American Medical Association, 279*, 381–383.

Schwartz, G. E. (1982). Testing the biopsychosocial model: The ultimate challenge facing behavioral medicine? *Journal of Consulting and Clinical Psychology, 50*(6), 1040–1053.

Schwartz, M. D., Peshkin, B. N., Tercyak, K. P., Taylor, K. L., & Valdimarsdottir, H. (2005). Decision making and decision support for hereditary breast-ovarian cancer susceptibility. *Health Psychology, 24*(4), 78–84.

Schwartz, M. D., Taylor, K. L., Willard, K. S., Siegel, J. E., Lamdan, R. M., & Moran, K. (1999). Distress, personality, and mammography utilization among women with a family history of breast cancer. *Health Psychology, 18*(4), 327–332.

Schwartzberg, S. S. (1993). Struggling for meaning: How HIV-positive gay men make sense of AIDS. *Professional Psychology: Research and Practice, 24*(4), 483–490.

Schwarzer, R. (1992). *Self-efficacy: Thought control of action*. Washington, DC: Hemisphere.

Schwarzer, R., & Leppin, A. (1992). The possible impact of social ties and social support on morbidity and mortality. In U. Baumann & H. Yeiel (Eds.), *The meaning and measurement of social support* (pp. 65–83). Washington, DC: Hemisphere.

Schwebel, D. C., & Gaines, J. (2007). Pediatric unintentional injury: Behavioral risk factors and implications for prevention. *Journal of Developmental & Behavioral Pediatrics, 28*(3), 245–254.

Schwebel, D. C., Severson, J., Ball, K. K., & Rizzo, M. (2006). Individual difference factors in risky driving: The roles of anger/hostility, conscientiousness, and sensation-seeking. *Accident Analysis & Prevention, 38*(4), 801–810.

Scott, J. C., & Hochberg, M. C. (1993). Arthritis and other musculoskeletal diseases. In R. C. Brownson, P. L., Remington, & J. R. Davis (Eds.), *Chronic disease epidemiology and control* (pp. 285–305). Washington, DC: American Public Health Association.

Scott-Sheldon, L. A. J., Kalichman, S. C., Carey, M. P., & Fielder, R. L. (2008). Stress management interventions for HIV+ adults: A meta-analysis of randomized controlled trials, 1989 to 2006. *Health Psychology, 27*(2), 129–139. http://doi.org/10.1037/0278-6133.27.2.129

Sears, S. F., Jr., Marhefka, S. L., Rodrigue, J. R., & Campbell, C. (2000). The role of patients' ability to pay, gender, and smoking history on public attitudes toward cardiac transplant allocation: An experimental investigation. *Health Psychology, 19*(2), 192–196.

Sears, S. R., & Stanton, A. L. (2001). Physician-assisted dying: Review of issues and roles for health psychologists. *Health Psychology, 20*(4), 302–310.

Seeman, T. E., Singer, B. H., Rowe, J. W., Horwitz, R. I., & McEwen, B. S. (1997). Price of adaptation – allostatic load and its health consequences: MacArthur studies of successful aging. *Archives of Internal Medicine, 157*(19), 2259–2269.

Seery, M. D., Holman, E. A., & Silver, R. C. (2010). Whatever does not kill us: Cumulative lifetime adversity, vulnerability, and resilience. *Journal of Personality and Social Psychology, 99*(6), 1025–1042.

Segerstrom, S. C. (2007). Stress, energy, and immunity: An ecological view.

Current Directions in Psychological Science, 16(6), 326–330. doi:10.1111/j.1467-8721.2007.00522.x

Segerstrom, S. C., & Miller, G. E. (2004). Psychological stress and the human immune system: A meta-analytic study of 30 years of inquiry. *Psychological Bulletin, 130*(4), 601–631.

Segerstrom, S. C., Taylor, S. E., Kemeny, M. E., & Fahey, J. L. (1998). Optimism is associated with mood, coping, and immune change in response to stress. *Journal of Personality and Social Psychology, 74*(6), 1646–1655.

Segerstrom, S. C., Taylor, S. E., Kemeny, M. E., Reed, G. M., & Visscher, B. R. (1996). Causal attributions predict rate of immune decline in HIV-seropositive gay men. *Health Psychology, 15*(6), 485–493.

Self, C. A., & Rogers, R. W. (1990). Coping with threats to health: Effects of persuasive appeals on depressed, normal, and antisocial personalities. *Journal of Behavioral Medicine, 13*(4), 343–357.

Seligman, M. E. P., & Csikszentmihalyi, M. (2000). Special issue on happiness, excellence, and optimal human functioning. *American Psychologist, 55*(1), 5–183.

Selye, H. (1956). *The stress of life.* New York, NY: McGraw-Hill.

Selye, H. (1974). *Stress without distress.* Philadelphia, PA: Lippincott.

Sen, B., & Panjamapirom, A. (2012). State background checks for gun purchase and firearm deaths: An exploratory study. *Preventive Medicine, 55*(4), 346–350.

Senecal, C., Nouwen, A., & White, D. (2000). Motivation and dietary self-care in adults with diabetes: Are self-efficacy and autonomous self-regulation complementary or competing constructs? *Health Psychology, 19*, 452–457.

Senn, C. Y., Eliasziw, M., Barata, P. C., Thurston, W. E., Newby-Clark, I. R., Radtke, H. L., & Hobden, K. L. (2015). Efficacy of a sexual assault resistance program for university women. *New England Journal of Medicine, 372*(24), 2326–2335.

Seth, P., Walker, T., Hollis, N., Figueroa, A., & Belcher, L. (2015). HIV testing and service delivery among Blacks or African Americans—61 health department jurisdictions, United States, 2013. *Morbidity and Mortality Weekly Report, 64*(4), 87–90.

Severeijns, R., Vlaeyen, J. W. S., van den Hout, M. A., & Picavet, H. S. J. (2004). Pain catastrophizing is associated with health indices in musculoskeletal pain: A cross-sectional study in the Dutch community. *Health Psychology, 23*(1), 49–57. https://doi.org/10.1037/0278-6133.23.1.49

Sevincer, A. T., & Oettingen, G. (2014). Alcohol myopia and goal commitment. *Frontiers in Psychology, 5*, 169.

Sewell, A. A. (2015). Disaggregating ethnoracial disparities in physician trust. *Social Science Research, 54*, 1–20. doi:10.1016/j.ssresearch.2015.06.020

Seybold, K. S., & Hill, P. C. (2001). The role of religion and spirituality in mental and physical health. *Current Directions in Psychological Science, 10*(1), 21–24.

Shackelton, R., Siegrist, J., Link, C., Marceau, L., von dem Knesebeck, O., & McKinlay, J. (2010). Work stress of primary care physicians in the US, UK and German health care systems. *Social Science & Medicine (1982), 71*(2), 298–304. http://doi.org/10.1016/j.socscimed.2010.03.043

Shaffer, J. W., Graves, P. L., Swank, R. T., & Pearson, T. A. (1987). Clustering of personality traits in youth and the subsequent development of cancer among physicians. *Journal of Behavioral Medicine, 10*(5), 441–447.

Shaffer, W. J., Duszynski, K. R., & Thomas, C. B. (1982). Family attitudes in youth as a possible precursor of cancer among physicians: A search for explanatory mechanisms. *Journal of Behavioral Medicine, 15*, 143–164.

Shai, D., & Lupinacci, P. (2003). Fire fatalities among children: An analysis across Philadelphia's census tracts. *Public Health Reports, 118*(2), 115–126.

Shanafelt, T. D., Dyrbye, L. N., Sinsky, C., Hasan, O., Satele, D., Sloan, J., & West, C. P. (2016). Relationship between clerical burden and characteristics of the electronic environment with physician burnout and professional satisfaction. *Mayo Clinic Proceedings, 91*(7), 836–848. http://dx.doi.org/10.1016/j.mayocp.2016.05.007

Shanahan, D. F., Bush, R., Gaston, K. J., Lin, B. B., Dean, J., Barber, E., & Fuller, R. A. (2016). Health benefits from nature experiences depend on dose. *Scientific Reports, 6*, 28551. doi:10.1038/srep28551

Shankar, A., McMunn, A., Demakakos, P., Hamer, M., & Steptoe, A. (2017). Social isolation and loneliness: Prospective associations with functional status in older adults. *Health Psychology, 36*(2), 179–187. doi:10.1037/hca0000437

Sharp, E. S., & Gatz, M. (2011). Relationship between education and dementia. *Alzheimer Disease & Associated Disorders, 25*(4), 289–304. doi:10.1097/wad.0b013e318211c83c

Shattuck, D., Kerner, B., Gilles, K., Hartmann, M., Ng'ombe, T., & Guest, G. (2011). Encouraging contraceptive uptake by motivating men to communicate about family planning: The Malawi Male Motivator project. *American Journal of Public Health, 101*(6), 1089–1095.

Shavitt, S., Cho, Y. I., Johnson, T. P., Jiang, D., Holbrook, A., & Stavrakantonaki, M. (2016). Culture moderates the relation between perceived stress, social support, and mental and physical health. *Journal of Cross-Cultural Psychology, 47*(7), 956–980. doi:10.1177/0022022116656132

Shaw, E. G., & Routh, D. K. (1982). Effect of mother presence on children's reaction to adverse procedures. *Journal of Pediatric Psychology, 7*, 33–42.

Shea, S., Ottman, R., Gabrieli, C., Stein, Z., & Nichols, A. (1984). Family history as an independent risk factor for coronary artery disease. *Journal of the American College of Cardiology, 4*(4), 793–801. https://doi.org/10.1016/S0735-1097(84)80408-8

Sheeran, P., & Orbell, S. (2000). Using implementation intentions to increase attendance for cervical cancer screening. *Health Psychology, 19*(3), 283–289.

Sheeran, P., Maki, A., Montanaro, E., Avishai-Yitshak, A., Bryan, A., Klein, W. M., . . . Rothman, A. J. (2016). The impact of changing attitudes, norms, and self-efficacy on health-related intentions and behavior: A meta-analysis. *Health Psychology, 35*(11), 1178–1188.

Sheets, E. S., & Craighead, W. E. (2014). Comparing chronic interpersonal and noninterpersonal stress domains as predictors of depression recurrence in emerging adults. *Behaviour Research and Therapy, 63*, 36–42. doi:10.1016/j.brat.2014.09.001

Shekelle, P. G., Adams, A. H., & Chassin, M. R. (1992). Spinal manipulation for low-back pain. *Annals of Internal Medicine, 117*, 590–595.

Shekelle, R. B., Gale, M., Ostfield, A. M., & Paul, O. (1983). Hostility, risk of coronary heart disease and mortality. *Psychosomatic Medicine, 45*, 109–114.

Shekelle, R. B., Raynor, W. J., Jr., Ostfeld, A. M., Garron, D. C., Bieliauskas, L. A., Livy, Sc. C., . . . & Paul, O. (1981). Psychological depression and 17-year risk of death from cancer. *Psychosomatic Medicine, 43*, 117–125.

Shekelle, R. B., Rossof, A. H., & Stamler, J. (1991). Dietary cholesterol and incidence of lung cancer: The Western Electric Study. *American Journal of Epidemiology, 134*(5), 480–484.

Sheppard, B. H., Hartwick, J., & Warshaw, P. R. (1988). The theory of reasoned action: A meta-analysis of past research with recommendations for modifications and future research. *Journal of Consumer Research, 15*(3), 325–343.

Shepperd, J. A., Maroto, J. J., & Pbert, L. A. (1996). Dispositional optimism as a predictor of health changes among cardiac patients. *Journal of Research in Personality, 30*(4), 517–534.

Shepperd, S. L., Solomon, L. J., Atkins, E., Foster, R. S., & Frankowski, B. (1990). Determinants of breast self-examination among women of lower income and lower education. *Journal of Behavioral Medicine, 13*(4), 359–371.

Sher, K. J., Gotham, H. J., Erickson, D. J., & Wood, P. K. (1996). A prospective, high-risk study of the relationship between tobacco dependence and alcohol use disorders. *Alcoholism: Clinical and Experimental Research, 20*(3), 485–492.

Sher, K. J., Trull, T. J., Bartholow, B. D., & Vieth, A. (1999). Personality and alcoholism: Issues, methods, and etiological processes. In K. E. Leonard & H. T. Blane (Eds.), *Psychological theories of drinking and alcoholism* (2nd ed., pp. 54–105). New York, NY: Guilford Press.

Sherbourne, C. D., Asch, S. M., Shugarman, L. R., Goebel, J. R., Lanto, A. B., Rubenstein, L. V., . . . Lorenz, K. A. (2009). Early identification of co-occurring pain, depression and anxiety. *Journal of General Internal Medicine, 24*(5), 620–625. https://doi.org/10.1007/s11606-009-0956-2

Sherbourne, C. D., Hays, R. D., Ordway, L., DiMatteo, M. R., Kravitz, R. L. (1992). Antecedents of adherence to medical recommendations: Results from the Medical Outcomes Study. *Journal of Behavioral Medicine, 15*, 447–468.

Sherman, D. A., Nelson, L. D., & Steele, C. M. (2000). Do messages about health risks threaten the self? Increasing the acceptance of threatening health messages via self-affirmation. *Personality and Social Psychology Bulletin, 26*(9), 1046–1058.

Sherman, D. K., & Cohen, G. L. (2002). Accepting threatening information: Self–affirmation and the reduction of defensive biases. *Current Directions in Psychological Science, 11*(4), 119–123.

Sherman, S. M., Cheng, Y. P., Fingerman, K. L., & Schnyer, D. M. (2015). Social support, stress and the aging brain. *Social Cognitive and Affective Neuroscience, 11*(7), 1050–1058.

Sherr, L. (1990). Fear arousal and AIDS: Do shock tactics work? *AIDS, 4*(4), 361–364.

Shiffman, S., Fischer, L. A., Paty, J. A., Gnys, M., Hickcox, M., & Kassel, J. D. (1994). Drinking and smoking: A field study of their association. *Annals of Behavioral Medicine, 16*(3), 203–209.

Shiffman, S., Gnys, M., Richards, T. J., Paty, J. A., Hickcox, M., & Kassel, J. D. (1996). Temptations to smoke after quitting: A comparison of lapsers and maintainers. *Health Psychology, 15*(6), 455–461.

Shiloh, S., Ben-Sinai, R., & Keinan, G. (1999). Effects of controllability, predictability, and information-seeking style on interest in predictive genetic testing. *Personality and Social Psychology Bulletin, 25*(10), 1187–1195.

Shinn, M., Rosario, M., Morch, H., & Chestnut, D. E. (1984). Coping with job stress and burnout in the human services. *Journal of Personality and Social psychology, 46*, 864–876.

Shipley, B. A., Weiss, A., Der, G., Taylor, M. D., & Deary, I. J. (2007). Neuroticism, extraversion, and mortality in the UK Health and Lifestyle Survey: A 21-year prospective cohort study. *Psychosomatic Medicine, 69*(9), 923–931.

Shnayderman, I., & Katz-Leurer, M. (2013). An aerobic walking programme versus muscle strengthening programme for chronic low back pain: A randomized controlled trial. *Clinical Rehabilitation, 27*(3), 207–214.

Shorey, R. C., Stuart, G. L., McNulty, J. K., & Moore, T. M. (2014). Acute alcohol use temporally increases the odds of male perpetrated dating violence: A 90-day diary analysis. *Addictive Behaviors, 39*, 365–368. https://doi.org/10.1177/0269215512453353

Shouksmith, G., & Taylor, J. E. (1997). The interaction of culture with general job stressors in air traffic controllers. *International Journal of Aviation Psychology, 7*(4), 343–352.

Siegel, I. (2010). Does body weight dissatisfaction change with age? A cross-sectional analysis of American women. *The New School Psychology Bulletin, 7*(1), 42–50.

Siegel, J. M. (1990). Stressful life events and use of physician services among the elderly: The moderating role of pet ownership. *Journal of Personality and Social Psychology, 58*(6), 1081–1086.

Siegel, K., Schrimshaw, E. W., & Pretter, S. (2005). Stress-related growth among women living with HIV/AIDS: Examination of an explanatory model. *Journal of Behavioral Medicine, 28*(5), 403–414.

Siegel, M., Albers, A. B., Cheng, D. M., Hamilton, W. L., & Biener, L. (2008). Local restaurant smoking regulations and the adolescent smoking initiation process: Results of a multilevel contextual analysis among Massachusetts youth. *Archives of Pediatrics & Adolescent Medicine, 162*(5), 477–483.

Siegel, M., Ross, C. S., Albers, A. B., DeJong, W., King, I. C., Naimi, T. S., & Jernigan, D. H. (2015). The relationship between exposure to brand-specific alcohol advertising and brand-specific consumption among underage drinkers-United States, 2011-2012. *The American Journal of Drug and Alcohol Abuse, 42*(1), 4–14.

Siegel, R. L., Miller, K. D., Fedewa, S. A., Ahnen, D. J., Meester, R. G., Barzi, A., & Jemal, A. (2017). Colorectal cancer statistics, 2017. *CA: A Cancer Journal for Clinicians, 67*(3), 177–193.

Siegler, I. C., Feaganes, J. R., & Rimer, B. K. (1995). Predictors of adoption of mammography in women under age 50. *Health Psychology, 14*(3), 274–278.

Siegman, A. W. (1993). Cardiovascular consequences of expressing, experiencing, and repressing anger. *Journal of Behavioral Medicine, 16*, 539–569.

Siegman, A. W., Anderson, R., Herbst, J., Boyle, S., & Wilkinson, J. (1992). Dimensions of anger-hostility and cardiovascular reactivity in provoked and angered men. *Journal of Behavioral Medicine, 15*(3), 257–272.

Sieman, D., & Hollander, E. (2001). *Self-injury behavior: Assessment and treatment.* Washington, DC: American Psychiatric Publishing.

Sieverding, M., Matterne, U., & Ciccarello, L. (2010). What role do social norms play in the context of men's cancer screening intention and behavior? Application of an extended theory of planned behavior. *Health Psychology, 29*(1), 72–81.

Sikkema, K. J., Hansen, N. B., Ghebremichael, M., Kochman, A., Tarakeshwar, N., Meade, C. S., & Zhang, H. (2006). A randomized controlled trial of a coping group intervention for adults with HIV who are AIDS bereaved: Longitudinal effects on grief. *Health Psychology, 25*(5), 563–570. https://doi.org/10.1037/0278-6133.25.5.563

Silberman, I. (2005). Religion as a meaning system: Implications for the new *millennium. Journal of Social Issues, 61*, 641–663. doi:10.1111/j.1540-4560.2005.00425.x

Silveira, M. J., Kim, S. Y. H., & Langa, K. M. (2010). Advance directives and outcomes of surrogate decision making before death. *New England Journal of Medicine, 362*(13), 1211–1218. http://doi.org/10.1056/NEJMsa0907901

Silver, L. D., Ng, S. W., Ryan-Ibarra, S., Taillie, L. S., Induni, M., Miles, D. R., . . . Popkin, B. M. (2017). Changes in prices, sales, consumer spending, and beverage consumption one year after a tax on sugar-sweetened beverages in Berkeley, California, US: A before-and-after study. *PLoS Medicine, 14*(4), e1002283. http://doi.org/10.1371/journal.pmed.1002283

Silverstein, B., Perdue, L., Peterson, B., & Kelly, E. (1986). The role of the mass media in promoting a thin standard of bodily attractiveness for women. *Sex Roles, 14*(9), 519–532.

Simon, N. (1977). Breast cancer induced by radiation: Relation to mammography and treatment of acne. *Journal of the American Medical Association, 237*(8), 789–790.

Simoni, J. M., Mason, H. R., Marks, G., Ruiz, M. S., & Al, E. (1995). Women's self-disclosure of HIV infection: Rates, reasons, and reactions. *Journal of Consulting and Clinical Psychology, 63*(3), 474–478. doi:10.1037//0022-006x.63.3.474

Simons-Morton, B., Chen, R., Abroms, L., & Haynie, D. L. (2004). Latent growth curve analyses of peer and parent influences on smoking progression among early adolescents. *Health Psychology, 23*(6), 612–621.

Simons-Morton, B., Lerner, N., & Singer, J. (2005). The observed effects of teenage passengers on the risky driving behavior of teenage drivers. *Accident Analysis & Prevention, 37*(6), 973–982.

Simpson, S., Hurtley, S. M., & Marx, J. (2000). Immune cell networks. *Science, 290*(5489), 79.

Sims, R., Gordon, S., Garcia, W., Clark, E., Monye, D., Callender, C., & Campbell, A. (2007). Perceived stress and eating behaviors in a community-based sample of African Americans. *Eating Behaviors, 9*(2), 137–143.

Sims, R., van der Lee, S. J., Naj, A. C., Bellenguez, C., Badarinarayan, N., Jakobsdottir, J., . . . Martin, E. R. (2017). Rare coding variants in PLCG2, ABI3, and TREM2 implicate microglial-mediated innate immunity in Alzheimer's disease. *Nature Genetics, 49*(9), 1373–1384. doi:10.1038/ng.3916

Sin, N. L., Moskowitz, J. T., & Whooley, M. A. (2015). Positive affect and health behaviors across five years in patients with coronary heart disease: The Heart and Soul Study. *Psychosomatic Medicine, 77*(9), 1058–1066. doi:10.1097/PSY.0000000000000238

Sinha, R., Dufour, S., Petersen, K. F., LeBon, V., Enoksson, S., Ma, Y. Z., . . . Caprio, S. (2002). Assessment of skeletal muscle triglyceride content by 1 H nuclear magnetic resonance spectroscopy in lean and obese adolescents. *Diabetes, 51*(4), 1022–1027.

Sinsky, C., Colligan, L., Li, L., Prgomet, M., Reynolds, S., Goeders, L, . . . Blike, G. (2016). Allocation of physician time in ambulatory practice: A time and motion study in 4 specialties. *Annals of Internal Medicine, 165,* 753–760. **doi:10.7326/M16-0961**

Sirin, S. R., Rogers-Sirin, L., Cressen, J., Gupta, T., Ahmed, S. F., & Novoa, A. D. (2015). Discrimination-related stress effects on the development of internalizing symptoms among Latino adolescents. *Child Development, 86*(3), 709–725.

Skaali, T., Fosså, S. D., Bremnes, R., Dahl, O., Haaland, C. F., Hauge, E. R., . . . Dahl, A. A. (2009). Fear of recurrence in long-term testicular cancer survivors. *Psycho-Oncology, 18*(6), 580–588. **https://doi.org/10.1002/pon.1437**

Skaer, T. L., Robison, L. M., Sclar, D. A., & Harding, G. H. (1996). Cancer-screening determinants among Hispanic women using migrant health clinics. *Journal of Health Care for the Poor and Underserved, 7*(4), 338–354.

Skelton, J. A., & Pennebaker, J. W. (1982). The psychology of physical symptoms and sensations. In G. S. Sanders & J. Suls (Eds.), *Social psychology of health and illness* (pp. 99–128). Hillsdale, NJ: Erlbaum.

Skinner, B. F. (1938). *The behavior of organisms.* New York, NY: Appleton.

Skinner, C. S., Campbell, M. K., Rimer, B. K., Curry, S., & Prochaska, J. O. (1999). How effective is tailored print communication? *Annals of Behavioral Medicine, 21*(4), 290–298.

Skinner, C. S., Strecher, V. J., & Hospers, H. (1994). Physicians' recommendations for mammography: Do tailored messages make a difference? *American Journal of Public Health, 84*(1), 43–49.

Sklar, L. S., & Anisman, H. (1981). Stress and cancer. *Psychological Bulletin, 89*(3), 369–406. **doi:10.1037/0033-2909.89.3.369**

Skogan, W. G., Hartnett, S. M., Bump, N., & Dubois, J. (2008). *Evaluation of CeaseFire-Chicago.* Washington, DC: U.S. Department of Justice.

Skrabanek, P. (1988). The debate over mass mammography in Britain. The case against. *BMJ: British Medical Journal, 297*(6654), 971–972.

Slater, S. J., Chaloupka, F. J., Wakefield, M., Johnston, L. D., & O'Malley, P. M. (2007). The impact of retail cigarette marketing practices on youth smoking uptake. *Archives of Pediatrics & Adolescent Medicine, 161*(5), 440–445.

Slattery, M. L., Boucher, K. M., Caan, B. J., Potter, J. D., & Ma, K.-N. (1998). Eating patterns and risk of colon cancer. *American Journal of Epidemiology, 148,* 4–16.

Slattery, M. L., Schumacher, M. C., Smith, K. R., West, D. W., & Abd-Elghany, N. (1990). Physical activity, diet, and risk of colon cancer in Utah. *American Journal of Epidemiology, 128,* 989–999.

Sloand, E. M., Pitt, E., Chiarello, R. J., & Nemo, G. J. (1991). HIV testing: State of the art. *Journal of the American Medical Association, 266*(20), 2861–2866.

Slochower, J., Kaplan, S. P., & Mann, L. (1981). The effects of life stress and weight on mood and eating. *Appetite, 2*(2), 115–125.

Smart Richman, L., Bennett, G. G., Pek, J., Siegler, I., & Williams, R. J. (2007). Discrimination, dispositions, and cardiovascular responses to stress. *Health Psychology, 26*(6), 675–683. **doi:10.1037/0278-6133.26.6.675**

Smart Richman, L., Pek, J., Pascoe, E., & Bauer, D. J. (2010). The effects of perceived discrimination on ambulatory blood pressure and affective responses to interpersonal stress modeled over 24 hours. *Health Psychology, 29*(4), 403–411.

Smeets, M. A. (1999). Body size categorization in anorexia nervosa using a morphing instrument. *International Journal of Eating Disorders, 25*(4), 451–455.

Smith, A. D., Crippa, A., Woodcock, J., & Brage, S. (2016). Physical activity and incident type 2 diabetes mellitus: A systematic review and dose–response meta-analysis of prospective cohort studies. *Diabetologia, 59*(12), 2527–2545. **doi:10.1007/s00125-016-4079-0**

Smith, C. A., & Pratt, M. (1993). Cardiovascular disease. In R. C. Brownson, P. L. Remington, & J. R. Davis (Eds.), *Chronic disease epidemiology and control* (pp. 83–107). Washington, DC: American Public Health Association.

Smith, G. T., Goldman, M. S., Greenbaum, P. E., & Christiansen, B. A. (1995). Expectancy for social facilitation from drinking: The divergent paths of high-expectancy and low-expectancy adolescents. *Journal of Abnormal Psychology, 104*(1), 32–40.

Smith, J. T., Barabasz, Z., & Barabasz, M. (1996). Comparision of hypnosis and distraction in severly ill children undergoing painful medical procedures. *Journal of Counseling Psychology, 43,* 187–195.

Smith, K. A., Harvath, T. A., Goy, E. R., & Ganzini, L. (2015). Predictors of pursuit of physician-assisted death. *Journal of Pain and Symptom Management, 49*(3), 555–561. **https://doi.org/10.1016/j.jpainsymman.2014.06.010**

Smith, S. G., Chen, J., Basile, K. C., Gilbert, L. K., Merrick, M. T., Patel, N., . . . Jain, A. (2017). *The National Intimate Partner and Sexual Violence Survey (NISVS): 2010-2012 State Report.* Atlanta, GA: Centers for Disease Control and Prevention.

Smith, T. J., Dow, L. A., Virago, F., Khatcheressian, J., Lyckholm, L. J., & Matsuyama, R. (2010). Giving honest information to patients with advanced cancer maintains hope. *Oncology (Williston Park), 24*(6), 521–525.

Smith, T. W. (1992). Hostility and health: Current status of a psychosomatic hypothesis. *Health Psychology, 11*(3), 139–150.

Smith, T. W., Orleans, C. T., & Jenkins, C. D. (2004). Prevention and health promotion: Decades of progress, new challenges, and an emerging agenda. *Health Psychology, 23*(2), 126–131.

Smith, T. W., Pope, M. K., Sanders, J. D., Allred, K. D., & O'Keefe, J. L. (1988). Cynical hostility at home and work: Psychosocial vulnerability across domains. *Journal of Research in Personality, 21*, 525–548.

Smith, T. W., & Williams, P. G. (1992). Personality and health: Advantages and limitations of the five-factor model. *Journal of Personality, 60*(2), 395–423.

Smith-Greenaway, E., & Clark, S. (2017). Variation in the link between parental divorce and children's health disadvantage in low and high divorce settings. *SSM–Population Health, 3,* 473–486. https://doi.org/10.1016/j.ssmph.2017.04.004

Smyth, J. M. (1998). Written emotional expression: Effect sizes, outcome types, and moderating variables. *Journal of Consulting and Clinical Psychology, 66*(1), 174–184. doi:10.1037//0022-006X.66.1.174

Smyth, J. M., Stone, A. A., Hurewitz, A., & Kaell, A. (1999). Effects of writing about stressful experiences on symptom reduction in patients with asthma or rheumatoid arthritis: A randomized trial. *Journal of the American Medical Association, 281*(14), 1304–1309.

Snyder, C. R., Sympson, S. C., Ybasco, F. C., Borders, T. F., Babyak, M. A., & Higgins, R. L. (1996). Development and validation of the State Hope Scale. *Journal of Personality and Social Psychology, 70*(2), 321–335.

Soames Job, R. F. (1988). Effective and ineffective use of fear in health promotion campaigns. *American Journal of Public Health, 78*(2), 163–167.

Sobell, L. C., Cunningham, J. A., & Sobell, M. B. (1996). Recovery from alcohol problems with and without treatment: Prevalence in two population surveys. *American Journal of Public Health, 86*(7), 966–972.

Sokol, D. J., Sokol, S., & Sokol, C. K. (1985). A review of nonintrusive therapies used to deal with anxiety and pain in the dental office. *The Journal of the American Dental Association, 110*(2), 217–222.

Solomon, G. F. (1991). Psychosocial factors, exercise, and immunity: Athletes, elderly persons, and AIDS patients. *International Journal of Sports Medicine, 12*(S 1), S50-S52.

Solomon, L. J., Secker-Walker, R. H., Skelly, J. M., & Flynn, B. S. (1996). Stages of change in smoking during pregnancy in low-income women. *Journal of Behavioral Medicine, 19*(4), 350–366.

Song, J., Floyd, F. J., Seltzer, M. M., Greenberg, J. S., & Hong, J. (2010). Long-term effects of child death on parents' health related quality of life: A dyadic analysis. *Family Relations, 59*(3), 269–282. https://doi.org/10.1111/j.1741-3729.2010.00601.x

Sorensen, G., Jacobs, D. R., Pirie, P., Folsom, A., Luepker, R., & Gillum, R. (1987). Relationships among Type A behavior, employment experiences, and gender: The Minnesota heart survey. *Journal of Behavioral Medicine, 10*(4), 323–336.

Sorensen, G., Pechacek, T., & Pallonen, U. (1986). Occupational and worksite norms and attitudes about smoking cessation. *American Journal of Public Health, 76*(5), 544–549.

Sosa, R., Kennell, J., Klaus, M., Robertson, S., & Urrutia, J. (1980). The effect of a supportive companion on perinatal problems, length of labor, and mother-infant interaction. *New England Journal of Medicine, 303*(11), 597–600.

Spanakis, E. K., & Golden, S. H. (2013). Race/ethnic difference in diabetes and diabetic complications. *Current Diabetes Reports, 13*(6), 814–823. doi:10.1007/s11892-013-0421-9

Spanos, N. P., & Katsanis, J. (1989). Effects of instructional set on attributions of nonvolition during hypnotic and non-hypnotic analgesia. *Journal of Personality and Social Psychology, 56,* 182–188.

Sparano, J. A., Gray, R. J., Makower, D. F., Pritchard, K. I., Albain, K. S., Hayes, D. F., . . . Sledge, G. W. (2015). Prospective validation of a 21-gene expression assay in breast cancer. *New England Journal of Medicine, 373*(21), 2005–2014. https://doi.org/10.1056/NEJMoa1510764

Speca, M., Carlson, L. E., Goodey, E., & Angen, M. (2000). A randomized, wait-list controlled clinical trial: The effect of a mindfulness meditation-based stress reduction program on mood and symptoms of stress in cancer outpatients. *Psychosomatic Medicine, 62,* 613–622.

Spector, P. (2002). Employee control and occupational stress. *Current Directions in Psychological Science, 11*(4), 133–136.

Speisman, J. C., Lazarus, R. S., Mordkoff, A., & Davison, L. (1964). Experimental reduction of stress based on ego-defense theory. *Journal of Abnormal and Social Psychology, 68,* 367–380.

Spencer, S. M., Lehman, J. M., Wynings, C., Arena, P., Carver, C. S., Antoni, M. H., Derhagopian, R. P., . . . Love, N. (1999). Concerns about breast cancer and relations to psychosocial well-being in a multiethnic sample of early-stage patients. *Health Psychology, 18,* 159–168.

Spiegel, D. (2001). Mind matters—Group therapy and survival in breast cancer. *New England Journal of Medicine, 345,* 1767–1768.

Spiegel, D., Bloom, J. R., Kraemer, H. C., & Gottheil, E. (1989). Effect of psychosocial treatment on survival of patients with metastatic breast cancer. *The Lancet, 2*(8668), 888–891.

Spiegel, D., & Kato, P. M. (1996). Psychosocial influences on cancer incidence and progression. *Harvard Review of Psychiatry, 4*(1), 10–26.

Spijkerman, M. P. J., Pots, W. T. M., & Bohlmeijer, E. T. (2016). Effectiveness of online mindfulness-based interventions in improving mental health: A review and meta-analysis of randomized controlled trials. *Clinical Psychology Review, 45*, 102–114.

Spring, B., King, A. C., Pagoto, S. L., Van Horn, L., & Fisher, J. D. (2015). Fostering multiple healthy lifestyle behaviors for primary prevention of cancer. *American Psychologist, 70*(2), 75–90. **http://doi.org/10.1037/a0038806**

Sproesser, G., Schupp, H. T., & Renner, B. (2014). The bright side of stress-induced eating: Eating more when stressed but less when pleased. *Psychological Science, 25*(1), 58–65.

Squires, D., & Blumenthal, D. (2016). *Mortality trends among working-age Whites: The untold story.* New York, NY: The Commonwealth Fund.

Stacy, A. W., Newcomb, M. D., & Bentler, P. M. (1991). Cognitive motivation and drug use. *Journal of Abnormal Psychology, 100*(4), 502–515.

Stagl, J. M., Bouchard, L. C., Lechner, S. C., Blomberg, B. B., Gudenkauf, L. M., Jutagir, D. R., . . . Antoni, M. H. (2015). Long-term psychological benefits of cognitive-behavioral stress management for women with breast cancer: 11-year follow-up of a randomized controlled trial. *Cancer, 121*(11), 1873–1881.

Stam, H. J., McGrath, P. A., & Brooke, R. I. (1984). The effects of a cognitive-behavioral treatment program on temporo-mandibular pain and dysfunction syndrome. *Psychosomatic Medicine, 46*, 534–545.

Stamler, J., Wenthworth, D., & Neaton, J. D. (1986). Is relationship between serum cholesterol and risk of premature death from coronary heart disease continuous and graded? Findings in 356, 222 primary screenees of the Multiple Risk Factor Intervention Trial (MRFIT). *Journal of the American Medical Association, 256*, 2823–2828.

Stampfer, M. J., Colditz, G. A., Willett, W. C., Manson, J. E., Rosner, B., Speizer, F. E., & Hennekens, C. H. (1991). Postmenopausal estrogen therapy and cardiovascular disease—Ten-year follow-up from the Nurses' Health Study. *New England Journal of Medicine, 325*, 756–762. **doi:10.1056/NEJM199109123251102**

Stampfer, M. J., Rimm, E. B., & Walsh, D. C. (1993). Commentary: Alcohol, the heart, and public policy. *American Journal of Public Health, 83*, 801–804.

Stanek, K., Abbott, D., & Cramer, S. (1990). Diet quality and the eating environment of preschool children. *Journal of the American Dietetic Association, 90*(11), 1582–1584.

Stanton, A. L. (1987). Determinants of adherence to medical regimens by hypertensive patients. *Journal of Behavioral Medicine, 10*, 377–394.

Stanton, A. L., Danoff-Burg, S., Sworowski, L. A., Collins, C. A., Branstetter, A. D., Rodriguez-Hanley, A., . . . Austenfeld, J. L. (2002). Randomized, controlled trial of written emotional expression and benefit finding in breast cancer patients. *Journal of Clinical Oncology, 20*(20), 4160–4168.

Stanton, A. L., Kirk, S. B., Camerson, C. L., & Danoff-Burg, S. (2000). Coping through emotional approach: Scale construction and validation. *Journal of Personality and Social Psychology, 78*, 1150–1169.

Stanton, A. L., Lobel, M., Sears, S., & DeLuca, R. S. (2002). Psychosocial aspects of selected issues in women's reproductive health: Current status and future directions. *Journal of Consulting and Clinical Psychology, 70*(3), 751–770.

Stanton, A. L., Parsa, A., & Austenfeld, J. L. (2002). The adaptive potential of coping through emotional approach. In C. R. Snyder & S. J. Lopez (Eds.), *Handbook of positive psychology* (pp. 148–158). New York, NY: Oxford University Press.

Stanton, A. L., & Snider, P. R. (1993). Coping with a breast cancer diagnosis: A prospective study. *Health Psychology, 12*(1), 16–23.

Staras, S. A., Livingston, M. D., & Wagenaar, A. C. (2016). Maryland alcohol sales tax and sexually transmitted infections: A natural experiment. *American Journal of Preventive Medicine, 50*(3), 73–80.

Stark, M. J. (1992). Dropping out of substance abuse treatment: A clinically oriented review. *Clinical Psychology Review, 12*(1), 93–116.

Stark, O., Atkins, E., Wolff, O. H., & Douglas, J. W. (1981). Longitudinal study of obesity in the National Survey of Health and Development. *British Medical Journal, 283*(6283), 13–17.

Steele, C. M., & Josephs, R. A. (1990). Alcohol myopia: Its prized and dangerous effects. *American Psychologist, 45*(8), 921–933.

Steers, M., Wickham, R., & Acitelli, L. (2014). Seeing everyone else's highlight reels: How Facebook usage is linked to depressive symptoms. *Journal of Social and Clinical Psychology, 33*(8), 701–731.

Steffens, D., Maher, C. G., Pereira, L. M., Stevens, M. L., Oliveira, V. C., Chapple, M., . . . Hancock, M. J. (2016). Prevention of low back pain: A systematic review and meta-analysis. *JAMA Internal Medicine, 176*(2), 199–208. **https://doi.org/10.1001/jamainternmed.2015.7431**

Stein, J. A., Newcomb, M. D., & Bentler, P. M. (1996). Initiation and maintenance of tobacco smoking: Changing personality correlates in adolescence and young adulthood. *Journal of Applied Social Psychology, 26*(2), 160–187.

Steingart, R. M., Packer, M., Hamm, P., Coglianese, M. E., Gersh, B., Geltman, E. M., . . . Lewis, S. J. (1991). Sex differences in the management of coronary artery disease. *New England Journal of Medicine, 325*(4), 226–230.

Stephens, A. N., & Sullman, M. J. (2015). Trait predictors of aggression and crash-related behaviors across drivers from the United Kingdom and the Irish Republic. *Risk Analysis, 35*(9), 1730–1745.

Stephenson, K. R., Simpson, T. L., Martinez, M. E., & Kearney, D. J. (2017). Changes in mindfulness and posttraumatic stress disorder symptoms among veterans enrolled in mindfulness-based stress reduction. *Journal of Clinical Psychology, 73*(3), 201–217.

Steptoe, A., Hackett, R. A., Lazzarino, A. I., Bostock, S., La Marca, R., Carvalho, L. A., & Hamer, M. (2014). Disruption of multisystem responses to stress in type 2 diabetes: Investigating the dynamics of allostatic load. *Proceedings of the National Academy of Sciences of the United States of America, 111*(44), 15693–15698.

Steptoe, A., & Molloy, G. J. (2007). Personality and heart disease. *Heart, 93*(7), 783–784. https://doi.org/10.1136/hrt.2006.109355

Steptoe, A., Owen, N., Kunz-Ebrecht, S. R., & Brydon, L. (2004). Loneliness and neuroendocrine, cardiovascular, and inflammatory stress responses in middle-aged men and women. *Psychoneuroendocrinology, 29*(5), 593–611. https://doi.org/10.1016/S0306-4530(03)00086-6

Steptoe, A., Wright, C., Kunz-Ebrecht, S. R., & Iliffe, S. (2006). Dispositional optimism and health behaviour in community-dwelling older people: Associations with healthy ageing. *British Journal of Health Psychology, 11*(1), 71–84.

Sternbach, R. A. (1986). Pain and 'hassles' in the United States: Findings of the Nuprin Pain Report. *Pain, 27*(1), 69–80. doi:10.1016/0304-3959(86)90224-1

Stevens, J., Cai, J., Pamuk, E. R., Williamson, D. F., Thun, M. J., & Wood, J. L. (1998). The effect of age on the association between body-mass index and mortality. *New England Journal of Medicine, 338*(1), 1–7.

Stevens, M. M. (1997). Psychological adaptation of the dying child. In D. Doyle, G. W. C. Hanks, & N. MacDonald (Eds.), *Oxford textbook of palliative medicine* (pp. 1046–1055). New York, NY: Oxford University Press.

Stevens, M. M., & Dunsmore, J. C. (1996). Adolescents who are living with a life-threatening illness. In C. A. Corr & D. E. Balk (Eds.), *Handbook of adolescent death and bereavement* (pp. 107–135). New York, NY: Springer.

Stewart-Williams, S. (2004). The placebo puzzle: Putting together the pieces. *Health Psychology, 23*, 198–206.

Stewart-Williams, S., & Podd, J. (2004). The placebo effect: Dissolving the expectancy versus conditioning debate. *Psychological Bulletin, 130*(2), 324–340.

Stice, E., Chase, A., Stormer, S., & Appel, A. (2001). A randomized trial of a dissonance-based eating disorder prevention program. *International Journal of Eating Disorders, 29*(3), 247–262.

Stice, E., Durant, S., Rohde, P., & Shaw, H. (2014). Effects of a prototype internet dissonance-based eating disorder prevention program at 1-and 2-year follow-up. *Health Psychology, 33*(12), 1558–1567.

Stice, E., Marti, C. N., Spoor, S., Presnell, K., & Shaw, H. (2008). Dissonance and healthy weight eating disorder prevention programs: Long-term effects from a randomized efficacy trial. *Journal of Consulting and Clinical Psychology, 76*(2), 329–340.

Stice, E., Mazotti, L., Weibel, D., & Agras, W. S. (2000). Dissonance prevention program decreases thin-ideal internalization, body dissatisfaction, dieting, negative affect, and bulimic symptoms: A preliminary experiment. *International Journal of Eating Disorders, 27*(2), 206–217.

Stice, E., Presnell, K., Groesz, L., & Shaw, H. (2005). Effects of a weight maintenance diet on bulimic symptoms: An experimental test of the dietary restraint theory. *Health Psychology, 24*(4), 402–412.

Stice, E., Rohde, P., Butryn, M. L., Shaw, H., & Marti, C. N. (2015). Effectiveness trial of a selective dissonance-based eating disorder prevention program with female college students: Effects at 2-and 3-year follow-up. *Behaviour Research and Therapy, 71*, 20–26.

Stice, E., Rohde, P., Gau, J., & Shaw, H. (2009). An effectiveness trial of a dissonance-based eating disorder prevention program for high-risk adolescent girls. *Journal of Consulting and Clinical Psychology, 77*(5), 825–834.

Stice, E., Rohde, P., Shaw, H., & Gau, J. (2011). An effectiveness trial of a selected dissonance-based eating disorder prevention program for female high school students: Long-term effects. *Journal of Consulting and Clinical Psychology, 79*(4), 500–508.

Stice, E., Rohde, P., Shaw, H., & Gau, J. M. (2017). Clinician-led, peer-led, and internet-delivered dissonance-based eating disorder prevention programs: Acute effectiveness of these delivery modalities. *Journal of Consulting and Clinical Psychology, 85*(9), 883–895. doi:10.1037/ccp0000211

Stice, E., Shaw, H., Burton, E., & Wade, E. (2006). Dissonance and healthy weight eating disorder prevention programs: A randomized efficacy trial. *Journal of Consulting and Clinical Psychology, 74*(2), 263–275.

Stice, E., Yokum, S., & Waters, A. (2015). Dissonance-based eating disorder prevention program reduces reward region response to thin models; how actions shape valuation. *PLOS ONE, 10*(12).

Stillion, J., & Wass, H. (1984). Children and death. In E. S. Shneidman (Ed.), *Death: Current perspectives* (pp. 225–246). Palo Alto, CA: Mayfield.

Stockwell, T., Zhao, J., Panwar, S., Roemer, A., Naimi, T., & Chikritzhs, T. (2016). Do "moderate" drinkers have reduced mortality risk? A systematic review and meta-analysis of alcohol consumption and all-cause mortality. *Journal of Studies on Alcohol and Drugs, 77*(2), 185–198.

Stokes, A., & Preston, S. H. (2017). Deaths attributable to diabetes in the United States: Comparison of data sources and estimation approaches. *PLOS ONE, 12*(1). **doi:10.1371/journal.pone.0170219**

Stolerman, I. P., & Jarvis, M. J. (1995). The scientific case that nicotine is addictive. *Psychopharmacology, 117*(1), 2–10.

Stolz, E., Burkert, N., Großschädl, F., Rásky, É., Stronegger, W. J., & Freidl, W. (2015). Determinants of public attitudes towards euthanasia in adults and physician-assisted death in neonates in Austria: A national survey. *PLOS ONE, 10*(4), e0124320. **https://doi.org/10.1371/journal.pone.0124320**

Stone, A. A., Mezzacappa, E. S., Donatone, B. A., & Gonder, M. (1999). Psychosocial stress and social support are associated with prostate-specific antigen levels in men: Results from a community screening program. *Health Psychology, 18*(5), 482–486.

Stone, A. A., Schwartz, J. E., Broderick, J. E., & Shiffman, S. S. (2005). Variability of momentary pain predicts recall of weekly pain: A consequence of the peak (or salience) memory heuristic. *Personality and Social Psychology Bulletin, 31*(10), 1340–1346. **https://doi.org/10.1177/0146167205275615**

Stone, A. L., & Wilson, A. C. (2016). Transmission of risk from parents with chronic pain to offspring: An integrative conceptual model. *Pain, 157*(12), 2628–2639.

Stoney, C. M., Davis, M. C., & Matthews, K. A. (1987). Sex differences in physiological responses to stress and in coronary heart disease: A causal link? *Psychophysiology, 24*(2), 127–131.

Stoney, C. M., Matthews, K. A., McDonald, R. H., & Johnson, C. A. (1988). Sex differences in lipid, lipoprotein, cardiovascular, and neuroendocrine responses to acute stress. *Psychophysiology, 25*, 645–656.

Story, M., & Faulkner, P. (1990). The prime time diet: A content analysis of eating behavior and food messages in television program content and commercials. *American Journal of Public Health, 80*(6), 738–740.

Strecher, V. J., Kreuter, M., Den Boer, D. J., Kobrin, S., Hospers, H. J., & Skinner, C. S. (1994). The effects of computer-tailored smoking cessation messages in family practice settings. *Journal of Family Practice, 39*(3), 262–270.

Strike, P. C., Magid, K., Whitehead, D. L., Brydon, L., Bhattacharyya, M. R., & Steptoe, A. (2006). Pathophysiological processes underlying emotional triggering of acute cardiac events. *Proceedings of the National Academy of Sciences of the United States of America, 103*(11), 4322–4327.

Strickhouser, J. E., Zell, E., & Krizan, Z. (2017). Does personality predict health and well-being? A metasynthesis. *Health Psychology, 36*, 797–810. **doi:10.1037/hea0000484**

Stroebe, M., & Schut, H. (1999). The dual process model of coping with bereavement: Rationale and description. *Death Studies, 23*(3), 197–224. **https://doi.org/10.1080/074811899201046**

Stroebe, M. S., & Schut, H. (2001). Models of coping with bereavement: A review. In M. S. Stroebe, R. O. Hansson, W. Stroebe, & H. Schut (Eds.), *Handbook of bereavement research: Consequences, coping, and care* (pp. 375–403). Washington, DC: American Psychological Association.

Stroebe, M. S., & Stroebe, W. (1983). Who suffers more? Sex differences in health risks of the widowed. *Psychological Bulletin, 93*, 279–301.

Stroebe, M. S., & Stroebe, W. (1991). Does "grief work" work? *Journal of Consulting and Clinical Psychology, 59*, 479–482.

Stroebe, W., & Stroebe, M. (1996). The social psychology of social support. In E. T. Higgins & A. W. Kruglanski (Eds.), *Social psychology: Handbook of basic principles* (pp. 597–621). New York, NY: Guilford.

Stroebe, W., Stroebe, M. S., & Abakoumkin, G. (1999). Does differential social support cause sex differences in bereavement outcome? *Journal of Community and Applied Social Psychology, 9*, 1–12.

Struckman-Johnson, C. J., Gilliland, R. C., Struckman-Johnson, D. L., & North, T. C. (1990). The effects of fear of AIDS and gender on responses to fear-arousing condom advertisements. *Journal of Applied Social Psychology, 20*(17), 1396–1410.

Stuckey, H. L., Mullan-Jensen, C. B., Reach, G., Burns, K. K., Piana, N., Vallis, M., . . . Peyrot, M. (2014). Personal accounts of the negative and adaptive psychosocial experiences of people with diabetes in the Second Diabetes Attitudes, Wishes and Needs (DAWN2) Study. *Diabetes Care, 37*(9), 2466–2474.

Stunkard, A. J., & Sorensen, T. I. (1993). Obesity and socioeconomic status—a complex relationship. *New England Journal of Medicine, 329*, 1036–1037.

Sturges, J. W., & Rogers, R. W. (1996). Preventive health psychology from a developmental perspective: An extension of protection motivation theory. *Health Psychology, 15*(3), 158–166.

Suarez, E. C., Kuhn, C. M., Schanberg, S. M., Williams, R. B., & Zimmermann, E. A. (1998). Neuroendocrine, cardiovascular, and emotional responses of hostile men: The role of interpersonal challenge. *Psychosomatic Medicine, 60*(1), 78–88.

Substance Abuse and Mental Health Services Administration. (2014). *Results from the 2013 National Survey on Drug Use and Health: Summary of national findings,* NSDUH Series H-48, HHS Publication No. (SMA) 14-4863. Rockville, MD: Substance Abuse and Mental Health Services Administration. Retrieved from **https://www.samhsa.gov/data/sites/default/files/NSDUHresultsPDFWHTML2013/Web/NSDUHresults2013.htm**

Substance Abuse and Mental Health Services Administration. (2016). *Results from the 2015 National Survey on*

Drug Use and Health. Rockville, MD: Substance Abuse and Mental Health Services Administration.

Suecoff, S. A., Avner, J. R., Chou, K. J., & Crain, E. F. (1999). A comparison of New York City playground hazards in high-and low-income areas. *Archives of Pediatrics & Adolescent Medicine, 153*(4), 363–366.

Suinn, R. M. (1975). The cardiac stress management program for Type A patients. *Cardiac Rehabilitation, 5*, 13–15.

Sullivan, M. J., & D'Eon, J. L. (1990). Relation between catastrophizing and depression in chronic pain patients. *Journal of Abnormal Psychology, 99*(3), 260–263.

Sullivan, M. J. L., Bishop, S. R., & Pivik, J. (1995). The Pain Catastrophizing Scale: Development and validation. *Psychological Assessment, 7*(4), 524–532.

Sullivan, M. J. L., Reesor, K., Mikail, S., & Fisher, R. (1992). The treatment of depression in chronic low back pain: Review and recommendations. *Pain, 50*, 5–13. **https://doi.org/10.1037/1040-3590.7.4.524**

Suls, J., & Bunde, J. (2005). Anger, anxiety, and depression as risk factors for cardiovascular disease: The problems and implications of overlapping affective dispositions. *Psychological Bulletin, 131*(2), 260–300. doi:10.1037/0033-2909.131.2.260

Suls, J., & Fletcher, B. (1985). The relative efficacy of avoidant and nonavoidant coping strategies: A meta-analysis. *Health Psychology, 4*(3), 249–288.

Suls, J., & Marco, C. A. (1990). Relationship between JAS-and FTAS-Type A behavior and non-CHD illness: A prospective study controlling for negative affectivity. *Health Psychology, 9*(4), 479–492.

Suls, J., & Rothman, A. (2004). Evolution of the biopsychosocial model: Prospects and challenges for health psychology. *Health Psychology, 23*(2), 119–125.

Sumartojo, E. (1993). When tuberculosis treatment fails: A social behavioral account of patient adherence. *American Review of Respiratory Disorders, 147*, 1311–1320.

Sumner, J. A., Kubzansky, L. D., Elkind, M. S. V., Roberts, A. L., Agnew-Blais, J., Chen, Q., . . . Koenen, K. C. (2015). Trauma exposure and posttraumatic stress disorder symptoms predict onset of cardiovascular events in women. *Circulation, 132*(4), 251–259. **https://doi.org/10.1161/CIRCULATIONAHA.114.014492**

Sumter, S. R., Bokhorst, C. L., Miers, A. C., Van Pelt, J., & Westenberg, P. M. (2010). Age and puberty differences in stress responses during a public speaking task: Do adolescents grow more sensitive to social evaluation? *Psychoneuroendocrinology, 35*(10), 1510–1516. doi:10.1016/j.psyneuen.2010.05.004

Sun, Q., Townsend, M. K., Okereke, O. I., Franco, O. H., Hu, F. B., & Grodstein, F. (2010). Physical activity at midlife in relation to successful survival in women at age 70 years or older. *Archives of Internal Medicine, 170*(2), 194–201.

Sunday, S. R., & Halmi, K. A. (1996). Micro-and macroanalyses of patterns within a meal in anorexia and bulimia nervosa. *Appetite, 26*(1), 21–36.

Sundquist, K., Winkleby, M., Li, X., Ji, J., Hemminki, K., & Sundquist, J. (2011). Familiar transmission of coronary heart disease: A cohort study of 80,214 Swedish adoptees linked to their biological and adoptive parents. *American Heart Journal, 162*(2), 317–323. **https://doi.org/10.1016/j.ahj.2011.05.013**

Sung, L., Klaassen, R. J., Dix, D., Pritchard, S., Yanofsky, R., Ethier, M.-C., & Klassen, A. (2009). Parental optimism in poor prognosis pediatric cancers. *Psycho-Oncology, 18*(7), 783–788. **https://doi.org/10.1002/pon.1490**

Sunitha Suresh, B. S., De Oliveira, G. S., & Suresh, S. (2015). The effect of audio therapy to treat postoperative pain in children undergoing major surgery: A randomized controlled trial. *Pediatric Surgery International, 31*(2), 197–201. **https://doi.org/10.1007/s00383-014-3649-9**

SUPPORT Principal Investigators. (1995). Controlled trial to improve care for seriously ill hospitalized patients: The study to understand prognoses and preferences for outcomes and risks of treatments (SUPPORT). *Journal of the American Medical Association, 274*(20), 1591–1598. **doi:10.1001/jama.1995.03530200027032**

Surtees, P. G., Wainwright, N. W., Luben, R., Khaw, K. T., & Day, N. E. (2006). Mastery, sense of coherence, and mortality: Evidence of independent associations from the EPIC-Norfolk Prospective Cohort Study. *Health Psychology, 25*(1), 102–110.

Sussman, S., Sun, P., & Dent, C. W. (2006). A meta-analysis of teen cigarette smoking cessation. *Health Psychology, 25*(5), 549–557.

Sutherland, G. T., Sheedy, D., & Kril, J. J. (2014). Using autopsy brain tissue to study alcohol-related brain damage in the genomic age. *Alcoholism: Clinical and Experimental Research, 38*(1), 1–8.

Sutherland, R. J., McDonald, R. J., & Savage, D. D. (1997). Prenatal exposure to moderate levels of ethanol can have long-lasting effects on hippocampal synaptic plasticity in adult offspring. *Hippocampos, 7*(2), 232–238.

Sutin, R., Terracciano, A., Milaneschi, Y., An, Y., Ferrucci, L., & Zonderman, A. B. (2013). The effect of birth cohort on well-being: The legacy of economic hard times. *Psychological Science, 24*, 379–385. **http://dx.doi.org/10.1177/0956797612459658**

Sutker, P. B., Davis, J. M., Uddo, M., & Ditta, S. R. (1995). War zones stress, personal resources, and PTSD in Persian Gulf war returnees. *Journal of Abnormal Psychology, 104*(3), 444–453.

Sutkowi-Hemstreet, A., Vu, M., Harris, R., Brewer, N. T., Dolor, R. J., & Sheridan, S. L. (2015). Adult patients' perspectives on the benefits and harms of overused screening tests: A qualitative study. *Journal of General Internal Medicine, 30*(11), 1618–1626.

Swami, V., Frederick, D. A., Aavik, T., Alcalay, L., Allik, J., Anderson, D., . . . Danel, D. (2010). The attractive female body weight and female body dissatisfaction in 26 countries across 10 world regions: Results of the International Body Project I. *Personality and Social Psychology Bulletin, 36*(3), 309–325.

Swanson, S. A., Crow, S. J., le Grange, D., Swendsen, J., & Merikangas, K. R. (2011). Prevalence and correlates of eating disorders in adolescents: Results from the national comorbidity survey replication adolescent supplement. *Archives of General Psychiatry, 68*(7), 714–723.

Sweat, M., Morin, S., Celentano, D., Mulawa, M., Singh, B., Mbwambo, J., . . . Richter, L. (2011). Community-based intervention to increase HIV testing and case detection in people aged 16–32 years in Tanzania, Zimbabwe, and Thailand (NIMH Project Accept, HPTN 043): A randomised study. *The Lancet Infectious Diseases, 11*(7), 525–532.

Swendsen, J. D., Tennen, H., Carney, M. A., Affleck, G., Willard, A., & Hromi, A. (2000). Mood and alcohol consumption: An experience sampling test of the self-medication hypothesis. *Journal of Abnormal Psychology, 109*(2), 198–204.

Szasz, T. S., & Hollender, M. H. (1956). A contribution to the philosophy of medicine. *Archives of Internal Medicine, 97*, 585–592.

Taddio, A., Katz, J., Ilersich, A. L., & Koren, G. (1997). Effects of neonatal circumcision on pain response during subsequent routine vaccination. *Lancet, 349*, 599–603.

Talbot, F., Nouwen, A., Gingras, J., Bélanger, A., & Audet, J. (1999). Relations of diabetes intrusiveness and personal control to symptoms of depression among adults with diabetes. *Health Psychology, 18*(5), 537–542.

Talbot, M. (2000). The placebo prescription. *The New York Times Magazine*, January 9.

Talmor, A., & Dunphy, B. (2015). Female obesity and infertility. *Best Practice & Research Clinical Obstetrics & Gynaecology, 29*(4), 498–506.

Tam, L., Bagozzi, R. P., & Spanjol, J. (2010). When planning is not enough: The self-regulatory effect of implementation intentions on changing snacking habits. *Health Psychology, 29*(3), 284–292.

Tang, D. W., Fellows, L. K., & Dagher, A. (2014). Behavioral and neural valuation of foods is driven by implicit knowledge of caloric content. *Psychological Science, 25*(12), 2168–2176.

Tang, S. T., Chang, W. C., Chen, J. S., Chou, W. C., Hsieh, C. H., & Chen, C. H. (2016). Associations of prognostic awareness/acceptance with psychological distress, existential suffering, and quality of life in terminally ill cancer patients' last year of life. *Psycho-Oncology, 25*(4), 455–462.

Tang, S. T., Lin, K. C., Chen, J. S., Chang, W. C., Hsieh, C. H., & Chou, W. C. (2015). Threatened with death but growing: Changes in and determinants of posttraumatic growth over the dying process for Taiwanese terminally ill cancer patients. *Psycho-Oncology, 24*(2), 147–154.

Taylor, C. A., Greenlund, S. F., McGuire, L. C., Lu, H., & Croft, J. B. (2017). Deaths from Alzheimer's Disease—United States, 1999–2014. *Morbidity and Mortality Weekly Report, 66*(20), 521–526.

Taylor, C. B., Bandura, A., Ewart, C. K., Miller, N. H., & DeBusk, R. F. (1985). Exercise testing to enhance wives' confidence in their husbands' cardiac capability soon after clinically uncomplicated acute myocardial infarction. *American Journal of Cardiology, 55*, 635–638.

Taylor, S. E. (1979). Hospital patient behavior: Reactance, helplessness, or control. *Journal of Social Issues, 35*(1), 156–184.

Taylor, S. E. (1990). Health psychology: The science and the field. *American Psychologist, 45*(1), 40–50.

Taylor, S. E., & Aspinwall, L. G. (1993). Coping with chronic illness. In L. Goldberger, S. Breznitz, L. Goldberger, & S. Breznitz (Eds.), *Handbook of stress: Theoretical and clinical aspects* (2nd ed., pp. 511–531). New York, NY: Free Press.

Taylor, S. E., Burklund, L. J., Eisenberger, N. I., Lehman, B. J., Hilmert, C. J., & Lieberman, M. D. (2008). Neural bases of moderation of cortisol stress responses by psychosocial resources. *Journal of Personality and Social Psychology, 95*(1), 197–211.

Taylor, S. E., Kemeny, M. E., Aspinwall, L. G., Schneider, S. G., Rodriguez, R., & Herbert, M. (1992). Optimism, coping, psychological distress, and high-risk sexual behavior among men at risk for acquired immunodeficiency syndrome (AIDS). *Journal of Personality and Social Psychology, 63*, 460–473.

Taylor, S. E., Klein, L. C., Lewis, B. P., Gruenewald, T. L., Gurung, R. R., & Updegraff, J. A. (2000). Biobehavioral responses to stress in females: Tend-and-befriend, not fight-or flight. *Psychological Review, 107*(3), 411–429.

Taylor, S. E., Lichtman, R. R., & Wood, J. V. (1984). Attributions, beliefs about control, and adjustment to breast cancer. *Journal of Personality and Social Psychology, 46*(3), 489–502.

Taylor, S. E., Welch, W. T., Kim, H. S., & Sherman, D. K. (2007). Cultural differences in the impact of social support on psychological and biological stress responses. *Psychological Science, 18*(9), 831–837.

Tedeschi, R. G., & Calhoun, L. G. (1996). The posttraumatic growth inventory: Measuring the positive legacy of trauma. *Journal of Traumatic Stress, 9*(3), 455–471.

Telzer, E. H., Ichien, N. T., & Qu, Y. (2015). Mothers know best: Redirecting adolescent reward sensitivity towards safe behavior during risk taking. *Social Cognitive and Affective Neuroscience, 10*(10), 1383–1391.

Teng, Y., & Mak, W. W. (2011). The role of planning and self-efficacy in condom use among men who have sex with men: An application of the Health Action Process Approach model. *Health Psychology, 30*(1), 119–128.

Tennen, H., & Affleck, G. (2002). Benefit-finding and benefit-reminding. In C. R. Snyder & S. J. Lopez (Eds.), *The handbook of positive psychology* (pp. 279–304). New York, NY: Oxford University Press.

Teno, J. M., Clarridge, B. R., Casey, V., Welch, L. C., Wetle, T., Shield, R., & Mor, V. (2004). Family perspectives on end-of-life care at the last place of care. *Journal of the American Medical Association, 291*(1), 88–93.

ter Kuile, M. M., Spinhoven, P., Linssen, A. C., Zitman, F. G., Van Dyck, R., & Rooijmans, H. G. (1994). Autogenic training and cognitive self-hypnosis for the treatment of recurrent headaches in three different subject groups. *Pain, 58,* 331–340.

Tercyak, K. P., Lerman, C., Peshkin, B. N., Hughes, C., Main, D., Isaacs, C., & Schwartz, M. D. (2001). Effects of coping style and BRCA1 and BRCA2 test results on anxiety among women participating in genetic counseling and testing for breast and ovarian cancer risk. *Health Psychology, 20*(3), 217–222.

Terracciano, A., Löckenhoff, C. E., Zonderman, A. B., Ferrucci, L., & Costa, P. T., Jr. (2008). Personality predictors of longevity: Activity, emotional stability, and conscientiousness. *Psychosomatic Medicine, 70*(6), 621–627.

Terry, D. J., & Hynes, G. J. (1998). Adjustment to a low-control situation: Reexamining the role of coping responses. *Journal of Personality and Social Psychology, 74*(4), 1078–1092.

Thakkar, J., Kurup, R., Laba, T.-L., Santo, K., Thiagalingam, A., Rodgers, A., . . . Chow, C. K. (2016). Mobile telephone text messaging for medication adherence in chronic disease. *JAMA Internal Medicine, 176*(3), 340–349.

Theorell, T., Ahlberg-Hulten, G., Sigala, F., Perski, A., Soderholm, M., Kallner, A.,

& Eneroth, P. (1990). A psychosocial and biomedical comparison between men in sex contrasting service occupations. *Work and Stress, 4,* 51–63.

Theorell, T., Blomkvist, V., Jonsson, H., Schulman, S., Berntorp, E., & Stigendal, L. (1995). Social support and the development of immune function in human immunodeficiency virus infection. *Psychosomatic Medicine, 57*(1), 32–36.

Thoits, P. A. (1986). Social support as coping assistance. *Journal of Consulting and Clinical Psychology, 54*(4), 416–423.

Thoits, P. A., Hohmann, A. A., Harvey, M. R., & Fletcher, B. (2000). Similar-other support for men undergoing coronary artery bypass surgery. *Health Psychology, 19*(3), 264–273.

Thomas, J. G., Bond, D. S., Phelan, S., Hill, J. O., & Wing, R. R. (2014). Weight-loss maintenance for 10 years in the National Weight Control Registry. *American Journal of Preventive Medicine, 46*(1), 17–23.

Thomas, K., Hudson, P., Trauer, T., Remedios, C., & Clarke, D. (2014). Risk factors for developing prolonged grief during bereavement in family carers of cancer patients in palliative care: A longitudinal study. *Journal of Pain and Symptom Management, 47*(3), 531–541.

Thomas, S. L., Olds, T., Pettigrew, S., Randle, M., & Lewis, S. (2014). "Don't eat that, you'll get fat!" Exploring how parents and children conceptualise and frame messages about the causes and consequences of obesity. *Social Science & Medicine, 119,* 114–122.

Thompson, D. C., Nunn, M. E., Thompson, R. S., & Rivara, F. P. (1996). Effectiveness of bicycle safety helmets in preventing serious facial injury. *Journal of the American Medical Association, 276*(24), 1974–1975.

Thompson, D. C., & Rivara, F. (2000). Pool fencing for preventing drowning in children. *Cochrane Database of Systematic Reviews, 2,* CD001047.

Thompson, D. C., Rivara, F. P., & Thompson, R. S. (1996). Effectiveness of bicycle safety helmets in preventing head injuries: A case-control study. *Journal of the American Medical Association, 276*(24), 1968–1973.

Thompson, M. D., & Kenna, G. A. (2015). Variation in the serotonin transporter gene and alcoholism: Risk and response to pharmacotherapy. *Alcohol and Alcoholism, 51*(2), 164–171.

Thompson, S. C., Nanni, C., & Levine, A. (1994). Primary versus secondary and central versus consequence-related control in HIV-positive men. *Journal of Personality and Social Psychology, 67*(3), 540–547.

Thompson, S. C., Nanni, C., & Schwankovsky, L. (1990). Patient-oriented interventions to improve communication in a medical visit. *Health Psychology, 9,* 390–404.

Thompson, S. C., Sobolew-Shubin, A., Galbraith, M. E., Schwankovsky, L., & Cruzen, D. (1993). Maintaining perceptions of control: Finding perceived control in low-control circumstances. *Journal of Personality and Social Psychology, 64*(2), 293–304.

Thoolen, B. J., Ridder, D. D., Bensing, J., Gorter, K., & Rutten, G. (2009). Beyond good intentions: The role of proactive coping in achieving sustained behavioural change in the context of diabetes management. *Psychology and Health, 24*(3), 237–254.

Thorndike, E. L. (1905). *The elements of psychology.* New York, NY: Seiler.

Thorpe, C. T., Lewis, M. A., & Sterba, K. R. (2008). Reactions to health-related social control in young adults with type 1 diabetes. *Journal of Behavioral Medicine, 31*(2), 93–103.

Thune, I., Brenn, T., Lund, E., & Gaard, M. (1997). Physical activity and the risk of breast cancer. *New England Journal of Medicine, 336,* 1269–1275.

Tian, Y., & Robinson, J. D. (2017). Predictors of cell phone use in distracted driving: Extending the theory of planned behavior. *Health Communication, 32*(9), 1066–1075.

Tibben, A., Timman, R., Bannink, E. C., & Duivenvoorden, H. J. (1997). Three-year follow-up after presymptomatic testing for Huntington's disease in tested individuals and partners. *Health Psychology, 16*(1), 20–35.

Tice, D. M., & Baumeister, R. F. (1997). Longitudinal study of procrastination, performance, stress, and health: The costs and benefits of dawdling. *Psychological Science, 8*(6), 454–458.

Tickle, J. J., Hull, J. G., Sargent, J. D., Dalton, M. A., & Heatherton, T. F. (2006). A structural equation model of social influences and exposure to media smoking on adolescent smoking. *Basic and Applied Social Psychology, 28*(2), 117–129.

Tickle, J. J., Sargent, J. D., Dalton, M. A., Beach, M. L., & Heatherton, T. F. (2001). Favourite movie stars, their tobacco use in contemporary movies, and its association with adolescent smoking. *Tobacco Control, 10*(1), 16–22.

Tilahun, T., Coene, G., Temmerman, M., & Degomme, O. (2015). Couple based family planning education: Changes in male involvement and contraceptive use among married couples in Jimma Zone, Ethiopia. *BMC Public Health, 15*(1), 682.

Tiller, J., Schmidt, U., Ali, S., & Treasure, J. (1995). Patterns of punitiveness in women with eating disorders. *International Journal of Eating Disorders, 17*(4), 365–371.

Timman, R., Roos, R., Maat-Kievit, A., & Tibben, A. (2004). Adverse effects of predictive testing for Huntington disease underestimated: Long-term effects 7–10 years after the test. *Health Psychology, 23*(2), 189–197.

Tinetti, M. E., Baker, D. I., King, M., Gottschalk, M., Murphy, T. E., Acampora, D., . . . Allore, H. G. (2008). Effect of dissemination of evidence in reducing injuries from falls. *New England Journal of Medicine, 359*(3), 252–261.

Tinsworth, D. K., & McDonald, J. E. (2001). *Special study: Injuries and deaths associated with children's playground equipment.* Washington, DC: US Consumer Product Safety Commission.

Tiro, J. A., Diamond, P. M., Perz, C. A., Fernandez, M., Rakowski, W., DiClemente, C. C., & Vernon, S. W. (2005). Validation of scales measuring attitudes and norms related to mammography screening in women veterans. *Health Psychology, 24*(6), 555–566.

Toker, S., Shirom, A., Melamed, S., & Armon, G. (2012). Work characteristics as predictors of diabetes incidence among apparently healthy employees. *Journal of Occupational Health Psychology, 17*(3), 259–267.

Tomar, S. L., & Giovino, G. A. (1998). Incidence and predictors of smokeless tobacco use among US youth. *American Journal of Public Health, 88*(1), 20–26.

Tomarken, A., Holland, J., Schachter, S., Vanderwerker, L., Zuckerman, E., Nelson, C., . . . Prigerson, H. (2008). Factors of complicated grief pre-death in caregivers of cancer patients. *Psycho-Oncology, 17*(2), 105–111.

Tomfohr, L. M., Pung, M. A., & Dimsdale, J. E. (2016). Mediators of the relationship between race and allostatic load in African and White Americans. *Health Psychology, 35*(4), 322–332.

Tomiyama, A. J., Hunger, J. M., Nguyen-Cuu, J., & Wells, C. (2016). Misclassification of cardiometabolic health when using body mass index categories in NHANES 2005–2012. *International Journal of Obesity, 40*(5), 883–886.

Tomkins, S. S. (1966). Psychological model for smoking behavior. *American Journal of Public Health and the Nations Health, 56*(12), 17–20.

Tomkins, S. S. (1968). A modified model of smoking behavior. In E. F. Borgatta & R. R. Evans (Eds.), *Smoking, health and behavior* (pp. 165–186). Chicago, IL: Aldine.

Toniolo, P., Ribloi, E., Protta, F., Charrel, M., & Coppa, A. P. (1989). Calorie-providing nutrients and risk of breast cancer. *Journal of the National Cancer Institute, 81*, 278–286.

Topa, G., & Moriano, J. A. (2010). Theory of planned behavior and smoking: Meta-analysis and SEM model. *Substance Abuse and Rehabilitation, 1*, 23–33.

Topic, I., Brkljacic, T., & Grahovac, G. (2006). Survey of medical students about attitudes toward organ donation. *Dialysis & Transplantation, 35*(9), 567, 571–574, 577–578.

Torpy, J. M., Campbell, A., & Glass, R. M. (2010). Chronic diseases of children. *Journal of the American Medical Association, 303*(7), 682.

Tosteson, D. C. (1990). New pathways in general medical education. *New England Journal of Medicine, 322*, 234–238.

Toth, P. L., Stockton, R., & Browne, R. (2000). College student grief and loss. In J. H. Harvey & E. D. Miller (Eds.), *Loss and trauma* (pp. 237–248). Philadelphia, PA: Brunner-Rutledge.

Toulany, A., Wong, M., Katzman, D. K., Akseer, N., Steinegger, C., Hancock-Howard, R. L., & Coyte, P. C. (2015). Cost analysis of inpatient treatment of anorexia nervosa in adolescents: Hospital and caregiver perspectives. *CMAJ Open, 3*(2), 192.

Towers, S., Gomez-Lievano, A., Khan, M., Mubayi, A., & Castillo-Chavez, C. (2015). Contagion in mass killings and school shootings. *PLOS ONE, 10*(7), e0117259.

Townsend, S. S. M., Major, B., Gangi, C. E., & Mendes, W. B. (2011). From "in the air" to "under the skin": Cortisol responses to social identity threat. *Personality & Social Psychology Bulletin, 37*(2), 151–164.

Tran, V., Wiebe, D. J., Fortenberry, K. T., Butler, J. M., & Berg, C. A. (2011). Benefit finding, affective reactions to diabetes stress, and diabetes management among early adolescents. *Health Psychology, 30*(2), 212–219.

Trice, A. D., & Price-Greathouse, J. (1986). Joking under the drill: A validity study of the Coping Humor Scale. *Journal of Social Behavior & Personality*, *1*(2), 265–266.

Tristano, A. G. (2014). Impact of rheumatoid arthritis on sexual function. *World Journal of Orthopedics*, *5*(2), 107–111.

Trobst, K. K., Herbst, J. H., Masters, H. L., & Costa, P. T. (2002). Personality pathways to unsafe sex: Personality, condom use, and HIV risk behaviors. *Journal of Research in Personality*, *36*(2), 117–133.

Troxel, W. M., Matthews, K. A., Bromberger, J. T., & Sutton-Tyrrell, K. (2003). Chronic stress burden, discrimination, and subclinical carotid artery disease in African American and Caucasian women. *Health Psychology*, *22*(3), 300–309.

Tsai, W.-I., Prigerson, H. G., Li, C.-Y., Chou, W.-C., Kuo, S.-C., & Tang, S. T. (2015). Longitudinal changes and predictors of prolonged grief for bereaved family caregivers over the first 2 years after the terminally ill cancer patient's death. *Palliative Medicine*, *30*(5), 495–503.

Tucker, J. S., Orlando, M., Burnam, M. A., Sherbourne, C. D., Kung, F. Y., & Gifford, A. L. (2004). Psychosocial mediators of antiretroviral nonadherence in HIV-positive adults with substance use and mental health problems. *Health Psychology*, *23*(4), 363–370.

Tugade, M. M., & Fredrickson, B. L. (2004). Resilient individuals use positive emotions to bounce back from negative emotional experiences. *Journal of Personality and Social Psychology*, *86*(2), 320–333.

Tulloch, H. E., Pipe, A. L., Els, C., Clyde, M. J., & Reid, R. D. (2016). Flexible, dual-form nicotine replacement therapy or varenicline in comparison with nicotine patch for smoking cessation: A randomized controlled trial. *BMC Medicine*, *14*(1), 80.

Tuong, W., & Armstrong, A. W. (2014). Effect of appearance-based education compared with health-based education on sunscreen use and knowledge: A randomized controlled trial. *Journal of the American Academy of Dermatology*, *70*(4), 665–669.

Turk, D. C. (1996). Biopsychosocial perspective on chronic pain. In R. J. Gatchel & D. C. Turk (Eds.), *Psychological approaches to pain management: A practitioner's handbook* (pp. 3–32). New York, NY: Guilford.

Turk, D. C., & Flor, H. (1999). Chronic pain: A biobehavioral perspective. In R. J. Gatchel & D. C. Turk (Eds.), *Psychosocial factors in pain: Critical perspectives* (pp. 18–34). New York, NY: Guilford.

Turk, D. C., Meichenbaum, D., & Genest, M. (1983). *Pain and behavioral medicine: A cognitive-behavioral perspective.* New York, NY: Guilford.

Turk, D. C., Sist, T. C., Okifuji, A., Miner, M. F., Florio, G., Harrison, P., . . . Zevon, M. A. (1998). Adaptation to metastatic cancer pain, regional/local cancer pain, and non-cancer pain: Role of psychological and behavioral factors. *Pain*, *74*(2–3), 247–256.

Turner, J. A., & Chapman, C. R. (1982). Psychological interventions for chronic pain: A critical review. I. Relaxation training and biofeedback. *Pain*, *12*(1), 1–21.

Turner, J. A., & Clancy, S. (1988). Comparison of operant behavioral and cognitive-behavioral group treatment for chronic low back pain. *Journal of Consulting and Clinical Psychology*, *56*(2), 261–266.

Turner, J. A., Clancy, S., McQuade, K. J., & Cardenas, D. D. (1990). Effectiveness of behavioral therapy for chronic low back pain: A component analysis. *Journal of Consulting and Clinical Psychology*, *58*(5), 573–579.

Tuschen-Caffier, B., Bender, C., Caffier, D., Klenner, K., Braks, K., & Svaldi, J. (2015). Selective visual attention during mirror exposure in anorexia and bulimia nervosa. *PLOS ONE*, *10*(12), e0145886.

Twisk, J. W. R., Kemper, H. C. G., van Mechelen, W., & Post, G. B. (1997). Tracking of risk factors for coronary heart disease over a 14-year period: A comparison between lifestyle and biologic risk factors with data from the Amsterdam Growth and Health Study. *American Journal of Epidemiology*, *145*(10), 888–898.

Uchino, B. N., Cacioppo, J. T., & Kiecolt-Glaser, J. K. (1996). The relationship between social support and physiological processes: A review with emphasis on underlying mechanisms and implications for health. *Psychological Bulletin*, *119*(3), 488–531.

Uchino, B. N., Cacioppo, J. T., Malarkey, W., & Glaser, R. (1995). Individual differences in cardiac sympathetic control predict endocrine and immune responses to acute psychological stress. *Journal of Personality and Social Psychology*, *69*(4), 736–784.

Uchino, B. N., Uno, D., & Holt-Lunstad, J. (1999). Social support, physiological processes, and health. *Current Directions in Psychological Science*, *8*(5), 145–148.

Ulrich, R. (1984). View through a window may influence recovery. *Science*, *224*(4647), 420–421.

Undén, A. L., Orth-Gomér, K., & Elofsson, S. (1991). Cardiovascular effects of social support in the work place: Twenty-four-hour ECG monitoring of men and women. *Psychosomatic Medicine*, *53*(1), 50–60.

Unger, J. B., Hamilton, J. E., & Sussman, S. (2004). A family member's job loss as a risk factor for smoking among adolescents. *Health Psychology*, *23*(3), 308–313.

Untas, A., Thumma, J., Rascle, N., Rayner, H., Mapes, D., Lopes, A. A., . . . Pisoni, R. L. (2010). The associations of social support and other psychosocial factors with mortality and quality of life in the dialysis outcomes and practice patterns study. *Clinical Journal of the American Society of Nephrology*, *6*(1), 142–152.

Updegraff, J. A., Taylor, S. E., Kemeny, M. E., & Wyatt, G. E. (2002). Positive and negative effects of HIV infection in women with low socioeconomic resources. *Personality and Social Psychology Bulletin, 28*(3), 382–394.

Ursin, H., Baade, E., & Levine, S. (1978). *Psychobiology of stress: A study of coping men.* New York, NY: Academic Press.

U.S. Department of Health and Human Services. (2014). *The health consequences of smoking—50 years of progress: A report of the Surgeon General.* Atlanta, GA: U.S. Department of Health and Human Services, Centers for Disease Control and Prevention, National Center for Chronic Disease Prevention and Health Promotion, Office on Smoking and Health.

U.S. Department of Health and Human Services. (2016). *E-cigarette use among youth and young adults: A report of the Surgeon General.* Atlanta, GA: Centers for Disease Control and Prevention.

U.S. Department of Justice, Federal Bureau of Investigation. (2011). *Crime in the United States, 2010.* Uniform Crime Reports. Washington, DC: Author.

Vable, A. M., Subramanian, S. V., Rist, P. M., & Glymour, M. M. (2015). Does the "widowhood effect" precede spousal bereavement? Results from a nationally representative sample of older adults. *Sexual Function, 23*(3), 283–292.

Vagi, K. J., Olsen, E. O. M., Basile, K. C., & Vivolo-Kantor, A. M. (2015). Teen dating violence (physical and sexual) among US high school students: Findings from the 2013 National Youth Risk Behavior Survey. *JAMA Pediatrics, 169*(5), 474–482.

Valent, P. (2000). Stress effects of the Holocaust. In G. Fisk (Ed.), *Encyclopedia of stress* (pp. 390–395). San Diego, CA: Academic Press.

Valente, T. W., Murphy, S., Huang, G., Gusek, J., Greene, J., & Beck, V. (2007). Evaluating a minor storyline on ER about teen obesity, hypertension, and 5

a day. *Journal of Health Communication, 12*(6), 551–566.

Valtorta, N. K., Kanaan, M., Gilbody, S., Ronzi, S., & Hanratty, B. (2016). Loneliness and social isolation as risk factors for coronary heart disease and stroke: Systematic review and meta-analysis of longitudinal observational studies. *Heart, 102*(13), 1009–1016.

Van Baal, P. H., Hoogenveen, R. T., de Wit, A. G., & Boshuizen, H. C. (2006). Estimating health-adjusted life expectancy conditional on risk factors: Results for smoking and obesity. *Population Health Metrics, 4*, 14.

Van de Bongardt, D., Reitz, E., Sandfort, T., & Deković, M. (2015). A meta-analysis of the relations between three types of peer norms and adolescent sexual behavior. *Personality and Social Psychology Review, 19*(3), 203–234.

Van Eerdewegh, M. M., Bieri, M. D., Parilla, R. H., & Clayton, P. J. (1982). The bereaved child. *American Journal of Psychiatry, 140*, 23–29.

van Koningsbruggen, G. M., Das, E., & Roskos-Ewoldsen, D. R. (2009). How self-affirmation reduces defensive processing of threatening health information: Evidence at the implicit level. *Health Psychology, 28*(5), 563–568.

Van Norman, G. A. (2014). Physician aid-in-dying: Cautionary words. *Current Opinion in Anaesthesiology, 27*(2), 177–182.

Van Zundert, R. M., Ferguson, S. G., Shiffman, S., & Engels, R. C. (2010). Dynamic effects of self-efficacy on smoking lapses and relapse among adolescents. *Health Psychology, 29*(3), 246–254.

Vanable, P. A., McKirnan, D. J., Buchbinder, S. P., Bartholow, B. N., Douglas, J. M., Jr., Judson, F. N., & MacQueen, K. M. (2004). Alcohol use and high-risk sexual behavior among men who have sex with men: The effects of consumption level and partner type. *Health Psychology, 23*(5), 525–532.

Vasiljevic, M., Petrescu, D. C., & Marteau, T. M. (2016). Impact of

advertisements promoting candy-like flavoured e-cigarettes on appeal of tobacco smoking among children: An experimental study. *Tobacco Control, 25*, e107–e112.

Vassen, O., Røysamb, E., Nielsen, C. S., & Czajkowski, N. O. (2017). Musculoskeletal complaints, anxiety-depression symptoms, and neuroticism: A study of middle-aged twins. *Health Psychology, 36*(8), 729–739.

Vasunilashorn, S., Lynch, S. M., Glei, D. A., Weinstein, M., & Goldman, N. (2015). Exposure to stressors and trajectories of perceived stress among older adults. *The Journals of Gerontology, Series B, 70*(2), 329–336.

Vaughan, E., Anderson, C., Agran, P., & Winn, D. (2004). Cultural differences in young children's vulnerability to injuries: A risk and protection perspective. *Health Psychology, 23*(3), 289–298.

Vaughan, P. W., Rogers, E. M., Singhal, A., & Swalehe, R. M. (2000). Supplementary entertainment-education and HIV/AIDS prevention: A field experiment in Tanzania. *Journal of Health Communication, 5*(Suppl 1), 81–100.

Vertosick, F. T., Jr. (2000). *Why we hurt: The natural history of pain.* New York, NY: Harcourt.

Vicary, A. M., & Fraley, R. C. (2010). Student reactions to the shootings at Virginia Tech and Northern Illinois University: Does sharing grief and support over the internet affect recovery? *Personality and Social Psychology Bulletin, 36*(11), 1555–1563.

Vickers, A. J., Till, C., Tangen, C. M., Lilja, H., & Thompson, I. M. (2011). An empirical evaluation of guidelines on prostate-specific antigen velocity in prostate cancer detection. *Journal of the National Cancer Institute, 103*(6), 462–469.

Victora, C. G., Bahl, R., Barros, A. J., França, G. V., Horton, S., Krasevec, J., . . . Group, T. L. B. S. (2016). Breastfeeding in the 21st century:

Epidemiology, mechanisms, and lifelong effect. *The Lancet, 387*(10017), 475–490.

Vieselmeyer, J., Holguin, J., & Mezulis, A. (2017). The role of resilience and gratitude in posttraumatic stress and growth following a campus shooting. *Psychological Trauma: Theory, Research, Practice, and Policy, 9*(1), 62–69.

Vigdor, E. R., & Mercy, J. A. (2006). Do laws restricting access to firearms by domestic violence offenders prevent intimate partner homicide? *Evaluation Review, 30*(3), 313–346.

Villanti, A., Boulay, M., & Juon, H. S. (2011). Peer, parent and media influences on adolescent smoking by developmental stage. *Addictive Behaviors, 36*(1), 133–136.

Villavicencio-Chávez, C., Monforte-Royo, C., Tomás-Sábado, J., Maier, M. A., Porta-Sales, J., & Balaguer, A. (2014). Physical and psychological factors and the wish to hasten death in advanced cancer patients. *Psycho-Oncology, 23*(10), 1125–1132.

Vincent, C. A., & Richardson, P. H. (1986). The evaluation of therapeutic acupuncture: Concepts and methods. *Pain, 24*(1), 1–13.

Vincent, M. L., Clearie, A. F., & Schluchter, M. D. (1987). Reducing adolescent pregnancy through school and community-based education. *Journal of the American Medical Association, 257*(24), 3382–3386.

Viney, L. L., Walker, B. M., Robertson, T., Lilley, B., & Ewan, C. (1994). Dying in palliative care units and in hospital: A comparison of quality of life of terminal cancer patients. *Journal of Consulting and Clinical Psychology, 62*, 157–164.

Virtanen, M., Jokela, M., Nyberg, S. T., Madsen, I. E. H., Lallukka, T., Ahola, K., . . . Kivimäki, M. (2015). Long working hours and alcohol use: Systematic review and meta-analysis of published studies and unpublished individual participant data. *BMJ, 350*, g7772. **http://doi.org/10.1136/bmj.g7772**

Vitlic, A., Khanfer, R., Lord, J. M., Carroll, D., & Phillips, A. C. (2014). Bereavement reduces neutrophil oxidative burst only in older adults: Role of the HPA axis and immunesenescence. *Immunity & Ageing, 11*(1), 13.

Voci, S. C., Zawertailo, L. A., Hussain, S., & Selby, P. L. (2016). Association between adherence to free nicotine replacement therapy and successful quitting. *Addictive Behaviors, 61*, 25–31.

Vodermaier, A., Caspari, C., Wang, L., Koehm, J., Ditsch, N., & Untch, M. (2011). How and for whom are decision aids effective? Long-term psychological outcome of a randomized controlled trial in women with newly diagnosed breast cancer. *Health Psychology, 30*(1), 12–19.

von Känel, R., Mausbach, B. T., Patterson, T. L., Dimsdale, J. E., Aschbacher, K., Mills, P. J., . . . Grant, I. (2008). Increased Framingham coronary heart disease risk score in dementia caregivers relative to non-caregiving controls. *Gerontology, 54*, 131–137.

Vorona, R. D., Szklo-Coxe, M., Lamichhane, R., Ware, J. C., McNallen, A., & Leszczyszyn, D. (2014). Adolescent crash rates and school start times in two central Virginia counties, 2009–2011: A follow-up study to a southeastern Virginia study, 2007–2008. *Journal of Clinical Sleep Medicine, 10*(11), 1169–1177.

Vrinten, C., Waller, J., von Wagner, C., & Wardle, J. (2015). Cancer fear: Facilitator and deterrent to participation in colorectal cancer screening. *Cancer Epidemiology and Prevention Biomarkers, 24*(2), 400–405.

Vuolo, M., Kadowaki, J., & Kelly, B. C. (2016). A multilevel test of constrained choices theory: The case of tobacco clean air restrictions. *Journal of Health and Social Behavior, 57*(3), 351–372.

Waber, R. L., Shiv, B., Carmon, Z., & Ariely, D. (2008). Commercial features of placebo and therapeutic. *Journal of the American Medical Association, 299*(9), 1016–1017.

Wadden, T. A. (1993). Treatment of obesity by moderate and severe caloric restriction: Results of clinical research trials. *Annals of Internal Medicine, 119*(7), 688–693.

Wadden, T. A., Brownell, K. D., & Foster, G. D. (2002). Obesity: Responding to the global epidemic. *Journal of Consulting and Clinical Psychology, 70*(3), 510–525.

Wade, D. T., & Halligan, P. W. (2004). Do biomedical models of illness make for good healthcare systems? *British Medical Journal, 329*(7479), 1398–1401.

Wagenaar, A. C., & Maldonado-Molina, M. M. (2007). Effects of drivers' license suspension policies on alcohol-related crash involvement: Long-term follow-up in forty-six states. *Alcoholism: Clinical and Experimental Research, 31*, 1399–1406.

Wager, T. D., Rilling, J. K., Smith, E. E., Sokolik, A., Casey, K. L., Davidson, R. J., . . . Cohen, J. D. (2004). Placebo-induced changes in fMRI in the anticipation and experience of pain. *Science, 303*(5661), 1162–1167.

Wagner, P. J., & Curran, P. (1984). Health beliefs and physician identified "worried well." *Health Psychology, 3*(5), 459–474.

Waitzkin, H. (1984). Doctor–patient communication. *Journal of the American Medical Association, 252*(17), 2441–2446.

Waitzkin, H. (1985). Information giving in medical care. *Journal of Health and Social Behavior, 26*, 81–101.

Waldrop, D., Meeker, M. A., & Kutner, J. S. (2015). The developmental transition from living with to dying from cancer: Hospice decision-making. *Journal of Psychosocial Oncology, 33*(5), 576–598.

Walitzer, K. S., Dermen, K. H., & Barrick, C. (2009). Facilitating involvement in Alcoholics Anonymous during out-patient treatment: A randomized clinical trial. *Addiction, 104*(3), 391–401.

Walker, E. A., Katon, W. J., Jemelka, R. P., & Roy-Bryne, P. P. (1992).

Comorbidity of gastrointestinal complaints, depression, and anxiety in the Epidemiologic Catchment Area (ECA) Study. *American Journal of Medicine*, *92*(1A):26S–30S.

Walker, L. S., Garber, J., Smith, C. A., Van Slyke, D. A., & Claar, R. L. (2001). The relation of daily stressors to somatic and emotional symptoms in children with and without recurrent abdominal pain. *Journal of Consulting and Clinical Psychology*, *69*, 85–91.

Walker, L. S., Smith, C. A., Garber, J., & Claar, R. L. (2005). Testing a model of pain appraisal and coping in children with chronic abdominal pain. *Health Psychology*, *24*(4), 364–374.

Walkup, J., Wei, W., Sambamoorthi, U., & Crystal, S. (2008). Antidepressant treatment and adherence to combination antiretroviral therapy among patients with AIDS and diagnosed depression. *Psychiatric Quarterly*, *79*(1), 43–53.

Wallace, R. K., & Benson, H. (1972). The physiology of meditation. *Scientific American*, *226*(2), 84–91.

Wallace, S., Nazroo, J., & Becares, L. (2016). Cumulative effect of racial discrimination on the mental health of ethnic minorities in the United Kingdom. *American Journal of Public Health*, *106*(7), 1294–1301.

Waller, G., & Hartley, P. (1994). Perceived parental style and eating psychopathology. *European Eating Disorders Review*, *2*(2), 76–92.

Wallston, B. S., Alagna, S. W., DeVellis, B. M., & DeVellis, R. F. (1983). Social support and physical health. *Health Psychology*, *2*(4), 367–391.

Walsh, B. T., & Devlin, M. J. (1998). Eating disorders: Progress and problems. *Science*, *280*(5368), 1387–1390.

Walters, S. T., Vader, A. M., Harris, T. R., Field, C. A., & Jouriles, E. N. (2009). Dismantling motivational interviewing and feedback for college drinkers: A randomized clinical trial. *Journal of Consulting and Clinical Psychology*, *77*(1), 64–73.

Wang, A. W.-T., Chang, C.-S., Chen, S.-T., Chen, D.-R., Fan, F., Carver, C. S., & Hsu, W.-Y. (2017). Buffering and direct effect of posttraumatic growth in predicting distress following cancer. *Health Psychology*, *36*(6), 549–559.

Wang, G. S., Le Lait, M. C., Deakyne, S. J., Bronstein, A. C., Bajaj, L., & Roosevelt, G. (2016). Unintentional pediatric exposures to marijuana in Colorado, 2009–2015. *JAMA Pediatrics*, *170*(9), e160971.

Wang, H., Wolock, T. M., Carter, A., Nguyen, G., Kyu, H. H., Gakidou, E., . . . Coates, M. M. (2016). Estimates of global, regional, and national incidence, prevalence, and mortality of HIV, 1980–2015: The Global Burden of Disease Study 2015. *Lancet HIV*, *3*(8), e361–387.

Wang, J., Cheng, Y., Wang, X., Hellard, E. R., Ma, T., Gil, H., . . . Ron, D. (2015). Alcohol elicits functional and structural plasticity selectively in dopamine D1 receptor-expressing neurons of the dorsomedial striatum. *Journal of Neuroscience*, *35*(33), 11634–11643.

Wang, S. S., Houshyar, S., & Prinstein, M. J. (2006). Adolescent girls' and boys' weight-related health behaviors and cognitions: Associations with reputation- and preference-based peer status. *Health Psychology*, *25*(5), 658–663.

Wang, Z., Zhou, Y. T., Kakuma, T., Lee, Y., Kalra, S. P., Kalra, P. S., . . . Unger, R. H. (1999). Leptin resistance of adipocytes in obesity: Role of suppressors of cytokine signaling. *Biochemical and Biophysical Research Communications*, *277*(1), 20–26.

Wansink, B., & Cheney, M. M. (2005). Super bowls: Serving bowl size and food consumption. *Journal of the American Medical Association*, *293*(14), 1727–1728.

Wansink, B., van Ittersum, K., & Painter, J. E. (2006). Ice cream illusions: Bowls, spoons, and self-served portion sizes. *American Journal of Preventive Medicine*, *31*(3), 240–243.

Ward, B. W., Schiller, J. S., & Goodman, R. A. (2014). Multiple chronic conditions among US Adults: A 2012 update. *Preventing Chronic Disease: Public Health Research, Practice, and Policy*, *11*, E62. **http://doi.org/10.5888/pcd11.130389**

Ward, E., DeSantis, C., Robbins, A., Kohler, B., & Jemal, A. (2014). Childhood and adolescent cancer statistics, 2014. *CA: A Cancer Journal for Clinicians*, *64*(2), 83–103.

Warda, L., Tenenbein, M., & Moffatt, M. E. (1999). House fire injury prevention update. Part I. A review of risk factors for fatal and non-fatal house fire injury. *Injury Prevention*, *5*(2), 145–150.

Wardle, J., Carnell, S., Haworth, C. M., & Plomin, R. (2008). Evidence for a strong genetic influence on childhood adiposity despite the force of the obesogenic environment. *American Journal of Clinical Nutrition*, *87*(2), 398–404.

Wardle, J., Robb, K. A., Johnson, F., Griffith, J., Brunner, E., Power, C., & Tovée, M. (2004). Socioeconomic variation in attitudes to eating and weight in female adolescents. *Health Psychology*, *23*(3), 275–282.

Wardle, J., Waller, J., & Jarvis, M. J. (2002). Sex differences in the association of socioeconomic status with obesity. *American Journal of Public Health*, *92*(8), 1299–1304.

Wass, H., & Stillion, J. M. (1988). Death in the lives of children and adolescents. In H. Wass, F. M. Berado, & R. A. Neimeyer (Eds.), *Dying: Facing the facts* (2nd ed., pp. 201–228). New York, NY: Hemisphere.

Watson, D. (1988). Intraindividual and interindividual analyses of positive and negative affect: Their relation to health complaints, perceived stress, and daily activities. *Journal of Personality and Social Psychology*, *54*(6), 1020–1030.

Watson, D., & Clark, L. A. (1984). Negative affectivity: The disposition to experience aversive emotional states. *Psychological Bulletin*, *96*(3), 465–490.

Watson, D., & Pennebaker, J. W. (1989). Health complaints, stress, and distress: Exploring the central role of negative affectivity. *Psychological Review*, *96*(2), 234–254.

Watson, J. D. (1990). The human genome project: Past, present, and future. *Science*, *248*(4951), 44–49.

Weafer, J., & Fillmore, M. T. (2012). Alcohol-related stimuli reduce inhibitory control of behavior in drinkers. *Psychopharmacology*, *222*(3), 489–498.

Weaver, K. E., Llabre, M. M., Durán, R. E., Antoni, M. H., Ironson, G., Penedo, F. J., & Schneiderman, N. (2005). A stress and coping model of medication adherence and viral load in HIV-positive men and women on highly active antiretroviral therapy (HAART). *Health Psychology*, *24*(4), 385–392.

Webel, A. R., Longenecker, C. T., Gripshover, B., Hanson, J. E., Schmotzer, B. J., & Salata, R. A. (2014). Age, stress, and isolation in older adults living with HIV. *AIDS Care*, *26*(5), 523–531.

Webster, D. W., Gainer, P. S., & Champion, H. R. (1993). Weapon carrying among inner-city junior high school students: Defensive behavior vs aggressive delinquency. *American Journal of Public Health*, *83*(11), 1604–1608.

Webster, D. W., Whitehill, J. M., Vernick, J. S., & Curriero, F. C. (2013). Effects of Baltimore's Safe Streets Program on gun violence: A replication of Chicago's CeaseFire Program. *Journal of Urban Health*, *90*(1), 27–40.

Wechsler, H., Dowdall, G. W., Davenport, A., & Castillo, S. (1995). Correlates of college student binge drinking. *American Journal of Public Health*, *85*(7), 921–926.

Weedon-Fekjær, H., Romundstad, P. R., & Vatten, L. J. (2014). Modern mammography screening and breast cancer mortality: Population study. *BMJ: British Medical Journal*, *348*, g3701.

Wegner, D. M. (1994). Ironic processes of mental control. *Psychological Review*, *101*(1), 34–52.

Wegner, D. M., Shortt, J. W., Blake, A. W., & Page, M. S. (1990). The suppression of exciting thoughts. *Journal of Personality and Social Psychology*, *58*(3), 409–418.

Weinstein, N. D. (1984). Why it won't happen to me: Perceptions of risk factors and susceptibility. *Health Psychology*, *3*(5), 431–457.

Weinstein, N. D. (1987). Unrealistic optimism about susceptibility to health problems: Conclusions from a community-wide sample. *Journal of Behavioral Medicine*, *10*(5), 481–500.

Weinstein, N. D. (1988). The precaution adoption process. *Health Psychology*, *7*(4), 355–386.

Weinstein, N. D., & Sandman, P. M. (1992). A model of the precaution adoption process: Evidence from home radon testing. *Health Psychology*, *11*(3), 170–180.

Weinstein, N. D., Rothman, A. J., & Sutton, S. R. (1998). Stage theories of health behavior: Conceptual and methodological issues. *Health Psychology*, *17*(3), 290–299.

Weisner, C., Greenfield, T., & Room, R. (1995). Trends in the treatment of alcohol problems in the US general population, 1979 through 1990. *American Journal of Public Health*, *85*(1), 55–60.

Weiss, A. J., & Elixhauser, A. (2014). Overview of hospital stays in the United States, 2012. *Healthcare Cost and Utilization Project (HCUP) Statistical Brief #180*. Rockville (MD): Agency for Healthcare Research and Quality.

Welin, L., Svärdsudd, K., Ander-Peciva, S., Tibblin, G., Tibblin, B., Larsson, B., & Wilhelmsen, L. (1985). Prospective study of social influences on mortality: The study of men born in 1913 and 1923. *The Lancet*, *325*(8434), 915–918.

Wellenius, G. A., Burger, M. R., Coull, B. A., Schwartz, J., Suh, H. H., Koutrakis, P., . . . Mittleman, M. A. (2012). Ambient air pollution and the risk of acute ischemic stroke. *Archives of Internal Medicine*, *172*(3), 229–234.

Wellisch, D., Kagawa-Singer, M., Reid, S. L., Lin, Y., Nishikawa-Lee, S., & Wellisch, M. (1999). An exploratory study of social support: A cross-cultural comparison of Chinese-, Japanese-, and Anglo-American breast cancer patients. *Psycho-Oncology*, *8*(3), 207–219.

Wenger, N. K., Speroff, L., & Packard, B. (1993). Cardiovascular health and disease in women. *New England Journal of Medicine*, *329*(4), 247–256.

Werner, R. M., & Pearson, T. A. (1998). What's so passive about passive smoking? Secondhand smoke as a cause of atherosclerotic disease. *Journal of the American Medical Association*, *279*(2), 157–158.

West, S. L., & O'Neal, K. K. (2004). Project D.A.R.E. outcome effectiveness revisited. *American Journal of Public Health*, *94*(6), 1027–1029.

Wetter, D. W., Fiore, M. C., Gritz, E. R., Lando, H. A., Stitzer, M. L., Hasselblad, V., & Baker, T. B. (1998). The Agency for Health Care Policy and Research Smoking Cessation Clinical Practice Guideline: Findings and implications for psychologists. *American Psychologist*, *53*(6), 657–669.

Whipple, B. (1987). Methods of pain control: Review of research and literature. *IMAGE: Journal of Nursing Scholarship*, *19*(3), 142–146.

Whisman, M. A. (2010). Loneliness and the metabolic syndrome in a population-based sample of middle-aged and older adults. *Health Psychology*, *29*(5), 550–554.

White, A. A., III, & Gordon, S. L. (1982). Synopsis: Workshop on idiopathic low-back pain. *Spine*, *13*, 1407–1410.

White, E., Jacobs, E. J., & Daling, J. R. (1996). Physical activity in relation to colon cancer in middle-aged men and women. *American Journal of Epidemiology*, *144*(1), 42–50.

White, E., Urban, N., & Taylor, V. (1993). Mammography utilization, public health impact, and cost-effectiveness in the United States. *Annual Review of Public Health, 14,* 605–633.

White, E. K., Warren, C. S., Cao, L., Crosby, R. D., Engel, S. G., Wonderlich, S. A., . . . le Grange, D. (2015). Media exposure and associated stress contribute to eating pathology in women with anorexia nervosa: Daily and momentary associations. *International Journal of Eating Disorders, 49*(6), 617–621.

Whitehead, W. E., Busch, C. M., Heller, B. R., & Costa, P. T. (1986). Social learning influences on menstrual symptoms and illness behavior. *Health Psychology, 5*(1), 13–23.

Whitlock, J., Muehlenkamp, J., Purington, A., Eckenrode, J., Barreira, P., Abrams, G. B., . . . Knox, K. (2011). Nonsuicidal self-injury in a college population: General trends and sex differences. *Journal of American College Health, 59*(8), 691–698.

Whittemore, R., Jaser, S., Chao, A., Jang, M., & Grey, M. (2012). Psychological experience of parents of children with type 1 diabetes: A systematic mixed-studies review. *The Diabetes Educator, 38*(4), 562–579.

Whittle, J., Conigliaro, J., Good, C. B., & Lofgren, R. P. (1993). Racial differences in the use of invasive cardiovascular procedures in the Department of Veterans Affairs medical system. *New England Journal of Medicine, 329*(9), 621–627.

Whooley, M. A., de Jonge, P., Vittinghoff, E., Otte, C., Moos, R., Carney, R. M., . . . Schiller, N. B. (2008). Depressive symptoms, health behaviors, and risk of cardiovascular events in patients with coronary heart disease. *Journal of the American Medical Association, 300*(20), 2379–2388.

Wickelgren, I. (1998). Obesity: How big a problem? *Science, 280*(5368), 1364–1367.

Wickens, C. M., Mann, R. E., Ialomiteanu, A. R., & Stoduto, G. (2016). Do driver anger and aggression contribute to the odds of a crash? A population-level analysis. *Transportation Research Part F: Traffic Psychology and Behaviour, 42,* 389–399.

Wickrama, K. S., Kwon, J. A., Oshri, A., & Lee, T. K. (2014). Early socioeconomic adversity and young adult physical illness: The role of body mass index and depressive symptoms. *Journal of Adolescent Health, 55*(4), 556–563.

Wickrama, K. S., Lee, T. K., O'Neal, C. W., & Kwon, J. A. (2015). Stress and resource pathways connecting early socioeconomic adversity to young adults' physical health risk. *Journal of Youth and Adolescence, 44*(5), 1109–1125.

Wiebe, J. S., & Christensen, A. J. (1997). Health beliefs, personality, and adherence in hemodialysis patients: An interactional perspective. *Annals of Behavioral Medicine, 19*(1), 30–35.

Wiens, A. N., & Menustik, C. E. (1983). Treatment outcome and patient characteristics in an aversion therapy program for alcoholism. *American Psychologist, 38*(10), 1089–1096.

Wiggins, S., Whyte, P., Huggins, M., Adam, S., Theilmann, J., Bloch, M., . . . Hayden, M. R. (1992). The psychological consequences of predictive testing for Huntingtons disease. *New England Journal of Medicine, 327*(20), 1401–1405.

Wight, R. G., LeBlanc, A. J., & Aneshensel, C. S. (1998). AIDS caregiving and health among midlife and older women. *Health Psychology, 17*(2), 130–137.

Wilcox, H. C., Conner, K. R., & Caine, E. D. (2004). Association of alcohol and drug use disorders and completed suicide: An empirical review of cohort studies. *Drug and Alcohol Dependence, 76,* 11–19.

Wilcox, H. C., Kuramoto, S. J., Lichtenstein, P., Långström, N., Brent, D. A., & Runeson, B. (2010). Psychiatric morbidity, violent crime, and suicide among children and adolescents exposed to parental death. *Journal of the American Academy of Child & Adolescent Psychiatry, 49*(5), 514–523.

Wilcox, H. C., Mittendorfer-Rutz, E., Kjeldgård, L., Alexanderson, K., & Runeson, B. (2015). Functional impairment due to bereavement after the death of adolescent or young adult offspring in a national population study of 1,051,515 parents. *Social Psychiatry and Psychiatric Epidemiology, 50*(8), 1249–1256.

Wildes, J. E., Marcus, M. D., Cheng, Y., McCabe, E. B., & Gaskill, J. A. (2014). Emotion acceptance behavior therapy for anorexia nervosa: A pilot study. *International Journal of Eating Disorders, 47*(8), 870–873.

Wildes, K. A., Miller, A. R., de Majors, S. S. M., & Ramirez, A. G. (2009). The religiosity/spirituality of Latina breast cancer survivors and influence on health-related quality of life. *Psycho-Oncology, 18*(8), 831–840.

Wilfond, B. S., & Fost, N. (1990). The cystic fibrosis gene: Medical and social implications for heterozygote detection. *Journal of the American Medical Association, 263*(20), 2777–2783.

Willenbring, M. L., Levine, A. S., & Morley, J. E. (1986). Stress induced eating and food preference in humans: A pilot study. *International Journal of Eating Disorders, 5*(5), 855–864.

Williams, D. A. (1996). Acute pain management. In R. J. Gatchel & D. C. Turk (Eds.), *Psychological approaches to pain management: A practitioner's handbook* (pp. 55–77). New York, NY: Guilford.

Williams, J. E., Paton, C. C., Siegler, I. C., Eigenbrot, M. L., Nieto, F. J., & Tyroler, H. A. (2000). Clinical investigation and reports: Anger proneness predicts coronary heart disease risk: Prospective analysis from the Atherosclerosis Risk in Communities (ARIC) Study. *Circulation, 101*(17), 2034–2039.

Williams, P. G., Wiebe, D. J., & Smith, T. W. (1992). Coping processes as mediators of the relationship between hardiness and health. *Journal of Behavioral Medicine*, *15*(3), 237–255.

Williams, R. B., Barefoot, J. C., Califf, R. M., Haney, T. L., Saunders, W. B., Pryor, D. B., . . . Mark, D. B. (1992). Prognostic importance of social and economic resources among medically treated patients with angiographically documented coronary artery disease. *Journal of the American Medical Association*, *267*(4), 520–524.

Williams, R. B., Jr., Haney, T. L., Lee, K. L., Kong, Y., Blumenthal, J. A., & Whalen, R. E. (1980). Type A behavior, hostility, and coronary arteriosclerosis. *Psychosomatic Medicine*, *42*(6), 539–549.

Williams, R. J., Herzog, T. A., & Simmons, V. N. (2011). Risk perception and motivation to quit smoking: A partial test of the Health Action Process Approach. *Addictive Behaviors*, *36*(7), 789–791.

Williams-Piehota, P., Pizarro, J., Schneider, T. R., Mowad, L., & Salovey, P. (2005). Matching health messages to monitor-blunter coping styles to motivate screening mammography. *Health Psychology*, *24*(1), 58–67.

Wills, T. A. (1985). Supportive functions of interpersonal relationships. In S. Cohen & S. L. Syme (Eds.), *Social support and health* (pp. 61–82). Orlando, FL: Academic Press.

Wills, T. A., Gibbons, F. X., Sargent, J. D., Gerrard, M., Lee, H. R., & Dal Cin, S. (2010). Good self-control moderates the effect of mass media on adolescent tobacco and alcohol use: Tests with studies of children and adolescents. *Health Psychology*, *29*(5), 539–549.

Wills, T. A., Resko, J. A., Ainette, M. G., & Mendoza, D. (2004). Role of parent support and peer support in adolescent substance use: A test of mediated effects. *Psychology of Addictive Behaviors*, *18*(2), 122–134.

Wills, T. A., Sargent, J. D., Stoolmiller, M., Gibbons, F. X., & Gerrard, M.

(2008). Movie smoking exposure and smoking onset: A longitudinal study of mediation processes in a representative sample of US adolescents. *Psychology of Addictive Behaviors*, *22*(2), 269–277.

Wills, T. A., Sargent, J. D., Stoolmiller, M., Gibbons, F. X., Worth, K. A., & Dal Cin, S. (2007). Movie exposure to smoking cues and adolescent smoking onset: A test for mediation through peer affiliations. *Health Psychology*, *26*(6), 769–776.

Wilson, H., Sheehan, M., Palk, G., & Watson, A. (2016). Self-efficacy, planning, and drink driving: Applying the health action process approach. *Health Psychology*, *35*(7), 695–703.

Wilson, R. S., Krueger, K. R., Gu, L., Bienias, J. L., de Leon, C. F. M., & Evans, D. A. (2005). Neuroticism, extraversion, and mortality in a defined population of older persons. *Psychosomatic Medicine*, *67*(6), 841–845.

Wilson, S. J., Martire, L. M., & Sliwinski, M. J. (2017). Daily spousal responsiveness predicts longer-term trajectories of patients' physical function. *Psychological Science*, *8*(6), 786–797.

Windle, M., & Windle, R. C. (2001). Depressive symptoms and cigarette smoking among middle adolescents: Prospective associations and intrapersonal and interpersonal influences. *Journal of Consulting and Clinical Psychology*, *69*(2), 215–226.

Windsor, R. A., Lowe, J. B., Perkins, L. L., Smith-Yoder, D., Artz, L., Crawford, M., . . . Boyd, N. R., Jr. (1993). Health education for pregnant smokers: Its behavioral impact and cost benefit. *American Journal of Public Health*, *83*(2), 201–206.

Winett, R. A. (1995). A framework for health promotion and disease prevention programs. *American Psychologist*, *50*(5), 341–350.

Wing, R. R., & Jeffery, R. W. (1999). Benefits of recruiting participants with friends and increasing social support for weight loss and maintenance. *Journal of*

Consulting and Clinical Psychology, *67*(1), 132–138.

Winkleby, M. A., Kraemer, H. C., Ahn, D. K., & Varady, A. N. (1998). Ethnic and socioeconomic differences in cardiovascular disease risk factors. *Journal of the American Medical Association*, *280*(4), 356–362.

Winkleby, M. A., Robinson, T. N., Sundquist, J., & Kraemer, H. C. (1999). Ethnic variation in cardiovascular disease risk factors among children and young adults: Findings from the Third National Health and Nutrition Examination Survey, 1988–1994. *Journal of the American Medical Association*, *281*(11), 1006–1013.

Winn, D. M., Blot, W. J., Shy, C. M., Pickle, L. W., Toledo, A., & Fraumeni, J. F., Jr. (1981). Snuff dipping and oral cancer among women in the southern United States. *New England Journal of Medicine*, *304*(13), 745–749.

Winning, A., Glymour, M. M., McCormick, M. C., Gilsanz, P., & Kubzansky, L. D. (2015). Psychological distress across the life course and cardiometabolic risk. *Journal of the American College of Cardiology*, *66*(14), 1577–1586.

Winslow, B. T., Onysko, M., & Hebert, M. (2016). Medication for alcohol use disorder. *American Family Physician*, *93*(6), 457–465.

Winters, R. (1985). Behavioral approaches to pain. In N. Schneiderman & J. T. Tapp (Eds.), *Behavioral medicine: The biopsychosocial approach* (pp. 565–587). Hillsdale, NJ: Erlbaum.

Winzelberg, A. J., Eppstein, D., Eldredge, K. L., Wilfley, D., Dasmahapatra, R., Dev, P., & Taylor, C. B. (2000). Effectiveness of an Internet-based program for reducing risk factors for eating disorders. *Journal of Consulting and Clinical Psychology*, *68*(2), 346–350.

Wise, P. H., Kotelchuck, M., Wilson, M. L., & Mills, M. (1985). Racial and socioeconomic disparities in childhood mortality in Boston. *New England Journal of Medicine, 313*(6), 360–366.

Wiseman, C. V., Gray, J. J., Mosimann, J. E., & Ahrens, A. H. (1992). Cultural expectations of thinness in women: An update. *International Journal of Eating Disorders, 11*(1), 85–89.

Wisocki, P. A., & Skowron, J. (2000). The effects of gender and culture on adjustment to widowhood. In R. M. Eisler & M. Hersen (Eds.), *Handbook of gender, culture, and health* (pp. 429–447). Mahwah, NJ: Erlbaum.

Witek-Janusek, L., Albuquerque, K., Chroniak, K. R., Chroniak, C., Durazo-Arvizu, R., & Mathews, H. L. (2008). Effect of mindfulness based stress reduction on immune function, quality of life and coping in women newly diagnosed with early stage breast cancer. *Brain, Behavior, and Immunity, 22*(6), 969–981.

Witt, W. P., Weiss, A. J., & Elixhauser, A. (2014). Overview of hospital stays for children in the United States, 2012. *Healthcare Cost and Utilization Project (HCUP) Statistical Brief #187*. Rockville (MD): Agency for Healthcare Research and Quality.

Witte, K., & Allen, M. (2000). A meta-analysis of fear appeals: Implications for effective public health campaigns. *Health Education & Behavior, 27*(5), 591–615.

Wnuk, S. M., Greenberg, L., & Dolhanty, J. (2014). Emotion-focused group therapy for women with symptoms of bulimia nervosa. *Eating Disorders, 23*(3), 253–261.

Wolf, L. L., Chowdhury, R., Tweed, J., Vinson, L., Losina, E., Haider, A. H., & Qureshi, F. G. (2017). Factors associated with pediatric mortality from motor vehicle crashes in the United States: A state-based analysis. *The Journal of Pediatrics, 187*, 295–302.e3.

Wolff, N. J., Darlington, A.-S. E., Hunfeld, J. A. M., Verhulst, F. C., Jaddoe, V. W. V., Moll, H. A., . . . Tiemeier, H. (2009). The association of parent behaviors, chronic pain, and psychological problems with venipuncture distress in infants: The Generation R study. *Health Psychology, 28*(5), 605–613.

Wolin, K. Y., Yan, Y., Colditz, G. A., & Lee, I. M. (2009). Physical activity and colon cancer prevention: A meta-analysis. *British Journal of Cancer, 100*(4), 611–616.

Wolpe, J. (1958). *Psychotherapy by reciprocal inhibition*. Stanford, CA: Stanford University Press.

Wonderlich, S., Klein, M. H., & Council, J. R. (1996). Relationship of social perceptions and self-concept in bulimia nervosa. *Journal of Consulting and Clinical Psychology, 64*(6), 1231–1237.

Wonderlich, S. A., Wilsnack, R. W., Wilsnack, S. C., & Harris, T. R. (1996). Childhood sexual abuse and bulimic behavior in a nationally representative sample. *American Journal of Public Health, 86*(8), 1082–1086.

Wong, J. M., Sin, N. L., & Whooley, M. A. (2014). A comparison of Cook-Medley hostility subscales and mortality in patients with coronary heart disease: Data from the Heart and Soul Study. *Psychosomatic Medicine, 76*(4), 311–317.

Woods, P. J., & Burns, J. (1984). Type A behavior and illness in general. *Journal of Behavioral Medicine, 7*(4), 411–415.

Woods, P. J., Morgan, B. T., Day, B. W., Jefferson, T., & Harris, C. (1984). Findings on a relationship between Type A behavior and headaches. *Journal of Behavioral Medicine, 7*(3), 277–286.

Woodward, W. A., Huang, E. H., McNeese, M. D., Perkins, G. H., Tucker, S. L., Strom, E. A., . . . Buchholz, T. A. (2006). African-American race is associated with a poorer overall survival rate for breast cancer patients treated with mastectomy and doxorubicin-based chemotherapy. *Cancer, 107*(11), 2662–2668.

Woolhandler, S., & Himmelstein, D. U. (1991). The deteriorating administrative efficiency of the US health care system. *New England Journal of Medicine, 324*(18), 1253–1258.

World Health Organization. (1964). *Basic documents* (15th ed.). Geneva, Switzerland: Author.

World Health Organization. (2017a). Number of people (all ages) living with HIV: Estimates by WHO region. Retrieved from **http://apps .who.int/gho/data/view.main.22 100WHO?lang=en**

World Health Organization. (2017b). Tobacco. Retrieved from **http://www .who.int/mediacentre/factsheets/ fs339/en/**

World Health Organization. (2018). Global Health Observatory (GHO) data. Retrieved from **http://www.who .int/gho/mortality_burden_disease/ en/**

Wortman, C. B., & Lehman, D. (1985). Reactions to victims of life crises: Support attempts that fail. In I. G. Sarason & B. R. Sarason (Eds.), *Social support: Theory, research, and application* (pp. 463–489). The Hague, NL: Martinus Nijhof.

Wright, A. A., Zhang, B., Ray, A., Mack, J. W., Trice, E., Balboni, T., . . . Prigerson, H. G. (2008). Associations between end-of-life discussions, patient mental health, medical care near death, and caregiver bereavement adjustment. *Journal of the American Medical Association, 300*(14), 1665–1673.

Wright, B., O'Brien, S., Hazi, A., & Kent, S. (2014). Increased systolic blood pressure reactivity to acute stress is related with better self-reported health. *Scientific Reports, 4*, 6882.

Writing Group for the Women's Health Initiative Investigators. (2002). Risks and benefits of estrogen plus progestin in healthy postmenopausal women: Principal results from the Women's Health Initiative Randomized Controlled Trial. *Journal of the American Medical Association, 288*(3), 321–333.

Xu, J., & Roberts, R. E. (2010). The power of positive emotions: It's a matter of life or death—Subjective well-being and longevity over 28 years in a general population. *Health Psychology, 29*(1), 9–19.

Xu, J. Q., Murphy, S. L., Kochanek, K. D., & Arias, E. (2016). Mortality in the United States, 2015. *National Center for Health Statistics Data Brief, No 267.* Hyattsville, MD: National Center for Health Statistics.

Xuan, Z., Naimi, T. S., Kaplan, M. S., Bagge, C. L., Few, L. R., Maisto, S., . . . Freeman, R. (2016). Alcohol policies and suicide: A review of the literature. *Alcoholism: Clinical and Experimental Research, 40*(10), 2043–2055.

Yamakawa, M., Yorifuji, T., Inoue, S., Kato, T., & Doi, H. (2013). Breastfeeding and obesity among schoolchildren: A nationwide longitudinal survey in Japan. *JAMA Pediatrics, 167*(10), 919–925.

Yamamoto, Y., Hayashino, Y., Akiba, T., Akizawa, T., Asano, Y., Saito, A., . . . Fukuhara, S. (2009). Depressive symptoms predict the subsequent risk of bodily pain in dialysis patients: Japan dialysis outcomes and practice patterns study. *Pain Medicine, 10*(5), 883–889.

Yang, Y. C., Boen, C., Gerken, K., Li, T., Schorpp, K., & Harris, K. M. (2016). Social relationships and physiological determinants of longevity across the human life span. *Proceedings of the National Academy of Sciences of the United States of America, 113*(3), 578–583.

Yang, Y. C., Schorpp, K., & Harris, K. M. (2014). Social support, social strain and inflammation: Evidence from a national longitudinal study of US adults. *Social Science & Medicine, 107,* 124–135.

Yarnold, P. R., Michelson, E. A., Thompson, D. A., & Adams, S. L. (1998). Predicting patient satisfaction: A study of two emergency departments. *Journal of Behavioral Medicine, 21*(6), 545–563.

Yarosh, H. L., Hyatt, C. J., Meda, S. A., Jiantonio-Kelly, R., Potenza, M. N., Assaf, M., & Pearlson, G. D. (2014). Relationships between reward sensitivity, risk-taking and family history of alcoholism during an interactive competitive fMRI task. *PLOS ONE, 9*(2), e88188.

Ybema, J. F., Kuijer, R. G., Buunk, B. P., DeJong, G. M., & Sanderman, R. (2001). Depression and perceptions of inequity among couples facing cancer. *Personality and Social Psychology Bulletin, 27*(1), 3–13.

Yedidia, M. J., Gillespie, C. C., Kachur, E., Schwartz, M. D., Ockene, J., Chepaitis, A. E., . . . Lipkin, M., Jr. (2003). Effect of communications training on medical student performance. *Journal of the American Medical Association, 290*(9), 1157–1165.

Yee, B. W. K., Castro, F. G., Hammond, W. R., John, R., Wyatt, G. E., & Yurg, B. R. (1995). Panel IV: Risk-taking and abusive behaviors among ethnic minorities. *Health Psychology, 14*(7), 622–631.

Yeh, E. S., Rochette, L. M., McKenzie, L. B., & Smith, G. A. (2011). Injuries associated with cribs, playpens, and bassinets among young children in the US, 1990–2008. *Pediatrics, 127*(3), 479–486.

Yehuda, R., Engel, S. M., Brand, S. R., Seckl, J., Marcus, S. M., & Berkowitz, G. S. (2005). Transgenerational effects of posttraumatic stress disorder in babies of mothers exposed to the World Trade Center attacks during pregnancy. *The Journal of Clinical Endocrinology & Metabolism, 90*(7), 4115–4118. **https://doi.org/10.1210/jc.2005-0550**

Yi, M. S., Mrus, J. M., Wade, T. J., Ho, M. L., Hornung, R. W., Cotton, S., . . . Tsevat, J. (2006). Religion, spirituality, and depressive symptoms in patients with HIV/AIDS. *Journal of General Internal Medicine, 21*(Suppl 5), S21–S27.

Yong, L.-C., Brown, C. C., Schatzkin, A., Dresser, C. M., Slesinshi, M. J., Cox, C. S., & Taylor, P. R. (1997). Intake of vitamins E, C, and A and risk of lung cancer: The NHANES I Epidemiologic Followup Study. *American Journal of Epidemiology, 146*(3), 231–243.

Yoon, H. H., Shi, Q., Alberts, S. R., Goldberg, R. M., Thibodeau, S. N., Sargent, D. J., & Sinicrope, F. A. (2015). Racial differences in BRAF/KRAS mutation rates and survival in stage III colon cancer patients. *Journal of the National Cancer Institute, 107*(10), djv186.

Younger, J., Aron, A., Parke, S., Chatterjee, N., & Mackey, S. (2010). Viewing pictures of a romantic partner reduces experimental pain: Involvement of neural reward systems. *PLOS ONE, 5*(10), e13309.

Yusuf, S., Hawken, S., Ôunpuu, S., Bautista, L., Franzosi, M. G., Commerford, P., . . . Tanomsup, S. (2005). Obesity and the risk of myocardial infarction in 27 000 participants from 52 countries: A case-control study. *The Lancet, 366*(9497), 1640–1649.

Zahran, S., Snodgrass, J. G., Maranon, D. G., Upadhyay, C., Granger, D. A., & Bailey, S. M. (2015). Stress and telomere shortening among central Indian conservation refugees. *Proceedings of the National Academy of Sciences of the United States of America, 112*(9), E928–E936.

Zarski, J. J. (1984). Hassles and health: A replication. *Health Psychology, 3*(3), 243–251.

Zashikhina, A., & Hagglof, B. (2007). Mental health in adolescents with chronic physical illness versus controls in Northern Russia. *Acta Paediatrica, 96*(6), 890–896.

Zaso, M. J., Park, A., Kim, J., Gellis, L. A., Kwon, H., & Maisto, S. A. (2016). The associations among prior drinking consequences, subjective evaluations, and subsequent alcohol outcomes. *Psychology of Addictive Behaviors, 30*(3), 367–376.

Zastowny, T. R., Kirschenbaum, D. S., & Meng, A. L. (1986). Coping skills training for children: Effects on distress before, during, and after hospitalization for surgery. *Health Psychology, 5*(3), 231–247.

Zavala, M. W., Maliski, S. L., Kwan, L., Fink, A., & Litwin, M. S. (2009). Spirituality and quality of life in low-income men with metastatic prostate cancer. *Psycho-Oncology, 18*(7), 753–761.

Zawertailo, L., Voci, S., & Selby, P. (2015). Depression status as a predictor of quit success in a real-world effectiveness study of nicotine replacement therapy. *Psychiatry Research*, *226*(1), 120–127.

Zebib, L., Stoler, J., & Zakrison, T. L. (2017). Geo-demographics of gunshot wound injuries in Miami-Dade County, 2002–2012. *BMC Public Health*, *17*, 174.

Zeidan, F., Emerson, N. M., Farris, S. R., Ray, J. N., Jung, Y., McHaffie, J. G., & Coghill, R. C. (2015). Mindfulness meditation-based pain relief employs different neural mechanisms than placebo and sham mindfulness meditation-induced analgesia. *The Journal of Neuroscience*, *35*(46), 15307–15325.

Zeidan, F., Martucci, K. T., Kraft, R. A., Gordon, N. S., McHaffie, J. G., & Coghill, R. C. (2011). Brain mechanisms supporting the modulation of pain by mindfulness meditation. *Journal of Neuroscience*, *31*(14), 5540–5548.

Zelman, D. C., Brandon, T. H., Jorenby, D. E., & Baker, T. B. (1992). Measures of affect and nicotine dependence predict differential response to smoking cessation treatments. *Journal of Consulting and Clinical Psychology*, *60*(6), 943–952.

Zeoli, A. M., & Webster, D. W. (2010). Effects of domestic violence policies, alcohol taxes and police staffing levels on intimate partner homicide in large US cities. *Injury Prevention*, *16*(2), 90–95.

Zhang, B., Cohen, J. E., Bondy, S. J., & Selby, P. (2015). Duration of nicotine replacement therapy use and smoking cessation: A population-based longitudinal study. *American Journal of Epidemiology*, *181*(7), 513–520.

Zhang, J., Walsh, M. F., Wu, G., Edmonson, M. N., Gruber, T. A., Easton, J., . . . Downing, J. R. (2015). Germline mutations in predisposition genes in pediatric cancer. *New England Journal of Medicine*, *373*(24), 2336–2346.

Zhang, S., Hunter, D. J., Forman, M. R., Rosner, B. A., Speizer, F. F., Colditz, G. A., . . . Willett, W. C. (1999). Dietary carotenoids and vitamins A, C, and E and risk of breast cancer. *Journal of the National Cancer Institute*, *91*(6), 547–556.

Zhu, S. H., Stretch, V., Balabanis, M., Rosbrook, B., Sadler, G., & Pierce, J. P. (1996). Telephone counseling for smoking cessation: Effects of single-session and multiple-session interventions. *Journal of Consulting and Clinical Psychology*, *64*(1), 202–211.

Zhu, S. H., Sun, J., Billings, S. C., Choi, W. S., & Malarcher, A. (1999). Predictors of smoking cessation in US adolescents. *American Journal of Preventive Medicine*, *16*(3), 202–207.

Zilioli, S., Slatcher, R. B., Ong, A. D., & Gruenewald, T. L. (2015). Purpose in life predicts allostatic load ten years later. *Journal of Psychosomatic Research*, *79*(5), 451–457.

Zisook, S., Schuchter, S. R., Sledge, P. A., & Judd, L. L. (1994). The spectrum of depressive phenomena after spousal bereavement. *Journal of Clinical Psychiatry*, *55*(Suppl), 29–36.

Zschucke, E., Renneberg, B., Dimeo, F., Wüstenberg, T., & Ströhle, A. (2015). The stress-buffering effect of acute exercise: Evidence for HPA axis negative feedback. *Psychoneuroendocrinology*, *51*, 414–425.

Zucker, R. A., & Gomberg, E. S. L. (1986). Etiology of alcoholism reconsidered. *American Psychologist*, *41*(7), 783–793.

Zucker, T. P., Flesche, C. W., Germing, U., Schroter, S., Willers, R., Wolf, H. H., & Heyll, A. (1998). Patient-controlled versus staff-controlled analgesia with pethidine after allogenic bone marrow transplantation. *Pain*, *75*(2–3), 305–312.

Zunhammer, M., Eichhammer, P., & Busch, V. (2014). Sleep quality during exam stress: The role of alcohol, caffeine and nicotine. *PLOS ONE*, *9*(10), e109490.

Zvolensky, M. J., Farris, S. G., Kotov, R., Schechter, C. B., Bromet, E., Gonzalez, A., . . . Moline, J. (2015). World Trade Center disaster and sensitization to subsequent life stress: A longitudinal study of disaster responders. *Preventive Medicine*, *75*, 70–74.

AUTHOR INDEX

Halmi, K. A., 259
Halpern, C. T., 260, 261
Halpern, M., 79
Halpern, S. D., 69
Halpern-Felsher, B. L., 204
Hamano, J., 385
Hambarsoomians, K., 214
Hamer, J., 363
Hamer, M., 139
Hamilton, J. E., 208
Hamilton, R. L., 28
Hamilton, W. L., 224
Hammon, S., 370
Hammond, S. K., 49
Hammond, S. L., 77, 81
Hampel, P., 327
Hampson, S. E., 148, 155
Hancock, J. T., 289
Hanisch, R., 363
Hanks, A. S., 448
Hannan, M. T., 213
Hannerz, H., 121, 244
Hanratty, B., 135, 354–55
Hansell, S., 150
Hansen, A. M., 395, 397
Hansen, N. B., 437
Hansen, W. B., 213, 215, 221
Hardesty, L. A., 416
Hardin, J. W., 459 (figure)
Harding, D. J., 186
Harding, G. H., 416
Harding, R., 394
Harding, S. V., 250
Hardison-Moody, A., 248
Hargreaves, W., 417
Harknett, K., 186
Harlow, B. L., 326
Harper, M., 401
Harrell, E., 101, 186
Harriger, J. A., 261
Harris, C., 151
Harris, G., 283
Harris, K. M., 10, 135, 141
Harris, M., 306
Harris, M. J., 151
Harris, P., 287
Harris, P. L., 411
Harris, P. R., 81
Harris, T. B., 143
Harris, T. R., 85, 184, 264
Harrop, E. N., 234
Hart M., 431
Hartley, P., 263
Hartmann, A. S., 258
Hartmann, L. C., 411
Hartnett, S. M., 195
Hartwick, J., 66, 362
Harvath, T. A., 388
Harvey, J. H., 395, 397

Harvey, M. R., 138
Harvey, W., 306
Hasan, O., 434
Hasegawa, T., 87
Hasenberg, N. M., 429
Hashibe, M., 363
Hashim, S. A., 243
Hashish, I., 306
Hasin, D., 188
Haskard, K. B., 433
Hassan, N.-H., 437
Hassler, M., 34
Hatchett, L., 324
Hatira, P., 299
Hatsukami, D., 201
Hatzenbuehler, M. L., 135, 178
Hauck, E. R., 286
Haviland, M. L., 223
Hawes, A. M., 137, 355
Hawkes, R. J., 300 (figure)
Hawkins, N. A., 463
Hawkley, L. C., 355
Haworth, C. M., 241
Hawrilenko, M., 166
Hawthorne, D. M., 402
Hay, P., 269
Haybittle, J. L., 367
Hayden, M. R., 412
Hayes, B. E., 121
Hayman, L., 99
Haynes, O. M., 145
Haynes, R. B., 431, 442
Haynie, D. L., 205
Hays, R. B., 136, 139, 153, 332
Hays, R. D., 436, 437
Hazi, A., 106
Hazuda, H. P., 389
He, L. F., 291
He, M., 158
He, Y., 121
Head, J., 106
Healton, C. G., 223
Heath, A. C., 202
Heath, C. W., 362
Heatherton, T. F., 205, 206, 244
Heaton, A., 176, 258, 259
Heaton, P., 451
Hebert, L. E., 320, 320 (figure), 321
Hebert, M., 225
Hecht, K., 322
Heckman, B. D., 413
Heckman, J. J., 18
Heckman, T., 326
Heckman, T. G., 333, 338, 437
Hedegaard, H., 179
Hedegaard, U., 442
Heemst, J. V., 392
Hegel, M. T., 441
Hehman, E., 114

Heinberg, L. J., 260
Heine, S. J., 243
Heinrichs, M., 106
Heisel, M. J., 183
Heishman, S. J., 191
Heisler-MacKinnon, J., 86
Heissel, J. A., 115
Helfer, S. G., 298
Helgeson, V. S., 88, 134, 136, 137, 148, 325 (table), 366, 367, 368, 369, 370, 373
Heller, B. R., 69
Helmick, C. G., 314, 317
Helmrich, S. P., 250
Helms, J. M., 290
Helsing, K., 398
Hemenover, S. H., 152
Hemenway, D., 188
Henderson, B. E., 363
Henderson, E., 68
Hendrickson, K. L., 252
Hendriks, E. H., 354
Henifin, M. S., 414
Henke, C. J., 417
Henley, S. J., 463
Hennekens, C. H., 213
Hennessy, E. V., 79
Hennigan, K. M., 204
Henningfield, J. E., 191
Hennrikus, D. J., 203
Henoch, I., 404
Henry, C. L., 319
Henry, J. L., 365
Henter, J.-I., 386
Herbert, T. B., 4, 5, 6, 115, 117, 135
Herbst, J., 154, 354
Herbst, J. H., 155
Herman, C. P., 243, 244
Hernandez, D. C., 245
Hernandez-Reif, M., 292
Herndon, J. E., 68
Heron, M., 166, 167, 168, 169, 170, 171, 171 (figure), 172, 173, 174, 178, 179, 180, 181, 182, 187, 189, 192, 319
Hersey, J., 204
Hershey, J. C., 223
Hertel, A. W., 203
Herzog, D. B., 255
Herzog, T. A., 73, 74, 76
Hester, R. R., 224, 225
Heuch, I., 363
Hewett, J. E., 329
Hewitt, J. K., 258
Hewitt, P. L., 101, 155, 183, 184
Hickson, G. B., 177
Higbee, K. L., 77, 440
Higgins, P., 150
Higginson, I. J., 394

Irvin, J. E., 232, 435
Irvine, K., 70
Irwin, M., 122
Isaacs, S. L., 381
Ismail, M., 106
Iturralde, E., 330
Itzkowitz, S. H., 333
Ivanova, I. V., 258
Iwamoto, D. K., 215
Iwashyna, T. J., 384
Izard, C. E., 145

Jaarsveld, C. H., 316
Jackson, E. R., 434
Jackson, J. S., 99, 121, 348, 461
Jackson, K. M., 58 (table)
Jackson, M. L., 173
Jackson, S. E., 433, 434
Jackson, T., 288
Jackson, T. C., 419
Jackson, V. P., 421
Jacob, J. A., 300
Jacobi, C., 265
Jacobi, F., 275, 288
Jacobs, E. J., 363
Jacobs, I. J., 412
Jacobs, L. M., 382
Jacobs, T. J., 97, 364
Jacobsen, B. K., 363
Jacobsen, L. A., 462
Jacobson, E., 157, 295
Jacobson, P. D., 191
Jaffe, A. J., 85
Jagusztyn, N. E., 114
Jahangiri, M., 147
Jakicic, J. M., 253
Jallo, N., 296
Jamal, A., 202, 452, 461, 463
James, V. A. W., 269
Jandorf, L., 333
Jang, M., 325
Janicki, D. L., 113
Janicki-Deverts, D.,
    4 (figure), 5, 110, 122
Janis, I. L., 77, 79, 80, 81, 440
Janoff-Bulman R., 325
Jansen, A., 244
Jansen, L., 367
Jansen-McWilliams, L., 152, 352
Jansma, B. M., 79, 86
Janssen, C., 433
Janz, N. K., 59, 60
Jaremka, L. M., 135
Jarlais, D. C. D., 78
Jarpe-Ratner, E., 63
Jarvis, M. J., 202, 461
Jaser, S., 325
Jay, S. M., 427
Jayanthi, N., 169

Jefferson, T., 151
Jeffery, R. W., 62, 121, 203, 252, 253
Jeitler, M., 158
Jemal, A., 384, 415
Jemelka, R. P., 288
Jemmott, J. B., 63 (figure), 117,
    135, 458, 466
Jemmott, J. I., 412
Jena, A. B., 356
Jenkins, C. D., 448
Jenkins, R. A., 370
Jenkinson, S., 415
Jennings, B., 470
Jennings, J. R., 135, 460
Jennings-Bey, T., 195
Jensen, A. B., 394
Jensen, M. D., 242
Jensen, M. P., 287, 299, 300, 302
Jenson, M. P., 298
Jeong, Y., 100, 100 (figure)
Jeong, Y. J., 145
Jepson, C., 414, 415, 416
Jewell, S. L., 140
Jilcott Pitts, S. B., 250
Jo, B., 268, 268 (figure)
Joffe, A., 191
Johns, S. A., 158
Johnson, A., 290
Johnson, B. T., 65, 66, 84, 152, 352
Johnson, C. A., 106, 205
Johnson, C. J., 437
Johnson, E. J., 471 (figure)
Johnson, J. A., 437, 438 (figure)
Johnson, J. H., 99
Johnson, J. R., 295, 296
Johnson, K. W., 95, 458
Johnson, L. M., 287
Johnson, M. O., 437
Johnson, R. A., 233 (figure)
Johnson, S. B., 455
Johnston, L. D., 223
Johnston, M., 426
Joiner, T., 152
Jokl, P., 283
Jones, A., 466
Jones, A. L., 193
Jones, B. L., 206
Jones, C. M., 178
Jones, F., 121, 244
Jones, J. L., 80
Jones, J. M., 458
Jones, R. C., 21
Jones, S., 80
Jones, S. A., 217
Jordan, J. R., 392
Jorenby, D. E., 84, 225
Jorgensen, R. S., 152, 352
Joscelyne, A., 404 (figure)
Josephs, R. A., 175, 212

Joshi, P., 347
Josipovic, Z., 229
Jouriles, E. N., 85
Judd, L. L., 399
Judge, T. A., 33
Julliard, K., 428, 433
Jung, M. Y., 415
Juon, H. S., 205, 415
Just, D. R., 448
Juster, R., 112
Juszczyk, D., 316
Jutagir, D. R., 372 (figure)
Juth, V., 402, 404

Kabat-Zinn, J., 300
Kaczor, L. M., 241
Kadden, R. M., 85
Kadowaki, J., 224
Kaell, A., 130, 334 (figure)
Kagawa-Singer, M., 95, 461
Kahana, B., 367
Kahler, C. W., 228
Kahn, R. L., 132
Kahn, S., 148
Kakkar, A. K., 254
Kalesan, B., 192
Kalichman, S. C., 31, 49, 83, 84, 89, 323,
    326, 338
Kalinowski, L., 88
Kallan, M. J., 175
Kallmes, D. F., 304
Kalungi, S., 421
Kamarck, T., 101, 232
Kamarck, T. W., 68, 113, 135, 225
Kamboh, M. I., 28
Kanaan, M., 135, 354–55
Kane, R. L., 383, 384
Kang, C. D., 439
Kang, Y., 81
Kangas, M., 365
Kaniasty, K., 134, 139
Kanim, L. E. A., 295
Kann, L., 209
Kannel, W. B., 213, 354
Kanner, A., 100
Kanner, A. D., 100
Kapadia, F., 319
Kaplan, A. S., 269
Kaplan, G. A., 136, 354, 369, 421
Kaplan, R. M., 69, 191,
    453, 455, 456, 462
Kaplan, S., 383, 433
Kaplan, S. H., 430, 433
Kaplan, S. P., 245
Kaprio, J., 253
Kaptchuk, T. J., 308 (figure)
Kapuku, G. K., 158
Karim, Q. A., 466
Karkabi, K., 439

Sapolsky, Robert, 108
Saquib, J., 413
Saquib, N., 413
Sarason, B. R., 121, 155
Sarason, I. G., 99, 121, 155, 204, 206
Sardaro, M., 301
Sargent, J. D., 70, 205, 206
Sarna, S., 253
Sassaroli, S., 258
Sasson, I., 393, 394
Satele, D. V., 434
Sauer, A. G., 415
Saunders, Cicely, 383
Savage, D. D., 52
Sawyer, K. S., 211
Sayette, M. A., 212
Sbarra, D. A., 32
Scarmeas, N., 321
Scesi, M., 287
Schachter, S., 207, 243
Schaefer, C., 100, 398
Schaen, E. R., 301
Schafer, M. H., 365
Schaffer-Neitz, R., 288
Schanberg, S. M., 154, 353
Scharff, D. P., 86
Schauer, G., 202
Schaumberg, K., 265
Scheier, M. F., 5, 5 (table), 128, 128–29
    (table), 146, 146 (table), 147, 153,
    155, 156, 329
Scherer, K. P., 106
Scherer, L. D., 417, 418 (table)
Scherr, P. A., 320, 320 (figure)
Scherwitz, L., 357
Schettler, P., 292
Scheyer, R. D., 441
Schiffer, A. A., 354
Schiller, J. H., 368
Schiller, J. S., 209, 311–12
Schilling, E., 94
Schlenger, W. E., 120
Schluchter, M. D., 450
Schmaling, K., 335
Schmidt, J. E., 370
Schmidt, U., 263
Schmitt, K., 89 (figure)
Schneider, D., 181, 186
Schneider, M., 251
Schneider, T. R., 83, 88
Schneiderman, L. J., 470
Schneiderman, N., 334, 338
Schnittjer, S. K., 82
Schnyer, D. M., 141
Schofield, T. J., 176
Scholer, S. J., 177
Scholz, U., 38, 203
Schonert-Reichl, K. A., 180
Schootman, M., 248

Schorpp, K., 10, 135, 141
Schorr, L., 398
Schreer, G. E., 152, 352
Schreiber, G. B., 260
Schrimshaw, E. W., 332
Schroeder, D. H., 97
Schroeder, D. M., 415
Schroevers, M. J., 369
Schuchter, S. R., 399
Schuckit, M. A., 217
Schug, R. A., 261
Schuler, J., 130
Schulman, K. A., 423, 463
Schultz, A. B., 456
Schulz, R., 324, 325 (table),
    370, 373, 393
Schumacher, M. C., 363
Schupp, H. T., 245
Schut, H., 400, 400 (figure), 402
Schut, H. A. W., 401
Schüz, B., 244, 437
Schüz, N., 244
Schwab, R. J., 425
Schwankovsky, L., 148, 433
Schwartz, B. S., 275
Schwartz, D., 259
Schwartz, G. E., 8, 9
Schwartz, J., 352
Schwartz, J. C., 114
Schwartz, J. E., 147, 280
Schwartz, L. M., 69
Schwartz, M. D., 156, 415
Schwartzberg, S. S., 326
Schwarz, N., 108
Schwarzer, R., 60, 76, 136
Schwebel, D. C., 174, 177
Sciara, A. D., 20
Sclar, D. A., 416
Scott, J. C., 322
Scott-Sheldon, L. A. J., 338
Seage, G. R., 430
Sears, S., 463
Sears, S. F., 253, 470
Sears, S. R., 387
Secker-Walker, R. H., 84
Seckl, J., 34
Seeman, T. E., 106
Seery, M. D., 108
Segerstrom, S. C., 105, 106, 115, 153,
    331, 332 (table)
Sehgal, A. R., 470
Seifer, R., 193
Selby, P., 207, 225
Selby, P. L., 225
Self, C. A., 80
Seligman, M. E., 147, 148, 149
Seligman, M. E. P., 11, 146
Seltman, H., 366
Seltzer, M. M., 393

Selye, H., 108
Selye, Hans, 103
Semega, J. L., 460
Sen, A., 396
Sen, B., 192
Senecal, C., 437
Senn, C. Y., 189, 190 (figure)
Seow, A., 432
Serrano, J., 363
Seth, P., 319
Severeijns, R., 286
Severson, J., 174
Seville, L., 421
Sevincer, A. T., 175, 212
Sewell, A. A., 18
Seybold, K. S., 143
Shacham, S., 427
Shackelton, R., 433
Shadel, W. G., 73
Shafer, D., 87, 88, 286
Shaffer, D., 185
Shaffer, J. W., 364
Shaffer, W. J., 364, 365
Shah, D., 233 (figure)
Shai, D., 177
Shanafelt, T. D., 434
Shanahan, D. F., 160
Shankar, A., 139
Shapiro, Dan, 131
Sharma, M., 158
Sharma, S., 63, 248
Sharp, E. S., 321
Sharpe, M., 183
Shattuck, D., 468
Shavitt, S., 134
Shaw, E. G., 285
Shaw, H., 265, 266
Shay, K. A., 159
Shea, S., 347
Shearin, E. N., 121, 155
Sheedy, D., 211
Sheehan, M., 76
Sheeran, P., 60, 65, 416
Sheets, E. S., 105
Shekelle, P. G., 291
Shekelle, R. B., 352, 364, 365
Shen, B. J., 338
Shen, S., 333
Shepherd, R. W., 303
Sheppard, B. H., 66, 362
Shepperd, J. A., 156
Shepperd, S. L., 415
Sher, K. J., 199, 215, 217
Sheras, P. L., 427
Sherbourne, C. D., 288, 437,
    438, 439, 442
Sheridan, M. A., 120
Sherina, M.-S., 437
Sherman, A. C., 143

Sorensen, G., 153, 232
Sorensen, T. I., 348, 461
Sørensen, T. I., 243
Sorter, M. T., 190
Sosa, R., 6, 136
Sosin, D. M., 192
Sox, H. C., 83
Spanakis, E. K., 315
Spangler, A. S., 292–93
Spanjol, J., 66
Spanos, N. P., 299
Sparano, J. A., 360
Sparrow, D., 354
Speca, M., 370
Spector, P., 94, 95
Speicher, C. E., 94, 116, 364
Speisman, J. C., 101
Spek, V., 354
Spencer, S. M., 366
Speroff, L., 463
Spezzaferri, R., 425 (figure)
Spicer, R. S., 175
Spiegel, D., 131, 137, 367, 371, 372
Spiegel, David, 372
Spiegel, N., 135
Spijkerman, M. P. J., 158
Spire, B., 323
Spiro, I. A., 100, 100 (figure)
Spoor, S., 265
Spraul, M., 240
Spreeuwenberg, P., 160
Spring, B., 361, 363
Sproesser, G., 245
Squires, D., 179
Stachow, R., 327
Stacy, A., 215
Stacy, A. W., 215
Stafford, R., 454
Stagl, J. M., 371, 372 (figure)
Stam, H. J., 299
Stamler, J., 350
Stampfer, M. J., 41, 143, 213, 350
Stanek, K., 249
Stansfeld, S. A., 350
Stanton, A. L., 7, 130, 131, 334, 370, 387, 438, 439, 463
Stanton, C., 207
Stapleton, J., 65
Staras, S. A., 43, 227
Stark, M. J., 211
Stark, O., 249
Stayton, L. E., 137
Steele, C. M., 79, 175, 212
Steenhuis, I., 84
Steers, M., 94
Steffens, D., 292
Stein, J. A., 65, 206
Stein, K. D., 367, 371
Stein, Z., 347

Steinberg, B. A., 159
Steinberg, L., 175
Steineck, G., 386
Steingart, R. M., 422, 463
Steinglass, J. E., 16
Steinhardt, M. A., 155
Steinley, D., 418 (table)
Stellar, E., 106
Stener-Victorin, E., 287
Stephens, A. N., 174
Stephens, M. A., 323
Stephens, M. A. C., 213
Stephens, M. A. P., 324
Stephenson, B. J., 442
Stephenson, K. R., 158
Steptoe, A., 11, 106, 113, 139, 147, 352, 353, 354, 355
Sterba, K. R., 324
Stern, R. M., 285
Sternbach, R. A., 113
Sterns, S., 367
Stetler, C., 107
Stevens, J., 240
Stevens, M. M., 385
Stevens, M. R., 170
Stewart, W. F., 275
Stewart-Williams, S., 307
Stice, E., 241, 265, 266
Stigsdotter, U. A., 160
Stillion, J., 386, 395, 397
Stillion, J. M., 395, 396
Stillwell, D., 29
Stockton, R., 400
Stockwell, T., 213
Stoddard, A. M., 75
Stoduto, G., 174
Stohl, M., 188
Stok, M. F., 245
Stokes, A., 313
Stoler, J., 186
Stolerman, I. P., 202
Stolz, E., 387
Stone, A. A., 130, 135, 280, 334 (figure)
Stone, A. L., 284
Stoney, C. M., 106, 113
Stoolmiller, M., 206
Storer, B. E., 364
Storey, K. E., 63
Stormer, S., 265
Story, M., 36, 249, 263
Stowe, R. P., 428
Strauman, E. C., 403
Strauss, C., 158
Strauts, E., 227
Strecher, V., 16
Strecher, V. J., 81, 83, 84, 86, 88
Strickhouser, J. E., 156
Striegel-Moore, R. H., 261, 266
Striepe, M., 244

Strike, P. C., 113
Stroebe, M., 141, 397, 400, 400 (figure)
Stroebe, M. S., 394, 398, 399, 401, 402
Stroebe, W., 141, 394, 398, 399, 401
Ströhle, A., 159
Struckman-Johnson, C. J., 86
Struckman-Johnson, D. L., 86
Struening, E. L., 97
Strunk, C. M., 190
Strycker, L. A., 253
Stuart, G. L., 184
Stuckey, H. L., 322, 323, 324, 326, 327, 330, 332, 333
Stuetzle, R., 144
Stunkard, A. J., 252, 348, 461
Sturges, J. W., 80
Stussman, B. J., 291, 423
Stutts, W., 101
Suarez, E. C., 154, 353
Suarez, S. D., 52
Subra, B., 212
Subramanian, S. V., 397
Substance Abuse and Mental Health Services Administration, 209, 218, 218 (figure)
Suchindran, C., 260
Sudman, S., 47
Suecoff, S. A., 177
Sui, X., 348
Suinn, R. M., 136, 151, 352
Sullivan, M. J., 448
Sullivan, M. J. L., 287 (table), 288
Sullivan, P. F., 288
Sullivan-Halley, J., 363
Sullman, M. J., 174
Suls, J., 8, 9, 131, 150, 151
Sumartojo, E., 436
Summerton, J., 417
Sumner, J. A., 120, 350
Sumter, S. R., 111
Sun, J., 202
Sun, P., 226
Sun, Q., 6, 250
Sun, Y. C., 79
Sun Y. C., 431
Sunday, S. R., 259
Sundin, Ö., 283
Sundquist, J., 361
Sundquist, K., 347
Sung, H., 313
Sung, L., 382
Sunitha Suresh, B. S., 301
SUPPORT Principal Investigators, 381
Suresh, S., 301
Surtees, P. G., 149
Sussman, S., 208, 226
Sutherland, G. T., 211
Sutherland, R. J., 52

Sutin, A., 241
Sutin, A. R., 250
Sutin, R., 32
Sutker, P. B., 119
Sutkowi-Hemstreet, A., 414
Sutton, S. R., 58
Sutton-Tyrrell, K., 113, 114, 152, 352
Sveticic, J., 194
Swalehe, R. M., 70
Swami, V., 261
Swan, P. D., 138
Swank, R. T., 364
Swanson, S. A., 257
Sweat, M., 466
Swendsen, J., 257
Swendsen, J. D., 213
Sworowski, L. A., 130
Syme, S. L., 136, 421, 458
Symister, P., 324
Szasz, T. S., 431
Szczypka, G., 249
Szecsenyi, J., 288
Szklo, M., 398
Szocs, C., 247 (figure)

Taddio, A., 294
Taenzer, P., 301
Taffel, S. M., 454
Talbot, F., 328
Talbot, M., 304, 306
Talmor, A., 240
Tam, L., 66
Tamiello, M., 135
Tanenbaum, M. L., 139
Tang, D. W., 16
Tang, M., 360
Tang, S. T., 380, 381
Tang, Y., 472
Tangen, C. M., 413
Tanney, F., 20
Tanski, S. E., 205
Tarr, K. L., 364
Tasca, A. G., 269
Taubman, O., 148
Tauras, J. A., 450
Taylor, A., 116
Taylor, A. G., 296
Taylor, C. A., 319
Taylor, C. B., 101, 302, 366
Taylor, D. M., 282
Taylor, J. E., 95
Taylor, K. C., 42, 464
Taylor, K. L., 415
Taylor, L., 178
Taylor, M. D., 150
Taylor, S. E., 7, 106, 128, 134, 137, 138,
   146, 147, 148, 153, 322, 323, 326,
   329, 330, 331, 332, 334, 335, 366,
   367, 368, 401, 425, 439

Taylor, V., 456
Taylor, W. C., 430
Tedeschi, R. G., 367
Tejada-Vera, B., 16, 169 (table), 343
Telzer, E. H., 177
Temmerman, M., 468
Temte, J. L., 13 (figure)
Tenenbein, M., 177
Teng, Y., 67, 76
Tennen, H., 146, 147, 150, 214, 367
Teno, J. M., 383, 384
ter Kuile, M. M., 299
Tercyak, K. P., 412, 415
Terracciano, A., 147
Terry, D. J., 132, 332
Teruya, S., 65
Terwilliger, R. F., 79
Tester, L., 292
Thakkar, J., 443
Tharps, Q. J., 419
Theakston, H., 292
Thee, S. L., 82
Theis, K. A., 314
Theorell, T., 95, 136, 333
Thiel, G., 441
Thoits, P. A., 138, 426
Thomas, C. B., 364
Thomas, G. I., 304
Thomas, J., 64
Thomas, J. G., 254
Thomas, K., 392
Thomas, M. G., 130
Thomas, S. A., 138, 138 (figure)
Thomas, S. L., 241
Thompson, D. A., 432
Thompson, D. C., 192, 194
Thompson, I. M., 413
Thompson, J. K., 206, 260
Thompson, M., 259, 421
Thompson, M. D., 217
Thompson, R. G., 188
Thompson, R. S., 192
Thompson, S. C., 130, 148, 331, 433
Thompson, W. D., 360
Thomson, J. B., 217
Thomtén, J., 283
Thoolen, B. J., 335
Thoresen, C., 143
Thorn, B. E., 364
Thorndike, E. L., 67
Thorpe, C. T., 324
Thorson, C., 252
Thorson, E., 77
Thun, M. J., 362
Thune, I., 363
Thurston, R. C., 354
Thurston, W. E., 190 (figure)
Tian, Y., 66
Tibben, A., 412

Tice, D. M., 129
Tice, T. N., 144
Tickle, J. J., 206
Tiemeier, H. W., 392
Tilahun, T., 468
Tildesley, E., 155
Till, C., 413
Tiller, J., 263
Timbers, D. M., 19, 422
Timman, R., 412
Timms, R. M., 69
Tinetti, M. E., 189
Tinney, F., 81
Tinsworth, D. K., 174
Tippetts, A. S., 191
Tiro, J. A., 415
Tison, J., 191
Tobin, J., 114
Tobler, N. S., 78, 221
Todd, M., 205
Toker, S., 4
Tomaka, J., 128, 131
Tomar, S. L., 203
Tomarken, A., 392
Tomasek, A. D., 179
Tomfohr, L. M., 114
Tomich, P. L., 366
Tomiyama, A. J., 240
Tomkins, S. S., 207
Tompson, S., 16, 449
Tong, Y., 158
Toniolo, P., 362
Topa, G., 65
Topic, I., 472 (table)
Torgerson, W. S., 280
Torpy, J. M., 312
Tosteson, D. C., 433
Toth, P. L., 400, 402
Tou, R. Y., 131, 373
Toulany, A., 269
Touyz, S. W., 269
Towers, S., 186
Towle, V. R., 463
Townsend, A. L., 395
Townsend, S. S. M., 115
Tracey, D. R., 421
Tran, V., 330
Trapl, E. S., 176
Trask, O. J., 116, 364
Trauer, T., 392
Trautner, C., 240
Trawalter, S., 294
Treanor, J. J., 146
Treasure, J., 263
Treasure, J. L., 258
Treiber, F. A., 158
Trentham-Dietz, A., 364
Trevisan, M., 135
Trice, A. D., 131

Wadhwa, N., 324, 339
Wagenaar, A. C., 43, 227, 451
Wagenknecht, L. E., 337 (figure)
Wager, T. D., 306, 424
Wagner, E. H., 435
Wagner, J. M., 292–93
Wagner, L. J., 367
Wagner, P. J., 417
Wagner, T. H., 228
Wahlberg, K. E., 185
Wainwright, N. W., 149
Waite, L., 333
Waits, J. B., 401
Waitzkin, H., 429, 430, 432
Wakefield, M., 223
Wakeland, W., 106
Walch, S. E., 65
Waldrop, D., 383
Waldstein, S. R., 114
Wales, J., 383
Walitzer, K. S., 229
Walker, A., 193
Walker, B. M., 383
Walker, E. A., 288
Walker, L. S., 283, 287
Walker, M., 393
Walker, T., 319
Walkup, J., 442
Wall, M., 263
Wall, P. D., 275, 276, 290, 292, 294, 295, 303, 359, 424
Wall, Patrick, 277
Wallace, G. S., 13 (figure)
Wallace, R., 143
Wallace, R. K., 299
Wallace, S., 119
Wallack, L., 214
Waller, G., 263
Waller, J., 415, 461
Wallston, B. S., 141
Wallston, K. A., 286, 333
Walsh, B. T., 16, 259, 267
Walsh, D. C., 350
Walsh, D. M., 290
Walsh, N. E., 291
Walt, L. C., 31
Walter, T., 85
Walters, S. T., 85
Waltz, W., 295
Wand, G. S., 213
Wang, A. W.-T., 368
Wang, D. B., 421
Wang, H., 173, 466
Wang, H. Y., 158
Wang, H. Y. J., 147, 331
Wang, J., 212
Wang, M. C., 232, 435
Wang, S. S., 260
Wang, Y., 352, 423

Wang, Z., 242
Wansink, B., 49 (figure), 245, 246, 247 (figure), 252
Wansink, Brian, 246
Ward, B. W., 311–12, 423, 462
Ward, E., 384
Ward, H. W., 121
Warda, L., 177
Wardle, J., 241, 261, 415, 461
Ware, J. E., 430, 433
Waring, E. J., 195
Warner, E., 363
Warner, M., 179
Warner, T. D., 182
Warren, J. L., 423
Warren, M. P., 264
Warshaw, P. R., 66, 362
Wartman, S. A., 437
Wass, H., 386, 395, 396, 397
Wasserman, J., 191
Waters, A., 266
Waters, S., 121
Watson, A., 76
Watson, D., 150, 156
Watson, J. D., 469
Watson, P., 413
Watts, D. D., 262
Watts, J. C., 78
Way, B. M., 106
Way, M., 120
Wayment, H. A., 155, 402
Waytz, A., 381
Weafer, J., 184
Wearing, J. R., 131
Weatherford, B., 186
Weaver, K. E., 437, 438
Webel, A. R., 323
Weber, E., 140
Weber, J., 229
Webster, D. W., 181, 192, 195
Wechsler, H., 47, 206
Wedel, H., 141
Wedlund, L. N., 356
Wee, C. C., 247
Weedon-Fekjær, H., 411
Wegner, Dan, 132
Wei, W., 442
Weibel, D., 265
Weidner, G., 357
Weinblatt, E., 136
Weingarten, M. A., 429
Weinstein, M., 99
Weinstein, N. D., 58, 74, 74 (figure), 75, 147
Weintraub, J. K., 128, 128–29 (table), 329
Weisner, C., 228
Weiss, A., 147, 150
Weiss, A. J., 425, 427

Weiss, D., 364
Weiss, H. B., 193
Weiss, S., 368
Weissberg-Benchell, J., 330
Welch, H. G., 69
Welch, W. T., 134
Welin, L., 136
Wellenius, G. A., 352
Wellisch, D., 373
Wellman, J. A., 298
Wells, C., 240
Wenger, N. K., 463
Wensing, M., 288
Wenthworth, D., 350
Werner, R. J., 435
Werner, R. M., 348
Wertheim, E. H., 262
West, D. W., 363
West, S. G., 415
West, S. L., 221
Westbrook, F., 227
Westenberg, P. M., 111
Wetter, D. W., 225, 226
Weuve, J., 320, 320 (figure)
Wewers, M. E., 206
Wheeler, L., 135
Whipple, B., 292
Whisman, M. A., 135, 262
Whitaker, R. C., 251
White, A. A., 283
White, D., 437
White, E., 363, 456
White, E. K., 260
White, M. J., 75
White, P., 299
Whitehead, D. L., 113
Whitehead, W. E., 69
Whitehill, J. M., 70, 195
Whitlock, J., 180
Whitlow, J. W., 244
Whittemore, R., 325
Whittle, J., 423
Whooley, M. A., 11, 122, 353
Wi, S., 398
Wickelgren, I., 240
Wickens, C. M., 174
Wickham, R., 94
Wickrama, K. S., 116
Widdershoven, J. W., 354
Wideman, M. V., 87, 87 (table), 442
Wiebe, D. J., 155, 159, 330, 417
Wiebe, J. S., 128, 131, 155, 437
Wiens, A. N., 225
Wiggins, S., 412, 413
Wight, R. G., 324
Wilcox, H. C., 179, 184, 188, 396
Wildes, J. E., 269
Wildes, K. A., 331
Wilfond, B. S., 456

depression and, 288

exercise and, 292

gate control theory of pain, 277 (figure), 277–79, 278 (figure)

impact of health psychology on, 6

impact of placebos on, 303–8, 305 (figure), 308 (figure)

impact of psychosocial factors on, 282–89

intractable-benign pain, 274

managing, 292

pattern theory of pain, 276

personalized health care messages for managing, 87–88

physical methods of managing, 290–95

physical stimulation and, 290

progressive pain, 274

psychological methods of managing, 295–303

psychophysiological measures of pain, 282

race and ethnicity and, 35, 274

recurrent acute pain, 274

self-report inventories and, 280–81, 281 (figure)

social support and, 289

specificity theory of pain, 276

stress and, 283–84

surgery and, 234–35

women and, 15

palliative care, 382

parasympathetic divisions, 110

Parkinson's disease (PD), 314, 336

participant observation, 29

participation, convenient, 48

patient cooperation, 44

patient-centered model, 432

patient–practitioner communication, 428–33, 430 (table)

pattern theory of pain, 276

perceived behavioral control, 64, 331

periaqueductal gray, 279

peripheral nervous system, 109 (figure), 109–10

personal relationships

bereavement and, 394–97

chronic disease and, 323

stress and, 94

personality. *See also* behavioral choices

alcohol use and, 215–16

cancer and, 364–65

coronary heart disease (CHD) and, 352–54

disordered eating and, 263–64

health and, 152–56, 153 (figure)

role of, 145–56

smoking and, 206

unintentional injuries and, 174–75

personalized health-promotion messages, 83–90

physical activity

cancer and, 363

chronic disease and, 336–37

coronary heart disease (CHD) and, 350

obesity and, 250

pain management and, 292

stress and, 159

physical stimulation, pain management and, 290

physical therapists, 22 (table)

physical therapy, 292

physician-assisted suicide, 387

physiological measures to assess stress, 101–2

physiological responses, impact of health psychology on, 3–5

placebo surgery, 303–4

placebos

impact on pain, 303–8, 305 (figure), 308 (figure)

use in research studies, 45–46

poisoning, 171–73

positive psychology, 11

positive reappraisal, 330–31

positive states, 146

post-traumatic growth, 367

posttraumatic stress disorder (PTSD), 118–20, 154 (figure)

poverty

intentional injuries and, 186–87

unintentional injuries and, 176–78

prayer. *See* religion and spirituality

precaution adoption process model, 74 (figure), 74–75, 75 (table)

precontemplation stage of change, 72, 72 (figure)

pregnancy, 15

preparation stage of change, 72, 72 (figure)

prevalence, epidemiological research and, 42

prevention

campaigns, 448–50

education and, 452

fire prevention, 192–93

injury prevention, 190–95

legislation and, 450–52

primary prevention, 14

secondary prevention, 6

socioeconomic status and, 452–56

tertiary prevention, 7

timing of, 449 (table)

primary appraisal, 107

primary prevention, 14

problem-focused coping, 128–30, 329

progressive muscle relaxation, 157–58, 291, 295

progressive pain, 274

Project DARE (Drug Abuse Resistance Education), 221

prospective studies, 42

prostaglandins, 279

psychedelics, 219

psychological realism, 40

psychological well-being, 119

psychology, research methods, 44 (table)

psychoneuroimmunology, 109, 117–18

psychophysiological measures of pain, 282

psychosomatic medicine, 16

public health

career options, 22 (table)

substance abuse and, 227

qualitative research, 28–29, 35 (table)

quality-adjusted life years (QALYs), 462

quasi-experiments, 40–41

quick-trajectory deaths, 392–93

race and ethnicity

alcohol use and abuse and, 209

cancer and, 360–61

coronary heart disease (CHD) and, 347

demographic factors and, 457–59

diabetes and, 315

health care seeking and, 422–23

HIV/AIDS and, 319

pain and, 274

suicide and, 179

random assignments, 37

randomized controlled trials (RCTs), 43–45

reaction stage of mourning, 391

realism, high mundane, 49

recurrent acute pain, 274

relapse, addiction and, 229, 230 (figure), 231–34, 233 (figure)

relational model, 106–7

relationships

bereavement and, 394–97

chronic disease and, 323

stress and, 94

relaxation, 157–58, 291, 295

religion and spirituality

advanced care directives and, 389

chronic disease and, 331

health care seeking and, 422

influence of, 142–45

meditation, 38, 158, 299, 300 (figure)

religiosity, 142

reorientation and recovery stage of mourning, 392

sympathetic adrenomedullary (SAM) system, 110
sympathetic divisions, 110
systematic desensitization, 157, 157 (table), 295

tangible support, 134.
    See also social support
task work model, 379
technology
    development of health psychology, 15–16
    reliance on, 454–55
    reproductive, 469
television viewing, obesity and, 249–50
tend-and-befriend response to stress, 106
tension-reducing imagery practice (TRIP), 296 (table)
tension-reduction theory, 213–14
tertiary prevention, 7.
    See also health care
tetrahydrocannabinol (THC), 219
theories, and the scientific method, 26
theory of planned behavior, 64–66, 65 (figure)
theory of reasoned action, 62–64
therapy, 160
tobacco use. *See* smoking
tolerance, addiction and, 201

training pathways, 19–20
transactional model, 106–7, 107 (table)
transcutaneous electrical nerve stimulation (TENS), 290
transtheoretical (stages of change) model, 71–74, 72 (figure)
Trauma Response Team, 195
traumatic events
    religion and spirituality and, 143–45, 145 (table)
    stress and, 95–96
treatment delay, 420 (figure), 421
Tuskegee experiment, 50
12 step programs, 227 (table), 227–29
Type 1 and Type 2 diabetes, 315
Type A behavior, 150–51, 352
Type D personality, 354

unintentional injuries, 166, 171–78.
    See also injuries
unintentional nonadherence, 436, 440–43. *See also* adherence
U.S. Air Force Biomedical Sciences Corps, 20–21 (table)
utilization delay, 419, 420 (figure)

vaccinations, 13 (figure)
validational support, 134.

See also social support
validity, internal vs. external, 46–49, 50 (table)
vapes. *See* smoking
vehicular accidents, 173, 191–92
vigilant coping, 130–31
vulnerability, 81

weapons
    access to, 187
    legislation on, 192
withdrawal symptoms, 201
women
    bereavement and, 394
    cancer and, 358 (figure), 410 (table)
    focus on, 463–64
    health care seeking and, 422
    maternal health of, 467–68
    pain and, 15
Women's Health Initiative study, 41
work, stress and, 94–95

yearning and searching stage of mourning, 392
young adulthood
    drug use during, 218 (figure)
    risk of injury during, 169–70, 170 (figure)